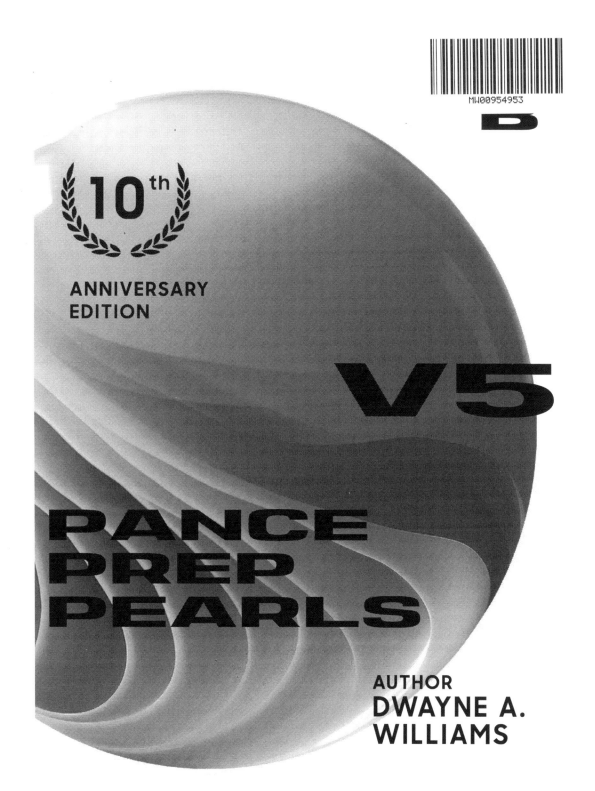

10th
ANNIVERSARY EDITION

V5

PANCE PREP PEARLS

AUTHOR
DWAYNE A. WILLIAMS

Copyright © 2024 Dwayne A. Williams
All rights reserved.
ISBN: 9798322880424
Imprint: Independently published

Printed by Kindle Direct Publishing Platform

Book cover design: Eli Ofel : Support @applocal.co

<u>DEDICATION</u>

Thanks to my foundation teachers Marion Masterson, Medea Valdez, Gerard Marciano. A very special thanks to Stacey Hughes (words can't describe my gratitude to you), Sharon Verity and William Ameres for being my inspirational teachers as a student.   To all those who contributed to making this profession great and to all my fellow educators who contribute to this field on so many levels.

Thanks to all of the owners of the photos. Your images helped to make this book a visual experience. Your contribution is invaluable. An extra special thanks to **Ian Baker**, the illustrator of most of the pictures in the book. You added a special touch to this project. Thanks Dr. Frank Gaillard and Jason Davis for your help during the process. Special thanks to **Kevin Young, Xiana Flowers & Kristen Risom** (the best illustrators I know!)

Special thanks to my parents Winifred & Robert Williams. Xiomara & Froylan Flowers (my second parents), Mercedes Avalon, Gilda Cain (the best nurse I know!) and my big brother Danilo Avalon.

To my gurus: Stacey Hughes, Tse-Hwa Yao, Ingrid Voigt, Dr. Antonio Dajer, & Dr. Kenneth Rose you guys have helped shaped the PA I became.

Thanks to Isaak Yakubov (my Akim) for the Ultimate Mnemonic Comic Book and the amazing journey we have embarked on together.

Pamela Bodley, the world's best manager. You are the real boss lady!

To Eli Ofel. Thank you for your friendship, partnership, and amazing covers.

Last but not least a very special thank you to my PPP warriors for rocking with me for 10 years! This book would have been nothing without the support of each and every one you! Thanks for being always being there!!!! YOU ARE PPP WARRIORS.....WARRIORS WIN!

PREFACE

STUDENTS

This book is designed for use in both didactic and clinical education. It is formatted to make you a rockstar on clinical rotations! It is a ***review book***, which means ***it is not meant to replace textbook-based education*** but as an additional study tool to enhance your knowledge base. Textbooks provide the foundation for understanding and learning medicine.

PRACTITIONERS

This book is purposed to increase your knowledge & retention of important clinical information and for use as a quick resource that is not time consuming.

THE STYLE OF PPP

Pance Prep Pearls is not written in the traditional style of a textbook but rather to feel like a collection of notes, drafts, charts, mnemonics and clinical pearls to make learning effective while entertaining. The use of bold and asterisks are to help you to organize the information and stress the importance of certain aspects of the disease states. The charts are designed for you to compare and contrast commonly grouped diseases and high-yield information. It is loaded with helpful algorithms to help you see the big picture on how to approach the disease.

I personally recommend that you use what I call the 6 P's of the ***Patient-Centered Learning Model*** as you study the different diseases:

1. **Pathophysiology:** imagine explaining the pathophysiology of a disease to your patient in 1 sentence (2 sentences maximum) in simple terms. Understanding the pathophysiology will often explain the clinical manifestations, physical examination findings, why certain tests are used and usually the treatment reverses the pathophysiology. This step is often skipped but is probably the most important (in terms of knowledge retention).
2. **People** be comfortable knowing the epidemiology of the diseases.
3. **Present** – based on the pathophysiology, how would this patient present? Know both the classic and the common findings and presentations (they aren't always the same).
4. **Pick it up**? – How would you diagnose the disease. Make sure to understand what is usually first line vs. gold standard (definitive diagnosis). Understand the indications and contraindications for each test.
5. **Palliate** – how do you treat (palliate) the disorder. Many people can list out the treatments but fail to remember first line treatments vs. alternative treatments. Make sure to understand the indications and contraindications of each treatment.
6. **Pharmacology** – understand the mechanism of action and understand why a medication is used for that disease. This helps to reinforce the pathophysiology as well as the presentation of the disease since the pharmacology often reverses the problem or treats the symptoms. A very important point is that if you see a medication that is used for different disorders, try to understand what connects the use of that drug to the different disorders.

PANCE PREP APP AVAILABLE ON IPHONE PLATFORMS!

EARN 20 CATEGORY 1 SELF-ASSESSMENT CME CREDITS

Go to Panceprepapp.io for more information

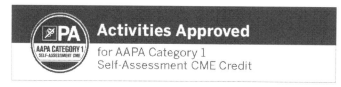
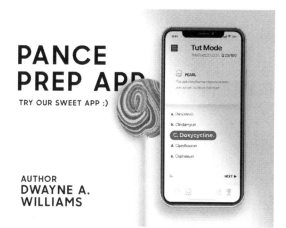
Over 15,000 clinically-based practice examination questions specifically formulated to enhance clinical skills and improve performance on examinations, such as the PANCE, PANRE, OSCES, USMLE, end of rotation examinations and comprehensive medical examinations.

PANCE PREP QUESTION BOOK

EARN 20 CATEGORY 1 SELF-ASSESSMENT CME CREDITS

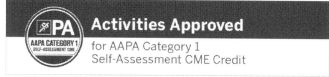
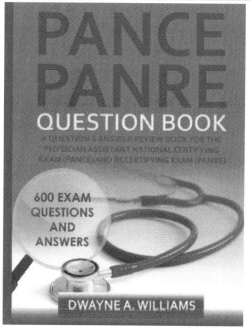

TABLE OF CONTENTS

CHAPTER 7 – ENDOCRINE SYSTEM

ADRENAL DISORDERS

Zona **G**lomerulosa:	**A**ldosterone (Controls Na⁺ balance)	Outer layer of cortex
Zona **F**asciculata:	**C**ortisol	Middle Layer of cortex
Zona **R**eticularis:	**E**strogens/Androgens	Inner Layer of Cortex

Think "GFR" for the layers of the cortex and "ACE" for the hormones they produce.

HYPOTHALAMIC-PITUITARY AXIS

The man (hypothalamus) turns on the thermostat (pituitary gland), which turns on the radiator (adrenal gland), which produces the heat (cortisol) to the desired temperature (homeostasis).

NEGATIVE FEEDBACK
When the heat (cortisol) becomes higher than the desired set temperature (homeostasis), this will cause the thermostat (pituitary gland) to shut off so that the radiator (adrenal gland) stops making heat (any new cortisol).

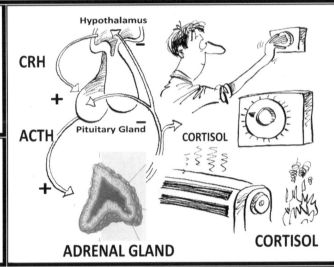

SECONDARY DISORDERS
Based on the feedback mechanisms, **secondary (pituitary gland)** & **tertiary (hypothalamic)** disorders have LABS IN THE SAME DIRECTION.
- **TSH-secreting PITUITARY adenoma**
  ↑TSH & ↑FreeT$_4$/T$_3$
- **Cushing disease (PITUITARY adenoma)**
  ↑ACTH & ↑cortisol
- **Hypopituitarism:** low pituitary hormones & low target organ hormones.

PRIMARY DISORDERS
Based on the feedback mechanisms, primary disorders have LABS IN OPPOSITE DIRECTIONS if the **problem is the target organ**:
Thyroid gland is the primary problem:
- **Graves', Toxic Goiter, Toxic adenoma**
  ↑FreeT$_4$/T$_3$ & ↓TSH

- **Hashimoto Thyroiditis**
  ↓FreeT$_4$/T$_3$ & ↑TSH

Ovaries are the primary problem:
- **Menopause:** ↓estrogen & ↑FSH/LH

Adrenal gland is the primary problem:
- **Addison's disease:** ↓cortisol & ↑ACTH
- **Adrenal adenoma:** ↑cortisol & ↓ACTH

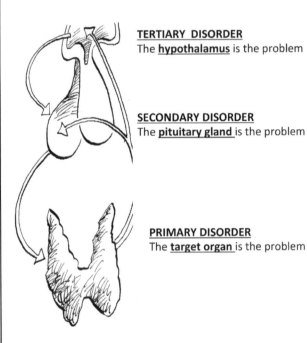

TERTIARY DISORDER
The **hypothalamus** is the problem

SECONDARY DISORDER
The **pituitary gland** is the problem

PRIMARY DISORDER
The **target organ** is the problem

Photo credit:
Shutterstock (used with permission).

PRIMARY HYPERALDOSTERONISM

Primary: renin-independent (autonomous) excessive & unregulated aldosterone production.
- **Idiopathic or idiopathic bilateral adrenal hyperplasia most common cause (60% of cases).**
- **Conn syndrome (unilateral adrenal aldosteronoma) 40%.** Located in the zona glomerulosa.
- Rare causes: unilateral adrenal hyperplasia, familial, or ectopic aldosterone secreting tumor.

Secondary Hyperaldosteronism: to increased renin. Increased renin leads to increased aldosterone via the RAAS (renin angiotensin aldosterone system):
- Renal artery stenosis most common cause of Secondary aldosteronism.
- Renal artery hypoperfusion (eg, CHF, hypovolemia, Nephrotic syndrome etc.).

PATHOPHYSIOLOGY
- Aldosterone is a mineralocorticoid that increases renal sodium reabsorption at the expense of increased potassium & hydrogen excretion to maintain blood pressure & regulate salt. Therefore, hyperaldosteronism leads to sodium retention and renal potassium & hydrogen ion wasting.

CLINICAL MANIFESTATIONS
- Usually asymptomatic. **Triad of [1] Hypertension + [2] Hypokalemia + [3] Metabolic alkalosis.**
- **Hypertension: may manifest as headache or flushing of the face** (edema is uncommon). Diastolic pressure is often more elevated than systolic pressure. Often moderate or resistant to medications.
- **Primary hyperaldosteronism is a cause of Secondary hypertension** — suspect in patients who develop Hypertension at extremes of age (<30 years or >60 years), not controlled on ≥3 blood pressure medications (including a diuretic), or with the classic triad.
- **Hypokalemia: proximal muscle weakness, polyuria (nephrogenic Diabetes insipidus),** fatigue, constipation, decreased deep tendon reflexes, Hypomagnesemia.

Step 1: SCREENING TESTS
- **Plasma renin activity & plasma aldosterone are the best initial screening tests for suspected Primary hyperaldosteronism. Primary: Elevated plasma and urine aldosterone levels** (plasma aldosterone often >15 ng/dL) **+ low (suppressed) plasma renin activity** in response.
- **Aldosterone to renin ratio: ARR > 20:1 (high aldosterone + low plasma renin levels) = Primary.** High plasma renin levels (ARR <20:1) = secondary Hyperaldosteronism.
- Labs: **Hypokalemia with Metabolic alkalosis [elevated bicarbonate level] classic** because aldosterone promotes sodium retention and increased potassium and hydrogen ion excretion.
- ECG may show signs of hypokalemia (eg, T wave flattening followed by prominent U wave).

Step 2: CONFIRMATORY TESTS
- **Lack of aldosterone suppression** aldosterone ≥8.5 ng/dL **(inappropriate aldosterone secretion) with any 1 of the following 4 tests**: [1] Oral sodium loading test, [2] Saline infusion test, [3] Fludrocortisone suppression test, or [4] Captopril challenge test. Sometimes, step 2 may be skipped.

STEP 3: Imaging after confirmation tests:
- **CT or MRI** to look for an adrenal or extra-adrenal mass AFTER laboratory tests:
- **Adrenal venous sampling: indicated in patients who are surgical candidates as the most accurate test (criterion standard) to distinguish between adenoma & bilateral hyperplasia** — if a unilateral adenoma is present, the plasma aldosterone concentration & aldosterone-to-cortisol ratio on one side is usually at least 5 times greater than the other indicating suppression. Bilateral hyperplasia tends to produce similar values on each side (little difference).

MANAGEMENT OF **BILATERAL** HYPERPLASIA
- **Medical: Mineralocorticoid antagonist: Spironolactone preferred** (more effective vs. Eplerenone).

MANAGEMENT OF **CONN SYNDROME OR UNILATERAL** HYPERPLASIA
- **Surgical: Laparoscopic unilateral adrenalectomy + Spironolactone** (blocks aldosterone).

CHRONIC ADRENOCORTICAL INSUFFICIENCY (AI)

- Disorder where the adrenal gland does not produce enough hormones.

SECONDARY (CENTRAL) ADRENOCORTICAL INSUFFICIENCY

Pituitary failure of ACTH secretion (lack of cortisol only). Aldosterone production is intact due to the Renin angiotensin aldosterone system (RAAS).

- Etiologies: **history of exogenous glucocorticoid use (especially without tapering) most common cause of secondary & overall adrenal insufficiency. Hypopituitarism. Sheehan syndrome:** postpartum pituitary infarction in the setting of obstetric hemorrhage complicated by hypotension.

PRIMARY ADRENOCORTICAL INSUFFICIENCY (ADDISON DISEASE)

Adrenal gland destruction (lack of cortisol AND aldosterone). Etiologies include:

- **Autoimmune most common cause in the US (80-90%),** often due to 21-hydroxylase antibodies.
- **Infection Tuberculosis** most common cause in developing countries; **HIV,** disseminated fungi.
- Vascular: thrombosis or hemorrhage in the adrenal gland **(Waterhouse-Friderichsen syndrome: bilateral adrenal hemorrhage & infarction due to meningococcemia),** anticoagulation.
- Trauma, metastatic disease, meds: **Ketoconazole, Metyrapone,** Rifampin, Phenytoin, Barbiturates.
- **Congenital adrenal hyperplasia:** 21 hydroxylase deficiency results in increased 17-ketosteroids, which have **weak androgen activity [virilization in male neonates, ambiguity of female genitalia at birth (or atypical appearance),** precocious puberty in both sexes, & variable effects of adrenal insufficiency].

CLINICAL MANIFESTATIONS

- Nonspecific symptoms due to lack of cortisol weakness, myalgias, fatigue, lethargy, arthralgia. Nonspecific GI symptoms — weight or appetite loss, anorexia, nausea, vomiting, abdominal pain, & diarrhea. Headache, sweating, abnormal menstruation, Hyponatremia, salt craving, hypotension.

Primary (Addison's disease):

- Additional symptoms due to lack of sex hormones & aldosterone — **hyperpigmentation** [increased ACTH production, leads to increased Melanocyte-stimulating hormone (MSH) as a byproduct because they are produced from the same precursor molecule, pro-opiomelanocortin (POMC)], **orthostatic hypotension.** Women may have loss of libido, amenorrhea, & loss of axillary pubic hair.

BASELINE LABS

- Early 8am ACTH, cortisol, & renin levels are obtained. **Increased renin, especially with Primary AI.**
- **Primary AI: elevated ACTH + decreased cortisol; Secondary AI: decreased ACTH + low cortisol.**
- Labs: **Hypoglycemia (more common in 2ry AI). Primary (Addison) — Hyponatremia, Hyperkalemia, & Non-anion gap metabolic acidosis** due to decreased aldosterone. Eosinophilia. **Autoimmune adrenalitis: 21-hydroxylase antibodies,** cytoplasmic & 17-hydroxylase antibodies.
- CT scan if negative antibodies: Autoimmune — small adrenal glands (atrophy), Infection — calcification or hemorrhage (eg, TB). METS or hemorrhage — bilateral adrenal enlargement.

SCREENING TEST

High-dose (250 mcg) ACTH (Cosyntropin) stimulation test

- **Adrenal insufficiency if insufficient or absent rise in serum cortisol** (<18 mcg/dL) after ACTH administration. Normal response is rise in serum cortisol to ≥20 mcg/dL after ACTH administration.

MANAGEMENT

- **Glucocorticoid replacement: Hydrocortisone first-line.** Prednisolone, Methylprednisolone.
- **Mineralocorticoid replacement (Fludrocortisone) often added only in Primary AI (Addison's).** Check daily weights. Increased weight may need a dose reduction in Fludrocortisone.

Patient education:

- Because cortisol is a "stress" hormone, people with chronic AI must be treated with IV glucocorticoids & IV isotonic fluids before & after surgical procedures (mimicking the body's natural response).
- During illness/surgery/high fever, oral dosing needs to be adjusted to recreate the normal adrenal gland response to "stress" (eg, triple the normal oral dosing for the first few days).
- Patients should wear a medical alert tag as well as carry an injectable form of cortisol for emergencies.

ADRENAL (ADDISONIAN) CRISIS [ACUTE ADRENOCORTICAL INSUFFICIENCY]

- **Sudden worsening of symptoms in diagnosed or undiagnosed chronic adrenal insufficiency precipitated by a "stressful" event (eg, infections are the most common precipitants,** sepsis, illness, surgery, trauma, volume loss, hypothermia, MI, hypoglycemia, etc.).

PATHOPHYSIOLOGY
- The normal response to "stress" is a 3-fold increase in cortisol. In Adrenal crisis, these patients are unable to increase cortisol during times of stress to meet the increased demand for cortisol.
- Normally aldosterone, a mineralocorticoid, promotes sodium retention and enhances vasoconstrictor responses of the vasculature. In Acute Adrenal crisis, patients are unable to maintain a normal blood pressure or an effective vasoconstrictor response, resulting in **distributive shock.**

TRIGGERS
Most commonly due to recent sudden change in glucocorticoid exposure:
- In patients with undiagnosed primary or secondary adrenal insufficiency, causes of a crisis include:
  - **Abrupt withdrawal of glucocorticoids (especially without tapering) most common cause.**
  - **Severe "stress" in previously undiagnosed patients with Addison's disease (eg, infections).** May be the primary manifestation in patients with chronic primary Adrenal insufficiency in the setting of a serious infection or other major stress. The stressor precipitates hypotension.
- In patients with known primary or secondary adrenal insufficiency who are under-replaced, due to:
  - (1) insufficient daily doses of glucocorticoid and/or mineralocorticoid
  - (2) failure to increase their glucocorticoid dose during an infection or other major illness (stress)
  - (3) persistent vomiting or diarrhea caused by viral gastroenteritis or other gastrointestinal disorders, leading to decreased absorption.
- **Pituitary or bilateral adrenal injury, hemorrhage, and infarction:**
  - **Sheehan syndrome: postpartum pituitary gland necrosis** due to pituitary gland ischemia.
  - **Waterhouse-Friderichsen Syndrome:** bilateral adrenal infarction, usually due to **hemorrhage, especially with Meningococcemia.**

CLINICAL MANIFESTATIONS
- **Shock primary manifestation — hypovolemia, orthostatic hypotension, or hypotension (often refractory to pressors).**
- Nonspecific symptoms: weakness, fatigue, nausea, vomiting, abdominal pain (mimicking acute abdomen), diarrhea, dizziness, arthralgia, apathy, syncope, confusion, altered mentation.
- **Fever indicates infection and the source should be identified and treated.**

DIAGNOSIS
- Labs: **Hyponatremia & Hyperkalemia (especially if primary AI), & Hypoglycemia. Cortisol & aldosterone confirms the diagnosis; cortisol levels will be low.** Order ACTH, renin, and CBC.
- **Primary AI: elevated ACTH + decreased cortisol; Secondary AI: low ACTH + decreased cortisol.**

MANAGEMENT
The mainstay of treatment of Acute adrenal insufficiency includes 3 major components:
- [1] early recognition of the underlying Adrenal insufficiency **(begin therapy immediately when suspected),**
- [2] **IV fluids: immediate administration of isotonic IV fluids — eg, 0.9% Normal saline to correct volume or Dextrose 5% in 0.9% saline [D5NS] to correct both volume and hypoglycemia, AND**
- [3] **IV glucocorticoid administration in supraphysiologic stress doses (eg, IV Hydrocortisone 100 mg IV bolus** followed by 50 mg IV every 6 hours **without waiting for laboratory results).** Hydrocortisone provides both glucocorticoid and mineralocorticoid effects. Dexamethasone can be used in undiagnosed Adrenal insufficiency because it doesn't interfere with cortisol assays.
- Other considerations: Reversal of electrolyte disorders. Identify and treat any underlying infection. Consider Vasopressor administration only after glucocorticoid therapy in patients unresponsive to aggressive fluid resuscitation (eg, Norepinephrine, Dopamine, or Phenylephrine).

CUSHING SYNDROME [CS] (HYPERCORTISOLISM)

Cushing syndrome = symptoms & signs related to cortisol excess. 4 main causes:

Exogenous:
- **[1] Iatrogenic long-term exogenous glucocorticoid** therapy most common overall cause of CS.

Endogenous:
- **[2] Cushing disease:** pituitary gland ACTH overproduction (hyperplasia or adenoma) — **most common endogenous cause of Cushing syndrome by far.** More common in women.
- **[3] Ectopic ACTH-producing tumor** (eg, **Small cell lung cancer**, thymus, Medullary thyroid cancer).
- **[4] Adrenal tumor (adenoma)** — autonomous **secretion of excess cortisol** (ACTH-independent).

CLINICAL MANIFESTATIONS
- **Proximal muscle weakness, weight gain,** headache, fatigue, oligomenorrhea, erectile dysfunction, polyuria, Osteoporosis. Psychological change (anxiety, depression, psychosis). Increased infections.

PHYSICAL EXAMINATION
- **Fat redistribution: central (truncal) obesity, "moon facies"** (roundly shaped faces with puffiness & facial redness), **buffalo hump, supraclavicular fat pads, thin extremities (muscle atrophy).**
- Skin changes: fragility [thin skin (atrophy), **pigmented (red or purple) striae ≥1 cm wide,** easy bruising], poor wound healing. Hyperpigmentation & androgen excess if markedly increased ACTH.
- **Acanthosis nigricans** epidermal hyperplasia & thickening of the skin with a velvety sensation on palpation, especially around the neck & armpit. Associated with hyperinsulinemia.
- **Increased ACTH: Androgen (DHEAS) excess:** hirsutism, oily skin, acne, menstrual irregularities.
- **Hypertension.**

LABORATORY EVALUATION
- **Hyperglycemia,** dyslipidemia. **Hypokalemia & Metabolic alkalosis** due to the aldosterone-like effects of cortisol. **Leukocytosis.**

Step 1: SCREENING TESTS: 3 options (often, at least 2 screening tests are performed to diagnose CS):
- **24-hour urinary free cortisol most specific** but often difficult to collect [≥2 measurements].
- **Late night (10-11 pm) salivary cortisol** 2 measurements. Convenient to obtain.
- **Low-dose (1 mg) overnight Dexamethasone suppression test:**
  - Cushing syndrome = elevated cortisol or no cortisol suppression after low dose Dexamethasone administration (serum cortisol does not decrease by ≥50%).

Step 2: DIFFERENTIATING TESTS: ordered once the diagnosis of CS is made on screening tests.
Baseline ACTH prior to high-dose testing. **If elevated ACTH, High-dose (8 mg) Dexamethasone suppression test helps to distinguish Cushing disease (↑ pituitary ACTH) from ectopic ↑ ACTH.**
- **Cushing disease: elevated ACTH + suppression of cortisol with high-dose Dexamethasone (Dex) (≥50% decrease in serum cortisol).** Cushing disease is the only 1 of the 4 major causes in which serum cortisol levels suppress ≥50% with high-dose Dexamethasone testing. **Increased DHEAS.**
- **Ectopic ACTH-producing tumor: elevated ACTH + no suppression of cortisol with high-dose Dex.**
- Adrenal tumor & steroids: **low ACTH** + no suppression of cortisol with high-dose Dex; low DHEAS.

Step 3: Imaging based on suspected cause: after lab confirmation suggests the possible etiology:
- Cushing disease: Pituitary MRI; sampling of the petrosal sinus performed if MRI is negative.
- Adrenal tumor: CT of the abdomen; Ectopic ACTH-producing lung tumor: chest imaging.

MANAGEMENT
- **Corticosteroid use: gradual taper (withdrawal) to prevent Addisonian crisis.**
- **Cushing disease: Transsphenoidal surgical resection of the pituitary tumor.**
  Radiation therapy or Pasireotide can be used in inoperable pituitary tumors. Mifepristone
- **Adrenal tumor tumor excision (adrenalectomy).** Mitotane reduces cortisol secretion. Ketoconazole.
- Ectopic tumor: resection if resectable. **If unresectable, Ketoconazole** or Metyrapone can be used.

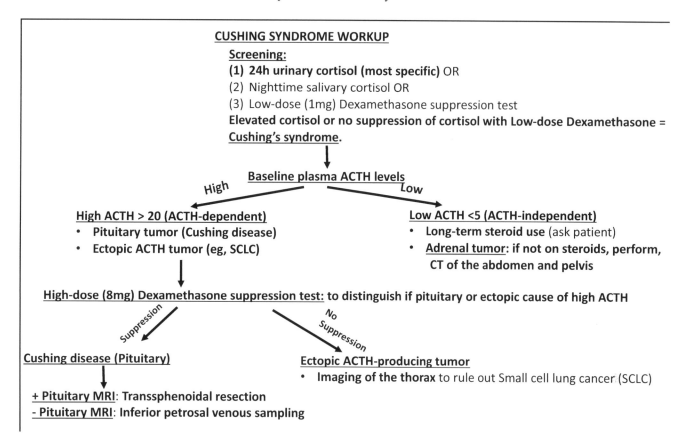

CUSHING SYNDROME WORKUP
Screening:
(1) **24h urinary cortisol (most specific)** OR
(2) Nighttime salivary cortisol OR
(3) Low-dose (1mg) Dexamethasone suppression test
Elevated cortisol or no suppression of cortisol with Low-dose Dexamethasone = Cushing's syndrome.

Baseline plasma ACTH levels
High   Low

High ACTH > 20 (ACTH-dependent)
• **Pituitary tumor (Cushing disease)**
• Ectopic ACTH tumor (eg, SCLC)

Low ACTH <5 (ACTH-independent)
• **Long-term steroid use** (ask patient)
• **Adrenal tumor:** if not on steroids, perform, CT of the abdomen and pelvis

High-dose (8mg) Dexamethasone suppression test: to distinguish if pituitary or ectopic cause of high ACTH

Suppression   No Suppression

Cushing disease (Pituitary)

Ectopic ACTH-producing tumor
• **Imaging of the thorax** to rule out Small cell lung cancer (SCLC)

+ Pituitary MRI: Transsphenoidal resection
- Pituitary MRI: Inferior petrosal venous sampling

CUSHING SYNDROME LAB VALUES

	Baseline ACTH	High-dose Dexamethasone suppression test
Exogenous corticosteroid use	Decreased	No suppression of cortisol
Adrenal Tumor: (cortisol producing)	Decreased	No suppression of cortisol
Cushing Disease: ACTH-secreting Pituitary adenoma	Increased	**Suppression of cortisol by ≥50%**
Ectopic ACTH-producing tumor	Increased	No suppression of cortisol (<50%)

Note that Cushing's disease is the only one that suppresses during high-dose suppression test.

ADRENAL INSUFFICIENCY LAB VALUES

	CRH	ACTH	Cortisol	CRH Stimulation Test	Aldosterone	Renin
Adrenal (Primary)	High	**HIGH**	**LOW**	↑ACTH response	Low	**High**
Pituitary (Secondary)	High	**LOW**	**LOW**	Absent/↓ ACTH Response	Low	Normal or low
Hypothalamus (Tertiary)	Low	Low	Low	Exaggerated, prolonged response	Low	Normal or low

Note that primary disorders, ACTH & cortisol go in opposite directions (same direction seen in 2ry/3ry).

PHEOCHROMOCYTOMA

- **Catecholamine-secreting tumor arising from the adrenal medulla** derived from chromaffin cells of neural crest origin from the sympathetic or parasympathetic system.
- Extra-adrenal locations of catecholamine-secreting Paragangliomas are the superior and inferior abdominal paraaortic areas (75% of extra-adrenal tumors). **90% are benign.**

EPIDEMIOLOGY
- Rare (causes 0.1-0.5% of Hypertension) but is the most common adrenal tumor in adults.
- May be associated with MEN syndrome 2, Neurofibromatosis type 1, & von Hippel-Lindau disease.
- Rule of 10s: 10% malignant, 10% bilateral, 10% seen in children, 10% extra-adrenal (paraganglioma).

PATHOPHYSIOLOGY
- **Secretes norepinephrine, epinephrine, & dopamine autonomously & intermittently.**

CLINICAL MANIFESTATIONS
- **Hypertension is the most consistent finding** — may be temporary or sustained.
- **"PHE": P**alpitations; **H**eadache (most common symptom); **E**xcessive sweating (diaphoresis).
- Chest or abdominal pain, weakness, fatigue, weight loss (despite increased appetite), tremor, & pallor.
- Triggers of paroxysms: exercise, bending, lifting, emotional stress, pregnancy, Decongestants, Amphetamines, Corticosteroids, Fluoxetine and other SSRIs, Tricyclic antidepressants, MAO inhibitors, opiates, Metoclopramide, glucagon, histamine, Cocaine, Epinephrine, Caffeine, Nicotine, and ionic intravenous contrast.

DIAGNOSIS
STEP 1: Biochemical testing:
- **Metanephrines: measurements for elevations in urinary and plasma fractionated metanephrines and catecholamines initial test of choice for suspected Pheochromocytoma** [24-hour urinary fractionated catecholamines, plasma fractionated catecholamines and catecholamine metabolites (eg, **metanephrines more sensitive and vanillylmandelic acid)].**
  - **High risk: Plasma fractionated metanephrines initial biochemical test (most sensitive) for high risk** for a Pheochromocytoma (eg, family history, familial tumor syndrome, history of previously resected pheochromocytoma, presence of adrenal mass found incidentally).
  - **Low risk: 24-hour urine fractionated metanephrines & catecholamines.**

STEP 2: Imaging:
- **Abdominal imaging: MRI or Noncontrast CT of abdomen & pelvis to locate the tumor after biochemical testing** (not the other way around). No further workup if negative + low suspicion.
- If Pheochromocytoma is still considered likely despite negative abdominal imaging, Iobenguane I-123 (metaiodobenzylguanidine [MIBG]) scintigraphy may be done. Fludeoxyglucose-positron emission tomography (PET) most sensitive.

MANAGEMENT
- **The order of management is [1] nonselective alpha blockade, followed by [2] beta blockade, followed by [3] surgery (definitive management) once medically stabilized.**
Preoperative management:
- **Nonselective alpha-blockade:** best initial therapy — **PHEnoxybenzamine (preferred) or PHEntolamine 1-2 weeks, followed by Beta blockers or Calcium channel blockers** to control blood pressure prior to surgery. Think "PHE" for symptoms & management.
- **DO NOT initiate therapy with beta-blockade to prevent unopposed alpha-1 receptor related vasoconstriction** during catecholamine release triggered by surgery or spontaneously, which could lead to life threatening hypertensive crisis.
Definitive management:
- **Complete adrenalectomy,** often laparoscopically, after at least 1-2 weeks of medical therapy.

CLINICAL MANIFESTATIONS OF THYROID DISORDERS

	HYPOTHYROIDISM	HYPERTHYROIDISM
ETIOLOGIES	• **Iodine deficiency (dietary),** Cretinism • **Hashimoto's Thyroiditis** • Thyroiditis: Postpartum, deQuervain, Silent (lymphocytic) **later stage** • Pituitary Hypothyroidism • Hypothalamic Hypothyroidism • Riedel's Thyroiditis • Medications: **Lithium, Amiodarone, Apha interferon**	• **Grave's Disease** • Iatrogenic thyrotoxicosis • Thyroiditis: Postpartum, deQuervain, Silent (lymphocytic) **earlier stage** • Toxic Multinodular Goiter • Toxic adenoma • **TSH-secreting pituitary adenoma** • Medications: **Amiodarone** • Excess intake of T3, T4
CLINICAL MANIFESTATIONS		
CALORIGENIC	• Decreased metabolic rate: in general, all metabolic processes are decreased, except for menstrual flow, which is increased. • **Cold intolerance** (↓heat production) • Weight gain (despite ↓appetite)	• Increased metabolic rate: In general, all metabolic processes are increased, except for menstrual flow, which is decreased. • **Heat intolerance** (↑heat production) • Weight loss (despite ↑appetite)
SKIN	• Dry, thickened rough skin • **loss of outer 1/3 of eyebrow** • Goiter • **Nonpitting edema (myxedema)**	• **Skin warm, moist, soft, fine hair,** alopecia, easy bruising • Goiter
CNS	• **Hypoactivity:** Fatigue, sluggishness, memory loss, depression, ↓*DTR* • Hoarseness of voice	• **Hyperactivity:** anxiety, **fine tremors, nervousness,** fatigue, weakness, increased sympathetic
GI	• Constipation, anorexia	• Diarrhea, hyperdefecation
CVS	• **Bradycardia, ↓ cardiac output** • Pericardial effusion	• **Tachycardia, palpitations** • **High-output heart failure**

IATROGENIC HYPOTHYROIDISM

• Often due to treatment for hyperthyroidism with radioactive iodine or surgery (total or subtotal thyroidectomy) without subsequent thyroid hormone replacement.

Medications:

• **Amiodarone: contains iodine and may induce hypothyroidism** (by the Wolff-Chaikoff effect) by inhibition of T4/T3 secretion and release; may cause thyroiditis, inhibits thyroid hormone entry into peripheral tissues. **May cause hyperthyroidism** (by the Jod-Basedow effect) depending on the underlying state of the patient.

• **Interferon alfa** may stimulate the immune system in patients with baseline thyroid autoimmune predisposition (eg, patients with anti-TPO or anti-TG antibodies). May cause thyroiditis.

• **Lithium** causes hypothyroidism by a poorly understood mechanism — may affect colloid and inhibits T4/T3 secretion and release.

• **Propylthiouracil and Methimazole** — inhibit T4 & T3 synthesis.

• Others include Thalidomide, oral tyrosine kinase inhibitors (eg, Imatinib), Stavudine, Interleukin-2, Rifampin, Anti-epileptics (eg, Carbamazepine, Phenytoin, Phenobarbital), and Sulfisoxazole.

Exogenous thyroid hormone use:

• **Increased free T4, decreased TSH, and low/undetectable thyroglobulin.**

THYROID FUNCTION TESTS

TEST	DESCRIPTION	CLINICAL UTILITY

TSH	Thyroid stimulating hormone	• **(1) BEST THYROID FUNCTION SCREENING TEST.** Initial test for suspected thyroid disease.
		
		• (2) Also used to adjust dosage of on thyroid hormone replacement therapy:
		   - Low TSH ⇨ decrease dose of Levothyroxine
		   - High TSH ⇨ increase dose of Levothyroxine
		   - Normal TSH ⇨ maintain the current dose
		
		• Used with T_4 to manage patients with Graves'.

Free T₄ (FT₄)	**Free thyroxine** levels (metabolically active hormone)	• **Performed by the lab when TSH is abnormal** to determine thyroid hyperfunction or hypofunction. Hyperthyroidism • Primary hyperthyroidism: ↓ TSH + ↑ FT4 • Secondary hyperthyroidism: ↑ TSH + ↑ FT4 • Subclinical hyperthyroidism: ↓ TSH + normal FT4 Hypothyroidism: • Primary hypothyroidism: ↑ TSH + ↓ FT4 • Secondary hypothyroidism: ↓TSH + ↓ FT4 • Subclinical hypothyroidism: ↑ TSH + normal FT4
THYROID ANTIBODIES	• **Anti-thyroid peroxidase Ab** • **Anti-Thyroglobulin Ab** • **Thyroid stimulating Ab (TSH receptor Ab)**	• **Both are used to diagnose Hashimoto's thyroiditis** or other **autoimmune thyroiditis** (eg, Silent lymphocytic or Postpartum thyroiditis). • **Specific for Graves' disease**
Free T₃	Serum triiodothyronine	• Useful to diagnose hyperthyroidism when TSH is low & T_4 is still normal.
FTI	Free Thyroxine Index	• Used in thyroid disease when the patient has protein abnormalities.

	TSH	FREE T4
PRIMARY Thyroid is the problem	• INCREASED	• DECREASED
	• In primary disorders, the labs are in OPPOSITE directions	
SECONDARY Pituitary gland is the problem	• DECREASED	• DECREASED
	• In secondary & tertiary disorders, the labs are in the SAME direction	
SUBCLINICAL	• INCREASED (hypothyroid)	• NORMAL (subclinical)
	• Management is to repeat TSH. • Thyroid hormone replacement may be needed if **TSH >10 mIU/L** to reduce cardiovascular risk.	

TERTIARY DISORDER
The **Hypothalamus** is the problem

SECONDARY DISORDER
The **Pituitary Gland** is the problem

PRIMARY DISORDER
The **target organ** is the problem

HYPOTHALAMUS

PITUITARY

TARGET ORGAN
(Thyroid, Adrenal Gland, Ovary)

TSH is the initial test of choice for suspected hypothyroid or hyperthyroid conditions

Radioactive uptake scan assesses for **new thyroid hormone synthesis** using radioactive iodine.

RADIOACTIVE IODINE SCAN (RAIU) [THYROID SCINTIGRAPHY] Iodine 131 nuclear medicine scan	POSSIBLE DIAGNOSIS
DIFFUSE increased uptake	**(1) Graves' disease or (2) TSH-secreting pituitary adenoma**
DIFFUSE decreased or absent uptake	**Thyroiditis** — eg, Hashimoto's, Postpartum, DeQuervain, Silent lymphocytic. Diffuse decreased or absent uptake due to release of preformed hormones from inflammation, which suppresses production of new thyroid hormone via negative feedback.
Hot Nodule (focal uptake in one area)	**Toxic Adenoma**
Multiple Nodules (multiple areas of increased uptake)	**Toxic Multinodular goiter**
Cold Nodules	May be a benign nodule but may need to rule out malignancy

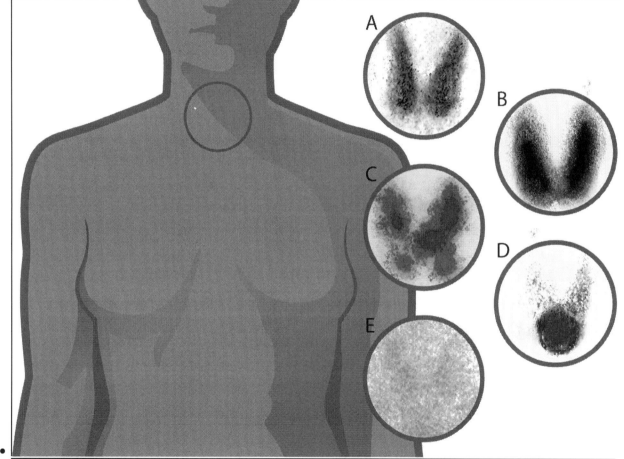

RADIOACTIVE UPTAKE SCAN (thyroid scintigraphy, Iodine 131 nuclear medicine scan)
A. Normal thyroid gland
B. Graves' disease or TSH-secreting adenoma (diffuse increased uptake)
C. Toxic multinodular goiter (multiple areas of increased and decreased uptake)
D. Toxic adenoma (focal area of increased uptake – hot nodule)
E. Thyroiditis (diffuse decreased uptake)

Petros Perros [CC BY-SA 3.0 (https://creativecommons.org/licenses/by-sa/3.0)]

CONGENITAL HYPOTHYROIDISM (CRETINISM)

- **Symptoms & signs due to untreated congenital deficiency of thyroid hormone (Hypothyroidism).**

ETIOLOGIES
- **Thyroid gland dysgenesis in 80–85% of neonatal hypothyroidism,** inborn errors of thyroid hormone synthesis in 10–15%, and TSHR antibody-mediated in 5% of affected newborns.
- May be acquired if maternal TSH-receptor blocking antibodies pass into fetal circulation via placenta.
- **Lack of maternal iodine intake in developing countries.**
- Transplacental passage of maternal thyroid hormone occurs before the fetal thyroid gland begins to function and provides partial hormone support to a fetus with congenital hypothyroidism.

CLINICAL MANIFESTATIONS
- The majority of infants appear normal at birth; may be detected with the use of biochemical screening.
- **Classic clinical features in neonates include prolonged jaundice, feeding problems, hypotonia, enlarged tongue, delayed bone maturation, and umbilical hernia.**
- **Symptoms of hypothyroidism:** decreased metabolic rate, cold intolerance, dry thickened rough skin, constipation, weight gain despite decreased oral intake, menorrhagia, myxedema (eyelid and facial edema), weakness, & lethargy. **Mental developmental delays,** short stature.
- Congenital malformations, especially cardiac, are 4x more common in congenital hypothyroidism.
- **Goiter symptoms** in older children — hoarseness and dyspnea (tracheal compression).

Physical examination:
- **Coarse facial features, macroglossia, umbilical hernia, hypotonia (decreased DTRs),** prolonged jaundice, feeding problems, & congenital malformations.

DIAGNOSIS
- **Primary hypothyroid profile: most common — increased TSH + decreased free T4 or T3.**

MANAGEMENT:
- **Levothyroxine (synthetic T4).** Early treatment with T4 results in normal IQ levels, but subtle neurodevelopmental abnormalities may occur in those with the most severe hypothyroidism at diagnosis or when treatment is delayed or suboptimal.

SUBCLINICAL HYPOTHYROIDISM

- **Hypothyroidism determined by laboratory tests (isolated increased TSH + normal T4 levels) in patients with little or no symptoms of Hypothyroidism.**
- Subclinical hypothyroidism may be associated with increased risk of cardiovascular disease (eg, coronary artery disease, CHF, stroke), especially when the serum TSH concentration is >10 mU/L.

CLINICAL MANIFESTATIONS
- **Most patients are asymptomatic;** may have nonspecific symptoms suggestive of hypothyroidism.

DIAGNOSIS
- **[1] Isolated increased TSH (hypothyroid) + [2] normal free T4 and/or free T3 (subclinical).**

MANAGEMENT
- **Observation with repeat TSH levels at least once after 3-6 months are recommended** because ~46% resolve spontaneously within 2 years. Most patients have TSH <10 mIU/L.
- **Levothyroxine may be given if TSH ≥10 mIU/L, women who wish to conceive or get pregnant, or Dyslipidemia to prevent cardiovascular complications,** in patients with a positive thyroid peroxidase antibody, the presence of hypothyroid symptoms, or cardiovascular risk factors. The goal of therapy is to normalize TSH levels. Treatment in other patients is controversial.
- In older adults with <u>mild</u> Subclinical hypothyroidism, treatment is generally not recommended, since TSH values in the upper limit of normal to 6.9 mU/L are considered age appropriate.

HASHIMOTO THYROIDITIS [CHRONIC AUTOIMMUNE (LYMPHOCYTIC) THYROIDITIS]

- **Most common cause of hypothyroidism in the US**. Increased incidence in **women 30-50 years.**
- **2 forms:** [1] **goitrous** thyroid gland enlargement (goiter); [2] **atrophic**: minimal residual tissue (late).

PATHOPHYSIOLOGY

- **Autoimmune thyroid cell destruction** by anti-thyroid peroxidase & anti-thyroglobulin antibodies (and TSH receptor-*blocking* antibodies to a lesser extent, which prevent binding of TSH).

CLINICAL MANIFESTATIONS

- **Symptoms of Hypothyroidism** — decreased metabolic rate, fatigue, cold intolerance, dry thickened rough skin, constipation, weight gain despite decreased oral intake, menorrhagia, myxedema (eyelid and facial edema), weakness, lethargy.
- Goiter symptoms: hoarseness and dyspnea (tracheal compression).
- Women may have galactorrhea (due to increased prolactin).

PHYSICAL EXAMINATION

- The thyroid gland may be normal, enlarged (goiter), or atrophic (later in the disease course).
- **Bradycardia,** decreased DTR (hyporeflexia), **loss of outer 1/3 of eyebrows.**
- **Myxedema** — nonpitting edema (eg, periorbital, peripheral) due to ↑ glycosaminoglycan deposition.

DIAGNOSIS

- **Primary hypothyroid pattern** — **increased TSH + decreased free T4 or T3 in response to the low T4 (most common).** May be normal or subclinical Hypothyroidism in early disease.
- ⊕ **Antithyroid peroxidase and/or anti-thyroglobulin antibodies** (>95% of patients).
- Radioactive uptake scan: diffuse decreased iodine uptake (thyroiditis). Usually not needed.
- Biopsy: rarely done — **lymphocytic infiltration with germinal centers & Hürthle cells** (enlarged epithelial cells with abundant eosinophilic granular cytoplasm).

MANAGEMENT: Levothyroxine therapy.
LEVOTHYROXINE
INDICATIONS

- **First-line management of Hashimoto thyroiditis** & Subclinical hypothyroidism if TSH ≥10 mIU/L. Thyroid hormone replacement after thyroidectomy or Radioactive iodine ablation.

MECHANISM OF ACTION:

- Synthetic thyroxine (T4). Half-life of 7 days and can be given daily.

MONITORING

- **Monitor TSH levels at ~6-week intervals when initiating or changing the dose.**
- Increase the dose if TSH is high and decrease the dose if TSH is low. The goal is a normal TSH.
- **Low doses with small incremental increases should be used to initiate therapy in the elderly and patients with cardiovascular disease.**
- During pregnancy, the dose needs to be increased by 30%.

INTERACTIONS

- Best taken in the morning on an empty stomach for optimal absorption.
- Multivitamins, aluminum, iron or calcium supplements, & proton pump inhibitors should be taken 4 hours apart from Levothyroxine as they can decrease its effectiveness.
- May need to decrease the dose with anticoagulants, insulin, and oral hypoglycemics. Cholestyramine may increase T4 requirements.

ADVERSE EFFECTS

- **Overtreatment increases risk for Atrial fibrillation & high-output Heart failure, reduces bone density resulting in Osteopenia,** worsening of Angina pectoris, and increased cardiovascular risk.

SICK EUTHYROID SYNDROME (NONTHYROIDAL ILLNESS)

- **Abnormal thyroid function tests in patients with normal thyroid function (absence of underlying thyroid disease) due any acute severe nonthyroidal illness,** making the measurements of TSH and free T4 potentially misleading.

PATHOPHYSIOLOGY
- **Most commonly seen with severe non-thyroidal illnesses** (eg, sepsis, cardiac, malignancies, etc.).
- Severe illness causes hormonal changes due to inflammatory cytokines and decreases peripheral conversion of T4 to T3.

DIAGNOSIS
- **Low T3 syndrome: decreased Free T3 & increased reverse T3 with normal TSH & free T4 most common pattern** — Low T3 due to illness-related decreased peripheral conversion of T4 into T3. Decreased clearance rather than increased production is major basis for increased reverse T3 (rT3).
- Free thyroxine (T4) often normal or decreased in more severe disease.
- **TSH may be normal, low, or high.** TSH usually low with severe disease & increased in the recovery phase.

MANAGEMENT
- **Because the cause is a nonthyroidal illness, treatment and management of underlying medical illness is the mainstay of treatment;** monitoring of patient's thyroid function. Endocrine consult.
- Thyroid hormone replacement is usually not indicated.
- Unless a thyroid disorder is suspected, routine thyroid testing should be avoided in severe acute illness.

FIBROUS (RIEDEL, INVASIVE) THYROIDITIS

- Extremely rare chronic autoimmune thyroiditis characterized by **[1] chronic inflammation (macrophage and eosinophil infiltration) & [2] dense fibrosis that invades the thyroid & adjacent neck structures.**
- May be part of the IgG4-related systemic disease. Most common in females 30-50 years of age.

CLINICAL MANIFESTATIONS
- **Presents similar to thyroid malignancy** — **"rock" hard, nontender, rapidly growing, asymmetric, fixed goiter** (moves poorly with swallowing). Often, not clearly separable from the adjacent tissues. Absence of cervical lymphadenopathy.
- **Compression symptoms:** neck tightness or pressure, hoarseness, dysphagia, choking, coughing, increased respiratory rate from **airway compression**.

DIAGNOSIS
- **IgG4 serum levels.** Hashimoto thyroiditis can occur concomitantly, and **thyroid peroxidase (TPO) antibodies are positive in about 90% of patients with Riedel thyroiditis.**
- **Open thyroid biopsy** — **extensive fibrosis;** macrophage and eosinophilic infiltration. Biopsy usually performed to rule out malignancy. FNA insufficient test if suspected.

MANAGEMENT
- **Glucocorticoids mainstay of treatment** (they lead to dramatic symptom improvement).
- Alternatives include Tamoxifen, Rituximab, or Mycophenolate.
- Hypothyroidism may be treated with Levothyroxine.
- Surgical management when all other alternatives have failed, or when the patient has symptoms of esophageal and/or tracheal compression.

EXAM TIP
- **A "rock hard" thyroid is either indicative of Anaplastic thyroid cancer or Riedel thyroiditis.**
- A biopsy is needed to distinguish between the two.

MYXEDEMA CRISIS OR COMA

- **<u>Rare form of severe hypothyroidism</u>** that results in an altered mental status, hypothermia, bradycardia, hypercarbia, and hyponatremia. High mortality rate (>40%).
- **Most commonly seen in elderly women with long standing hypothyroidism during the winter.**

PATHOPHYSIOLOGY
- Usually an acute precipitating factor (eg, infection, CVA, CHF, sedative/narcotic use) in a patient with longstanding hypothyroidism, discontinuation or noncompliance with Levothyroxine therapy, or failure to start Levothyroxine after treatment for hyperthyroidism.

CLINICAL MANIFESTATIONS
<u>Severe signs of hypothyroidism</u>:
- The hallmarks of myxedema coma are **[1] altered mental status and [2] hypothermia, but obtundation, hypotension, bradycardia, hyponatremia, hypoglycemia, and hypoventilation (hypercarbia) are often present.**
- **<u>Neurologic manifestations</u>** — altered consciousness such as confusion with lethargy and obtundation, and if left untreated, patients will progress to coma. Focal or generalized seizures.
- **<u>Pericardial effusion</u>** due to the accumulation of fluid rich in mucopolysaccharides may occur.
- Patients with Myxedema coma have an increased risk of bleeding due to an acquired Von Willebrand syndrome Type 1 and a decrease in factors V, VII, VIII, IX, and X.

PHYSICAL EXAMINATION
- **The two most common findings will be [1] altered mental status and [2] hypothermia, along with common findings of hypothyroidism.**
- **<u>Vital signs</u>: hypothermia, bradycardia, hypoventilation, diastolic hypertension (early) followed by hypotension (late).** Severe hypothyroidism is associated with bradycardia, decreased myocardial contractility, and a low cardiac output. Decreased delayed deep tendon reflexes.

DIAGNOSIS
- **<u>Primary hypothyroid profile most common</u>** — **increased TSH + decreased free T4** (free T4 and T3 levels may so low that it may be undetectable). Hyponatremia, Hypoglycemia.

MANAGEMENT
- Glucocorticoids, Thyroid hormone, supportive management, ICU admission, and sufficient management of coexisting factors (eg, infection) should be instituted <u>without waiting</u> for laboratory confirmation when Myxedema coma is suspected due to high mortality rate.
- **<u>IV Glucocorticoids</u>:** IV Glucocorticoids often given at stress doses until coexisting Adrenal insufficiency can be excluded via cortisol levels (eg, high-dose Hydrocortisone 100 mg IV every 8 hours). **Hydrocortisone is recommended to be administered prior to thyroid hormone therapy, especially if the patient is hypotensive to avoid adrenal crises.** This is because Levothyroxine will increase cortisol metabolism.
- **<u>IV Thyroid hormone</u>: Replacement thyroid hormone therapy with IV Levothyroxine (T4)** 200-400 mcg. Liothyronine (T3) may be added to Levothyroxine, however proper dosing is essential to prevent increased mortality from over metabolism due to T3.
- **<u>Hypothermia</u>: <u>passive</u> rewarming with a blanket is preferred for correction of hypothermia.** Active rewarming may cause peripheral vasodilatation, worsening hypotension.
- **<u>IV fluid resuscitation</u>** essential. If hypoglycemia is present, 5-10% Dextrose with half normal saline should be administered carefully. Hypotension, if present and not caused by volume depletion, will be corrected by thyroid hormone therapy and management of hyponatremia, hypoglycemia, and hypothermia. If hypotension is refractory to IV fluid resuscitation, then vasopressors should be initiated until Levothyroxine has time to act.
- <u>Empiric antibiotics</u>: should be considered until appropriate cultures are proven negative.

SUBACUTE GRANULOMATOUS (DEQUERVAIN) THYROIDITIS

- **Inflammation of the thyroid gland** characterized by **neck pain, a tender diffuse goiter**, and transient thyrotoxicosis, often occurring **after a viral infection**.

PATHOPHYSIOLOGY
- **Unknown but often follows antecedent <u>viral</u> respiratory tract infection or post-viral inflammation** (but it is <u>not</u> an autoimmune disease).
- **Hyperthyroidism is typically the initial presentation,** followed by euthyroidism, then hypothyroidism, followed by resolution & restoration of normal thyroid function within 6 months.

CLINICAL MANIFESTATIONS
- **Neck pain or discomfort:** pain most common symptom and chief complaint (96%) — **painful and tender thyroid gland or neck pain and sore throat,** aggravated with head movements, coughing, & swallowing. May radiate to the jaw, throat, ears, or upper chest.
- **Viral symptoms: low-grade fever, myalgias, malaise, fatigue, anorexia are common.**
- 50% of patients usually present in (1) <u>hyperthyroid phase</u> due to acute neck pain (even though many have little, if any, symptoms of thyroid excess). Later in the disease, they may present in the (2) <u>hypothyroid phase </u>with symptoms and signs of hypothyroidism. (3) <u>Recovery phase</u> after 6 months.

Physical examination:
- **Diffusely tender small goiter.** May have a fever.

DIAGNOSIS
- **High ESR + negative thyroid antibodies.**
- **Hyperthyroid profile early in the disease (decreased TSH + increased free T4).** May present in a euthyroid or later in a transient hypothyroid state.
- <u>Adjunctive:</u> Radioactive uptake scan — diffuse decreased or absent iodine uptake (thyroiditis) due to release of preformed hormones from inflammation and decreased production of new hormones.
- <u>Biopsy:</u> granulomatous inflammation with multinucleated giant cells (rarely performed).

MANAGEMENT
- **Supportive: reassurance it is self-limiting** (95% return to euthyroid state with complete resolution).
- **NSAIDs or Aspirin for pain & inflammation.** Aspirin avoided if significant hyperthyroidism phase.
- <u>Corticosteroids</u> (eg, Prednisone) in <u>severe</u> disease (marked local or systemic symptoms) or if no response to NSAIDs or Salicylates in 2-3 days.
- Antithyroid medications play no role in the management of Subacute thyroiditis.

PANCE PREP PEARL OF THE WEEK
DEQUERVAIN THYROIDITIS
- AKA **Subacute** or **Granulomatous** Thyroiditis.
- **Most common in women.**

HALLMARKS
She has **DquerPAINS**
- **D**iffuse decreased uptake on Radioactive uptake scan
    (also seen with Hashimoto and Postpartum thyroiditis)
- **Painful thyroid hallmark! Diffusely tender thyroid** on examination
- **After VIRAL illness**
- **Increased ESR & CRP**
- **Negative thyroid antibodies**
- **Self-limiting. Salicylates or NSAIDs for pain.** Prednisone if severe.

Biopsy: Granulomas and Multinucleated Giant cells (not usually done).
Natural course: **Hyperthyroid initially -> Hypothyroid -> Resolution**

TOXIC THYROID GLAND ADENOMA (SOLITARY HYPERFUNCTIONING NODULE)

- **Single hyperfunctioning autonomous nodule.**
- Nontoxic usually asymptomatic. Toxic = symptoms of thyrotoxicosis.
- Risk factors: Iodine deficiency is a well-known environmental risk factor. Genetic mutations in BRAF, RET, KRAS, and genetic rearrangement of the PAX8-PPAR gene. More common in females.

CLINICAL MANIFESTATIONS
- The majority of the thyroid adenomas (nontoxic) are asymptomatic, or a **palpable nodule** is detected.
- **Signs of hyperthyroidism** — anxiety, heat intolerance, weight loss despite increased appetite, fatigue, weakness, increased sympathetic output (tachycardia, palpitations, atrial fibrillation, fine tremor), diarrhea, increased metabolic rate, high-output heart failure, & oligomenorrhea.
- **Obstructive symptoms (enlarged goiter)** — dyspnea (eg tracheal compression), dysphagia (esophageal compression), stridor, **hoarseness** (recurrent laryngeal nerve compression).

DIAGNOSIS
- **Primary hyperthyroid profile** decreased TSH + increased free T4 or T3. Normal or subclinical.
- Radioactive iodine scan: **single focal area of increased iodine uptake (hot nodule),** with decreased uptake in the remaining surrounding normal tissue (activity of the normal thyroid gland is reduced).

MANAGEMENT
- **Solitary toxic nodule: radioiodine-131 ablation & surgery are the 2 most effective treatment options for permanently decreasing the production of thyroid hormone.**
- Thionamide therapy (Methimazole, Propylthiouracil) may be used if patients prefer to avoid both radioiodine & surgery; they may also be used prior to these therapies to treat hyperthyroidism.
- Beta blockers can be used in patients with moderate-to-severe hyperadrenergic symptoms until euthyroidism is achieved by thionamides, radioiodine, or surgery.
- Surgery: (thyroid lobectomy or isthmusectomy) can relieve from compressive symptoms, immediate resolution of hyperthyroidism, & avoidance of radiation exposure but preserve thyroid function.

PITUITARY TSH-SECRETING ADENOMA

- **Benign pituitary adenoma that secretes TSH in an autonomous (independent) fashion.**
- Rare cause of hyperthyroidism (<1% of all cases).

CLINICAL MANIFESTATIONS
- **Diffuse goiter** (95%).
- **Signs of hyperthyroidism** — anxiety, heat intolerance, weight loss despite increased appetite, fatigue, weakness, increased sympathetic output (tachycardia, palpitations, atrial fibrillation, fine tremor), diarrhea, increased metabolic rate, high-output heart failure, & oligomenorrhea.
- Compression of local structures: **bitemporal hemianopsia (loss of outer visual fields of both eyes) due to compression of the optic chiasm. Headache,** mental disturbances.

DIAGNOSIS
- **Secondary hyperthyroid profile: increased free T4 AND inappropriately increased TSH** (both in the **same direction,** indicating a secondary cause). Elevated TSH β subunit levels.
- **Radioactive uptake scan: diffuse increased uptake** (same as Graves').
- **Pituitary MRI** to detect the adenoma.

MANAGEMENT
- **Transsphenoidal surgery — definitive management.** Beta blockers used for symptom control.
- **Somatostatin analogs (eg, Octreotide) may be used prior to surgery** to restore euthyroidism. Dopamine agonists (eg, Cabergoline) are alternatives to Somatostatin analogs. Sella radiation.

GRAVES' DISEASE

- Autoimmune disease which primarily affects the thyroid gland, characterized by Hyperthyroidism due to an increase in synthesis and release of thyroid hormones (due to thyroid-stimulating autoantibodies).

EPIDEMIOLOGY
- **Graves' is the most common cause of hyperthyroidism in the US** (causes 60-80% of thyrotoxicosis).
- Highest incidence in women 20-40 years of age. Associated with other autoimmune disorders.

PATHOPHYSIOLOGY
- **TSH-receptor autoantibodies [thyroid stimulating immunoglobulins (TSIs)]** bind to & stimulate the TSH receptor on the thyroid gland, leading to **[1] increased thyroid hormone production, [2] thyroid gland enlargement (growth), & [3] hyperthyroidism.**
- Ophthalmopathy: TSH-receptor autoantibodies activate retroocular fibroblasts and adipocytes, leading to muscle swelling by trapping water & fat growth orbitopathy (specific to Graves').
- Graves' dermopathy (pretibial myxedema): Glycosaminoglycans accumulation and lymphoid infiltration occur in affected skin, which becomes erythematous with a thickened, rough texture.

CLINICAL MANIFESTATIONS
- Symptoms of hyperthyroidism common to any cause of thyrotoxicosis — eg, heat intolerance, tremors, weight loss despite increased appetite, palpitations from tachycardias, warm moist skin, diarrhea (increased bowel movements), oligomenorrhea or amenorrhea in women, etc.
- **Specific to Graves':**
  - **Ophthalmopathy: proptosis, exophthalmos, lid lag or retraction causing staring gaze appearance,** diplopia, vision changes, conjunctival injection, grittiness, eye discomfort.
  - **Pretibial myxedema (dermopathy):** swollen red or brown patches on legs; non-pitting edema.

PHYSICAL EXAMINATION
- **Diffusely enlarged firm palpable nontender goiter with or without a thyroid bruit or thrill.**

DIAGNOSIS:
- **Primary hyperthyroid profile: decreased TSH + increased free T4 or T3.**
- ⊕ **Thyroid-stimulating immunoglobulins (TSH-receptor antibodies) hallmark;** Thyrotropin-binding inhibiting (TBI) immunoglobulin or thyrotropin-binding inhibitory immunoglobulin (TBII).
- **Radioactive uptake scan: diffuse, increased iodine uptake** (due to increased new hormone synthesis) may be used in equivocal cases to distinguish Graves' from thyroiditis. US: hypervascular.

MANAGEMENT
Treatment consists of rapid symptom control and reduction of thyroid hormone secretion.
Treatment for Graves' disease depends on its presentation & the 3 options include:
- **[1] Radioactive iodine (RAI) ablation of the thyroid gland — most common therapy used, OR**
- **[2] Antithyroid drugs Methimazole or Propylthiouracil (PTU), OR**
- **[3] Thyroidectomy total or subtotal thyroidectomy.**
- Radioactive iodine and Thyroidectomy are considered definitive management options.
All 3 options have pros and cons, and there is no consensus on which one is the best option.

Symptomatic management:
Beta-adrenergic blockers (eg, Propranolol ER, Atenolol)
- **Beta blockers can be used to rapidly ameliorate symptoms, such as tremor, hypertension, diaphoresis, anxiety, Atrial fibrillation, & tachycardia until hyperthyroidism is resolved or other treatments take effect.** Also useful if history of cardiovascular disease & in elderly patients.
- Beta blockers are the initial treatment of choice for thyrotoxic crisis and effectively treats Thyrotoxic hypokalemic periodic paralysis.

RADIOACTIVE IODINE ABLATION

- Indications: **131I (RAI) is the most common therapy used for the management of Graves' disease,** especially in non-pregnant adult patients >21 years, patients not planning to get pregnant within the next 6-12 months after treatment, patients with risky comorbid conditions for surgery.
- Mechanism of action: RAI is taken up by thyroid gland, destroying the thyroid gland within 6-18 weeks.
- Monitoring: The patient should be provided with a written radiation safety precautions after RAI treatment to avoid exposure to household members or community members, especially children, and pregnant women. **TFTs should be monitored every 4-6 weeks for 6 months or until the patient becomes hypothyroid. The patient is then placed on lifelong Levothyroxine.**
- Adverse reactions: **Radioactive iodine may exacerbate ophthalmopathy initially. Pretreatment with Glucocorticoids may be used to reduce worsening ophthalmopathy.**
- Contraindications: **pregnant & lactating women** (can damage fetal or neonatal thyroid tissue). Women are advised to avoid pregnancy for at least 4 months following 131I therapy. **Moderate to severe Graves orbitopathy (RAI can worsen ophthalmopathy initially).**

ANTITHYROID THIONAMIDES Methimazole or Propylthiouracil (PTU).

- Mechanism of action: **[1] Inhibition of thyroid hormone synthesis and release** by inhibiting thyroid peroxidase-mediated iodination of thyroglobulin, blocking synthesis of T3 and T4. **[2] They also reduce thyroid antibody levels. Propylthiouracil also blocks peripheral conversion (deiodination) of T4 to T3.** They often achieve a euthyroid state within 3-8 weeks.
- Indications: May be used in older patients or patients with cardiovascular disease (they respond well) and young adults with mild thyrotoxicosis, small goiters, or fear of radioactive iodine. May also be used prior to more definitive treatment (eg, thyroidectomy or radioactive iodine). **In nonpregnant patients, Methimazole is preferred** due to less frequent adverse effects (especially hepatotoxicity), once-daily dosing [longer half-life (6h) compared to PTU (90 min) given q6-8h], & more rapid achievement of normal thyroid function. Methimazole is teratogenic in the first trimester. **Propylthiouracil is preferred [1] in the first trimester of pregnancy and lactation & [2] for Thyroid storm** (due to the added benefit of inhibition of peripheral conversion of T4 to T3).
- Adverse effects: common: skin rash, pruritus, allergic dermatitis, nausea, alopecia, dyspepsia. Antihistamines may control mild pruritus without discontinuation of the drug. **Severe: Agranulocytosis or Aplastic anemia (pancytopenia)** in 0.4%, **hypoprothrombinemia, and hepatotoxicity; fulminant hepatitis with PTU.** These effects are usually reversible. Cholestasis.
- Follow-up & monitoring: **Monitor thyroid function tests every 4-6 weeks for dose adjustment.** Goal in Primary hyperthyroidism is normalization of TSH levels. Monitor LFTs with PTU.

THYROIDECTOMY Total or subtotal thyroidectomy.

- Indications: **Surgery for definitive treatment is usually recommended for very large goiters (>80g), large thyroid nodules (>4 cm), nodules suspicious for malignancy, symptoms or signs of anterior neck compression/obstruction, rapid & definitive resolution of Hyperthyroidism.**
- Complications: [1] permanent hypoparathyroidism, [2] **hoarseness (recurrent laryngeal nerve damage due to vocal cord involvement).** Bleeding & laryngeal edema.

ORBITOPATHY

- Mild to moderate ophthalmopathy may not require active treatment (usually spontaneous improvement with treatment). **Radioactive iodine & smoking may worsen orbitopathy.**
- **Glucocorticoids best initial therapy for Ophthalmopathy when therapy is needed (IV Methylprednisolone preferred over oral Prednisone).**
- Other options include orbital irradiation, Rituximab, and emergency orbital decompression.
- Teprotumumab is an IGF-IR inhibitor that reduces proptosis in about 80% of patients.

GRAVES' DERMOPATHY

- **Does not usually require treatment but topical high potency glucocorticoids may be used.**

THYROIDITIS

- **Inflammation of the thyroid gland with transient hyperthyroidism due to release of preformed hormone from the colloid space.** Includes Silent lymphocytic and Postpartum thyroiditis.

Thyroid function evolution:
- **Variable triphasic course:** Thyroid function tests characteristically evolve through 3 distinct phases over about 6 months: [1] thyrotoxic phase, followed by transient euthyroidism, [2] hypothyroid phase, and [3] recovery phase. Each phase usually lasts 2-8 weeks with the possible exception of the initial transition through euthyroidism, which may be shorter.
- **[1] Hyperthyroid (thyrotoxic) phase** Thyroid inflammation and attack by cytotoxic T lymphocytes damage thyroid follicles and activate proteolysis of the thyroglobulin stored within the follicles. **This inflammation results in unregulated release of large amounts of preformed thyroxine (T4) and triiodothyronine (T3) into the circulation from destroyed follicles, instead of the synthesis of new T3 and T4, resulting in biochemical (and in some cases, clinical) hyperthyroidism.**
- **[2] hypothyroid phase** There is usually a period of rapid evolution through euthyroidism and **then into transient often asymptomatic hypothyroidism.** Hypothyroidism occurs due to follicular cell damage, leading to **reduction of new hormone synthesis and the depletion of hormone stores.** The hypothyroidism lasts until the thyroid gland can generate sufficient thyroid hormone synthesis and secretion so that the patient regains normal homeostasis
- **[3] recovery phase,** As the inflammation subsides, thyroid follicles regenerate and thyroid hormone synthesis & secretion resume, with **resolution & restoration of normal thyroid function in most.**

DIAGNOSIS
Thyroid function tests:
- **Hyperthyroid profile (thyrotoxic phase): decreased TSH** typically <0.1 mU/L **+ increased free FT4 &/or FT3),** even though many have little, if any, symptoms of thyroid excess.
- Thyroid function tests characteristically evolve through three distinct phases over about 6 months: [1] thyrotoxic phase, where FT4 and FT3 levels are increased, reflecting their discharge from the damaged thyroid cells, and TSH is suppressed. [2] hypothyroid phase, where FT3 and FT4 may be low with increased TSH, and [3] recovery phase.

Radioactive uptake scan
- **Findings: — diffuse, decreased (low) iodine uptake.** There is decreased iodine uptake (decreased synthesis of new T3 and T4) because it is associated with release of preformed thyroid hormone from destroyed follicles instead of the synthesis of new T3 and T4.

Ultrasonography
- Indications: For patients in whom the clinical presentation is less obvious (eg, thyroid tenderness not as prominent), thyroid ultrasonography may be useful to assess for cystic and/or solid masses.

MANAGEMENT
- **Supportive: reassurance it is self-limiting (most return to euthyroid state).**

Symptomatic hyperthyroidism:
- **Therapy for hyperthyroidism is not often necessary** because symptoms, if present, are mild and short-lived. Short-term Beta blocker use if severe hyperthyroidism (it is transient if present).
- **Thionamides (eg, Methimazole, Propylthiouracil) should not be used** because the hyperthyroidism results from preformed hormone release of not excess hormone synthesis).
- **Radioactive iodine therapy is neither indicated nor effective,** since uptake of radioiodine is low.

Hypothyroidism:
- **Therapy for hypothyroidism is not often needed, because symptoms, if present, are usually mild, and transient (short duration).**
- Levothyroxine: If hypothyroidism is prolonged or severe (TSH >10 mU/L) or associated with more than mild symptoms, Levothyroxine for 6-8 weeks may be used and then discontinued with follow-up to ensure the hypothyroidism is not permanent because complete recovery occurs in most.

SILENT (SUBACUTE LYMPHOCYTIC; PAINLESS) THYROIDITIS

- Accounts for 1-5% of cases of Hyperthyroidism and is considered a variant of Chronic autoimmune thyroiditis (Hashimoto's thyroiditis). Has a clinical course similar to Subacute thyroiditis.
- Three times more common in women with type 1 Diabetes mellitus.

Etiologies:
- It can occur spontaneously or can be caused by medications.
- **Medications:** chemotherapeutic agents (eg, **tyrosine kinase inhibitors**; Denileukin Diftitox; Alemtuzumab; **Interferon alfa**; Interleukin2; and immune checkpoint inhibitors). Other drugs can cause silent thyroiditis, including **Lithium and Amiodarone.**
- **The key clinical findings are mild hyperthyroidism of short duration, little or no thyroid enlargement, and no Graves' ophthalmopathy or pretibial myxedema.**

Antibodies:
- **~50% have antithyroid antibodies** eg, antithyroid peroxidase (TPO) antibodies &/or **antithyroglobulin antibodies.** Silent (Subacute lymphocytic) is associated with a painless nontender thyroid, the presence of TPO antibodies antepartum, and normal ESR, which can distinguish it from Subacute granulomatous thyroiditis, which presents with a painful thyroid, thyroid tenderness, elevated ESR, and negative thyroid antibodies.

Radioactive uptake scan
- **Findings:** — **diffuse, decreased (low) iodine uptake** due to decreased synthesis of new T3 and T4 resulting from preformed thyroid hormone instead of the synthesis of new T3 and T4.

Clinical course:
- In those with spontaneous silent thyroiditis, ~10–20% remain hypothyroid after 1 year.
- There is a recurrence rate of 5–10%; this rate is higher in Japan.

POSTPARTUM THYROIDITIS

- **Autoimmune thyroiditis that occurs in the first 12 months postpartum and occasionally after spontaneous or induced abortion**, otherwise similar clinically and pathogenetically to Painless (Subacute lymphocytic) thyroiditis.

Thyroid antibodies:
- **>80% have antithyroid antibodies (antithyroglobulin or antithyroid peroxidase antibodies).**

Radioactive uptake scan
- **Findings:** — **diffuse, decreased (low) iodine uptake** due to decreased synthesis of new T3 and T4 resulting from preformed thyroid hormone instead of the synthesis of new T3 and T4.

Clinical course:
- About 22% of affected women experience hyperthyroidism followed by hypothyroidism, whereas 30% of such women have isolated thyrotoxicosis and 48% have isolated hypothyroidism. The thyrotoxic phase typically occurs 2–6 weeks postpartum and lasts 2–3 months.
- Most women progress to a hypothyroid phase that usually lasts 4-12 weeks before complete resolution but may become permanent in some.

AMIODARONE

Amiodarone is an anti-arrhythmic drug that contains 37% iodine. As a result, it can affect thyroid function in several different ways:
- [1] **Amiodarone can cause hyperthyroidism.** There are two types of Amiodarone-induced thyrotoxicosis (AIT). In **Type 1**, there is **increased synthesis of thyroid hormone** (usually in patients with a preexisting underlying thyroid abnormality) with increased uptake on RAIU and **increased vascularity on ultrasound**, whereas in **Type 2**, there is excess release of T4 and T3 due to a **destructive thyroiditis** (decreased iodine uptake on RAIU and normal gland with **decreased vascularity on ultrasound**). These types differ in their pathogenesis, management, and outcome.
- [2] **Amiodarone can cause hypothyroidism** via the antithyroid action of iodine (especially in patients with preexisting thyroid disease).
- Amiodarone thyrotoxicosis occurs in 3% taking Amiodarone during treatment or even several months after discontinuation. **Amiodarone is the leading cause of Thyrotoxic crisis "Thyroid storm".**

541

HYPERTHYROID DISORDERS

TYPE	CAUSE	CLINICAL MANIFESTATIONS	DIAGNOSIS (not all tests need to be done)	MANAGEMENT
GRAVE'S DISEASE	**Autoimmune** MC women 20-40y. Circulating **TSH receptor antibodies** cause ↑thyroid hormone synthesis, release & thyroid gland growth **worse with stress (ex. pregnancy, illness)**. **Graves MC cause of hyperthyroidism*** (90%)	Clinical Hyperthyroidism • Diffuse, enlarged thyroid. • **THYROID BRUITS*** • **OPHTHALMOPATHY*: lid lag, exophthalmos/proptosis (exclusive to Grave)*** Hyaluronic acid deposition. **Tx c steroids.** Smoking & iodine may make ophthalmopathy worse. • **PRETIBIAL MYXEDEMA*** Nonpitting, edematous, pink to brown plaques/nodules on shin (exclusive to Grave)	• ⊕ **Thyroid-Stimulating Immunoglobulins (Ab)* most spp.** ± Thyroid peroxidase & anti-TG Ab • Hyperthyroid TFTs: ↑FT_4/FT_3 & ↓TSH (± be subclinical) • RAIU: ↑ **DIFFUSE uptake*** Normal ┃ Grave's Diffuse uptake seen in TSH-secreting pituitary adenoma also.	• **Radioactive Iodine: MC therapy used.*** Destroys thyroid gland. Will need hormone replacement • **Methimazole or PropylThioUracil** • **Beta blockers (ex. Propranolol) for symptomatic relief:*** tremors, anxiety, tachycardia, diaphoresis, palpitations, etc • **Thyroidectomy:** if compressive sx, no response to meds, If RAI is contraindicated (ex pregnancy)
TOXIC MULTINODULAR GOITER (TMG) (Plummer's Disease)	Autonomous functioning nodules **MC in elderly**	BOTH TMG & TA Clinical Hyperthyroidism • Diffuse, enlarged thyroid • **No skin/eye changes!** • Palpable nodule(s)	• Hyperthyroid TFTs: ↑FT_4/T_3; ↓TSH (± be subclinical) • RAIU: (PATCHY areas of both ↑ & ↓ uptake) in TMG TMG	BOTH TMG & TA • **Radioactive Iodine:** MC therapy • Surgery (subtotal thyroidectomy) if compressive symptoms present • **Methimazole or PTU:** - MOA: *inhibit hormone synthesis.* Methimazole preferred (less S/E) - S/E of both: *agranulocytosis** (so monitor WBC) & *hepatitis.** • PTU preferred in pregnancy. (especially 1st trimester) • **Beta blockers for symptoms of thyrotoxicosis**
TOXIC ADENOMA (TA)	One autonomous functioning nodule	Compressive sx: • **Dyspnea, dysphagia, stridor, hoarseness** (laryngeal compression).	• RAIU: ↑LOCAL uptake (hot nodule) in TA TA	
TSH SECERETING PITUITARY ADENOMA	Autonomous TSH secretion by pituitary adenoma	Clinical Hyperthyroidism • Diffuse, enlarged thyroid • **Bitemporal Hemianopsia*** • Mental disturbances	• TFT's: ↑FT_4/T_3 + ↑TSH* (inappropriate TSH elevation in the setting of elevated FT_4/T_3 (same direction)* • RAIU: DIFFUSE uptake • Pituitary MRI: adenoma	• Transsphenoidal Surgery to remove the pituitary adenoma

HYPOTHYROID DISORDERS

TYPE	CAUSE	CLINICAL MANIFESTATIONS	DIAGNOSIS	DURATION
HASHIMOTO'S thyroiditis (CHRONIC LYMPHOCYTIC) MC cause of hypothyroidism in the US* – 6x MC in women	**Autoimmune** (Anti-thyroid Antibodies) (Ab)	Clinical Hypothyroidism • Painless, enlarged thyroid • May present in euthyroid state (rarely in hyperthyroid state)	• ⊕**Thyroid Ab present: thyroglobulin Ab, antimicrosomial & Thyroid Peroxidase Ab** • **TFTs** *(usually **HypOthyroid**)* • ↓Radioactive I- uptake (usually not needed) • Bx: lymphocytes, germinal follicles, Hurthle	• Hypothyroidism usually permanent. • **Levothyroxine therapy*** *Thyroid hormone replacement*
SILENT (LYMPHOCYTIC) THYROIDITIS	**Autoimmune** (Anti-thyroid Ab)	Painless, enlarged thyroid. Thyrotoxicosis ⇨ hypothyroid (depends on when they present)	• ⊕**Thyroid Ab present:** thyroglobulin Ab, antimicrosomial & Thyroid Peroxidase Ab • TFTs: Hyper/Hypothyroid (depends on when they present) • ↓Radioactive Iodine uptake on RAIU scan	• Return to euthyroid state within 12-18 months without treatment. **Aspirin** • *No anti-thyroid meds** • 20% possible permanent hypothyroidism
POSTPARTUM THYROIDITIS	**Autoimmune** (Anti-thyroid Ab)	Painless, enlarged thyroid. Thyrotoxicosis ⇨ hypothyroid (depends on when they present)	• ⊕**Thyroid Ab present:** thyroglobulin Ab, antimicrosomial & Thyroid Peroxidase Ab • TFTs (Hyper/Hypothyroid) (depends on when they present) • ↓Radioactive Iodine uptake on RAIU scan	• Return to euthyroid state in 12-18 months without treatment. **Aspirin, NSAIDs** • *No anti-thyroid meds** • 20% possible permanent hypothyroidism
de QUERVAIN'S THYROIDITIS (GRANULOMATOUS) PAINFUL SUBACUTE	**MC POST VIRAL *** or viral inflammatory reaction. Associated with HLA-B35	**PAINFUL, tender neck/thyroid*** **Clinical Hyperthyroidism** (due to neck pain in acute phase) Thyrotoxicosis ⇨ hypothyroid (depend on when they present)	• ↑**ESR (hallmark)*** • **NO thyroid Ab*** • **TFTs (usually HypERthyroid)** (depends on when they present) • ↓Radioactive Iodine uptake on RAIU scan	• Return to euthyroid state in 12-18 months without treatment. **Aspirin (for pain, inflammation,** ↑'es T4) • *No anti-thyroid meds** • 5% possible permanent hypothyroidism
MEDICATION-INDUCED	**AMIODARONE** (contains iodine), **LITHIUM** **Alpha interferon**	Painless, enlarged thyroid. Thyrotoxicosis ⇨ hypothyroid (depend on when they present)		Often returns to euthyroid states when med is stopped, Corticosteroids
ACUTE THYROIDITIS (Suppurative)	**S. aureus MC** (any organism may cause it)	May have **PAINFUL, fluctuant** thyroid. Usually very ill, **febrile.**	Increased WBC count with left shift. Usually **euthyroid**	Antibiotics Drainage if abscess present
RIEDEL'S THYROIDITIS	**Fibrous** thyroid	**Firm hard 'woody' nodule (similar to anaplastic cancer)***	May develop hypothyroidism	Surgery may be needed

LEVOTHYROXINE: *synthetic T4.* Monitor TSH levels @ 6 week intervals when initiating/changing dose. *Slow, small increases in >50y & patients with cardiovascular disease. Monitor elderly, patients with angina, MI, or CHF for adverse reactions* due to increased metabolic rate or withhold until cardiovascular status is stabilized. May need to lower doses of anticoagulants, insulin, and oral antihyperglycemics. Oral cholestyramine may increase T4 requirements.

The MC cause of hypothyroidism in the US is Hashimoto's thyroiditis. * *The MC cause of hypothyroidism worldwide is iodine deficiency.* *

TOXIC MULTINODULAR GOITER [TMG] (PLUMMER DISEASE)

- **Autonomous hyperfunctioning thyroid nodules that produce biochemical and clinical hyperthyroidism (thyrotoxicosis)**. 3-10% may be associated with Thyroid cancer.
- **Toxic adenoma & TMG are the result of focal hyperplasia of thyroid follicular cells whose functional capacity is independent of regulation by TSH.**
- TMG is most common <u>in increasing age and regions where iodine deficiency is common</u>.

CLINICAL MANIFESTATIONS
- **Palpable nodular goiter or a thyroid ultrasound showing multiple nodules**.
- <u>**Signs of hyperthyroidism**</u> — anxiety, heat intolerance, weight loss despite increased appetite, fatigue, weakness, increased sympathetic output (tachycardia, palpitations, atrial fibrillation, fine tremor), diarrhea, increased metabolic rate, high-output heart failure, & oligomenorrhea.
- <u>**Obstructive symptoms (enlarged goiter)**</u> — dyspnea (eg tracheal compression), dysphagia (esophageal compression), stridor, **hoarseness** (recurrent laryngeal nerve compression).

DIAGNOSIS
- <u>**Primary hyperthyroid profile**</u> **decreased TSH + increased free T4 or T3 if toxic.**
- <u>Ultrasound</u>: may be used to assess the characteristics of the multiple nodules visualized on US.
- <u>**Radioactive iodine scan**</u>: **>1 focal areas of increased heterogenous radioiodine uptake.**

MANAGEMENT
- Treatment options include surgery, radioiodine, or prolonged (probably lifelong) thionamide therapy.
- Patients with symptoms or signs of compression/obstruction, a need for rapid return to euthyroidism, or coexisting thyroid cancer require surgery (near total or total thyroidectomy).

INFECTIOUS (SUPPURATIVE) THYROIDITIS

- <u>**Bacterial infection of the thyroid gland**</u> by Gram-positive bacteria **(*Staphylococcus aureus* most common)** or Streptococcus. Gram-negative organisms. Pneumocystis, Mycobacterial, etc.
- Rare. Usually occurs in children.

CLINICAL MANIFESTATIONS
- <u>**Thyroid pain & tenderness:**</u> sudden onset of neck pain & tenderness to the thyroid gland. The pain is often worse with hyperextension and improves slightly with neck flexion. May radiate to the mandible, ears, or posteriorly. **May have overlying erythema to the skin.**
- **Fever, chills, pharyngitis,** dysphagia, dysphonia, hoarseness.

DIAGNOSIS
- <u>Labs:</u> **both leukocytosis & increased ESR.** Thyroid function testing usually normal.
- **Fine needle aspiration** of the mass with Gram stain and culture. Neutrophilia seen with FNA.
- <u>Thyroid ultrasonography</u>: diffuse heterogeneous thyroid density and reduced echogenicity.

MANAGEMENT
- Antibiotics.
- Surgical drainage if fluctuance is very significant.

- **EXAM TIP**
- The only 2 causes of a **painful** thyroid are Subacute (Granulomatous, DeQuervain) and Suppurative thyroiditis. Most other thyroid diseases are usually painless.

THYROTOXIC CRISIS (THYROID STORM)

- **Rare, potentially fatal complication of untreated (or partially treated) thyrotoxicosis usually after a precipitating event** (eg, surgery, trauma, infection, pregnancy). High mortality (75%).

TRIGGERS
- Systemic insults: infection, trauma, burns, surgery, acute illness. Endocrine insults: DKA, Hyperosmolar coma, Graves'. Cardiovascular insults: MI, CVA, PE. Drug or hormonal: abrupt withdrawal of antithyroid medications, ingestion of thyroid hormone, Amiodarone, salicylates, anesthetics, Iodine administration. Obstetrics related: Eclampsia, labor and delivery.

CLINICAL MANIFESTATIONS
Exaggerated manifestations of Hyperthyroid symptoms & hypermetabolic state:
- **Thermoregulatory: high fever (eg, 104-106°F) with diaphoresis is a key feature.**
- **Cardiovascular: hyperadrenergic state — tachycardia (often >140 beats/min), palpitations,** Atrial fibrillation, arrhythmia, hypertension, dyspnea, Heart failure.
- **CNS dysfunction mild: agitation, tremors;** moderate: **altered mentation,** delirium, lethargy, psychosis; severe: seizures, stupor, coma, & hypotension.
- **GI symptoms:** eg, nausea, vomiting, diarrhea, abdominal pain, intestinal obstruction, hepatic failure.
Physical examination:
- Fever, tachycardia, systolic hypertension. May reveal goiter, hand tremor, lid lag, moist and warm skin, hyperreflexia, and jaundice. Orbitopathy may be seen if Graves' disease is present.

DIAGNOSIS:
- **Thyroid storm is primarily a clinical diagnosis based upon the presence of severe and life-threatening symptoms** (hyperpyrexia, cardiovascular dysfunction, Atrial fibrillation, altered mentation) in a patient with biochemical evidence of hyperthyroidism.
- Except for pregnancy test, initiate treatment on suspicion of the diagnosis without waiting for labs.
Laboratory evaluation:
- **Primary hyperthyroid profile — increased free T4 or T3 + decreased TSH most common** (may be so low it may be undetectable) but other patterns may be seen, depending on the cause.
- Mild hyperglycemia, mild hypercalcemia, elevated alkaline phosphatase, elevated cortisol.

MANAGEMENT
Obtain pregnancy testing before beginning ED treatment; obtain consult if pregnant or breastfeeding.
- **[1] Supportive management:** general: oxygen cardiac monitoring; **fever: external cooling with ice packs or cooling blanket, Acetaminophen. Avoid Aspirin** because it can increase T3 and T4 levels by displace them off of carrier proteins; **dehydration: IV fluids** (fluid losses could result from the combination of fever, diaphoresis, vomiting, and diarrhea). IV saline with 5% Dextrose may be used to replace glycogen depletion if blood sugar is low; **Admit to ICU.**
- **[2] Beta-adrenergic blocker:** After initial supportive measures, immediate treatment with a Beta-blocker (eg, Propranolol) to control symptoms and signs due to increased adrenergic tone.
- [3] Inhibition of new hormone synthesis: **Antithyroid medications (thionamide) — Propylthiouracil often preferred because it has a small but additional benefit of blocking peripheral conversion of T4 to T3.** Avoid Methimazole in pregnant women in the first trimester.
Secondary management:
- [4] Inhibition of thyroid hormone release: **Initial management may be followed by Iodine (eg, Iodine Lugol solution, Potassium iodide, or Ipodate) to stop thyroid hormone release at least 1 hour after beta blockers and antithyroid medications** to prevent the iodine from being used as substrate for new hormone synthesis.
- [5] Block peripheral conversion of T4 to T3: **IV Glucocorticoids (eg, Hydrocortisone or Dexamethasone) to block peripheral conversion of T4 to T3.**
- Bile acid sequestrants: (eg, Cholestyramine) may be used in severe cases to inhibit thyroid hormone reabsorption (reduces enterohepatic recycling of thyroid hormone).

THYROID NODULE

- Discrete lesion within the thyroid gland that may be solitary, multiple, cystic, or solid.
- **>90% of palpable thyroid nodules (≥1 cm) are benign, such as benign adenomas, colloid nodules, or cysts.**
- 4-6.5% of thyroid nodules are Thyroid cancer. Less frequently, metastatic malignancy is the cause.

BENIGN ETIOLOGIES
- **Follicular adenoma (colloid) most common type of thyroid nodule (50-60%).** While most Follicular adenomas are benign, they share characteristics with Follicular carcinomas.
- Adenomas, cysts, localized thyroiditis.

RISK FACTORS
- **The risk of a nodule being malignant is higher in men, extremes of age (children and adults <30 years or >60 years), history of head &/or neck ionizing radiation.**
- Smoking, obesity, alcohol consumption, uterine fibroids, female gender, iron deficiency.

CLINICAL MANIFESTATIONS
- **Most are asymptomatic & most individuals with a thyroid nodule are euthyroid.**
- **Most patients present with a palpable nodule in the anterior neck**, or an incidental nodule found on imaging studies performed for other reasons.
- Compressive symptoms: difficulty swallowing or breathing, neck pressure or pain, jaw or ear pain, hoarseness (recurrent laryngeal nerve impingement).
- Functional nodules: rare — presents with thyrotoxicosis.

PHYSICAL EXAMINATION
- **Benign: varied — smooth, soft,** sharply outlined, discrete, irregular, painless, **freely mobile,** painful or tender nodule all suggest benign nature.
- **Malignant: rapid growth, firm-hard mass, fixed in place to adjacent tissues, nonmobile or no movement with swallowing** (Riedel's thyroiditis may also present like this), large >4 cm size, **obstructive symptoms,** cervical adenopathy (>1 cm), and vocal cord paralysis all suggest increased possibility of cancer.

WORKUP
- **Initial evaluation for patients with a thyroid nodule should include [1] history, physical examination, [2] measurement of TSH, and [3] thyroid ultrasound to characterize the nodule.** Thyroid nodules ≥1 cm warrant follow-up.

Thyroid function testing:
- **Often the initial test done as part of the nodule workup.**
- **If TSH is subnormal (indicating subclinical or overt hyperthyroidism), thyroid scintigraphy (radioactive iodine uptake scan) should be performed next** because the possibility that the nodule is hyperfunctioning (hyperthyroidism) is increased and that it is cancer is decreased.
- **If TSH is normal or high & meets US criteria for sampling, FNA with biopsy may be indicated (often ultrasound-guided)** because the risk of malignancy increases in parallel with the level of serum TSH.

Thyroid ultrasound:

- **Usually performed after thyroid function testing (TFTs) in patients with known or suspected nodules (high-resolution ultrasound is the best modality for the <u>initial</u> evaluation of thyroid nodules after TFTs)** as it gives more details about the size and anatomy of the thyroid gland.
- <u>**High-risk nodules**</u> **(80% malignancy risk) — solid hypoechoic nodule, irregular margins, central vascularity, microcalcifications,** abnormal cervical lymphadenopathy, taller-than-wide shape, documented nodule growth, or evidence, extrathyroidal extension.
- <u>Intermediate-risk:</u> (15% malignancy risk) hypoechoic or isoechoic, solid, spongiform appearance, comet-tail artifact within a cystic nodule.
- <u>Low risk:</u> (7% malignancy risk) are partially cystic with eccentric solid areas.

Thyroid scintigraphy (Radioactive iodine uptake scan, Iodine 131 nuclear medicine scan):

- <u>**Radioactive iodine uptake scan:**</u> usually performed if the FNA is indeterminate or if TSH is low or subnormal to rule out hyperthyroidism and determine the functional status of a nodule.
- <u>**Functioning (normal) or hot nodules**</u> **(hyperfunctioning) have lower malignant potential, and FNA is usually <u>not</u> indicated.**
- <u>**Cold nodules**</u> **(no or low iodine uptake) may require FNA with biopsy to rule out malignancy.**

Fine needle aspiration:

- <u>**Fine needle aspiration:**</u> **most accurate test to evaluate if a nodule is benign vs. malignant) & identify the need for surgical resection** (often guided by ultrasound).
- **US-FNA performed in nodule with normal TSH in highly suspicious nodules** (eg, via ultrasound, examination, risk factors), **solid and hypoechoic nodules ≥1.5 cm on US, solid and hypoechoic nodules ≥1 to 1.5 cm with one of these suspicious sonographic features** [eg, irregular margins (≥1.5 cm), Microcalcifications (≥1 cm), Taller-than-wide shape (≥1 cm), Macrocalcifications (≥1.5 cm), Peripheral (rim) calcifications (≥1.5 cm), Any combination (≥1 cm)].

MANAGEMENT

- <u>Non-diagnostic FNA:</u> FNA is usually repeated in 4 to 6 weeks. Surgical excision if an indeterminate FNA + cold nodule seen on RAIU scan (no uptake) or if suspicious.
- <u>**Benign nodules:**</u> **Observation + follow-up Ultrasound if surgery is not performed** - usually every 6-12 months for subcentimeter nodules with suspicious characteristics; 12 to 24 months for nodules with low to intermediate suspicion on ultrasound or FNA. 2-3 years for very-low-risk nodules.
- <u>**Suspicious for malignancy:**</u> **Treatment should include surgical excision.**
- <u>Autonomous nodules:</u> Options include radioiodine, surgery, or long-term antithyroid drugs.

EVALUATION OF THE THYROID NODULE

PAPILLARY THYROID CARCINOMA

- **Most common type of thyroid cancer.** Pure papillary and mixed papillary with follicular carcinoma comprises ~80-85% of all thyroid cancers. They are well-differentiated.
- More common in women but the prognosis is worse in men.
- Least aggressive type of thyroid cancer & excellent prognosis (high cure rate).
- Metastasis usually occurs local (cervical lymph nodes most common). Distant METS uncommon (when present, it usually involves the lungs or bone).

RISK FACTORS
- **Most common after ionizing radiation exposure of the head & neck, especially in childhood.**
- **Increasing age,** family history of thyroid cancer. Genetics: ~45% of papillary thyroid carcinomas are caused by over expression of the ret protooncogene (RET). Mutations in *RET*/PTC, *NTRK1*, *RAS*, or *BRAF* occur in as many as 70% of well-differentiated thyroid cancers. Familial adenomatous polyposis — Gardner syndrome, Werner syndrome, and Carney complex type 1.

WORKUP
- Usually presents as a painless thyroid nodule. Thyroid function tests usually normal.
- **Fine needle aspiration: test of choice — the 2 hallmark morphological features of conventional PTC are the papillae and nuclear changes.** Neoplastic epithelial lining & cells organized into papillary "fingers". Nuclear grooves, ground glass/empty nuclei ('orphan Annie" nuclei), & the **presence of psammoma bodies (calcifications).**

MANAGEMENT
- **Thyroidectomy** (total or near total) **often followed by postoperative Levothyroxine** to replace normal hormone production and/or to suppress tumor regrowth (most tumors are TSH-responsive).
- Post-surgery radioiodine in high-risk (some intermediate) to ablate residual normal thyroid tissue.
- Post-treatment: may monitor Thyroglobulin levels, TSH, and ultrasound of the neck.

FOLLICULAR THYROID CARCINOMA

- Second most common type of thyroid cancer (~5-10%). Well-differentiated cancer.
- **Generally, more aggressive than Papillary but also slow-growing** (relatively good prognosis). Most common in adults 40-60 years of age & females.
- **Distant METS more common than local METS (hematogenous spread) — lung most common** and, less commonly, the brain, liver, bladder, and skin. Think **Follicular** goes **FAR.**
- **Usually presents as a single asymptomatic (painless) thyroid nodule with or without thyroid gland enlargement.**

RISK FACTORS
- Increased incidence with iodine deficiency. Less often associated with radiation exposure.

DIAGNOSIS
- FTC is difficult to diagnose because FNA with biopsy alone often cannot distinguish between follicular adenoma and carcinoma so definitive diagnosis is often made with postsurgical histologic testing.

MANAGEMENT
- **Thyroidectomy (total or near total) usually followed by postoperative Levothyroxine** to replace normal hormone production and/or to suppress tumor regrowth.
- Post-surgery radioiodine in some patients (high-risk and some intermediate risk disease).
- Post-treatment: may monitor Thyroglobulin levels, TSH, and ultrasound of the neck.
- Metastasis to bones & soft tissue: Total thyroidectomy followed by either radiotherapy or chemotherapy (eg, tyrosine kinase inhibitor — sorafenib, lenvatinib, vandetanib, cabozantinib).

MEDULLARY THYROID CARCINOMA

- **Neuroendocrine tumor derived from <u>Calcitonin-synthesizing parafollicular (C) cells</u> of the thyroid gland (of neural crest origin).**
- <u>Rare</u> — Medullary thyroid carcinoma represents 1–3% of thyroid cancers

<u>CHARACTERISTICS</u>
- **<u>75% sporadic</u>** — 40-50% of sporadic Medullary thyroid cancers have acquired *RET* mutations.
- **Men 2 syndrome: 25% associated with MEN 2A or 3 (formerly 2B)** due to activation or mutation of the ret protooncogene on chromosome 10. Familial medullary thyroid carcinoma.
- **Medullary thyroid carcinoma arises from thyroid parafollicular cells that can secrete calcitonin,** prostaglandins, serotonin, ACTH, corticotropin releasing hormone (CRH), and other peptides. These peptides can cause symptoms and can be used as tumor markers.

<u>CLINICAL MANIFESTATIONS</u>
- Solitary thyroid nodule. Mets may present with cervical lymphadenopathy or compressive symptoms.
- <u>Carcinoid syndrome</u>: **Tumor secretion of calcitonin or other substances (eg, serotonin and prostaglandins) can cause diarrhea or facial flushing in patients with advanced disease.**
- <u>Cushing syndrome</u>: **some tumors secrete corticotropin (ACTH), causing Cushing's syndrome (via ectopic ACTH production).** May also associated with melanin production.

<u>DIAGNOSIS</u>
- **<u>FNA with biopsy</u>** is the test of choice to establish the diagnosis. <u>Findings:</u> Nests of round or ovoid cells and spindle-shaped cells without follicle development. Amyloid deposits.
<u>Serum calcitonin and CEA:</u>
- **<u>Increased Calcitonin</u> — The production of Calcitonin is a characteristic feature of Medullary thyroid carcinoma & used to monitor for recurrence or residual disease after treatment.** Calcitonin measurements often correlate with tumor mass.
- <u>Carcinoembryonic antigen</u> (CEA) levels often elevated.
- Perform testing for germline *RET* mutation (to rule out MEN2 syndrome).

<u>MANAGEMENT</u>
- **<u>Surgical resection</u> (eg, Total thyroidectomy) is the primary treatment for Medullary thyroid carcinoma** (may include dissection of lymph nodes and surrounding fatty tissue on the ipsilateral side). MTC does not take up iodine so Radioactive iodine ablation treatment is not an option.
- **<u>Urinary metanephrine levels</u> to rule out Pheochromocytoma (MEN2) prior to surgery.**
- <u>Prognosis:</u> worse than Papillary or Follicular.

ANAPLASTIC THYROID CARCINOMA

- **An undifferentiated, highly aggressive malignant tumor — most aggressive thyroid carcinoma; often metastasizes early to surrounding nodes and distant sites (poor prognosis).**
- Rare. Most commonly seen in the elderly > 65 years of age. TP53 gene inactivation.

<u>CLINICAL MANIFESTATIONS</u>
- **Rapid growth of neck mass, compressive symptoms** — dyspnea (trachea invasion), dysphagia.

<u>PHYSICAL EXAMINATION</u>
- **"Rock" hard thyroid mass.** May be fixed.

<u>MANAGEMENT</u>
- **Most are not amenable to resection and treatment should be directed toward securing the airway (palliative tracheostomy) and ensuring access for nutritional support.**
- Everolimus (for mTOR mutations). In BRAFV600E mutant Anaplastic thyroid cancer, combined BRAF and MEK inhibition with Dabrafenib and Trametinib has induced prolonged responses.

DIABETES MELLITUS

Type I DIABETES MELLITUS
- **Insulin deficiency due to pancreatic beta cell destruction. Prone to development of ketosis.**
- These patients require exogenous Insulin. Type I represents 10% of Diabetes mellitus; type II DM (90%).
- **Early onset usually <30 years of age (3/4 are diagnosed in childhood).** Peaks at 4-6 years of age then **10-14 years.** Not associated with obesity. Type I DM is a catabolic disorder. ↑ Glucagon levels.

ETIOLOGIES
- **Type 1A (Autoimmune): most common.** Often triggered by environmental factors (eg, infection). Increased with HLA DR3-DQ2 & DR4 genes. Islet autoantibodies frequently present: Glutamic acid decarboxylase (GAD65), insulin, tyrosine phosphatase IA2, & zinc transporter 8 (ZnT8) autoantibodies.
- **Type 1B: non-autoimmune beta cell destruction.**

CLINICAL MANIFESTATIONS
- **[1] Hyperglycemia without acidosis: most common initial presentation — polyuria, polydipsia, polyphagia; weight loss,** paresthesias, blurred vision (lens exposed to hyperosmolar fluids).
- **[2] Diabetic ketoacidosis second most common initial presentation.** Ketonemia & ketonuria.
- [3] Silent (asymptomatic) incidental discovery. Lethargy, weakness, or fatigue.

Type II DIABETES MELLITUS
- **Combination of insulin insensitivity (resistance) & relative impairment of insulin secretion** (increased insulin levels early in the disease but often diminishes with disease progression).
- **Hypertension, Dyslipidemia, and Atherosclerosis often associated with type II DM.**

RISK FACTORS
- **Likely due to genetic & environmental factors: obesity greatest risk factor (especially visceral) & decreased physical activity.** 90% of type II diabetics are overweight.
- **Most common in adults >40y;** however, seen with increased incidence in children & adolescents.
- History of impaired glucose tolerance, **family history, first degree relative with DM**, Hispanic, African American, Pacific Islanders, hypertension, dyslipidemia, delivery of baby >9 lbs., syndrome X, & insulin resistance: "CHAOS" — Chronic HTN, Atherosclerosis, Obesity (central), & Stroke.

CLINICAL MANIFESTATIONS
- **Most are asymptomatic** (may be an incidental finding).
- Classic symptoms: polyuria, polydipsia, & polyphagia. May have symptoms of complications.
- **Poor wound healing, increased infections (eg, Candidiasis, candida vulvovaginitis).**
- Hyperglycemic hyperosmolar syndrome (HHS). Acanthosis nigricans.

DIAGNOSIS

GLUCOSE TEST	PRE DIABETES	DIABETES MELLITUS	COMMENTS
FASTING PLASMA GLUCOSE	110-125 mg/dL	≥ 126 mg/dL	- Fasting at least 8 hours **on at least 2 occasions.** - **CRITERION STANDARD.**
2-HOUR GLUCOSE TOLERANCE TEST	≥140-199 mg/dL	≥ 200 mg/dL	- **Oral glucose tolerance test (GTT)** after 75g of glucose. - **3h GTT criterion standard in Gestational diabetes.**
HEMOGLOBIN A$_{1C}$	5.7–6.4%	≥ 6.5%	**Indicates average glucose 10-12 weeks prior** to testing
RANDOM PLASMA		≥200 mg/dL	Patients with classic diabetic symptoms or complications.

SCREENING: ADA: [1] Any adult with a BMI ≥25 kg/m^2 and at least 1 risk factor (eg, triglycerides >250 mg/dL, HDL <35 mg/dL, physical inactivity, HTN, 1history of cardiovascular disease, 1st degree relative with DM, PCOS). **[2] Screen adults aged ≥35 years if normal BMI and no risk factors.** For normal results, screen every 3 years (35-70). Those with high risk factors may need annual screening.
USPSTF: adults 35-70 years who have overweight or obesity should be screened.

INITIAL MANAGEMENT OF TYPE II DIABETES MELLITUS

- **Diet, exercise, & lifestyle changes are the initial management of type II DM. Goal Hgb A1C ≤7%.**
  - No universal percentages: Carbohydrates 50-60%; Protein 15-20%, 10% unsaturated fats.

BIGUANIDES (METFORMIN)
Mechanisms of action:

- **Primary mechanism of action is decreased <u>hepatic glucose production</u> by inhibition of hepatic gluconeogenesis and lipogenesis** [via activation of the enzyme AMP-activated protein kinase (AMPK) in hepatocytes]. Also inhibits renal gluconeogenesis. Can be used alone or with other agents.
- Increases insulin-mediated glucose utilization, including stimulation of glucose uptake and glycolysis in peripheral tissues (eg, muscle and liver), decreases intestinal absorption, reduces postprandial and fasting plasma glucose and insulin levels, and reduces plasma glucagon levels.
- <u>Benefits</u>: **Not usually associated with hypoglycemia** (it has no effect on pancreatic beta cells), **not associated with weight gain (causes mild weight reduction). Metformin reduces the risk of all-cause and cardiovascular mortality in patients with T2DM & established cardiovascular disease.** Decreases triglycerides and LDL, increases HDL. Possible decreased cancer risk.
- <u>Decreased CVD risk</u>: In people with type 2 diabetes and established cardiovascular disease (CVD), Metformin, GLP-1 receptor agonists (Liraglutide, Semaglutide, Dulaglutide), and SGLT2 inhibitors reduce the risk of all-cause and cardiovascular mortality as well as reduced diabetic kidney disease.

Indications:

- **Usually the first-line oral medication in Type II DM**. Can decrease Hgb A1C by 1.5%.

Adverse reactions:

- **<u>GI complaints</u> most common** — metallic taste, diarrhea, abdominal discomfort, anorexia, nausea.
- **<u>Vitamin B12 deficiency</u>** — decreased calcium-dependent B12 absorption with long-term use.
- **<u>Lactic acidosis</u> rare but serious adverse effect** — tends to occur in patients predisposed to hypoxemia, hypoperfusion, heart failure, and severe renal or hepatic impairment.

Contraindications:

- **Severe renal or hepatic impairment**, heart failure, & excessive alcohol intake.
- **Metformin held before giving iodinated contrast** & may be resumed 48 hours with monitoring of creatinine because of **increased risk of Acute kidney injury** (prerenal or Acute tubular necrosis).

SULFONYLUREAS

- **2nd-generation: Glipizide, Glyburide. Glimepiride** (long duration of action, no active metabolites).
- 1st-generation: Tolbutamide, Chlorpropamide (not used as often due to higher adverse effect profile).

Mechanism of action:

- **<u>Stimulates pancreatic beta cell insulin release</u> (insulin secretagogue) via mimicking the action of glucose, leading to closure of the K-ATP channel of the SUR1 receptor.**
- **2nd-generation preferred because they are associated with less adverse effects** & shorter duration of action.

Indications:

- In addition to Metformin or as initial therapy in patients with contraindications to Metformin.
- Similar glycemic efficacy compared to Metformin.
- Glimepiride or Glipizide safer in patients with chronic renal disease.

Adverse effects:

- **<u>Hypoglycemia</u> most common adverse effect,** especially with the long-acting 1st-generation, because insulin release is non-glucose dependent. Avoid Glyburide in the elderly.
- **<u>Weight gain</u>** — insulin is anabolic, so it promotes lipogenesis (the metabolic formation of fat).
- GI upset (reduced incidence if taken with food). Cardiac dysrhythmias; Hematologic toxicity.
- Dermatitis (including photosensitivity, pruritus, erythema, rash, urticaria). Sulfonamide allergies.
- <u>CP450 system inducer</u> may decrease levels of other medications; can lead to drug interactions.
- **<u>Chlorpropamide</u> has 2 unique adverse effects: [1] <u>Hyponatremia</u>** (increases ADH secretion) & **[2] <u>Disulfiram reaction</u>** — **flushing reaction after alcohol ingestion** due to inhibition of the metabolism of acetaldehyde.

MEGLITINIDES
Repaglinide, Nateglinide
Mechanism of action:
- **Stimulates pancreatic beta cell insulin release** (insulin secretagogue) by closure of the K-ATP channel but is more glucose dependent, leading to postprandial insulin release.

Indications:
- May be used as monotherapy in patients with contraindications to Metformin or in combination with Metformin.
- Similar benefits of Sulfonylureas without the sulfa component (safe with sulfa allergies).

Adverse effects:
- **Hypoglycemia lower incidence compared to Sulfonylureas.** Often administered with meals to decrease postprandial hyperglycemia.
- **Weight gain** — insulin is anabolic, so it promotes lipogenesis (the metabolic formation of fat).
- Nateglinide should not be used in chronic renal or liver disease because it is metabolized by the liver with active metabolites renally excreted.
- **Repaglinide is safer in patients with chronic renal disease** (principally metabolized by the liver).

THIAZOLIDINEDIONES
Pioglitazone, Rosiglitazone
Mechanism of action:
- **Increase insulin sensitivity** at the peripheral receptor sites (adipose tissue, muscle, & liver), leading to increased glucose utilization & decreased glucose production. They bind & activate the nuclear receptor peroxisome proliferator-activated receptor gamma (PPAR-gamma), having effects on the expression of a number of genes related to glucose and lipid metabolism.
- No effect on pancreatic beta cells (they do not cause Hypoglycemia as monotherapy) and are not contraindicated in patients with renal disease. Hemoglobin A1C falls 2% with monotherapy.
- Improved lipid profile: Pioglitazone also lowers triglycerides and increases HDL.

Adverse effects:
- **Peripheral edema, weight gain, fluid retention, decompensated (Congestive) Heart failure**.
- Hepatotoxicity LFTs should be monitored while on therapy. **Increased fractures (females).**
- **Rosiglitazone is associated with higher incidence of cardiovascular events (eg, MI stroke) & atherogenic lipid profiles**; Pioglitazone is usually preferred if TZD therapy is needed.
- **Pioglitazone associated with increased Bladder cancer risk.** Macular edema.

Contraindications:
- **Heart failure** (symptomatic, Class III or IV), history of Bladder cancer, active liver disease, high-risk for fractures, pregnancy, Type I Diabetes mellitus.

ALPHA-GLUCOSIDASE INHIBITORS
Acarbose, Miglitol
Mechanism of action:
- **Carbohydrate analogs that delay intestinal glucose & carbohydrate absorption from the small intestine** (inhibit pancreatic alpha amylase and intestinal alpha-glucosidase hydrolase).
- They increase GLP-1 release. No effect on insulin secretion, so no hypoglycemia as monotherapy.
- Less potent than Metformin & Sulfonylureas. Can be used in patients with renal insufficiency.

Adverse effects:
- **GI:** most common — **flatulence (most common), diarrhea, abdominal pain, & bloating** due to increased fermentation and degradation of undigested carbohydrates by intestinal bacteria.
- **Hepatitis rare adverse effect reported with Acarbose** (reversible with discontinuation). Liver function tests (LFTs) should be monitored before and during treatment with Acarbose.

CONTRAINDICATIONS
- **Patients with excess gas or increased risk of intestinal obstruction (eg, gastroparesis, inflammatory bowel disease, patients on bile acid resins).** Advanced kidney disease.

GLUCAGON-LIKE PEPTIDE 1 (GLP-1) RECEPTOR AGONIST

Mechanism of action: **Liraglutide, Exenatide, or Dulaglutide** injection. **Semaglutide** (oral or injection).

- **Mimics incretin, leading to increased glucose-dependent insulin secretion, decreased glucagon secretion, delayed gastric emptying, and reduced food intake.**
- Decreased CVD risk: **In people with type 2 diabetes and established cardiovascular disease (CVD), Metformin, GLP-1 receptor agonists (Liraglutide, Semaglutide, Dulaglutide), and SGLT2 inhibitors reduce the risk of all-cause and cardiovascular mortality as well as reduced diabetic kidney disease.** GLP-1 agonists improve LV ejection fraction, myocardial contractility, coronary blood flow, cardiac output, & endothelial function. **Associated with weight loss.**

Adverse effects:
- **GI: nausea, vomiting, diarrhea, & constipation common;** gallbladder disease. **Acute Pancreatitis.**
- Small risk of hypoglycemia (usually in the setting of other hypoglycemic agents). Not used in T1DM.

Contraindications:
- **History of Gastroparesis or Pancreatitis. Medullary thyroid carcinoma or MEN 2 syndrome.**

DPP4 INHIBITORS Sitagliptin, Linagliptin, Alogliptin

Mechanism of action:
- **Dipeptidyl peptidase-4 (DPP-4) inhibition causes decreased degradation and prolonged action of endogenously released Glucagon-like peptide-1 (GLP-1) & GIP, increasing levels of both.**
- Increased GLP1 levels lead to increased insulin release, decreased glucagon, decreased hepatic glucose production, & increased uptake of glucose in the peripheral tissues.
- Not associated with hypoglycemia if not used with insulin secretagogues.

Indications:
- Monotherapy in patients who are intolerant of or have contraindications to other oral medications.
- Can be adjunctive therapy to those medications. **Weight neutral.**

Adverse effects:
- **The most common adverse effects are headache, upper respiratory tract infections, and nasopharyngitis. Acute pancreatitis,** hepatitis, skin changes, joint pain, & renal dysfunction.

SGLT-2 INHIBITORS "flozin" — Empagliflozin, Canagliflozin, Dapagliflozin, Ertugliflozin

Mechanism of action:
- **Osmotic diuresis: Sodium-glucose transport (SGLT-2) inhibition lowers renal glucose excretion threshold, leading to increased urinary glucose excretion.**
- SGLT2 is expressed in the proximal tubule & mediates reabsorption of ~90% of the filtered glucose load. They are relatively weak glucose-lowering agents.
- Not associated with hypoglycemia in the absence of therapies that otherwise cause hypoglycemia.

Indications:
- Most often used in combination with Metformin, Pioglitazone, Sitagliptin, or Insulin.
- Cardiovascular risk reduction: **improves cardiovascular outcomes and decreases the risk of heart failure (especially Empagliflozin). Added benefit of blood pressure & weight reduction.**
- Decreased CVD risk: In people with type 2 diabetes and established cardiovascular disease (CVD), Metformin, GLP-1 receptor agonists (Liraglutide, Semaglutide, Dulaglutide), and **SGLT2 inhibitors reduce the risk of all-cause and cardiovascular mortality & reduce diabetic kidney disease.**

Adverse effects:
- Transient nausea, vomiting, abdominal pain. **Hypovolemia:** thirst, Acute kidney injury, **hypotension.**
- **Increased infections: UTIs & yeast infections** (↑urinary glucose), **Fournier gangrene. Bone fractures.**

Contraindications & cautions:
- Not used in Type I DM, type II with estimated GFR <60 mL (reduced efficacy in chronic renal disease).
- Canagliflozin & Ertugliflozin may be associated with **increased risk of amputation & foot ulcers.**
- **Cautious use with other medications that can cause dehydration (eg, NSAIDs, ACE inhibitors, ARBs, diuretics — may need dose adjustments of these medications due to lower blood pressures).** Cautious use in patients with low bone mineral density (**may decrease bone density**).
- **Patients with ketosis prone T2DM because of increased of DKA (including euglycemic DKA).**

DUAL GLP-1 & GIP RECEPTOR AGONIST (TIRZEPATIDE)

Mechanism of action:

- **Dual-acting GLP-1 and GIP receptor agonist:** Dual incretin [glucose-dependent insulinotropic polypeptide (GIP) and GLP-1 receptor] agonist that has glycemic and weight-reducing efficacy. Acylation results in albumin binding, allowing for prolonged action & once-weekly dosing.
- Treatment with Tirzepatide resulted in dose-dependent HbA$_{1c}$ reductions of 1.9%-2.6%. The average weight loss ranged from 6.2 kg-12.9 kg.
- **Beneficial effects include weight loss, improved lipid profile, lowering of blood pressure, and reduction of fatty liver.**

Adverse effects

- **GI**: most common — **nausea, vomiting, diarrhea** (may result in dehydration), constipation, **early satiety. Acute Pancreatitis.**
- GLP-1 receptor agonist therapy has been associated with increased risk of gallbladder and biliary diseases including cholelithiasis and cholecystitis.
- Small risk of hypoglycemia (usually in the setting of other hypoglycemic agents).

Contraindications:

- **History of Gastroparesis or Pancreatitis. Medullary thyroid carcinoma or MEN 2 syndrome.**
- Type 1 Diabetes mellitus

HYPOGLYCEMIA

- **Blood glucose level ≤70 mg/dL.**
- A complication of the management of Diabetes mellitus. Usually due to too much insulin use, too little food, or excess exercise.

CLINICAL MANIFESTATIONS

- **Autonomic:** sweating, tremors, palpitations, nervousness, tachycardia, pallor, cool clammy skin.
- **CNS (neuroglycopenic symptoms):** headache, lightness, confusion, slurred speech, dizziness, irritability, difficulty concentrating, blurred vision, nausea, syncope.

Management of mild to moderate:

- **Ingest 15-20 grams of fast-acting carbohydrate (eg, fruit juice), hard candies.**
- Recheck in 10-15 minutes.

Severe, unconscious, <40 mg/dL:

- **IV Dextrose (bolus of D50) or IV Glucagon.** No IV access: Glucagon SQ or IM.
- If unknown cause, order C-peptide, plasma insulin levels & anti-insulin antibodies as part of the workup.
- **Elevated C-peptide seen in endogenous insulin production.** C-peptide is normal with exogenous insulin administration.

ANTI-HYPERGLYCEMIC AGENTS

	MECHANISM OF ACTION	SIDE EFFECTS/CAUTION
BIGUANIDES Metformin	• Mainly ↓'es hepatic glucose production, ↑'es peripheral glucose utilization • ↓GI intestinal glucose absorption, ↑insulin sensitivity (no effect on pancreatic beta cells ⇨ no hypoglycemia, no weight gain • Usually 1st line PO medication used to control Type II DM. ↓'es triglycerides.	• Lactic acidosis, Not given in patients c̄ hepatic or renal impairment Cr >1.5 • GI complaints common. Macrocytic anemia (↓B12), metallic taste. • Metformin should be d/c'ed 24h before given iodinated contrast & resumed 48 hours afterwards with monitoring of creatinine.
SULFONYLUREAS 1st gen: Tolbutamide, Chlorpropamide 2nd gen: Glipizide, Glyburide, Glimepiride	• Stimulates pancreatic beta cell insulin release (insulin secretagogue – non glucose dependent) • 2nd generation: less S/E (so preferred), shorter half-lives	• Hypoglycemia most common. • GI upset (reduced if taken c̄ food). Dermatitis • Disulfiram reaction sulfa allergy • Cardiac dysrhythmias, weight gain • CP450 inducer (drug-drug interactions)
MEGLITINIDES Repaglinide, Nateglinide	• Stimulates pancreatic beta cell insulin release* (insulin secretagogue)	• Hypoglycemia (less than sulfonylureas) • Weight gain
c̄ - GLUCOSIDASE INHIBITORS: Acarbose Miglitol	• Delays intestinal glucose absorption (inhibits pancreatic alpha amylase and intestinal α - glucosidase hydrolase). • Does not affect insulin secretion.	• Hepatitis (↑LFT's), flatulence, diarrhea, abdominal pain. • Cautious use in patients c̄ gastroparesis, inflammatory bowel disease, on bile acid resins.
THIAZOLIDINEDIONES Pioglitazone Rosiglitazone	• ↑insulin sensitivity at the peripheral receptor site adipose & muscle. • No effect on pancreatic beta cells.	• Fluid retention & edema (CHF), hepatotoxicity, bladder CA, fractures. • Cardiovascular toxicity with Rosiglitazone.
GLUCAGON-LIKE PEPTIDE 1 (GLP-1) AGONISTS: Exenatide, Liraglutide	• Mimics incretin ⇨ ↑insulin secretion, delays gastric emptying, ↓ glucagon secretion. No weight gain.	• Hypoglycemia (less than sulfonylureas b/c glucose dependent), pancreatitis. • CI if history of gastroparesis
DPP-4 INHIBITOR: Sitagliptin, Linagliptin	• Dipeptidylpeptase inhibition ⇨inhibition of degradation of GLP-1 ⇨ ↑ GLP-1	• Pancreatitis, renal failure, GI symptoms
SGLT-2 INHIBITOR: Canagliflozin Dapagliflozin	• SGLT-2 inhibition lowers renal glucose threshold ⇨ ↑urinary glucose excretion SGLT = Sodium-Glucose Transport	• Thirst, nausea, abdominal pain, UTIs

TYPE OF INSULIN	APPROX. ONSET OF ACTION	EFFECTIVE PEAK	APPROXIMATE DURATION OF ACTION	INSULIN COVERAGE
Preprandial				

Rapid-acting
• Lispro
  U-100, U-200
• Lispro-aabc
  U-100, U-200
• Aspart
• Faster Aspart
• Glulisine
	15-30 minutes	1-3 hours	4-6 hours	**Given at the same time of meal (10-15 minutes before** and up to no later than immediately after meals).
				
				Often used with intermediate or long-acting Insulin to maintain glycemic control.

Short-acting • Regular U-100	30 minutes	1.5-3.5 hours	8 hours	**Given 30-45 minutes prior to meal.** Often used with intermediate or long-acting Insulin.
Basal				
Insulin type	**Half-life**	**Effective peak**	**Approximate duration of Action**	
Intermediate • NPH	4.4 hours	4-6 hours	**12 hours**	**Covers Insulin for about half day (or overnight).** Often combined with rapid or short-acting Insulin. NPH often given at bedtime.
Longer acting **Glargine** • U-100 • U-300 **Detemir** **Degludec** • U-100 • U-200	12 hours 19 hours 5-7 hours 25 hours	No peak No peak 3-9 hours No peak	20 to >24 hours 20 to >24 hours 6-24 hours >24 hours	**Glargine causes fewer hypoglycemic episodes than NPH.** Once daily glargine caused less weight gain than NPH once daily.

Glucose-reducing action can vary significantly in different individuals or within the same individual; the duration of action is dose dependent.

The choice of basal insulin & preprandial insulin depends on many factors, including patient preference.

Basal insulins:
- Glargine, degludec, and detemir have little peak activity at steady state.
- **U-100 insulin glargine:** can be used as a single daily injection in the morning or evening. Some people with type 1 diabetes achieve better glycemic control with U-100 glargine given twice daily. Glargine once daily caused less weight gain than NPH once daily.
- **U-300 insulin glargine** a more concentrated formulation of insulin glargine prolongs its duration of action (given once daily). Similar to Insulin degludec, U-300 insulin glargine has little peak effect and may reduce hypoglycemia in individuals with type 1 diabetes.
- **Insulin detemir:** Like NPH, twice-daily injections appear to be necessary in most people with type 1 diabetes. Duration of action is shorter when lower doses are used. **Slightly lower risk of severe hypoglycemia & nocturnal hypoglycemia with detemir compared with NPH.**
- **Insulin degludec:** very long-acting basal insulin administered once daily at any time of day. **In contrast to U-100 glargine and detemir insulins, degludec may be mixed with rapid-acting insulins without appreciably altering the kinetics of the degludec or the rapid-acting insulin.**

Prandial (pre-meal or preprandial) Insulin bolus options:
- **Rapid-acting insulin advantages**: ability to inject them 10 to 15 minutes before and no later than immediately after meals (compared to regular Insulin, which is given 30 to 45 minutes or more before meals to maximally coincide with postprandial glycemic movement. They have a shorter duration of action, decreasing hypoglycemia several hours after the dose is administered (they lower glucose levels more rapidly and without the prolonged effect of regular Insulin).
- **Ultra-rapid-acting insulin**: **insulin aspart** [with added niacinamide (vitamin B6)] has more rapid initial onset of action than insulin aspart, with a similar time to peak concentration.
- **Insulin lispro** as well as the faster-acting insulin lispro are available in pens in more concentrated formulations (U-200). Lispro-aabc formulation has more rapid onset of action than insulin lispro.
- **Regular insulin** U-100 regular insulin.

SOMOGYI PHENOMENON
- **Nocturnal hypoglycemia followed by rebound hyperglycemia.**

PATHOPHYSIOLOGY
- Hyperglycemia occurs due to surge in growth hormone after early AM hypoglycemia.

MANAGEMENT

Prevent hypoglycemia with any 1 of the following 3:
- **[1] Decreasing nighttime NPH dose**
- **[2] Move the evening NPH dose earlier**
- **[3] Give a bedtime snack.**

DAWN PHENOMENON
- Normal glucose **until rise in serum glucose levels between 2am-8 am**.

PATHOPHYSIOLOGY
- Results from decreased insulin sensitivity & **nightly surge of counterregulatory hormones** (during nighttime fasting).

MANAGEMENT

Reduce early morning hyperglycemia with any one of the following:
- **[1] Bedtime injection of NPH** (to blunt morning hyperglycemia)
- **[2] Increase the evening NPH dose**
- **[3] Avoiding carbohydrate snack late at night**
- [4] Insulin pump usage early in the morning.

INSULIN WANING
- Progressive rise in glucose from bed to morning (seen when NPH dose evening dose is administered before dinner).
- Due to ineffective dosing of NPH insulin.

MANAGEMENT:
- Move NPH insulin dose to bedtime or increase the evening dose.

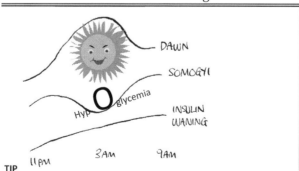

TIP
- In answering these questions, the 11pm dose is usually normal and the 8 am preprandial dose will be high.
- The key is what is the 3 am dose? If it rises with the sun at 3 am, it's the Dawn phenomenon
- If the 3am dose is lOw (HypOglycemia, then it is the SOmOgyi

DIABETIC KETOACIDOSIS (DKA)

- **Consequence of insulin deficiency & counterregulatory hormone excess (eg, glucagon) characterized by the triad of [1] hyperglycemia + [2] acidosis + [3] ketonemia &/or ketonuria.**
- Insulin deficiency and counterregulatory hormone excess lead to increased gluconeogenesis & glycogenolysis as well as impaired glucose utilization, resulting in hyperglycemia. Excess counterregulatory hormones release free fatty acids which oxidize into ketone bodies (beta-hydroxybutyrate and acetoacetate), resulting in ketonemia, ketonuria, and metabolic acidosis.
- Epidemiology: **DKA most commonly seen in Type I Diabetes mellitus due to insulin deficiency.**

ETIOLOGIES

DKA is often a response to <u>stressful triggers</u>:
- **Infection** — **most common cause (eg, UTI or pneumonia) 30-40%.**
- **Discontinuation or inadequate insulin therapy.** New-onset DM, MI, CVA, Pancreatitis, etc.
- **SGLT-2 inhibitors** can predispose to DKA via multiple mechanisms (may even precipitate a euglycemic DKA with a high anion gap, positive serum & urine ketones, glucose <250 mg/dL).

CLINICAL MANIFESTATIONS

- **Symptoms of hyperglycemia: most common early symptoms — eg, polyuria, nocturia, polydipsia, and polyphagia with marked fatigue, nausea, or vomiting.**
- Nonspecific: malaise, generalized weakness, fatigue, drowsiness, altered mental status changes, anorexia, nausea, vomiting, chest pain, **abdominal pain,** weight loss.
- **Hypovolemia** eg, tachycardia, hypotension, decreased skin turgor, dry mouth and mucous membranes, poor capillary refill.
- **Fruity (acetone) breath, & Kussmaul respirations (deep, continuous, tachypneic respirations).**

DIAGNOSIS

- **D:iabetes — plasma glucose >250 mg/dL** (usually not >600 mg/dL); increased serum osmolarity.
- **K:etones — serum >5 mEq/L &/or urine** due to ↑ lipolysis. Beta hydroxybutyrate >4 nmol/L.
- **A:cidosis — decreased arterial pH (<7.3) & bicarbonate (<15)** [high anion gap metabolic acidosis].
- Serum potassium: Despite serum K+, DKA is associated with depletion of total body K+ due to cellular potassium shift & losses through urine, so close attention paid to serum K+ levels during treatment. With Insulin treatment, K+ will shift intracellularly, which may cause dangerous Hypokalemia.

MANAGEMENT

SIPS — <u>S</u>aline, <u>I</u>nsulin (regular), <u>P</u>otassium repletion, <u>S</u>earch for underlying cause. Admit to ICU.
- **IV fluids: critical initial step** to correct hypovolemia, fluid deficit, and hyperosmolality.
    - **Isotonic (0.9% Normal saline or Lactated ringers)** until hypotension & orthostasis resolves.
    - **Switch to ½ normal saline (0.45% sodium chloride) once volume is repleted.**
    - **When glucose levels become ≤250 mg/dL, use the D5 version of the current solution** to prevent hypoglycemia from continued Insulin therapy.
- **Insulin (regular): lowers serum glucose & switches body from catabolic to anabolic state** (reduces ketones, fatty acid production, & gluconeogenesis). Insulin given until the anion gap closes.
    - **In patients with initial serum potassium <3.3 mEq/L, insulin therapy should be delayed until the serum K+ is ≥3.3 mEq/L to avoid complications of Hypokalemia** (Insulin shifts potassium intracellularly, which can result in or worsen Hypokalemia).
- **Potassium repletion:** despite serum K+ levels, patients are always in a total body potassium deficit. **Correction of DKA will invariably cause Hypokalemia. Check serum K+ levels hourly.**
    - **Unless serum K+ is >5.3 mEq/L, K+ repletion is recommended.**
    - **If serum K+ is 3.3–5.3 mEq/L:** IV KCl (20-30 mEq/L) added to each liter of IV fluid **+ Insulin.**
    - **If serum K+ is <3.3 mEq/L,** IV potassium chloride (KCl 20-40 mEq/L); **hold Insulin.**
    - **If serum K+ >5.3:** hold (delay) K+ replacement until K+ falls below 5.3 mEq/L; **give Insulin.**
- **Treatment goals: closing the anion gap in DKA determines complete management.**
    Serum bicarbonate levels more important than glucose levels in determining the severity of DKA.
- Bicarbonate administration used only if severe because may cause overcorrection or cerebral edema.

HYPEROSMOLAR HYPERGLYCEMIC STATE (HHS)

- **Consequence of Insulin deficiency and/or resistance & counterregulatory hormone excess (eg, glucagon);** similar to DKA.

EPIDEMIOLOGY
- **HHS is more common with type II DM** & seen in older patients (fifth and sixth decades of life).
- HHS is associated with more severe dehydration and a higher mortality compared to DKA (10 times higher than DKA at a mortality rate of 20%).

ETIOLOGIES:
- HHS is a response to <u>stressful triggers</u> — **infection is the most common cause eg, UTI, pneumonia, GI** (50-60%).
- **Newly diagnosed, previously unknown Diabetes** (15%).
- Catabolic stress of acute illness (eg, trauma, surgery, MI, CVA, pancreatitis, etc.).

PATHOPHYSIOLOGY
- Illness leading to reduced fluid intake (infection most common), **profound dehydration**, increased osmolarity, hyperglycemia, total body potassium deficit, and shrinkage of brain cells.
- **HHS is not usually associated with severe ketosis or acidosis** because although there is relative insulin deficiency; patients with type II DM make enough insulin to prevent significant ketogenesis (Insulin inhibits ketogenesis). Therefore, ketonemia and acidemia are absent or very mild in HHS.

CLINICAL MANIFESTATIONS
- <u>**Hyperglycemia**</u> increased thirst, polyuria, nocturia, weakness, fatigue, nausea, vomiting.
- <u>**Neurologic symptoms:**</u> **mental status changes, lethargy, confusion.** Depressed mental status and coma are more frequent in HHS than DKA due to the greater degree of hyperosmolality in HHS (often > 320-330 mOsmol/kg in HHS).

PHYSICAL EXAMINATION
- Tachycardia, tachypnea, hypotension, decreased skin turgor (dehydration), dry mouth, & increased capillary refill time.
- **Due to shrinkage of the brain cells from dehydration & decreased cerebral flow** — focal neurological deficits, visual acuity deficits, delirium, coma.

DIAGNOSIS
- <u>**Increased osmolarity (>320)**</u> **& increased serum glucose (>600** mg/dL).
- <u>Absence of significant acidosis/ketosis</u>: arterial pH >7.30 & serum bicarbonate >15 mEq/L.

MANAGEMENT
- **SIPS — <u>S</u>aline most important component of treatment, <u>I</u>nsulin (regular), <u>P</u>otassium repletion, <u>S</u>earch for the underlying cause.** See DKA for treatment details.
- **Resolution of HHS is achieved when patients are mentally alert, the effective plasma osmolality has fallen <315 mOsmol/kg,** & the patient is able to eat.

	HHS	Mild DKA	Moderate DKA	Severe DKA
Plasma Glucose (mg/dL)	**>600**	**>250**	>250	>250
Arterial pH	**>7.30**	**<7.30**	7.0-7.24	<7.0
Serum Bicarbonate (mEq/L)	>15	**15-18**	10 to <15	<10
Ketones (Urine/Serum)	Small	**Positive**	Positive	Positive
Serum Osmolarity	**>320**	Variable	Variable	Variable

COMPLICATIONS OF DIABETES MELLITUS

- Morbidity from Diabetes is a consequence of both macrovascular disease (atherosclerosis) and microvascular disease (eg, retinopathy, nephropathy, and neuropathy).

CARDIOVASCULAR COMPLICATIONS
- Atherosclerosis — **Diabetes mellitus is considered a Coronary artery disease equivalent.**
- Peripheral arterial disease, Acute decompensated heart failure (CHF), Cardiomyopathy.
- Stroke — risk 2-4 times greater than the general population. Hypertension common.

MANAGEMENT:
- **Hypertension** blood pressure goals in Diabetes mellitus <140/90 mm Hg. **ACE inhibitors or Angiotensin receptor blockers if blood pressure ≥140/90 mm Hg** or urine is positive for **microalbuminuria.**
- Decreased CVD risk: In people with type 2 diabetes and established cardiovascular disease (CVD), **Metformin, GLP-1 receptor agonists** (Liraglutide, Semaglutide, Dulaglutide), **& SGLT2 inhibitors reduce the risk of all-cause and cardiovascular mortality & reduce diabetic kidney disease.**

Cardiovascular risk reduction:
- Statin medication indicated with LDL goal <100 mg/dL.
- Reduce other cardiac risks. Hemoglobin A1C <7.0% goal.

DIABETIC NEUROPATHY
[1] DISTAL SYMMETRIC POLYNEUROPATHY:
- **Most common type of diabetic neuropathy & most common complication of Diabetes mellitus.**
- **Progressive distal sensory loss in a "stocking-glove" pattern (involving the <u>distal lower extremities at first</u>,** progressing to the hands) — loss of vibratory, proprioception, light touch, & temperature. **May lead to foot ulcer formation.** Charcot arthropathy.
- Decreased or absent ankle reflexes, gait abnormalities, and motor dysfunction can occur.

[2] AUTONOMIC NEUROPATHY:
- **Blood pressure changes: eg, Orthostatic (postural) hypotension;** heart rate variability.
- **GI: Gastroparesis** (occurs after many years). Enteropathy (constipation or diarrhea).
- Erectile dysfunction and retrograde ejaculation.

[3] CRANIAL NERVE MONONEUROPATHY
- Most commonly affecting extraocular muscles — **cranial nerve III (oculomotor): diplopia & ptosis with sparing of the pupils** (unlike other CN III palsies), VI (abducens), & IV (trochlear).
- CN VII (facial nerve) palsy.

[4] PERIPHERAL MONONEUROPATHY
- **Median neuropathy most common (Carpal tunnel syndrome),** ulnar neuropathy.

MANAGEMENT OF DIABETIC NEUROPATHY
- **Optimal glycemic control** slows progression of neuropathy & microvascular disease. **Foot care.**
First-line pharmacotherapy options for painful diabetic neuropathy include:
- **[1] SNRIs:** Serotonin-norepinephrine reuptake inhibitors [Duloxetine > Venlafaxine], **OR**
- **[2] Tricyclic antidepressants** eg, Amitriptyline, Desipramine, Nortriptyline, **OR**
- **[3] Gabapentinoid antiseizure medications eg, Pregabalin Gabapentin.**
- Selection of a specific agent individualized based on comorbidities, medication interactions, adverse effect profiles, & cost. **Foot care.** Gabapentinoids preferred in patients with Restless legs syndrome over SNRIs.
- Second-line: topical agents (eg, Capsaicin cream & Lidocaine patches), alpha-lipoic acid, Neuromodulation (transcutaneous electrical nerve stimulation). Carbamazepine, Valproate, Tramadol.

SCREENING
- **After initial screening, all diabetics should be <u>screened annually</u>** by examining sensory function in the feet and assessing ankle reflexes.

DIABETIC GASTROPARESIS

- **Decreased GI motility & delayed gastric emptying** due to decreased ability of the gut to sense the stretch of the bowel walls in the absence of a mechanical obstruction (diabetic neuropathy).
- Normally, stretch is the main stimulant for gastric motility.

CLINICAL MANIFESTATIONS

- **Nausea, vomiting, bloating, early satiety, upper abdominal discomfort, & constipation in the setting of longstanding Diabetes mellitus (years).**
- May have epigastric distention or tenderness with a **succussion splash** but no rigidity or guarding.

DIAGNOSIS

- **Upper endoscopy usually performed initially to rule out other causes of symptoms**.
- **CT/MR enterography (CTE/MRE): Upper endoscopy is followed, if clinically indicated, by CTE/MRE** to exclude mechanical obstruction or mucosal disease as a cause of impaired gastric emptying.
- **Nuclear gastric emptying scintigraphy: delayed gastric emptying in the absence of structural obstruction is required to establish the diagnosis of Gastroparesis.**

MANAGEMENT

- **Dietary modifications: initial management consists of dietary modification, optimization of glycemic control, and hydration** — small, frequent meals low in fat and contain only soluble fiber. If solids are not tolerated, meals can be homogenized and liquid meals supplemented with vitamins.
- **Prokinetics: In patients who fail to respond to dietary modification, prokinetics are used to increase the rate of gastric emptying & GI motility — Metoclopramide initially;** Domperidone if no response to Metoclopramide, and subsequently oral Erythromycin. H2RAs and PPIs for acid.
- Avoid medications that delay gastric emptying [eg, GLP1 agonists (eg, Exenatide & DPP4 inhibitors)].

DIABETIC KIDNEY DISEASE [DKD] (NEPHROPATHY)

- **The presence of albuminuria, decreased estimated glomerular filtration rate (eGFR), or both.**
- **Proteinuria is the single best predictor of disease progression.**
- **Diabetes mellitus is the most common cause of end stage renal disease in the US.**

PATHOPHYSIOLOGY

- Progressive kidney deterioration leading to **microalbuminuria** (first sign of Diabetic nephropathy).

DIAGNOSIS

- **Spot urine albumin: creatinine: on early morning urine samples to estimate excretion. A value that lies between 30 mg/g to 300 mg/g indicates microalbuminuria.** 24-hour urine protein.
- Histology: **Kimmelstiel-Wilson lesion:** nodular glomerulosclerosis **(pink hyaline material** around the glomerular capillaries from protein leakage) — **pathognomonic of Diabetic nephropathy.**

MANAGEMENT

- **Uncontrolled hypertension and poor glycemic control are the 2 main causes of the progression of Diabetic nephropathy.** Early treatment can delay or prevent the progression of DKD.
- **Glycemic control:** In patients with type 2 diabetes and DKD who have not achieved glycemic control despite initial glucose-lowering therapy (which is typically Metformin), **addition of an SGLT2 inhibitor or GLP-1 receptor agonist can improve glycemic control.** Hemoglobin A1C goal ≤7%.
- **Hypertension:** Patients with type 2 Diabetes and Diabetic kidney disease (DKD) should generally be treated with either an **Angiotensin converting enzyme (ACE) inhibitor or Angiotensin receptor blocker (ARB)** to reduce intraglomerular pressure **[often with sodium-glucose cotransporter 2 (SGLT2) inhibitor if T2DM].** ADA recommends BP <140/90 mmHg (<130/80 in higher risk patients).
- **Finerenone useful in individuals with Diabetes and Chronic kidney disease with albuminuria.**
- Monitoring: Patients with DKD should ideally be monitored every three to six months.

Screening for Diabetic kidney disease:
- **Yearly screening for microalbuminuria**, BUN, & creatinine.

SYNDROME OF INAPPROPRIATE ADH (SIADH)

- **Non-physiologic excess & unsuppressed ADH release** from the pituitary gland or ectopic source, leading to **[1] free water retention** (& secondary solute loss), **[2] dilutional Hyponatremia due to impaired kidney water excretion, [3] a concentrated urine, & [4] a reduced urine volume.**
- Inappropriate ↑ADH in absence of appropriate physiologic stimuli (eg, hypovolemia or hyperosmolality).

ETIOLOGIES

- **CNS: most common** — hemorrhage (eg, subarachnoid), stroke, head trauma, infection (eg, meningitis, encephalitis), CNS tumors, post-op, hydrocephalus, mental illness, and psychosis.
- **Pulmonary: Small-cell lung cancer** (ectopic ADH), infection (eg, **Legionella pneumonia,** viral). HIV.
- **Medications: anticonvulsants, Carbamazepine, Hydrochlorothiazide,** NSAIDs, Chlorpropamide, **antidepressants** (TCAs, SSRIs), high-dose **IV Cyclophosphamide, ecstasy (MDMA),** narcotics.
- Endocrine: hypothyroidism, hypopituitarism, & Conn syndrome. Tumors. Vincristine, Vinblastine.
- **SIADH is also more prevalent in hospitalized, post-operative, and older patients** due to the administration of hypotonic fluids, drugs, and the body's response to stress.

CLINICAL MANIFESTATIONS

- **Neurologic symptoms due to cerebral edema** (decreased osmolality shifts water into the cells).
- Mild symptoms (sodium usually 125-130 mEq/L) — nausea and malaise earliest symptoms.
- Moderate: (115-125 mEq/L) — headache, weakness, lethargy, confusion, disorientation.
- Severe: (<120 mEq/L) — seizures, coma, respiratory arrest.
- Chronic Hyponatremia: nonspecific neurological symptoms — nausea, vomiting, gait disturbances, memory and cognitive problems, fatigue, dizziness, confusion, and muscle cramps.

PHYSICAL EXAMINATION

- **Usually euvolemic (normovolemic) fluid status — absence of edema, normal skin turgor,** blood pressure within normal range, moist mucous membranes, no evidence of jugular venous pulsation.

DIAGNOSIS

- Diagnosis made in the absence of renal, adrenal, pituitary, thyroid disease, or diuretic use.

Dilutional labs: due to free water retention:

- **[1] Hyponatremia: Normovolemic hypotonic Hyponatremia** absence of volume depletion or hypervolemia (eg, normal skin turgor, moist membranes, normal BP, **no signs of edema**).
- **[2] Decreased serum osmolality <280-275 mOsm/kg, sodium <135 mEq/L,** Hypouricemia (<4 mg/dL), & ↓BUN (<5-10 mg/dL) — all are dilutional due to excess free water. **Increased ADH.**

Urine studies:

- **[3] Increased urine osmolality >100 mOsm/kg (concentrated urine) & decreased urine volume.**
- **[4] Urine sodium >40 mEq/L** because they are euvolemic (no stimuli for renal Na⁺ reabsorption).

MANAGEMENT

- Treat the underlying cause. Rapid correction >0.5 mEq/L/hour may lead to rapid shrinkage of neurons in the brain, resulting in central pontine myelinolysis (osmotic demyelination).
- **Mild or asymptomatic: Water & fluid restriction mainstay (eg, <800 cc daily or 500 cc below the urine output).** Salt tablets or IV saline, high solute intake, or Loop diuretics are adjuvant.
- **Severe Hyponatremia (eg, obtunded, coma, seizure, SAH): IV hypertonic saline (3% saline)** boluses or infused ≤0.05 mL/kg body weight IV per minute, with hourly sodium levels measured until Na⁺ increases by 12 mEq/L or to 130 mEq/L, whichever occurs first. Furosemide may be added.
- **ADH receptor antagonists — Conivaptan (IV), Tolvaptan (oral) reserved for some patients with severe persistent SIADH.** They prevent ADH-mediated free water retention and increase urinary water excretion by antagonizing V2 receptors. Tolvapatan is hepatotoxic and is not given for ≥30 days.

Chronic:

- **ADH receptor antagonists — Tolvaptan** (oral) prevents ADH-mediated free water retention & increase urinary water excretion. Not used for >30 days or with liver disease due to hepatotoxicity.
- **Demeclocycline** inhibits ADH, inducing reversible form of nephrogenic DI in 7-14 days. Nephrotoxic.

ARGININE VASOPRESSIN DEFICIENCY OR RESISTANCE [DIABETES INSIPIDUS (DI)]

- **Inability of the kidney to concentrate urine, leading to production of large volumes (amounts) of dilute (hypotonic) urine** — eg, >3 liters/24 hours + urine osmolality <300 mOsm/kg.
- Due to abnormalities with **antidiuretic hormone (ADH; also called Arginine vasopressin or AVP).**

2 TYPES
- **[1] AVP deficiency (Central) most common type.** Etiologies: **Idiopathic most common**, damage to the hypothalamus or posterior pituitary, CNS surgery or tumor, head trauma, infection, Sarcoidosis.
- **[2] Partial or complete renal resistance to AVP (Nephrogenic):** Etiologies: Medications: **Lithium,** Amphotericin B, Demeclocycline, Foscarnet, **Hypokalemia or Hypercalcemia** (disrupt the kidney's concentrating ability), Acute tubular necrosis, Hereditary causes in children.
  Lithium & Hypercalcemia are the most common causes of AVP resistance (Nephrogenic).

CLINICAL MANIFESTATIONS
- **Polyuria (3-20 liters daily), nocturia + polydipsia (excessive thirst** to maintain water balance).
- High-volume nocturia & enuresis. Infants: may present with crying, irritability, & hyperthermia.
- **Neurologic symptoms of Hypernatremia can occur when water intake is less than urinary water loss** (eg, fatigue, weakness, myalgias, confusion, lethargy, disorientation, seizures, or coma).
- **Physical examination: normal if mild.** Severe: dehydration, hypotension, & rapid vascular collapse.

DIAGNOSIS
- Labs reflect production of **large amounts of dilute urine & increased urinary free water excretion:**
  - **[1] Increased serum osmolality (>300 mOsm)** due to increased urinary free water loss.
    Serum (plasma) osmolality ≤280 mOsm/kg implies Primary polydipsia.
  - **[2] Decreased urine osmolality (≤300 mOsm/kg), decreased specific gravity** (≤1.005), **increased urine volume (3-20 L/24h)**, & decreased urine Na+ (↑ urinary H$_2$O excretion).
  - **[3] Hypernatremia & dehydration if severe** (when inadequate free water intake doesn't keep up with urinary free water loss). **Serum sodium is often in the high-normal or high range.**

- **STEP 1 (Screening): Fluid deprivation test: establishes the diagnosis of Diabetes insipidus.**
  - Normal response = progressive urine concentration. Same results also seen in Primary polydipsia.
  - **DI = continued production of large amounts of dilute urine (low urine osmolality).**

- **STEP 2 Desmopressin (ADH/AVP) stimulation test: distinguishes central vs. nephrogenic DI.**
  - Normal response = progressive urine concentration (↑ in urine osmolality) after ADH is given.
  - **Central: reduction in urine output + >50% increase in urine osmolality (response to ADH).** Central DI is associated with urine osmolality of ≥300 mosmol/kg after Desmopressin is given. **Plasma copeptin; ≤4.9 pmol/L suggests Central DI** (terminal fragment of pre-pr AVP/ADH).
  - **Nephrogenic: continued production of large amounts of dilute urine (well below 300 mosmol/kg, indicating lack of response to ADH)** with no or minimal elevation (eg, <15%) in urine osmolality in complete nephrogenic DI or small (up to 45%) if partial nephrogenic DI.
- **MRI pituitary:** Central DI — normal posterior "bright spot" on T1 image is undetectable or small.

MANAGEMENT OF **ARGININE VASOPRESSIN DEFICIENCY (AVP-D)/CENTRAL DI:**
- **Desmopressin (DDAVP) first-line** — intranasal injection, subcutaneous, or oral. **Synthetic ADH/AVP analog that increases the urinary concentration ability.** Correct underlying abnormalities.
- **Low-solute (mostly low-sodium, low-protein) diet** causes excretion of a low amount of solute in the urine in a smaller volume of urine in Arginine vasopressin deficiency. Thiazides may be added.
- Not commonly used: Thiazides, NSAIDs; Chlorpropamide, Carbamazepine, and Clofibrate.

MANAGEMENT OF **ARGININE VASOPRESSIN RESISTANCE (AVP-R)]/NEPHROGENIC DI**
- **Initial step: correct the underlying cause + Low-solute (mostly low-sodium, low-protein) diet.**
- **Thiazide diuretic may be used if symptoms persist despite low solute diet, with subsequent addition of Amiloride if needed.** Discontinue the offending drug, if feasible.
- **Patients continued on Lithium: low sodium diet & Thiazide &/or Amiloride (with subsequent addition of Indomethacin if symptoms persist)** if Lithium discontinuation is not the best option.

CALCIUM DISORDERS

- 99% of calcium is found in the bone; 1% in extracellular fluid. 50% of ECF Ca^{2+} is ionized (active) form.
- Normal calcium level: 8.5-10 mg/dL. **Vitamin D is required for intestinal Ca^{2+} absorption.**
- Ca^{2+} is important for bone, blood clotting, normal cellular function, & neuromuscular transmission.
- Calcium is maintained within a normal range via 3 major hormones:
  - **Hypocalcemia** stimulates ❶ **↑parathyroid hormone (PTH) & ❷↑calcitriol (Vitamin D)** secretion: ↑'es blood Ca^{2+} via ↑GI Ca^{2+} absorption & kidney Ca^{2+} reabsorption & ↑bone Ca^{2+} resorption (via ↑osteoclast activity). PTH also inhibits renal phosphate reabsorption, **so phosphate is usually in the opposite direction of the PTH levels in Primary parathyroid disorders.**
  - **Hypercalcemia** stimulates ❸↑**Calcitonin secretion:** ↓'es blood Ca^{2+} (↓Ca^{2+} GI absorption & kidney Ca^{2+} reabsorption & ↑'es bone mineralization (calcium deposition into the bone).

HYPERCALCEMIA

ETIOLOGIES
90% of Hypercalcemia is due to [1] Primary hyperparathyroidism or [2] malignancy (inpatient).
- **[1] Primary hyperparathyroidism most common overall cause of Hypercalcemia (parathyroid adenoma, Lithium,** Multiple endocrine neoplasia). Familial hypocalciuric hypercalcemia [FHH].
- **[2] Malignancy second most common cause.** Due to increased PTH-related protein production.
- **Thiazides,** Hyperthyroidism, Vitamin D or A intoxication. Granulomas (eg, Sarcoidosis, Tuberculosis) result in overproduction of active vitamin D (1,25-dihydroxyvitamin D_3). Milk-alkali syndrome.

CLINICAL MANIFESTATIONS
- **Most patients are asymptomatic, especially if mild** (Ca^{+2} <12 mg/dL).
- **Stones** — Nephrolithiasis (calcium oxalate & phosphate), **bones** — bone pain & fractures, **abdominal groans** — ileus (constipation, nausea), Peptic ulcers, Pancreatitis. ↓**DTR & weakness** (↑Ca^{+2} increases excitation threshold & decreases muscle contraction), **psychic moans** (eg, depression, anxiety, confusion, lethargy); **thrones** — polyuria; **increased vascular tone** (**Hypertension**).
- **Polyuria, polydipsia, dehydration:** from Hypercalcemia-induced Nephrogenic Diabetes insipidus.

DIAGNOSIS
- **Step 1: repeat measurement to verify in asymptomatic patients & correct calcium for albumin** (low albumin falsely elevates Ca). Ionized serum calcium more accurate than Total serum calcium.
- **Intact PTH: second step once Hypercalcemia is confirmed to rule out 1ry Hyperparathyroidism. Elevated iPTH makes Primary hyperparathyroidism most likely, especially if ↓phosphate.**
- **PTH-related protein often ordered if intact PTH is low normal or low to rule out malignancy.** Symptomatic severe Hypercalcemia (>14 mg/dL) + low iPTH + ↑PTHrP usually due to malignancy.
- Vitamin D metabolites [eg, 25(OH)D & 1,25-dihydroxyvitamin D_3] & 24-h urinary calcium. Calcium excretion is usually elevated or high-normal in Hyperparathyroidism & malignancy (low if FHH). ↑25(OH)D is indicative of vitamin D intoxication; ↑1,25-dihydroxyvitamin $(OH)_2D$ due to granulomatous diseases (eg, Sarcoidosis) or Lymphoma (chest radiograph may evaluate for both).
- **ECG: may show shortened QTc interval**, prolonged PR interval, & QRS widening.

MANAGEMENT OF MILD (<12 mg/dL):
- **No immediate treatment is needed.** Management consists of identifying and treating the underlying cause, in addition to increasing water intake to promote renal calcium excretion.

MANAGEMENT OF MODERATE (12-13.9 mg/dL):
- **IV fluids (eg, 0.9% saline) initial management of choice** if associated with significant symptoms. IV Normal saline promotes urinary calcium excretion & corrects dehydration due to Hypercalcemia.
- **IV Calcitonin may be helpful adjunct for rapid serum calcium reduction if no response to fluids** (faster onset of action compared to Bisphosphonates). Limited duration of action (24-48 hours).
- **Bisphosphonates** (eg, Zoledronic acid or Pamidronate) **adjunct if associated with malignancy — achieves a prolonged, sustained reaction with attained maximum effect in 2-4 days.**
- **If severe (Ca^{+2} ≥14 mg/dL), give IV saline (first-line) + IV Calcitonin + Bisphosphonates.**
- Denosumab an adjunct in malignancy-related Hypercalcemia. Steroids in granulomatous disease.

HYPOCALCEMIA

ETIOLOGIES

- **Hypoparathyroidism** most common cause overall — autoimmune destruction or inadvertent removal of the parathyroid gland during neck surgery (eg, thyroid or parathyroid surgery).
- **Secondary Hyperparathyroidism:** increased PTH in response to Hypocalcemia — **Chronic renal disease,** chronic liver disease, or **Vitamin D deficiency or resistance** (Osteomalacia & Rickets).
- Electrolyte abnormalities: **Hypomagnesemia** (induces PTH resistance & decreases PTH function, or PTH deficiency); Hyperphosphatemia, Hypoalbuminemia. **Alkalemia** (↑calcium protein binding).
- Medications: **diuretics,** calcium chelators (eg, high citrate during blood transfusion), Inhibitors of bone resorption: Bisphosphonates, Denosumab, or Calcitonin, especially with vitamin D deficiency.
- **Acute pancreatitis** — Hypocalcemia may occur due to saponification (precipitation of calcium soaps in the abdominal cavity). Hungry bone syndrome after parathyroidectomy. Bony metastases.

CLINICAL MANIFESTATIONS

- **Most are asymptomatic,** especially if mild.
- **Increased muscular contractions** occur because Hypocalcemia decreases excitation threshold & increases muscle & nerve excitability. **The hallmark of acute Hypocalcemia is tetany, characterized by neuromuscular irritability.**
- **Neuromuscular irritability** mild: **perioral numbness, paresthesias of the feet or hands, myalgias, muscle cramping with tetany.** Severe: carpopedal spasm, laryngospasm, seizures.
- Cardiovascular: CHF (S3 gallop), arrhythmias, bradycardia, **prolonged QT interval.**
- Dermatologic: dry, rough, and puffy skin with chronic Hypocalcemia; dry hair; scalp and eyebrow hair loss; and brittle fingernails with transverse grooves. Psoriasis.
- **Gastrointestinal: diarrhea, abdominal pain, or cramps** (↓Ca^{+2} decreases excitation threshold).
- Skeletal: abnormal dentition, defective enamel, teeth hyopoplasia, Osteomalacia, Osteodystrophy.
- Respiratory: **bronchospasm or laryngospasm** that can cause respiratory stridor.
- **Neuropsychiatric symptoms:** irritability, fatigue, cognitive impairment, anxiety, depression, mental status or behavioral changes, psychosis, seizures. Parkinsonian, & extrapyramidal symptoms.
- **Chvostek sign facial spasm and twitching and contraction of the ipsilateral facial muscles on tapping of the facial nerve in front of the tragus.**
- **Trousseau's sign inflation of blood pressure cuff above systolic blood pressure for 3 minutes causes painful carpal spasms** (flexion of the wrists & MCP joints with adduction of the fingers).
- Hyperactive reflexes: **Increased deep tendon reflexes (hyperreflexia) and Hypotension.**

DIAGNOSIS

- Order intact PTH, magnesium, phosphate, BUN, creatinine, & vitamin D metabolites.
- **Serum calcium: The first step in the evaluation of Hypocalcemia is to repeat the measurement to confirm that there is a true decrease in the serum calcium concentration (Ca <8.5 mg/dL).**
- Albumin levels may be needed to correct calcium for hypoalbuminemia:
  Corrected Ca = [0.8 x (normal albumin 4.0 – patient's serum albumin)] + serum Ca.
- **Intact PTH: Measurement of serum intact parathyroid hormone (PTH) is the most valuable laboratory test for determining the etiology of Hypocalcemia.** Low PTH: **a suppressed or "inappropriately normal" PTH level + Hypocalcemia establishes Hypoparathyroidism.** Elevated PTH level: (Secondary hyperparathyroidism) — vitamin D axis most likely cause (eg, kidney disease, vitamin D deficiency).
- Serum phosphate elevated in Hypoparathyroidism or Chronic kidney disease; ↓in vitamin D deficiency.
- **ECG: prolonged QT interval classic finding of Hypocalcemia.**

MANAGEMENT

- **Mild, chronic: oral Calcium + Vitamin D.** K+ & Mg+ repletion may be needed. Recombinant human PTH 1-84 (rhPTH 1 84) is an option for patients with refractory chronic Hypoparathyroidism.
- **Severe or symptomatic: IV calcium gluconate,** IV calcium carbonate. K+ & Mg+ repletion if needed.

PRIMARY HYPERPARATHYROIDISM

- Excessive uncontrolled parathyroid hormone (PTH) release. **Most common cause of Hypercalcemia.**

ETIOLOGIES
- **Parathyroid adenoma most common cause (80-85%).** More common in women & >50 years.
- Parathyroid hyperplasia or enlargement (15%).
- **Lithium.** Thiazide therapy.
- Rare causes: MEN 1 and 2A; Parathyroid carcinoma <1% of cases.

MEN 1	Hyperparathyroidism	Pituitary Tumors	Pancreatic Tumors
Men 2A	Hyperparathyroidism	Pheochromocytoma	Medullary Thyroid Carcinoma

CLINICAL MANIFESTATIONS
- **Most are asymptomatic** (asymptomatic Hypercalcemia) often found incidentally on routine testing.
- **Signs of Hypercalcemia:** "stones, bones, abdominal groans, psychic moans." – **Nephrolithiasis**, bone pain, fractures, ileus, constipation, nausea, vomiting, **weakness, decreased deep tendon reflexes.**

DIAGNOSIS
- **Triad: [1] Hypercalcemia + [2] increased serum intact PTH + [3] decreased serum phosphate.**
- **24-hour urinary calcium excretion: usually elevated or high-normal in Primary Hyperparathyroidism;** Low urinary calcium excretion + normal or minimally elevated PTH seen in Familial hypocalciuric hypercalcemia [FHH] in the absence of Thiazide diuretics.
- Alkaline phosphatase normal or elevated. Increased vitamin D. Check Serum 25-OH vitamin D.
- Ancillary: Presurgical imaging studies to detect parathyroid adenoma (**ultrasound & nuclear scanning**; CT scan). Osteopenia on bone scan. Osteitis fibrosis cystica rarely seen on radiographs.

MANAGEMENT
- **Parathyroidectomy definitive management** — recommended if signs &/or symptoms of Hyperparathyroidism, Nephrolithiasis, parathyroid bone disease, <50y, fractures, T-score <-2.5.
- Vitamin D & Calcium supplementation post parathyroidectomy to prevent Hypocalcemia. DEXA screen.
- **Bisphosphonates: can increase bone mineral density in those with Osteoporosis or Osteopenia.**
- **Cinacalcet in patients that are not surgical candidates** (Calcimimetic that inhibits PTH release).
- **Mild truly asymptomatic cases: may be closely monitored** + increase fluids + increased activity.
- **Severe Hypercalcemia: IV fluids (0.9% saline)** ± Calcitonin or Bisphosphonates in some.

HYPOPARATHYROIDISM

ETIOLOGIES
- **The 2 most common causes are [1] post neck surgery (eg, thyroidectomy, parathyroidectomy)** damaging all 4 parathyroid glands or **[2] autoimmune destruction of the parathyroid gland.**
- DiGeorge syndrome: congenital parathyroid hypoplasia. Congenital Pseudohypoparathyroidism: resistance to PTH: ↓serum Ca + ↑phosphate + ↑PTH + shortened 4th & 5th digits + shortened stature.
- **Hypomagnesemia** causes reversible parathyroid gland dysfunction. Radiation therapy.

CLINICAL MANIFESTATIONS
- **Most patients with Hypocalcemia are asymptomatic.**
- **Signs of Hypocalcemia: increased muscle contraction** — carpopedal spasm, perioral numbness, tetany, Trousseau sign (carpopedal spasms when the blood pressure cuff is inflated), Chvostek sign (tapping of the cheek causes facial spasm), irritability, increased deep tendon reflexes, tetany.

DIAGNOSIS
- **Classic triad of [1] Hypocalcemia + [2] decreased intact PTH + [3] increased serum phosphate.**
- **ECG:** prolonged QT interval (increased risk of arrhythmias). T wave abnormalities.

MANAGEMENT
- **Calcium + active Vitamin D supplementation [eg, Calcitriol (1,25-dihydroxyvitamin D_3)].**
- **Acute symptomatic hypocalcemia: IV Calcium gluconate** plus oral Calcitriol.

	HYPOcalcemia	HYPERcalcemia
ETIOLOGIES	**HYPOCALCEMIA with ↓PTH:** *Hypoparathyroidism MC overall cause* of ↓Ca⁺² * - Hypoparathyroidism: parathyroid gland destruction *(autoimmune, post surgical)* * **HYPOCALCEMIA with ↑PTH:** - *Chronic renal dz MC cause if ↑PTH,* * Liver dz.* - *Vitamin D deficiency* (Osteomalacia & Rickets). ↑PTH in response to hypocalcemia - *Hypomagnesemia,* ↑phosphate. Hypoalbuminemia - High citrate states: ex. blood transfusion - Acute pancreatitis, rhabdomyolysis. Meds: PPIs	• 90% of cases of hypercalcemia are due to: *PRIMARY HYPERPARATHYROIDISM OR MALIGNANCY!* * • **PTH-mediated:** - *Primary hyperparathyroidism:* * MC cause overall* *Triad:* ❶ ↑Ca + ❷ ↑intact PTH + ❸ ↓phosphate* - *MEN I & IIa,* 3ry hyperparathyroidism • **PTH-independent:** - *Malignancy (secretes ↑PTH-related protein),* ↓intact PTH - Vitamin D excess (granulomatous dz, vitamin intoxication) - Vitamin A excess, milk alkali syndrome, *thiazides*, lithium* *
CLINICAL MANIFESTATIONS	Hypocalcemia ↓'es excitation threshold for heart, nerves & muscle ⇨ *less stimulus needed for activation/contraction.* • **Neuromuscular:** muscle cramping, bronchospasm, syncope, seizures, *finger/circumoral paresthesias* • **Tetany:** *Chvostek's sign:* facial spasm with tapping of the facial nerve. *Trousseau's sign:* inflation of BP cuff above systolic BP causes carpal spasms. ↑DTR • **Cardio:** CHF, arrhythmias. **Skin:** dry skin, psoriasis • **GI:** *diarrhea, abdominal pain/cramps.* • **Skeletal:** abn. dentition, osteomalacia, osteodystrophy	Hypercalcemia ↑'es excitation threshold for heart, nerves & muscle ⇨ *stronger stimulus needed for activation/contraction.* • **Most patients are asymptomatic.** ±Arrhythmias • **Stones:** *kidney stones* (hypercalciuria ⇨ calcium oxalate & phosphate stones), *Nephrogenic DI: polyuria,* nocturia. • **Bones:** *painful bones, fractures* (due to ↑bone remodeling). • **Abdominal groans:** *ileus, constipation,* * (decreased contraction of the muscles of the GI tract), nausea, vomiting. • **Psychic moans:** weakness, fatigue, AMS, ↓DTR, depression or psychosis may develop. Blurred vision.
LAB FINDINGS	• ↓*ionized Ca²⁺* & total serum Ca²⁺ (<8.5mg/dL) • ±↑Phosphate, ↓Magnesium. Check PTH, BUN/Cr	• ↑*ionized Ca²⁺* (most accurate), ↑Total serum Ca²⁺ (>10mg/dL) • PTH-related protein, 1,25 vitamin D levels, 24h urinary calcium
ECG FINDINGS	• *PROLONGED QT INTERVAL* *	• *SHORTENED QT INTERVAL,* * prolonged PR interval, QRS widening.*
MANAGEMENT	**Severe/symptomatic:** • *Calcium gluconate IV* * or IV calcium carbonate - Ca²⁺ carbonate must be given via central line **Mild:** • *PO Calcium + Vitamin D (Ergocalciferol, Calcitriol)* Calcitriol if renal disease b/c no renal conversion needed - K⁺ & Mg⁺² repletion may be needed in some cases. - Corrected Ca²⁺ in patients with low serum albumin: [0.8 x (nml albumin(4.4) - pts albumin)] + serum Ca²⁺	**Severe/symptomatic:** • *IV saline* * ⇨ *Furosemide* (Lasix) *1st line.* Loop diuretics enhance renal Ca²⁺ excretion. *Avoid Hydrochlorothiazide* * (causes ↑Ca)* • *Calcitonin, Bisphosphonates in severe cases (IV Pamidronate)* • Steroids: Vitamin D excess, malignancy (ex. myeloma), granulomas. **Mild:** • No treatment needed for mild hypocalcemia. Tx underlying cause.

ANTERIOR PITUITARY TUMORS

PROLACTINOMA (LACTROTROPH ADENOMA)

- **Mostly benign tumors (adenomas) due to monoclonal expansion of pituitary lactotroph cells that secrete prolactin.** <u>Epidemiology:</u> More common in women; peak prevalence 25-34 years.
- **Prolactinoma is the most common type of pituitary adenoma** (40% of all pituitary adenomas).

ETIOLOGIES
- <u>Sporadic:</u> Most pituitary adenomas are isolated but may rarely be familial as part of MEN type 1 or 4.
- <u>MEN 1:</u> 15%-60% of patients with Multiple endocrine neoplasia type 1 (MEN 1) may develop a pituitary adenoma, and the majority of them are Prolactinomas.

PROLACTIN FUNCTIONS
- Prolactin is responsible for lactation, suppression of pregnancy during lactation, & suppression of gonadotropin-releasing hormone (GnRH), leading to decreased FSH & LH secretion.
- **Dopamine normally inhibits prolactin release** (which is the premise of therapy for Prolactinoma).

CLINICAL MANIFESTATIONS
- **Prolactinomas cause a wide variety of symptoms either due to [1] mass effect of the tumor &/or [2] due to hypersecretion of prolactin.**
- Pituitary Prolactinomas may cosecrete growth hormone (10%) and cause Acromegaly (in adults) or Gigantism (in children). Larger tumors may cause hyposecretion of other pituitary hormones.
- Other features like osteopenia, anxiety, depression, fatigue, emotional instability may be seen in both sexes.

<u>Women:</u>
- **Hypogonadism: oligomenorrhea, amenorrhea, infertility, and decreased libido.**
- <u>Estrogen deficiency</u> can cause decreased vaginal lubrication, irritability, anxiety, and depression.
- **Galactorrhea** (lactation in the absence of nursing) in premenopausal women is less often seen.
- <u>Local compression</u> — headache & visual changes (eg, bitemporal hemianopsia, decreased acuity).

<u>Men:</u>
- **Secondary hypogonadism: decreased libido, erectile dysfunction, infertility, oligozoospermia** & rarely gynecomastia.
- **Unlike women, men tend to present with CNS symptoms (eg, headache, visual changes, blurred vision) in the presence of a Prolactinoma.** This is because the diagnosis is often delayed in men, allowing for the pituitary Prolactinoma to grow large and present with compressive symptoms.

PHYSICAL EXAMINATION
- Pituitary tumors can compress the optic chiasm, leading to **bitemporal hemianopsia.**

DIAGNOSIS
- <u>Endocrine labs:</u> **increased prolactin** level >200 ng/mL initial test of choice. Decreased FSH & LH.
- **TSH**, growth hormone, & ACTH levels ordered because Prolactinomas can cause hypersecretion or hyposecretion of other hormones. Order serum pregnancy to rule it out as cause of amenorrhea.
- **Pituitary MRI study of choice to look for sellar lesions & pituitary tumors.** Small adenomas may not be visible. Macroadenomas are >1 cm [>10 mm].

MANAGEMENT
- **Medical therapy: Dopamine agonists (eg, Cabergoline or Bromocriptine) first line. Unlike other pituitary tumors, most Prolactinomas are managed with medical therapy** [both symptomatic macro and microadenomas], **with surgery and radiotherapy reserved for refractory cases.** Cabergoline usually better tolerated & causes more tumor shrinkage; Bromocriptine if pregnant.
- <u>Watchful waiting</u> may be employed if asymptomatic or incidental finding.
- **Transsphenoidal surgery usually reserved for [1] Prolactinomas refractory to medical management** or [2] large adenomas (>3 cm) in women who wish to become pregnant.
- <u>Radiation therapy</u> may be used for residual tumors after surgery & resistance to Cabergoline therapy.

SOMATOTROPH ADENOMA

- **Growth hormone-secreting pituitary adenoma that leads to [1] <u>Acromegaly</u> in adults (excessive growth) or [2] <u>Gigantism</u> in children** if it occurs before epiphyseal closure.

PATHOPHYSIOLOGY
- Growth hormone (GH) is a counterregulatory hormone that increases glucose & postnatal growth.
- Increased GH stimulates increased hepatic production of insulin-like growth factor (IGF-1).

CLINICAL MANIFESTATIONS
- **Diabetes mellitus or glucose intolerance (Insulin resistance).**
- **<u>Enlargement of soft tissues, cartilage, and bone</u> over years** — hands, feet, skull, tongue, forehead, & enlarged jaw (macrognathia); **increased ring, shoe, & hat size**; Carpal tunnel syndrome, Obstructive sleep apnea, increased spaced between teeth, coarse facial features. Kidney stones.
- **Deepened voice, thickened moist skin (doughy).** Skin tags, weight gain, arthralgias. **Colon polyps.**
- **<u>Cardiovascular disease</u> most common cause of death. Hypertension (50%) & Left ventricular hypertrophy common in Acromegaly.** Heart failure, Aortic or Mitral regurgitation.
- <u>Compressive symptoms</u>: **Headache common**, visual symptoms (eg, **bitemporal hemianopsia)**,
- <u>Gigantism</u>: dramatic linear growth acceleration (tall stature) & obesity (rapid weight gain).

DIAGNOSIS
- <u>Screening</u>: **insulin-like growth factor (IGF-1) initial test: increased in Acromegaly & Gigantism, so proceed to MRI;** If IGF-1 is normal, Acromegaly is ruled out. If equivocal, assess GH suppression.
- <u>Confirmatory</u> **if the serum IGF-1 concentration is equivocal, <u>oral glucose suppression test</u>** — **failure of GH suppression [growth hormone >1 ng/mL (especially if >2 ng/mL)] within 1-2 hours of an oral glucose load (75g).** <u>Normal response</u>: GH suppression (≤1 ng/mL within 2 hours).
- **<u>MRI</u> imaging test of choice** to evaluate for sellar or pituitary lesions (after laboratory confirmation).

MANAGEMENT
- **<u>Transsphenoidal surgery</u> management of choice** for removal of active or compressive tumors.
<u>Medical management indications</u>: either an adjunct to surgery or when surgery is not possible.
- **<u>Somatostatin analogs</u>: Octreotide or Lanreotide first-line medical management. They inhibit GH release,** control hormonal overproduction, as well as control tumor growth.
- **<u>Pegvisomant</u> — GH receptor antagonist** that inhibits IGF-1 release if refractory to other treatment.
- <u>Dopamine agonist</u>: Cabergoline or Bromocriptine to inhibit GH release if mild [GH >1 but <1.3 ng/mL].
<u>Radiation therapy (stereotactic)</u>: Reserved for cases not responsive to surgical or medical management.

CORTICOTROPH ADENOMA (CUSHING DISEASE)

- **ACTH-secreting pituitary adenoma that leads to Hypercortisolism (Cushing syndrome).**
- **The presence of an ACTH-producing pituitary adenoma is also known as <u>Cushing disease</u>.**
- Second most common cause of Cushing syndrome, the first cause being exogenous use of steroids.

CLINICAL MANIFESTATIONS
- <u>Cushing syndrome symptoms</u>: proximal muscle weakness, **weight gain,** headache, oligomenorrhea, erectile dysfunction, polyuria, osteoporosis, mental disturbances, Hypertension, Diabetes mellitus.

DIFFERENTIATING TESTS
- **The presence of [1] an increased baseline ACTH + [2] suppression of cortisol by ≥50% after high-dose Dexamethasone suppression test distinguishes Cushing disease** from Ectopic ACTH.
- **<u>MRI of the pituitary</u> imaging test of choice** after laboratory confirmation.
- Sampling of the petrosal sinus if MRI is negative because MRI may miss small tumors.

MANAGEMENT: **<u>Transsphenoidal resection</u> of the pituitary tumor is the treatment of choice.**
- Radiation therapy alternative if refractory to surgery.

HYPERPROLACTINEMIA

ETIOLOGIES
- Pathologic: **Prolactinoma most common cause, Hypothyroidism (increased TRH stimulates prolactin)**, acromegaly, cirrhosis, & renal failure.
- Pharmacologic: **dopamine antagonists — [1st and 2nd-generation antipsychotics** (eg, **Risperidone, Haloperidol)**, Metoclopramide, Promethazine, & Prochlorperazine] because dopamine is an inhibitor of prolactin. SSRIs, TCAs, Cimetidine, Verapamil, & estrogen.
- **Physiologic: pregnancy, breastfeeding, stress, & exercise.**

PATHOPHYSIOLOGY: prolactin inhibits gonadotropin-releasing hormone, leading to hypogonadism.

MANIFESTATIONS IN WOMEN
- **Hypogonadism — oligomenorrhea, amenorrhea,** infertility, vaginal dryness. **Galactorrhea** (rare).

MANIFESTATIONS IN MEN
- **Hypogonadism —** erectile dysfunction, decreased libido, **infertility,** & rarely gynecomastia.

WORKUP:
- **Serum prolactin (often elevated, repeat to verify), TSH,** beta-hCG, BUN, creatinine, & LFTs.
- Pituitary MRI: Patients with hyperprolactinemia not induced by drugs, hypothyroidism, or pregnancy should be examined by pituitary MRI.

MANAGEMENT
- Depends on cause. Hyperprolactinemia due to hypothyroidism is corrected by Levothyroxine.
- **Medication-induced: discontinue offending drugs when possible.**
- **Prolactinoma: Dopamine agonists (eg, Cabergoline or Bromocriptine) inhibit prolactin.** Surgical or radiation therapy may be needed in some cases of refractory Prolactinomas.

ANTERIOR HYPOPITUITARISM

- Pituitary destruction or deficient hypothalamic pituitary stimulation.

ETIOLOGIES
- **Hypopituitarism can be caused by either [1] hypothalamic dysfunction** affecting the production of trophic hormones that act on the pituitary or **[2] direct pituitary dysfunction.**
- Pituitary tumors are the most common cause of hypopituitarism (61%).
- Congenital or acquired — tumor, infiltrative disease, pituitary infarction, radiation therapy.
- **Sheehan syndrome: postpartum pituitary necrosis,** usually following severe postpartum uterine hemorrhage. It is usually characterized by **postpartum amenorrhea and inability to lactate.**

CLINICAL MANIFESTATIONS
- Can be any combination of Growth hormone deficiency (Dwarfism, metabolic derangements in adults), Hypothyroidism, & gonadotropin deficiency.
- Headaches or visual defects (eg, bitemporal hemianopsia) may be seen when hypopituitarism is caused by a pituitary mass lesion or hypophysitis.

DIAGNOSIS
- **Both target hormones and pituitary hormones are decreased — same direction = secondary (pituitary) problem or tertiary (hypothalamus) problem.**
    - TSH and Free T4 are both decreased if secondary hypothyroidism is present.
    - ACTH and cortisol are both decreased if secondary Adrenal insufficiency is present.
    - ↓ Insulin-like growth factor (IGF-1) if Growth hormone deficiency is present.

MANAGEMENT
- **Hormone replacement therapy** depending on the deficient hormone.

MALE HYPOGONADISM

- **Decrease in either or both of the primary function of the testes (testosterone & sperm production).**

ETIOLOGIES

[1] Primary hypogonadism:

- **Hypergonadotropic hypogonadism** due to disease of the testes (<u>testicular failure</u>) — **(1) low serum testosterone &/or sperm count below normal + (2) elevated serum LH &/or FSH.**
- **Testicular failure: decreased Leydig cell function & testosterone synthesis, Klinefelter syndrome, seminiferous tubule dysfunction (spermatogenesis cannot be augmented),** Alcohol liver disease, radiation therapy, chemotherapy (eg, alkylating agents).
- In Primary hypogonadism, spermatogenesis is often impaired to a greater degree than Leydig cell function (testosterone production), especially early on because seminiferous tubules are damaged to greater extent than the Leydig cells. In contrast, both functions are impaired similarly in Secondary hypogonadism (testosterone and sperm production).

[2] Secondary hypogonadism:

- **Hypogonadotropic hypogonadism**: **disorder of the pituitary gland or the hypothalamus** (eg, pituitary adenoma, craniopharyngioma, Prader-Willi syndrome) — **(1) low serum testosterone &/or sperm count below normal + (2) low or normal serum LH &/or FSH.**

CLINICAL MANIFESTATIONS

- <u>Adolescents:</u> failure to undergo or complete puberty (decreased secondary male sex characteristics).
- **Adults: decreased libido, energy, body hair, & muscle mass**; gynecomastia (more common in primary hypogonadism), **infertility** (may have decreased sperm count), weight gain due to an increase in subcutaneous fat, **erectile dysfunction, and Osteopenia or Osteoporosis.**
- Eunuchoid proportions if hypogonadism developed prepubertally — lower body segment (floor to pubis) >2 cm longer than upper body segment (pubis to crown); arm span >5 cm longer than height.

DIAGNOSIS

- **[1] Morning (8-10 am) serum total testosterone: decreased**.
- **[2] Serum LH and FSH** — If the serum testosterone is below normal on at least 2 occasions, serum luteinizing hormone (LH) and follicle stimulating (FSH) concentrations should be measured to distinguish primary from secondary hypogonadism.
  - **Primary hypogonadism: decreased testosterone &/or subnormal sperm count + compensatory increase in LH &/or FSH** [normal FSH if limited to Leydig cells or high FSH if seminiferous tubule dysfunction is also present]. Karyotyping if Klinefelter is suspected.
  - **Secondary hypogonadism: subnormal testosterone &/or subnormal sperm count + normal or decreased FSH and LH** (same direction). **Perform serum prolactin levels** (to screen for prolactinoma). **Pituitary MRI to assess for masses** (eg, pituitary adenoma).
- <u>Sex hormone-binding globulin (SHBG) + Serum free testosterone</u>: only useful when it is suspected that an abnormality in testosterone binding to sex hormone-binding globulin (SHBG) coexists with hypogonadism. The two most common causes of abnormal testosterone binding are (1) <u>obesity</u>, which decreases SHBG concentrations, and (2) <u>normal aging</u>, which increases SHBG.
- <u>Semen analysis</u> (sperm count & motility) if hypogonadism is part of a fertility workup. A significantly low sperm count, eg, <5 million sperm/ejaculate, can occur with either primary or secondary. A mildly subnormal sperm count associated with markedly abnormal sperm motility is much more likely to be associated with either a sperm function abnormality or Primary hypogonadism.

MANAGEMENT

- **Testosterone replacement therapy (eg, gel)** if testosterone deficiency seen on 3 separate occasions. Formulations include gel, transdermal patches, intramuscular, or depot injection, buccal, or oral. <u>Adverse effects</u>: erythrocytosis, venous thromboembolism, increased cardiovascular events. <u>Contraindications</u>: Prostate or breast cancers, untreated severe sleep apnea or hematocrit >50%.
- <u>Infertility:</u> in vitro fertilization with sperm extracted from the testes if Primary. Gonadotropin therapy or pulsatile gonadotropin releasing hormone therapy (if pituitary function is normal).

DWARFISM

ETIOLOGIES
Achondroplasia:
- **Achondroplasia accounts for 70% of Dwarfism; this is a genetic mutation of cartilage and bone growth (mutations in FGR3 [fibroblast growth receptor] genes).** FGFR3 activity impairs chondrocyte proliferation and differentiation; this in turn leads to **impaired long bone formation (via endochondral ossification)** & enlarged head relative to limbs (via membranous ossification), with a normal axial skeleton.
- **Associated with normal life span, intelligence, and reproduction.**
- It is an autosomal dominant condition that frequently occurs due to spontaneous mutation; thus, many cases will not have an associated family history despite the autosomal dominant transmission.

Growth hormone deficiency:
- **Growth hormone deficiency** for most other cases. Often, a specific etiology cannot be identified.

CLINICAL MANIFESTATIONS
- **Children or infancy: short stature,** growth delays, **dwarfism, fasting hypoglycemia**.
- **Dwarfism: short height**: average height of an adult with achondroplasia is 4 feet 4 inches. Features include disproportionate short stature [eg, short limbs, long and narrow trunks, brachydactyly (shortening of the fingers and toes), large heads with midface hypoplasia, and prominent brows (frontal bossing), accentuated lumbar lordosis, kyphoscoliosis. Delayed motor milestones.
- **Adults: short height**: average height of an adult with achondroplasia is 4 feet 4 inches. Decreased muscle mass, weakness, poor exercise tolerance, decreased bone density, increased subcutaneous fat & weight gain, poor cognition, mental fatigue, memory impairment.

DIAGNOSIS
- Hypothyroidism should be excluded first by performing thyroid function tests.
- **Patients with suspected Growth hormone deficiency (GHD) should be screened with** radiographic measurement of bone age, insulin-like growth factor 1 (IGF-1), & insulin-like growth factor binding protein-3 (IGFBP-3).
- **Low IGF-1 & IGFBP-3: Moderately or severely reduced IGF-1 (eg, SD <-2) and IGFBP-3 with delayed bone age – Strong suspicion of GHD** & should be explored by provocative growth hormone (GH) testing, if other causes of low IGF-1 and IGFBP-3, such as poor nutrition, have been excluded.
- **Mutations in the FGFR3 gene,** including the classical 1138 variant in the *FGFR3* gene.
- Provocative Growth hormone (GH) testing has a number of limitations. Measurements of basal GH levels do **not** distinguish between normal and subnormal GH secretion. In children, Clonidine, Arginine, and Glucagon are common choices to attempt to stimulate GH in children.

Radiographs:
- Shortening of the long bones with metaphyseal abnormalities and hand films to look for shortening, brachydactyly, and trident deformity.

MANAGEMENT
Conservative
- **Monitoring, preventing, and addressing complications mainstay of therapy in most (eg, leg bowing is managed with physical therapy).**

Human growth hormone replacement:
- Children: In children, synthetic growth hormone replacement may be used for children with short stature, such as somatotropin, but its use is controversial. Replacement therapy is titrated against IGF1 levels. The goal of treatment is to ensure that adult height is obtained. Further evaluation is made post-puberty to determine whether GH replacement should continue into adulthood.
- Adults: Unlike in children with short stature due to GH deficiency, the role of GH replacement in the treatment of adult GH deficiency has not been well established.

GROWTH HORMONE DEFICIENCY

- Deficiency in pituitary production of growth hormone (GH).

Etiologies:

Congenital or acquired

- **Pituitary related most common (76%) — A pituitary tumor or the consequences of treatment of the tumor, including surgery and/or radiation therapy.** Infiltrative disease, bleeding into pituitary (Sheehan's syndrome), pituitary infarction, or radiation therapy.
- An extrapituitary tumor (eg, craniopharyngioma) — 13%
- Idiopathic — 8%
- Sarcoidosis — 1%

CLINICAL MANIFESTATIONS

Children or infancy:

- **Short stature,** growth delays, **Dwarfism,** **fasting hypoglycemia**.

Adults:

- Central obesity, increased blood pressure, **dyslipidemia**, decreased bone mass in men, decreased cardiac output, muscle wasting, increased inflammatory markers and impaired concentration.
- Individuals who develop GH deficiency in adulthood experience decrease in lean body mass, decrease in bone mineral density (BMD), an increase in fat mass, and increased rate of fractures, cardiovascular disease, and mortality.

DIAGNOSIS

- Measurements of basal Growth hormone (GH) levels do **not** distinguish between normal and subnormal GH secretion.
- **Serum IGF-1 — A serum insulin-like growth factor-1 (IGF-1) concentration lower than the sex- and age-specific lower limit of normal in a patient who has organic pituitary disease confirms the diagnosis of GH deficiency.**
- Provocative tests: If IGF-1 is equivocal, a subnormal GH response to a provocative test will confirm the diagnosis — (1) insulin tolerance test, (2) A combination of Arginine and GH-releasing hormone (GHRH). A subnormal increase in the serum GH concentration in a patient who has organic pituitary disease confirms the diagnosis of GH deficiency in those whose serum IGF-1 was equivocal. Macimorelin stimulation test.

Imaging:

- If GHD is confirmed, MRI of the hypothalamic-pituitary area is recommended to rule out tumors, investigate for structural causes of GHD, and evaluate the severity and prognosis of the deficiency.

HUMAN GROWTH HORMONE REPLACEMENT

- Children: In children, synthetic growth hormone replacement is used for children with short stature, such as somatotropin. Replacement therapy is titrated against IGF1 levels. The goal of treatment is to ensure that adult height is obtained. Further evaluation is made post-puberty to determine whether GH replacement should continue into adulthood.
- Unlike in children with short stature due to GH deficiency, the role of GH replacement in the treatment of adult GH deficiency has not been well established.

METABOLIC SYNDROME (SYNDROME X, INSULIN RESISTANCE SYNDROME)

- Syndrome of co-occurrence multiple metabolic abnormalities that increase the risk for complications such as type 2 Diabetes mellitus & cardiovascular disease, specifically abdominal obesity, hyperglycemia, dyslipidemia, and Hypertension.

PATHOPHYSIOLOGY
- **Insulin resistance is the key component.**
- Free fatty acids are released, which causes an increase in triglyceride & glucose production as well as reduction in insulin sensitivity, leading to insulin resistance & hyperinsulinemia.
- The high levels of insulin cause sodium reabsorption, leading to hypertension.

DIAGNOSIS
- There are several definitions for metabolic syndrome. The National Cholesterol Education Program (NCEP) Adult Treatment Panel III (ATP III) is the most widely used:

ATP III criteria: at least 3 of the following 5:
1. ↓HDL: <40 mg/dL in men & < 50 mg/dL in women or treatment for low HDL cholesterol.
2. Blood pressure ≥130/85 mm Hg or drug treatment for elevated blood pressure.
3. ↑Fasting triglyceride levels: ≥150 mg/dL or drug treatment for high triglycerides.
4. ↑Fasting blood sugar: ≥ 100 mg/dL (or drug treatment for high glucose).
5. ↑Abdominal obesity: waist circumference >40 inches in men & >35 inches in women.

MANAGEMENT
Lifestyle modification:
- **Aggressive lifestyle modification via weight reduction, exercise, & increased physical activity.**
- Diet rich in fruits, vegetables, lean poultry, fish, whole grains. **The Mediterranean or low-fat diet are preferred, rather than other diets.**
- Exercise programs that combine aerobic exercise and resistance training are preferred.
- All patients considered overweight (body mass index [BMI] ≥25 kg/m^2) or with obesity (BMI ≥30 kg/m^2) should receive counseling on diet, lifestyle, and goals for weight loss.

WEIGHT LOSS MEDICATIONS:
- Candidates for pharmacotherapy include individuals with a BMI ≥30 kg/m^2, or a BMI of 27-29.9 kg/m^2 with comorbidities, who have not attained weight loss goals (weight loss of ≥5% of total body weight at three to six months) with a comprehensive lifestyle intervention. The decision to initiate drug therapy should be individualized and made only after evaluation of risks and benefits of all treatment options.

Anti-obesity agents
- **Incretin-based therapy**: Tirzepatide or Semaglutide often used as initial agents when pharmacologic agents are used.
- **Phentermine can be used for a short term** (3 months short-term use only). Phentermine is a sympathomimetic with unknown mechanism of action.
- **Phentermine/Topiramate** has no restriction on treatment duration.
  Adverse effects: insomnia, constipation, palpitations, headache, paresthesias.
- **Lorcaserin:** selective serotonin agonist (5-HT2C receptor) that induces satiety.
- **Orlistat:** inhibits fat absorption.
- Combination Bupropion-Naltrexone.

Bariatric surgery:
- **For patients who do not have an adequate response to pharmacotherapy, Bariatric surgery is an option for those who meet surgical criteria.**

MULTIPLE ENDOCRINE NEOPLASIA 1 (WERMER SYNDROME)

- Rare autosomal dominant disorder with predisposition to ≥1 overactive endocrine gland tumors — **3 Ps: Parathyroid, Pancreas (gastro-entero-pancreatic), & Pituitary (anterior).**
- **Associated with MEN1 or *menin* gene defect on chromosome 11** on the long arm of chromosome 11 (11q13); *menin* is a tumor suppressor gene. Autosomal dominant in ~90%. 10% sporadic.
- Most tumors are benign (especially before 30 years).

CLINICAL MANIFESTATIONS
- **Parathyroid tumors Hyperparathyroidism most common (parathyroid adenoma) in 90%.**
- **Pancreatic tumors** (2nd most common) — **Gastrinomas (ZES) most common GI endocrine tumor** (60%), Insulinomas, Glucagonomas, VIPomas, Somatostatinomas. Pancreatic tumors are the most common cause of death from MEN 1.
- **Pituitary tumors: Prolactinoma (most common pituitary tumor).** Somatotroph, Corticotroph.
- Other tumors include carcinoid tumors, nonfunctioning polypeptide malignant tumors, lipomas.

DIAGNOSIS
- **DNA testing for *MEN1* gene** Germline *MEN1* mutation identification to establish the diagnosis positive in 60-95% of cases (also used to screen family members). Studies for suspected tumors.

MANAGEMENT
- Tumor specific similar to sporadic adenomas) — eg, parathyroidectomy for Parathyroid adenomas; Proton pump inhibitors for Gastrinomas; Dopamine agonist (eg, Cabergoline) for Prolactinomas.
Screening in patients with MEN 1:
- **[1] PTH + calcium (Hyperparathyroidism), [2] gastrin (ZES), & [3] prolactin (Prolactinoma) are used for routine monitoring in patients with the diagnosis of MEN1.**

MULTIPLE ENDOCRINE NEOPLASIA 2 (FORMERLY 2A) & MEN 3 (FORMERLY 2B)

- Rare inherited disorder of ≥1 overactive endocrine gland tumors due to a defect (gain of function) in the *RET* **proto-oncogene** localized to chromosome 10cen-10q11.2.

MEN 2 (2A) (90%)	Medullary thyroid carcinoma	Pheochromocytoma	Hyperparathyroidism
MEN 3 (2B) (5%)	Medullary thyroid carcinoma	Pheochromocytoma	Neuromas, Marfanoid
Familial MTC:	Medullary thyroid carcinoma		

MEN 2 (formerly 2A)
- Medullary thyroid carcinoma (>90%), Pheochromocytoma (>50%), Hyperparathyroidism (10-25%).
- **Hirschsprung disease** chronic aganglionic megacolon due to loss of Auerbach plexus.

MEN 3 (Formerly 2B):
- **Medullary thyroid carcinoma, Pheochromocytoma, Neuromas, & Marfanoid habitus.**
- **Men 3 (2B) associated with more aggressive form of Medullary thyroid carcinoma (may present in infancy).** Prophylactic total thyroidectomy may be performed in these patients.
- **Mucosal (bumpy) neuromas** of the lips, tongue, eyelids, conjunctiva, nasal & laryngeal mucosa.
- **Marfanoid habitus**, including high arched palate, pectus excavatum, & scoliosis.

DIAGNOSIS
- **Genetic testing for RET proto-oncogene.**
- Imaging depends on tumor presentation.

SCREENING:
- **Annually — [1] Calcitonin & neck ultrasound** (for Medullary thyroid cancer), **[2] plasma and urine 24-hour urinary fractionated metanephrines** (for Pheochromocytoma), **and [3] intact PTH + calcium** (for Primary hyperparathyroidism) as indicated.

INSULINOMA

- **Islet cell tumor (beta cell adenoma) that develops from pancreatic beta cells & produces insulin, leading to hypoglycemia as a result of inappropriately high insulin levels**.
- While most are sporadic, 4% are associated with Multiple endocrine neoplasia type 1 (MEN1).
- **Insulinomas are generally small (>90% are <2 cm), solitary (90% are solitary benign adenomas**; 7% are benign multiple tumors; only 5-15% are malignant), and **almost invariably occur in the pancreas.** Multiple Insulinomas tend to be associated with MEN1.

PATHOPHYSIOLOGY
- **In Insulinoma, insulin is secreted inappropriately despite low plasma glucose concentration.**
- When endogenous insulin is made, pro-insulin contains a connecting segment C-peptide. **Endogenous hyperinsulinemia (Insulinoma) is associated with <u>increased C-peptide</u>** (both produced in equal amounts). Decreased C-peptide is associated with exogenous insulin use (Factitious hypoglycemia).

CLINICAL MANIFESTATIONS
Whipple's triad:
- **[1] fasting or exertional episodes of hypoglycemia, such as <u>sympathetic autonomic activation</u>** (eg, diaphoresis, weakness, tremulousness, & palpitations) or **<u>neuroglycopenic symptoms</u>** (eg, blurred vision diplopia, headache, confusion, weakness, amnesia, disorientation, feelings of detachment, behavioral changes), especially with fasting, early in the morning, or missing a meal +
- **[2] <u>low plasma glucose</u> <40-50 mg/dL during attack** +
- **[3] symptom improvement with fast-acting carbohydrate (glucose) intake within 15 minutes.**
- **<u>Weight gain</u>** due the effect of Insulin (increased lipogenesis).

DIAGNOSIS
STEP 1: BIOCHEMICAL TESTING: when there is high clinical suspicion for Insulinoma:
- **The critical diagnostic test is to demonstrate <u>inappropriately elevated serum insulin, proinsulin, and C peptide levels</u>, at a time when plasma glucose level is <45 mg/dL.**
Diagnostic criteria for Insulinoma after a monitored 72-hour fast:
- **<u>Low plasma glucose</u> <45 mg/dL.**
- **<u>Concomitant increased insulin</u>** ICMA ≥ 3 microU/mL; or RIA ≥6 microunits/mL (36 pmol/L).
- **<u>Increased C-peptide level</u>** ≥0.6 ng/mL, 200 pmol/L, or 0.2 nmol/L
- **<u>Increased plasma pro-insulin level</u>** ≥5 pmol/L (sensitive and specific).
- **<u>Decreased beta-hydroxybutyrate</u>** level ≤2.7 mmol/L due to the antiketogenic effect of insulin.
- Simultaneous absence of sulfonylurea & meglitinide metabolites, indicating that the hypoglycemia induction is by endogenous hyperinsulinemia and not due to factitious hypoglycemia (exogenous).

STEP 2 TUMOR LOCALIZATION: localize the tumor after the diagnosis is made based on laboratory findings.
- After Insulinoma has been unequivocally diagnosed via clinical and laboratory findings, studies to localize the tumor should be initiated to characterize the tumor prior to surgical resection.
- **<u>Noninvasive testing</u>: spiral CT scan of the abdomen with contrast most frequently used noninvasive test after lab confirmation. Transabdominal Ultrasound** or MRI are alternatives.
- **<u>Endoscopic ultrasonography</u> test of choice if noninvasive testing is negative.**

MANAGEMENT
- **<u>Surgical resection</u>: Surgery is curative in >75% of cases** — recommended for local disease and also considered for advanced disease. **<u>Preoperative</u>: control of hypoglycemia with frequent small carbohydrate meals + medications (eg, Diazoxide) often used prior to surgery.**
Medical therapy:
- **<u>Diazoxide</u> in patients who are not candidates for or refuse surgery,** unresectable metastatic disease. Diazoxide is a thiazide diuretic that decreases insulin secretion and has a hyperglycemic effect by promoting glycogenolysis. <u>Adverse effects</u> sodium retention, gastric irritation, hirsutism.
- Octreotide & Lanreotide can be used in patients not responsive to Diazoxide. Everolimus, Sunitinib.

GLUCAGONOMA

- Rare neuroendocrine tumor of the <u>pancreatic islet alpha cells</u> that results in overproduction of glucagon, characterized by dermatitis, glucose intolerance or diabetes, and weight loss.

<u>CHARACTERISTICS</u>
- **Most are malignant, solitary, and located in the distal pancreas** (50-80% in the pancreatic tail) and are generally large at diagnosis (5-10 cm).
- **Slow growing but 50-80% are metastatic at the time of diagnosis, often to the liver.**
- Most glucagonomas are sporadic. **10% associated with the MEN syndrome type 1 (MEN1).**

<u>PATHOPHYSIOLOGY</u>
- Glucagonomas usually present with weight loss caused by glucagon stimulated protein hepatic gluconeogenesis and related protein catabolism. Diabetes mellitus develops in ~35% of patients.
- <u>Glucagonoma syndrome</u>: diarrhea, nausea, peptic ulcer, hypoaminoacidemia (due to the use of amino acids to make glucose in gluconeogenesis), weight loss, Necrolytic migratory erythema.

<u>CLINICAL MANIFESTATIONS</u>
- **Classic Glucagonoma syndrome consists of 5 "D"s: <u>D</u>ecreased weight (weight loss), <u>D</u>ermatitis [Necrolytic migratory erythema (NME)], <u>D</u>iabetes (glucose intolerance), <u>D</u>epression, & <u>D</u>iarrhea.**
Classic symptoms:
- <u>**Weight loss: often significant, is the most common presenting feature**</u>, occurring in 80%. **Muscle wasting and proximal muscle weakness** (hypoaminoacidemia), cachexia. **Stomatitis (cheilitis).**
- <u>**Glucose intolerance: including Hyperglycemia & Type II Diabetes mellitus**</u> (75–95%).
- <u>**Necrolytic migratory erythema**</u> (67-90%) — **The characteristic rash usually starts as annular erythema at intertriginous and periorificial sites**, especially in the groin or buttock. It subsequently becomes raised, with bullae formation; when the bullae rupture, eroded areas form. **Migratory spread of erythematous pruritic and/or painful papules, plaques, or swelling across areas with increased friction & pressure** (eg, extremities, face, and perineum).
- <u>Chronic diarrhea</u> is the most frequent gastrointestinal manifestation of Glucagonoma (~30%).
- <u>**Venous thrombosis**</u> up to 50% — unexplained Deep vein thrombosis (DVT) or Pulmonary embolism.
- <u>Neuropsychiatric</u> 20-50% — irritability, depression, hyperreflexia, psychosis, dementia.

<u>DIAGNOSIS:</u>
- <u>**Increased plasma glucagon: Inappropriately elevated fasting plasma glucagon level >500 pg/mL or 10- to 20-fold**</u> (normal fasting plasma glucagon level is < 150 pg/mL). **Hyperglycemia.**
- <u>**Hypoaminoacidemia is a characteristic laboratory finding of a Glucagonoma**</u> due to targeting of amino acids into metabolic pathways in the liver for gluconeogenesis by excessive hyperglucagonemia.
- **DNA testing**: *MEN-1* gene if MEN 1 is suspected.
<u>Tumor imaging:</u>
- <u>**Helical CT scan (abdomen)**</u> **initial imaging of choice after lab confirmation.** MRI may be performed if CT is indeterminate (MRI has a higher sensitivity for detecting liver metastases vs. CT).
- <u>Functional PET imaging</u>: performed to localize the tumor and determine extent. Somatostatin-receptor scintigraphy (SRS) using Octreotide may also be used.

<u>MANAGEMENT:</u>
Medical management
- <u>**Medical management:**</u> **In 50–80% of patients, hepatic metastases are present, and so curative surgical resection is not possible. <u>Somatostatin analogues</u> (eg, <u>Octreotide, Lanreotide</u>) are the treatment of choice to control symptoms related to glucagon hypersecretion.**
- Antibiotics, zinc replacement, and steroids may help with the improvement of NME.
<u>Surgical resection:</u>
- **Surgery is the only curative option for a minority of cases in which the tumor is localized to the pancreas at the time of diagnosis** (most are unresectable at presentation).

CHAPTER 8 – RENAL SYSTEM

DIURETICS

MANNITOL

MECHANISM OF ACTION
- **Osmotic diuretic** — nonreabsorbable solute that **increases urine volume by drawing fluid from the intracellular compartment into the tubular lumen by increasing tubular osmolarity** (Mannitol is freely filtered but minimally reabsorbed); reduces luminal Na^+ concentration so that net Na^+ absorption diminishes. Administration: **Given IV** (poor oral absorption).
- **The proximal tubule is the main site of action of Mannitol.** Mannitol also works at the loop of Henle. Mannitol increases urinary excretion of nearly all electrolytes, including Na^+, K^+, Ca^{2+}, Mg^{2+}, Cl^-, HCO_3^-, and phosphate.

4 MAIN INDICATIONS
- **(1) Treatment of increased intracranial pressure (ICP) in the management of Cerebral edema.** Mannitol draws water from the extravascular space into the central circulation for renal elimination.
- **(2) Treatment of refractory increased intraocular pressure (IOP)** during acute Glaucoma attacks.
- (3) Promotes diuresis in the oliguric phase of Acute kidney injury.
- (4) Increases excretion of toxic metabolites (increases urine output within 5-10 min. of administration).

ADVERSE EFFECTS
- Headache, nausea, and vomiting are common.
- **Hyponatremia & pulmonary edema** due to increased fluid shifts and movement of water from the intracellular compartment to the extracellular compartment.
- **Volume depletion & Hypernatremia** — osmotic diuresis leads to increased urinary losses of both sodium and electrolyte-free water. Lack of replacement of the fluid losses can lead to both volume depletion and Hypernatremia that may be profound. **This may precipitate Acute kidney injury.**
- **Volume expansion, Hyponatremia, Hyperkalemia, Hypokalemia, and Metabolic acidosis.**
- Monitoring: input, urine output, blood pressure, pulse, & electrolytes during administration.
- Contraindications: anuria, dehydration, Heart failure, severe electrolyte abnormalities, active CNS bleed.

ACETAZOLAMIDE

MECHANISM OF ACTION
- **Carbonic anhydrase inhibitor** in the **proximal tubule, leading to sodium & bicarbonate diuresis.**

INDICATIONS
- **Glaucoma: reduces intraocular pressure (IOP) in patients with Acute angle-closure as well as Open glaucoma** (decreases the rate of aqueous humor production).
- **Reduces intracranial pressure (ICP):** Normal pressure hydrocephalus, Intracranial hypertension.
- Mild diuretic; High altitude or mountain sickness (symptomatic relief).
- Acidifies the blood in patients with Metabolic alkalosis, **Alkalinizes the urine.**

ADVERSE EFFECTS
- **Digital or oral paresthesias and drowsiness are commonly reported after oral therapy.**
- **Hyperchloremic (normal gap) metabolic acidosis** due to increased urinary loss of bicarbonate.
- Hypokalemia. Numbness, tinnitus, vomiting, metallic taste.
- **Sulfonamide allergies** (Acetazolamide is a sulfonamide derivative), skin toxicity.
- **Kidney stones** (calcium phosphate) and other calcium salt precipitation resulting from alkalinization of the urine by Acetazolamide.

CONTRAINDICATIONS
- **Severe kidney or hepatic dysfunction** — Patients with hepatic impairment often excrete large amounts of ammonia in the urine in the form of ammonium ion, making them prone to developing hepatic encephalopathy.

LOOP DIURETICS

- **Sulfonamides: Furosemide & Bumetanide** (oral & IV forms). **Torsemide** (oral)
- **Nonsulfonamides: Ethacrynic acid** (oral tablet); **Ethacrynate sodium** (injectable solution).

MECHANISM OF ACTION

- **Strongest class of diuretics:** inhibits water, sodium, potassium, & chloride transport via inhibition of the $Na^+-K^+-2Cl^-$ transporter in the luminal membrane as well as Ca^+ and Mg^+ absorption across the thick ascending limb (TAL) of the Loop of Henle, leading to a dilute urine. They are efficacious because they affect 25% of the filtered Na^+ load that normally occurs at the TAL.
- Diuresis usually occurs over a 4-hour period following a dose.
- Increased prostaglandin synthesis, improving renal blood flow. **They decrease LV filling pressure.**

INDICATIONS

- **Pulmonary or peripheral edema** (eg, CHF, Nephrotic syndrome, & Cirrhosis). Hypertension.
- **Severe Hypercalcemia or Hypermagnesemia** — Furosemide lowers serum calcium and magnesium levels, often combined with parenteral fluids to enhance renal calcium &/or magnesium excretion.

ADVERSE EFFECTS

- **Decreased electrolytes (hypokalemia, hypocalcemia, hypomagnesemia, hypochloremia, & hyponatremia), Dyslipidemia, Ototoxicity** [especially with high-doses, rapid IV administration, or renal insufficiency (manifests as tinnitus, hearing impairment, vertigo, & sense of ear fullness)]; **sulfa allergy,** Acute interstitial nephritis, **hypochloremic metabolic alkalosis, Hyperuricemia** (can precipitate Gout), **and Hyperglycemia.**
- Interactions: NSAIDs may decrease their efficacy. May increase plasma Lithium & Propranolol levels.
- **Ethacrynic acid is a medication similar to Furosemide that can be used in patients with a sulfa allergy (does not contain sulfonamide) & safe in patients with Gout. However, Ethacrynic acid is associated with higher risk of ototoxicity** compared to Furosemide.

THIAZIDE DIURETICS

Hydrochlorothiazide, Chlorothiazide. Thiazide-like: Indapamide, Metolazone, Chlorthalidone.

MECHANISM OF ACTION

- **Inhibit Na^+-Cl^- import: Blocks NaCl & water reabsorption** by actively pumping sodium & chloride out of the nephron lumen via the **Na+/Cl- symport carrier at the early distal convoluted tubule (diluting segment).** This leads to diuresis and inability to produce a dilute urine.
- **Thiazides also decrease urinary calcium excretion and increase reabsorption of calcium.**

INDICATIONS

- **Hypertension** (eg, HTN with comorbidities, blacks, Osteoporosis, & in the elderly), peripheral edema.
- **AVP resistance [Nephrogenic diabetes insipidus]** — decreases ability to produce dilute urine.
- Nephrolithiasis **Calcium oxalate & phosphate stone prevention** (decreases urinary Ca^{+2} excretion).

ADVERSE EFFECTS

- **Electrolyte disorders:** most common — Hypokalemia, Hypomagnesemia, Hypochloremia, **Hypercalcemia. Thiazides are the diuretics most likely to cause Hyponatremia.** Hypovolemia.
- Increased **GLUC**ose (**increased Glucose, Lipids, Uric acid, Calcium**). Erectile dysfunction.
- **Metabolic alkalosis:** potassium & H^+ wasting from increased sodium delivery to the collecting duct.
- **Serum potassium levels should be closely monitored in patients who are predisposed to cardiac arrhythmias** (individuals with left ventricular hypertrophy, coronary artery disease, and congestive heart failure) and who are concurrently being treated with Thiazide diuretics & Digoxin.
- Contraindications: anuria and **sulfonamide allergies** (Thiazides contain a sulfa component).

POTASSIUM-SPARING DIURETICS

MINERALOCORTICOID RECEPTOR ANTAGONISTS (MRA): SPIRONOLACTONE, EPLERENONE, FINERENONE

MECHANISM OF ACTION
- **Aldosterone receptor antagonist** in the distal cortical collecting tubule (increasing sodium and water excretion while conserving potassium & hydrogen ions). Spironolactone & Eplerenone are steroidal Mineralocorticoid receptors antagonists (MRAs); Finerenone is a nonsteroidal MRA.

INDICATIONS
- **Primary hyperaldosteronism (Spironolactone preferred** vs. Eplerenone). Nephrotic syndrome.
- **Cirrhosis-related ascites,** weak diuretic (used in combination with loop or thiazide diuretic to minimize potassium loss). **Hypertension. Spironolactone anti-androgenic (female hirsutism).**
- **Heart failure with reduced & preserved EF: (decreased mortality) — beneficial in patients with Heart failure.** Decreased mortality with these agents is due to aldosterone antagonism.
- **Finerenone:** improves cardiovascular and renal outcomes in Chronic kidney disease associated with type 2 Diabetes mellitus. However, contraindicated in severe renal disease.

ADVERSE EFFECTS
- **Hyperkalemia (main adverse effect). Normal anion gap (hyperchloremic) metabolic acidosis.**
- **Anti-androgen effects (Spironolactone): gynecomastia, erectile dysfunction, decreased libido, and menstrual irregularities due to antagonism of androgen & progesterone receptors.**
- Eplerenone is more selective, so it is associated with lower incidence of anti-androgenic effects.

RENAL EPITHELIAL SODIUM ION CHANNEL (ENaC) BLOCKERS: AMILORIDE, TRIAMTERENE

MECHANISM OF ACTION
- **Directly decrease sodium channel activity by inhibiting the epithelial sodium ion channels (ENaC) in the luminal membrane of the principal cells of the cortical collecting duct, leading to decreased sodium and chloride reabsorption.** They do not affect the aldosterone receptor.

INDICATIONS
- **Potassium-sparing effect: often used in combination with other diuretics for their antikaliuretic effects to offset the actions of other diuretics that increase renal K+ excretion.**
- Hypertension, CHF. **Lithium-induced polyuria due to AVP resistance [Nephrogenic DI], especially Amiloride** because Amiloride blocks Lithium transport into the collecting tubule cells.
- Not associated with anti-androgenic effects. Used in the management of Liddle syndrome.

ADVERSE EFFECTS
- **Hyperkalemia** (not used in anyone with increased risk for Hyperkalemia, such as Acute kidney injury or patients on ACE inhibitors). Nausea, vomiting, diarrhea, headache.
- **Non-anion gap metabolic acidosis.** Triamterene is associated with urine crystal formation.

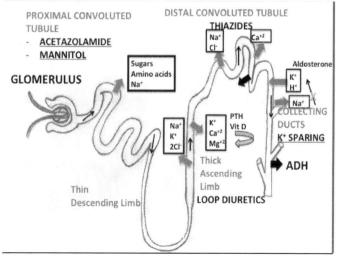

DIURETIC	MECHANISM OF ACTION	INDICATIONS	SIDE EFFECTS & CONTRAINDICATIONS
PROXIMAL TUBE DIURETIC			
MANNITOL	*Osmotic diuretic:* ↑es urine volume by ↑ing tubular fluid osmolarity (since mannitol is filtered but not easily reabsorbed).	• *Intracranial HTN* (↓'es intracranial CSF pressure) • Oliguria (trauma, shock) • Glaucoma, Acute kidney injury	**S/E:** *PULMONARY EDEMA** (due to ↑fluid shift) **CI:** anuria
ACETAZOLAMIDE	*CARBONIC ANHYDRASE INHIBITOR* in the *proximal tubule* ⇨ *NaHCO₃* diuresis. *Mild diuretic, acidifies the blood* in patients with metabolic alkalosis	• *Glaucoma* (↓'es intraocular pressure), • *Intracranial HTN* (↓'es intracranial CSF pressure) • Urinary alkalinization • Metabolic alkalosis	• *Hyperchloremic metabolic acidosis* (due to loss of bicarbonate). • Hypokalemia, *sulfa allergies* • *Kidney stones* (calcium & phosphate)
LOOP DIURETICS			
FUROSEMIDE (Lasix) **BUMETANIDE** (Bumex) TORSEMIDE	Inhibits water, *Na⁺-K⁺-Cl⁻* transport across thick ascending *LOOP OF HENLE* ⇨ dilute urine *(strongest class of diuretics)* ↑*PG synthesis* ⇨ ↑*renal blood flow*	• *HTN* • *Edema:* pulmonary edema, CHF, nephrotic syndrome, cirrhosis. • *Hypercalcemia*	• *Hypokalemia/hypocalcemia/↓ Mg* • *Hyperglycemia & Hyperuricemia (caution in DM, gout).** • *Ototoxicity, Sulfa allergy* • Acute Interstitial Nephritis (all sulfa drugs) • Hypochloremic metabolic alkalosis • NSAIDs decrease its efficacy
ETHACRYNIC ACID	*Similar action to furosemide (but does not contain sulfonamide)*	• *Diuresis in pts c sulfa allergy* • *Can be used in pts with gout*	• *More ototoxicity compared to Lasix*
THIAZIDE DIURETICS			
HYDROCHLOROTHIAZIDE Chlorthalidone Indapamide Metolazone Chlorothiazide	*Blocks NaCl & water reabsorption* at the early *distal diluting tubule.* ⇨ *diuresis & inability to produce dilute urine** Lowers urinary Ca⁺² excretion.	• *HTN* (if no comorbidities, elderly, African Americans). • Nephrolithiasis • *Nephrogenic DI* HCTZ ↓'es ability to dilute urine*	• *HypOnatremia,* *HYPERCALCEMIA,* hypokalemia, hyperlipidemia. • *Hyperuricemia & hyperglycemia,* therefore *caution in pts c DM, gout.* • *Sulfa allergies,* Metabolic alkalosis. Sexual dysfunction
POTASSIUM SPARING			
SPIRONOLACTONE **EPLERENONE**	*Inhibits aldosterone-mediated Na/H₂O absorption in cortical collecting tubule* while facilitating the reabsorption of K⁺ (potassium-sparing). Weak diuretic	• *CHF (reduces mortality)* • Most useful in combo with loop to minimize K loss. • *Hyperaldosteronism*	• *Hyperkalemia,** *metabolic acidosis* (K⁺ & H⁺ not exchanged for Na⁺) • *Spironolactone causes gynecomastia** *(anti-androgen effects)*
TRIAMTERENE **AMILORIDE**	*Blocks Na⁺ within cortical collecting tubule*	• Lithium-induced nephrogenic DI	• *Hyperkalemia,* metabolic acidosis

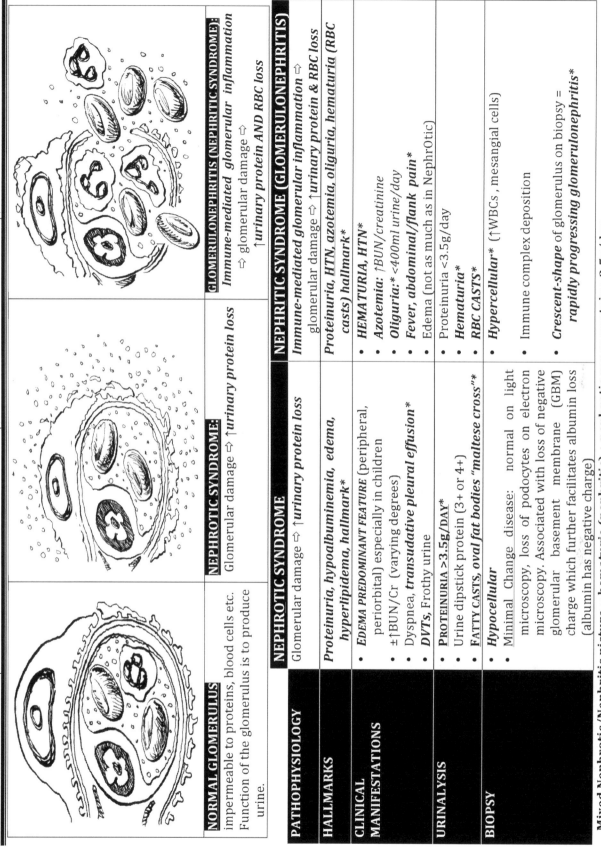

NORMAL GLOMERULUS impermeable to proteins, blood cells etc. Function of the glomerulus is to produce urine.

NEPHROTIC SYNDROME: Glomerular damage ⇨ ↑*urinary protein loss*

GLOMERULONEPHRITIS (NEPHRITIC SYNDROME): *Immune-mediated glomerular inflammation* ⇨ *glomerular damage* ⇨ ↑*urinary protein AND RBC loss*

	NEPHROTIC SYNDROME	NEPHRITIC SYNDROME (GLOMERULONEPHRITIS)
PATHOPHYSIOLOGY	Glomerular damage ⇨ ↑*urinary protein loss*	*Immune-mediated glomerular inflammation* ⇨ glomerular damage ⇨ ↑*urinary protein & RBC loss*
HALLMARKS	*Proteinuria, hypoalbuminemia, edema, hyperlipidemia, hallmark**	*Proteinuria, HTN, azotemia, oliguria, hematuria (RBC casts) hallmark**
CLINICAL MANIFESTATIONS	• *EDEMA PREDOMINANT FEATURE* (peripheral, periorbital) especially in children • ±↑BUN/Cr (varying degrees) • Dyspnea, *transudative pleural effusion** • *DVTs*, Frothy urine	• *HEMATURIA, HTN** • *Azotemia:* ↑*BUN/creatinine* • *Oliguria:* *<400ml urine/day* • *Fever, abdominal/flank pain** • Edema (not as much as in NephrOtic)
URINALYSIS	• **PROTEINURIA >3.5g/DAY*** • Urine dipstick protein (3+ or 4+) • *FATTY CASTS, oval fat bodies "maltese cross"**	• Proteinuria <3.5g/day • *Hematuria** • *RBC CASTS**
BIOPSY	• *Hypocellular* • <u>Minimal Change disease:</u> normal on light microscopy, loss of podocytes on electron microscopy. Associated with loss of negative glomerular basement membrane (GBM) charge which further facilitates albumin loss (albumin has negative charge)	• *Hypercellular** (↑WBCs , mesangial cells) • Immune complex deposition • *Crescent-shape* of glomerulus on biopsy = *rapidly progressing glomerulonephritis**

Mixed Nephrotic/Nephritic picture = hematuria (nephritic) + nephrotic range protein >3.5g/day.

NEPHROTIC SYNDROME

- **Kidney disease characterized by [1] proteinuria (>3.5 grams/24 hours, mostly albuminuria), [2] hypoalbuminemia, [3] edema, [4] hyperlipidemia, and [5] thromboembolic disease.**

PATHOPHYSIOLOGY
- **Increased glomerular permeability**: noninflammatory damage to the basement membrane of the renal glomerulus leads to increased glomerular permeability, followed by proteinuria (eg, albumin) & hypoalbuminemia. Loss of albumin decreases oncotic pressure, resulting in edema.
- The liver tries to compensate for the loss of albumin by producing other proteins, such as lipoproteins (resulting in hyperlipidemia and hypercholesterolemia) and clotting proteins (hypercoagulable state due to increased clotting proteins and loss of antithrombin and plasminogen proteins).

ETIOLOGIES
[1] Primary glomerular disease:
- **Minimal change disease (MCD) — most common cause of Nephrotic syndrome in children.**
- **Focal segmental glomerulosclerosis (FSGS).**
- **Membranous nephropathy (MN).**

[2] Secondary causes: glomerular damage secondary to a systemic disease:
- **Diabetic nephropathy: most common overall cause of Nephrotic syndrome in the US.**
- **Immune diseases:** eg, **Systemic lupus erythematosus,** Sjögren syndrome, Sarcoidosis.
- **Amyloidosis:** common cause of Nephrotic syndrome in older adults without Diabetes mellitus.
- **Viral hepatitis (eg, HBV, HCV)** and other infections (eg, **HIV,** Syphilis, Malaria, Schistosomiasis)
- Medications. Malignancy.

CLINICAL MANIFESTATIONS
- **Edema (especially periorbital edema in children) usually worse in the morning. Periorbital, lower extremity, or genital edema in adults.** Edema occurs secondary to salt and water retention and hypoalbuminemia. Ascites & anasarca may be seen in severe disease.
- **Frothy (foamy) urine due to proteinuria.**
- Nonspecific symptoms: lack of appetite, fatigue, weight gain, dyspnea (pleural effusion may be seen).
- Hematologic: Anemia. **Hypercoagulable state: DVT and PE** due to loss of anticoagulant proteins (eg, proteins C & S, plasminogen, & antithrombin III) and relative increase in clotting proteins.

PHYSICAL EXAMINATION
- **Hypertension, edema.** Leukonychia white streaking on the fingernails suggestive of low albumin.

DIAGNOSIS
[1] Urinalysis (UA):
- **Initial test — proteinuria**, lipiduria, often with a bland urine sediment. **Dipstick: ≥3+ protein.**
  Fatty casts represent lipids in the urine that take the shape of the tubule as the lipoproteins travel through the tubules of the nephron.
  Oval fat bodies represent lipids enclosed by the plasma membrane of degenerated epithelial cells.
  Oval Maltese cross-shaped fat bodies may be seen on light microscopy of the urine.

[2] Protein measurements:
- **24-hour urine protein >3-3.5 g/day criterion standard for nephrotic-range proteinuria.**
- **Spot urine protein to creatinine:** >300-350 mg/mmol on spot urine protein to creatinine ratio **may be easier to obtain than a 24-hour urine protein specimen.**

[3] Serologic studies:
- **Laboratory evaluation: Hypoalbuminemia:** albumin <3 mg/dL. **Hyperlipidemia (50%).**
- Based on suspected cause — antinuclear antibodies (ANA), complement (C3/C4 & total hemolytic complement), serum protein electrophoresis & immunofixation & serum free light chains, Syphilis serology, Hepatitis B & Hepatitis C serologies, HIV, PLA2R antibody titers, & cryoglobulins.

Renal biopsy: Definitive diagnosis (criterion standard). May be required to establish the etiology.

- **Minimal change disease: Electron microscopy: diffuse effacement of epithelial cell foot process & fusion**; Light microscopy: no change. Biopsy usually not performed in children with suspected MCD. Immunofluorescent staining negative for immune complexes. Loss of negative charge of the GBM.

- **Focal segmental glomerulosclerosis: Light microscopy: scarring or sclerosis in parts (segmental) of selected (focal) glomeruli.** May progress into global glomerular sclerosis and tubular atrophy. **Primary FSGS is associated with diffuse effacement of the epithelial foot processes** (similar to MCD); Secondary FSGS may have segmental foot process effacement.

- **Membranous nephropathy: Light microscopy: uniform thickening of the basement membrane along the peripheral capillary loops with little or no cellular proliferation or infiltration** (this thickening needs to be distinguished from that seen in Diabetes and Amyloidosis). Immunofluorescence: diffuse granular deposits of IgG and C3. Electron microscopy: **electron-dense subepithelial dense deposits with a "spike & dome" appearance.**
  Lupus nephritis: subendothelial deposits or tubuloreticular inclusions.

MANAGEMENT

- **Edema reduction: dietary sodium restriction** (~2g/day). **Thiazides &/or Loop diuretics** to reduce salt and water retention, avoiding intravascular depletion.

- **Proteinuria reduction: ACE inhibitors or Angiotensin receptor blockers reduce urinary protein excretion** & lower blood pressure in hypertensive patients. SGLT-2 inhibitors, MRAs.

- **Hyperlipidemia: diet modifications** to reduce the risk for cardiovascular disease until disease resolution. Lipid-lowering agents (eg, Statin therapy) may be required.

- Venous complications secondary to the hypercoagulable state may be managed with anticoagulation.

Minimal change disease:

- **Glucocorticoids: first line for Minimal change disease. 90-95% of children will develop complete remission after 8 weeks of corticosteroid therapy.** Severe anasarca or edema: active mobilization of fluid with IV loop diuretic in conjunction with salt-poor 25% albumin.

- Second-line agents: eg, Levamisole, Mycophenolate, Cyclophosphamide, Cyclosporine, Tacrolimus.

Focal segmental glomerulosclerosis (FSGS)

- Renin-angiotensin (RAAS inhibitors): eg, **ACE inhibitors or ARBs to reduce proteinuria.**

- **Glucocorticoids (eg, Prednisone) first line for Primary FSGS** — Patients with nephrotic-range proteinuria are treated with steroids but respond much less often & after a longer course of therapy than with MCD **(steroid responsiveness important determinant of prognosis in FSGS).**

- Immunomodulators — **Calcineurin inhibitors [Cyclosporine or Tacrolimus (with or without low-dose glucocorticoids)] second line** but avoid if severe renal disease. Rituximab, Mycophenolate.

Amyloidosis:

- Primary Amyloidosis: Melphalan and Autologous hematopoietic stem cell transplantation can delay the course of disease in ~30% of patients.

- Secondary Amyloidosis treat the primary chronic inflammatory disease, infection, or malignancy.

Diabetic nephropathy:

- Risk-factor modification: tobacco cessation, low sodium diet, strict glucose control (Hgb A1C <7%), and optimal lipid control are crucial for cardiovascular risk reduction in Diabetes mellitus.

- **Hypertension: Patients with type 2 Diabetes & Diabetic kidney disease (DKD) should generally be treated with either an Angiotensin converting enzyme (ACE) inhibitor OR Angiotensin receptor blocker (ARB) plus a Sodium-glucose cotransporter 2 (SGLT-2) inhibitor.**

- **Finerenone,** nonsteroidal selective mineralocorticoid receptor antagonist (MRA) may be added to SGLT2 therapy if the patient has a normal serum potassium while taking an ACE inhibitor or ARB.

- Kidney protective therapy: In patients with type 2 diabetes and DKD who have not achieved glycemic control despite initial glucose-lowering therapy (which is typically Metformin), addition of an SGLT2 inhibitor or a GLP-1 receptor agonist can improve glycemic control with additional benefits for DM.

MINIMAL CHANGE DISEASE (MCD) [NIL DISEASE]

- **Most common cause of Nephrotic syndrome in children** (~90% of children <10 years of age; >50% in older children); 10-15% of cases of Nephrotic syndrome in adults. Male predominance.

ETIOLOGIES
- **Idiopathic (Primary) most common.**
- **Secondary: May be associated with viral infections, allergies** (eg, insect stings), **immunizations, malignancies** (eg, **Hodgkin lymphoma**, Non-Hodgkin lymphoma, Leukemia), **Systemic lupus erythematosus, & medications (most commonly NSAIDs**. Antimicrobials, Lithium, etc.).

PATHOPHYSIOLOGY
- **Podocyte damage & loss of negative electric charge of the glomerular basement membrane, leading to proteinuria.** T cell dysfunction increases circulating factor, which damages the glomerular capillary wall & podocytes, leading to marked proteinuria and foot process effacement.

DIAGNOSIS
- **Presumptive diagnosis based on clinical findings & UA. Biopsy reserved if severe or refractory** (most children are treated with steroids; children who are nonresponders may be biopsied).

Renal biopsy:
- **Light microscopy: normal appearing — no obvious visible cellular changes seen.**
- Immunofluorescent microscopy: negative for deposits; ± small amounts of IgM in the mesangium.
- **Electron microscopy: podocyte fusion (diffuse and complete effacement of the epithelial foot processes** supporting the epithelial podocytes) with weakening of slit-pore membranes. The spaces between flattened podocyte foot processes are reduced in number, which may play a role in the excess albumin loss into the urinary space & loss of the net negative charge of the GBM.

MEMBRANOUS NEPHROPATHY (MN)

PATHOPHYSIOLOGY
- **Immune deposits: Antibody-immune complex deposition in the subepithelial space** either [1] in situ — eg, movement across the glomerular basement membrane (GBM) of circulating IgG antibodies targeting endogenous antigens expressed on or in close proximity to podocyte foot processes or [2] against circulating cationic or low-molecular-weight antigens that have crossed the anionic charge barrier in the GBM. Complement-mediated podocyte injury.
- **In Primary (idiopathic) MN, autoantibodies to the M-type phospholipase A2 receptor (PLA2R), a major antigen expressed on podocytes, are found in abundance** (70% cases of MN).

EPIDEMIOLOGY
- Membranous nephropathy (MN) is among the most common causes of the Nephrotic syndrome in nondiabetic adults, accounting for up to one-third of biopsy diagnoses.
- **Primary MN: Membranous nephropathy (MN) is the most common Primary cause of Nephrotic syndrome (NS) in nondiabetic White adults** (20-30% of NS). **2 times more common in men**, with a **peak incidence between 30-50 years of age**. Most common cause of NS in the elderly.
- **Secondary MN: May be seen with rheumatologic disorders (eg, Systemic lupus erythematosus**, Rheumatoid arthritis, IgG4 diseases); **medications (eg, meds used to treat Rheumatoid arthritis, such as NSAIDs, Penicillamine, gold)**, Captopril; **Viral hepatitis (HBV, HCV); malignancy** (solid tumors of the breast, lung, colon); infection (eg, Syphilis, Malaria, Schistosomiasis).

BIOPSY
- **Light microscopy: [1] Uniform thickening of the glomerular basement membrane along the peripheral capillary loops with [2] little or no cellular proliferation or infiltration.**
- **Immunofluorescence: immune complex deposition (eg, IgG & C3) leads to a diffuse granular appearance.** SLE nephritis: subendothelial deposits or the presence of tubuloreticular inclusions.
- Electron microscopy: **electron-dense subepithelial dense deposits ("spike & dome" appearance).**

MANAGEMENT OF PRIMARY MN:
- **High risk: Rituximab if stable renal function; Glucocorticoids + Cyclophosphamide if declining kidney function.** Moderate: Rituximab, Cyclophosphamide, Cyclosporine or Tacrolimus, Chlorambucil.

FOCAL SEGMENTAL GLOMERULOSCLEROSIS (FSGS)

- Focal segmental glomerulosclerosis (FSGS) is a histologic lesion, rather than a specific disease entity.
- **Podocyte damage**: FSGS represents a pattern of renal injury characterized by segmental glomerular scarring involving some but not all glomeruli, resulting from damage to the podocytes.
- **FSGS is more common in people of African ancestry** (>50% of Nephrotic syndrome in Blacks due to increased *APOL1* locus expression). FSGS causes 1/3 of cases of NS in adults in general.

TYPES

- **Primary FSGS: permeability factor-related podocyte damage** (which most often presents with Nephrotic syndrome), glomerular hypertrophy, toxin-mediated, and/or genetic predisposition.
- **Secondary FSGS**: adaptive response to glomerular hypertrophy or hyperfiltration. Most often presents with non-nephrotic proteinuria and, commonly, some degree of kidney function impairment. **Causes of Secondary FSGS include Hypertension, toxins (eg, Heroin), viral (collapsing form with HIV),** obesity. Other toxins: Interferon & **Bisphosphonates** (Pamidronate).

CLINICAL MANIFESTATIONS

- **FSGS can present with hematuria, Hypertension, any level of proteinuria, & renal insufficiency.**
- Nephrotic-range proteinuria, Black race, and renal insufficiency are associated with a poor outcome, with 50% of patients reaching Chronic renal failure in 6–8 years.

DIABETIC NEPHROPATHY

- **Diabetes mellitus most common overall cause and secondary cause of Nephrotic syndrome in adults, eventually resulting in Chronic kidney disease.** Higher prevalence in T2DM (90%).
- **Diabetic nephropathy is the single most common cause of Chronic kidney disease in the US.**

PATHOPHYSIOLOGY

- At the onset of Diabetes, renal hypertrophy as well as **glomerular hyperperfusion and hyperfiltration are present, result in leakage of albumin.** The glomerulus responds to these conditions via glomerular basement membrane thickening due to non-enzymatic glycosylation, ultimately leading to **hypertrophy, sclerosis, and podocyte injury.**

RENAL BIOPSY

- Diabetic nephropathy is usually diagnosed without a renal biopsy if longstanding Diabetes mellitus.
- **The initial abnormality of classical diabetic glomerulopathy is thickening of the glomerular basement membrane** (may be seen as early as 2 years following the diagnosis of DM).
- Other major diabetic glomerular changes include **mesangial expansion, with glomerulosclerosis which can be diffuse or nodular [often termed "Kimmelstiel-Wilson nodules" (pink hyaline material around the glomerular capillaries from protein leakage) is pathognomonic of Diabetic nephropathy]**, podocyte injury.
- **Tubulointerstitial fibrosis usually occurs after the initial glomerular lesions and is a final pathway-mediating progression to advanced CKD and ESKD.** Findings are more varied in type 2 diabetes than in type 1 Diabetes, with most patients having dominant vascular and tubulointerstitial disease compared to glomerular involvement.

RENAL AMYLOIDOSIS

- **Pathophysiology: Amyloid deposition in the mesangium of the kidney.** Either the result of (1) primary fibrillar deposits of immunoglobulin (Ig) **light chains known as amyloid L (AL),** or (2) secondary to fibrillar deposits of acute phase reactant serum **amyloid A (AA)** protein fragments.
- **Primary amyloidosis (AL): due to excess Ig light chain deposition. ~10% of these patients have overt Multiple myeloma with lytic bone lesions and infiltration of the bone marrow with >30% plasma cells;** Nephrotic syndrome is common, and ~20% of patients progress to dialysis.
- **Secondary (AA): Chronic inflammatory disease:** eg, Rheumatoid arthritis, IBD, Chronic osteomyelitis.

DIAGNOSIS

- Electron microscopy: **AA and AL amyloid fibrils are detectable as apple-green birefringence on Congo red stain under polarized light.** Screening tests: serum & urine protein electrophoresis; if a monoclonal spike is found, serum free light chains & kappa: lambda ratio should be ordered.

ACUTE GLOMERULONEPHRITIS (AGN) [ACUTE NEPHRITIC SYNDROME]

- **Immunologic inflammation of the glomeruli,** leading to protein & RBC leakage into the urine.
- **Characterized by Hypertension, hematuria (RBC casts), azotemia, & proteinuria (edema).**

ETIOLOGIES
- **Immunoglobulin A (IgA) Nephropathy (Berger's);** IgA Vasculitis (Henoch–Schönlein purpura).
- **Postinfectious glomerulonephritis (eg, poststreptococcal AGN)**
- **Membranoproliferative glomerulonephritis (including Lupus Nephritis);** Cryoglobulinemia.
- **Rapidly progressive glomerulonephritis (RPGN):** may include **Anti-GBM disease (Goodpasture syndrome), Microscopic polyangiitis (MPA), Granulomatosis with polyangiitis (GPA), & Eosinophilic GPA (EGPA),** but any cause of AGN may lead to RPGN.

CLINICAL MANIFESTATIONS
- **Hematuria hallmark (eg, cola, dark-colored, or tea-colored urine):** microscopic or macroscopic.
- **Edema:** peripheral & periorbital — fluid & salt retention results in edema and Hypertension.
- Nonspecific symptoms of uremia: fever, abdominal or flank pain, malaise, anorexia, headache.
- **Oliguria:** decreased urine output due to Acute kidney injury.
- Physical examination: **Hypertension common,** periorbital & facial edema, or peripheral edema.

DIAGNOSIS
- **UA: hematuria, RBC casts, dysmorphic RBCs hallmark of glomerular origin** (acanthocytes), **proteinuria** (often <3g/day but can be in nephrotic range), pyuria, **high specific gravity** (>1.020 osm).
- **Acute kidney injury (AKI): Increased BUN & creatinine.** Hyperkalemia may be seen with AKI.
- Serologies as needed: viral (HCV, HBV), HIV; Liver function tests. CRP, complement, SLE testing.
- Proteinuria: 24-hour urine collection or single specimen ratio of protein to creatinine ratio.
- **Renal biopsy criterion standard to establish the etiology.** Not required in all cases.
  - Ig A nephropathy: **IgA mesangial deposits** on immunostaining.
  - Poststreptococcal: hypercellularity, ↑monocytes/lymphocytes, **immune humps** of IgG, IgM, & C3.
  - Anti-GBM (Goodpasture syndrome): **linear IgG deposits** in the glomerular basement membrane.
  - **Membranoproliferative: thickening of the glomerular basement membrane & hypercellularity on light microscopy.**
  - **Rapidly progressive: extensive glomerular crescents** in Bowman's space (usually >50%).
  - **GPA, EGPA, & MPA: focal necrotizing, often crescentic, pauci-immune glomerulonephritis (associated with few or no immune complexes) + positive ANCA.**

MANAGEMENT
- Edema, hypervolemia, or Hypertension: **salt & water restriction in conjunction with diuretics (eg, Furosemide) for edema;** Hypertension: Beta-blockers, Calcium channel blockers, ACEIs, ARBs.
- **IgA nephropathy or proteinuria: ACE inhibitors or ARBs.** ± Corticosteroids.
- Post streptococcal AGN: Supportive (control of hypertension & edema), Antibiotics if active infection.
- **Lupus nephritis: Corticosteroids + either Mycophenolate or Cyclophosphamide** for induction.
- Membranoproliferative: Primary MPGN: Corticosteroids in children; Corticosteroids in adults with severe disease. Secondary MPGN: treat the underlying disease, which often resolves the MPGN.
- **Rapid progressive AGN or severe disease: Corticosteroids + either Rituximab or Cyclophosphamide.**

IgA NEPHROPATHY (BERGER DISEASE)

- Pathophysiology: immune-complex deposition in glomerular mesangial cells that results from **proliferation of IgA in response to upper respiratory tract or gastrointestinal infections.**
- Epidemiology: **Most common cause of AGN in the US, especially young males (teens and 20s).**
- Clinical manifestations: **[1] gross or microscopic hematuria (single or recurrent) 1-2 days after onset of URI or GI infection** (synpharyngitic); [2] Asymptomatic persistent microscopic hematuria.
- Renal biopsy: **IgA mesangial deposits on immunofluorescence microscopy.** Not usually done.
- Management: **ACE inhibitors or ARBs for Hypertension &/or proteinuria.** Supportive treatment. Glucocorticoids reserved for refractory or severe disease in high-risk patients.

POSTINFECTIOUS GLOMERULONEPHRITIS (including Poststreptococcal glomerulonephritis)

- PATHOPHYSIOLOGY: **Streptococcus GN is a Type III hypersensitivity reaction (immune antigen-antibody complex disease)** characterized by inflammation with IgA & complement C3 deposition.
- EPIDEMIOLOGY: **can occur after any infection but most commonly 1–3 weeks after streptococcal pharyngitis or 2–6 weeks after skin infection (Impetigo).** The risk of PSGN is greatest in children between 5-12 years of age, and in older adults >60 years of age. Not preventable with antibiotics.
- LABS: **low serum complement (C3) and recent GAS infection [eg, positive throat or skin culture or serologic tests for Group A streptococci (anti-streptolysin/ASO) or streptozyme test].**
- RENAL BIOPSY: **Light microscopy: enlarged, hypercellular glomeruli with neutrophil infiltration.** Immunofluorescence: diffuse granular pattern on glomerular capillary walls and mesangium **deposition of IgG, IgM, & complement (C3,** C4, C_{5-9}).
  Electron microscopy: electron-dense, **glomerular dome-shaped subepithelial immune complex deposits ("humps")** of IgG, IgM, & C3. Biopsy seldomly needed because most spontaneously resolve).
- MANAGEMENT: **supportive — diuretics for fluid overload.** Antibiotics if active infection still present.

MEMBRANOPROLIFERATIVE GLOMERULONEPHRITIS (MPGN)

- PATHOPHYSIOLOGY: inflammatory reaction due to immune complexes (Type 1), complement-mediated C3 glomerulopathy [dense deposit disease (Type II) & monoclonal Ig-mediated (Type III)].
- ETIOLOGIES: **Type 1 (immune complex) associated with viral hepatitis (HCV, HBV), autoimmune diseases (eg, Systemic lupus erythematosus,** Sjögren syndrome, cryoglobulinemia), malignancy.
- LABS: Usually associated with **mixed nephrotic-nephritic picture (red blood cells, RBC casts + nephrotic range protein >3.5g/day). Hypocomplementemia** is common (70% of MPGN).
- BIOPSY FINDING: **thickened basement membrane hallmark** [mesangial proliferation with lobular segmentation of glomerular tuft; mesangial interposition between the capillary basement membrane and endothelial cells, splitting the GBM, producing a double contour (tram-tracking)].

LUPUS NEPHRITIS

- EPIDEMIOLOGY: **Lupus nephritis is a common & serious complication of Systemic lupus erythematosus (SLE)** and most severe in Black female adolescents (30-50% of patients will have clinical manifestations of renal disease at the time of diagnosis). 60% of adults and 80% of children develop renal abnormalities at some point in the course of their disease.
- PATHOPHYSIOLOGY: **Lupus nephritis results from the deposition of circulating immune complexes,** which activate the complement cascade, resulting in complement-mediated damage, leukocyte infiltration, activation of procoagulant factors, and release of various cytokines.
- CLINICAL MANIFESTATIONS: **Proteinuria most common clinical sign of renal disease,** but hematuria, Hypertension, varying degrees of renal failure, & active urine sediment may also occur.
- LABS: **Anti-dsDNA antibodies** that fix complement correlate best with the presence of renal disease. **Hypocomplementemia is seen in 70-90%.**
- BIOPSY: **Light microscopy: "wire-looping" appearance of the capillaries,** mesangial proliferation (hypercellularity with expansion of the mesangial matrix), endocapillary infiltration.
  Immunofluorescence: **granular appearance** (diffuse proliferative glomerulonephritis).
- MANAGEMENT: Glucocorticoids in combination with either Mycophenolate or Cyclophosphamide.

ANTIGLOMERULAR BASEMENT MEMBRANE (ANTI-GBM) DISEASE [GOODPASTURE'S SYNDROME]

- PATHOPHYSIOLOGY: **type II hypersensitivity — antiglomerular basement membrane (GBM) antibodies against type IV collagen in the [1] alveolar basement membrane in the lungs and [2] glomeruli in the kidney.** Seen in 2 groups: men in their twenties & people in their 60s & 70s.
- **Goodpasture's syndrome: [1] glomerulonephritis (rapidly progressive,** associated with crescent formation) >90% **&/or [2] hemoptysis: pulmonary (alveolar) hemorrhage.** Dyspnea.
- BIOPSY: **immunofluorescence: Linear IgG deposition (anti-GBM antibodies** & complement) and staining with focal or segmental necrosis. Urgent kidney biopsy is important in suspected cases of Goodpasture's syndrome to confirm the diagnosis and determine prognosis.
- MANAGEMENT: **Glucocorticoids PLUS Cyclophosphamide + Plasmapheresis.**

GRANULOMATOSIS WITH POLYANGIITIS [GPA] (formerly WEGENER'S GRANULOMATOSIS)

- **Predominantly small-sized artery vasculitis associated with C-ANCA positivity.**
- PATHOPHYSIOLOGY: Cell-mediated immune reactions [⊕ **anti-proteinase 3 (PR3) PR3-ANCA, C-ANCA**], leading to necrotizing vasculitis. Silica exposure & α_1-antitrypsin deficiency increases risk.

CLINICAL MANIFESTATIONS

- **Triad of [1] <u>upper respiratory tract involvement</u>** — eg, sinusitis, saddle nose deformity, nasal ulcers, nasal crusting, otitis media, rhinorrhea, purulent or bloody nasal discharge, **[2] <u>lower tract involvement</u>** — pulmonary infiltrates or nodules, cough, dyspnea, stridor, wheezing, hemoptysis, pleuritic pain, and **[3] <u>nephritis</u>** — hematuria, proteinuria, increase in serum creatinine.
- **Cutaneous involvement**: purpura (especially involving the lower extremities), nodules, urticaria.
- **Neurologic involvement** may include multiple mononeuropathy (Mononeuritis multiplex), sensory neuropathy, cranial nerve abnormalities, central nervous system mass lesions, external ophthalmoplegia, and sensorineural hearing loss. Polyarthralgias or arthritis.

KIDNEY HISTOLOGY

- **Focal necrotizing, often crescentic (rapidly progressive),** pauci-immune glomerulonephritis (small-vessel vasculitis & adjacent noncaseating granulomas without immune complex deposits).

MANAGEMENT

- <u>Organ- or life-threatening:</u> **Glucocorticoids PLUS either Rituximab or Cyclophosphamide.**
- Non-organ- & non-life-threatening GPA not involving the kidney: initial therapy with Glucocorticoids combined with Methotrexate (rather than Cyclophosphamide or Rituximab).

MICROSCOPIC POLYANGIITIS (MPA)

- **MPA is a predominantly small-sized artery vasculitis associated with P-ANCA positivity.**
- PATHOPHYSIOLOGY: cell-mediated immune reactions [⊕ **myeloperoxidase MPO-ANCA/P-ANCA**].

CLINICAL MANIFESTATIONS:

- **Presents similar to GPA, except MPA is rarely associated with significant lung disease, has less ENT involvement (eg, no destructive sinusitis), ⊕ P-ANCA, and no granulomas on biopsy.**
- The 5 most common manifestations of MPA are [1] glomerulonephritis (~80%), [2] weight loss (>70%), [3] mononeuritis multiplex (60%), [4] fevers (55%), & [5] cutaneous vasculitis (>60%).
- Nonspecific constitutional symptoms, including fever, malaise, anorexia, weight loss, myalgias, and arthralgias. **Cutaneous involvement** include purpura (especially the lower extremities), papules; **Neurologic involvement** may include multiple mononeuropathy (Mononeuritis multiplex), sensory &/or motor neuropathy, cranial nerve abnormalities, central nervous system mass lesions, external ophthalmoplegia, and sensorineural hearing loss.

KIDNEY HISTOLOGY:

- **Focal necrotizing, often crescentic, pauci-immune glomerulonephritis, and small vessel vasculitis <u>without</u> granulomas** (unlike granulomas seen in GPA & EGPA).

MANAGEMENT: **same as GPA** (see above). Maintenance: Azathioprine after induction (or Methotrexate).

RAPIDLY PROGRESSIVE GLOMERULONEPHRITIS (RPGN)

- **Associated with poor prognosis: rapid progression** to end stage renal disease in days to months. **Crescent formation on biopsy** crescents formed due to fibrin & plasma protein deposition collapsing the crescent shape of Bowman's capsule.
- Any condition can present with RPGN but Microscopic polyangiitis (MPA), Anti-GBM disease, Granulomatosis with polyangiitis (GPA), & EGPA classically present with RPGN.
- MANAGEMENT: **Corticosteroids + either Rituximab or Cyclophosphamide.**

NEPHROTIC GLOMERULONEPHRITIS

- Any cause of Nephrotic syndrome may develop into glomerulonephritis: eg, Minimal change disease, Focal segmental glomerulosclerosis, Membranous nephropathy, HIV-associated nephropathy, Diabetic nephropathy, Amyloidosis.

BIOPSY FINDINGS IN NEPHROTIC SYNDROME

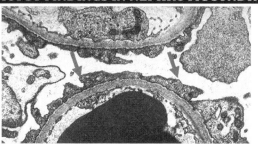

MINIMAL CHANGE DISEASE
- **Podocyte fusion (diffuse and complete effacement of the epithelial foot processes** supporting the epithelial podocytes) with weakening of slit-pore membranes

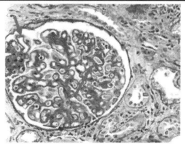

MEMBRANOUS NEPHROPATHY
- Light microscopy: **basement membrane thickening**/spike formation. Double contour.
- Electron microscopy: subepithelial deposits are seen.

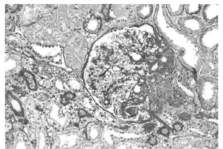

FOCAL SEGMENTAL GLOMERULOSCLEROSIS
scarring or sclerosis in parts (segmental) of selected (focal) glomeruli on light microscopy.

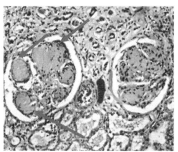

DIABETIC NEPHROPATHY
"Kimmelstiel-Wilson nodules" (pink hyaline material around the glomerular capillaries from protein leakage

BIOPSY FINDINGS IN NEPHRITIC SYNDROME (GLOMERULONEPHRITIS)

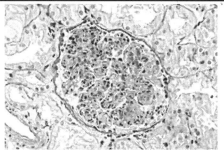

POSTINFECTIOUS GLOMERULONEPHRITIS
Light microscopy: Hypercellularity

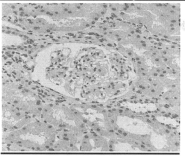

IgA NEPHROPATHY
IgA mesangial deposition

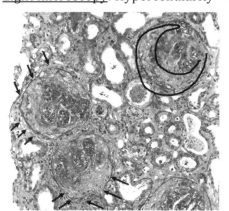

RAPIDLY PROGRESSIVE GLOMERULONEPHRITIS
Crescent-shaped lesions

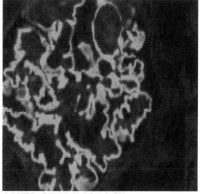

ANTI-GBM DISEASE
Linear IgG deposition

ACUTE KIDNEY INJURY (AKI)

- ❶ ↑ in serum creatinine >50% (≥0.3 mg/dL) in 48 hours or ❷ ↑ in blood urea nitrogen/BUN (azotemia).
- RIFLE Criteria: 3 progressive levels of AKI:
  Risk, Injury, Failure with 2 outcome determinants: Loss & End stage renal disease.
- Phases of AKI: **oliguric (maintenance) phase: ↓urine output <400 mL/d**, azotemia, hyperkalemia, metabolic acidosis ⇨ diuretic phase ↑ urine output, hypotension, hypokalemia ⇨ recovery phase.
- Symptoms of Uremia: nausea, vomiting, malaise, headache, altered sensorium. Metabolic acidosis.

3 MAJOR TYPES: ❶ PRErenal & ❷ POSTrenal (BOTH rapidly reversible); or ❸ INTRArenal (intrinsic).

PRERENAL AZOTEMIA

- **Characterized by decreased renal perfusion with nephrons still structurally intact.**
- If not corrected, Prerenal azotemia may lead to intrinsic injury [Acute tubular necrosis (ATN)].
- **Prerenal AKI most common type of Acute kidney injury overall (40-80%) in outpatients but Acute tubular necrosis (ATN) is the most common type in hospitalized patients.**

ETIOLOGIES
Reduced renal perfusion hallmark:
- **Hypovolemia** renal volume loss (eg, diuretic therapy), GI loss (diarrhea or vomiting), or blood loss.
- **Afferent arteriole** vasoconstriction — **Nonsteroidal anti-inflammatory drugs (NSAIDs) due to inhibition of prostaglandins, which minimize protective afferent arteriolar vasodilation** (normally, prostaglandins are recruited to increase renal blood flow via afferent arteriolar dilation). Calcineurin inhibitors (Cyclosporine, Tacrolimus), **IV radiocontrast media.**
- **Efferent arteriole** dilation — **eg, RAAS blockers, such as ACE inhibitors, Angiotensin receptor blockers** may limit efferent renal arteriolar constriction out of proportion to afferent arteriolar constriction, diminishing GFR.
- **Hypotension.** Relative hypovolemia in edematous states (eg, CHF with decreased pump function).

DIAGNOSIS
Evidence of water & electrolyte conservation since the renal parenchyma is still intact:
- Increased BUN > increased creatinine (**BUN: creatinine ratio >20:1**).
- Sodium conservation: Fractional excretion of sodium (**FENa) <1% & urine sodium <20 mEq/L.**
- Water conservation: **concentrated urine: high urine specific gravity** (>1.020) & **increased urine osmolarity (>500 mOsm/kg).** Serum cystatin C is a nonspecific marker of AKI.

MANAGEMENT
Volume repletion:
- **Volume repletion (eg, Normal saline) to restore volume & renal perfusion is the mainstay of treatment of Prerenal AKI** (unlike ATN, Prerenal azotemia rapidly responds to treatment).
- **With sufficient IV fluid replacement, return of the serum creatinine to the previous baseline within 24-72 hours is considered to represent correction of Prerenal disease,** whereas persistent Acute kidney injury is considered to represent Acute tubular necrosis (ATN).
- The aim is the achieve a positive fluid balance of 500 ml/day.

	PRERENAL AZOTEMIA	ACUTE TUBULAR NECROSIS (ATN)
Creatinine (Cr)	Increases slower than 0.3 mg/dL/day	Increases at ≥0.3-0.5 mg/dL/day
Urine sodium (UNa), FENa	↓Urine Na⁺ <20 mEq/L; FENa⁺ <1%	Urine Na⁺ >40 mEq/L; FENa⁺ >2%
URINALYSIS (UA)	Normal UA or bland sediment HIGH SPECIFIC GRAVITY (>1.020) (↑ Uosm >500)	**Casts: epithelial, granular, or muddy brown casts.** LOW SPECIFIC GRAVITY (<1.015) ↓Uosm (<500, often 200-500)
Response to volume replacement	Creatinine rapidly improves with IVF	Creatinine won't improve much
Blood Urea Nitrogen (BUN)/Cr	↑BUN: Cr >20:1	BUN: Cr ≤10-15:1

INTRINSIC RENAL FAILURE

ACUTE TUBULAR NECROSIS (ATN)
- A type of intrinsic Acute kidney injury characterized by acute destruction & necrosis of the renal tubules of the nephron.
- **Most common type of <u>intrinsic</u> Acute kidney injury** (50%). Most common cause of AKI in hospitals.

Ischemic:
- **<u>Prolonged Prerenal azotemia</u> associated with hypotension or hypovolemia. Sepsis.**

Nephrotoxic:
- **<u>Exogenous:</u> radiocontrast dye (immediate) Aminoglycosides &/or Vancomycin ~5-10 days after exposure** (incidence reduced with IV fluids). Calcineurin inhibitors (eg, Cyclosporine, Tacrolimus), NSAIDs, Amphotericin B, Methotrexate, Cisplatin, Foscarnet, Cidofovir, Tenofovir.
- **<u>Endogenous:</u>** uric acid precipitation (**Tumor lysis syndrome**), pigments [myoglobinuria (**Rhabdomyolysis**), hemoglobin], Lymphoma, Leukemia, Bence-Jones proteins (**Multiple myeloma**).

DIAGNOSIS
<u>Distinguishing Prerenal vs. ATN:</u> UA, response to IV fluid, & fractional excretion of sodium (FENa).
- **<u>Urinalysis (UA):</u> renal tubular epithelial cell casts & granular (muddy brown) casts:** sloughing off of tubular cells into the nephrons. Labs may show Hyperkalemia and Hyperphosphatemia.
- Unlike Prerenal, sodium & water reabsorptive abilities are lost in ATN, resulting in **low urine specific gravity** (**isosthenuria** inability to concentrate urine), **low urine osmolarity** <500 mOsm/kg, **<u>increased FENa >2%,</u> increased urine sodium >40 mEq/L, & BUN: creatinine ratio ≤15:1.**

MANAGEMENT
- **<u>Remove offending agent(s) & IV fluids</u> first-line.** IV fluids given before and after IV contrast.
- No other therapy proven to benefit ATN. N-acetylcysteine may be added to in contrast-induced cases.
- Furosemide used only when clinically indicated (critical AKI with volume overload).
- <u>Prognosis:</u> Most patients return to baseline within 7-21 days after injury.

<u>URINALYSIS:</u> most important noninvasive test regarding the possible etiologies.

URINARY PATTERN	
RBC CASTS, with hematuria, dysmorphic red cells	**Acute glomerulonephritis (AGN) or vasculitis.**
MUDDY BROWN (GRANULAR) OR EPITHELIAL CELL CASTS	**ATN (Acute tubular necrosis)**
WHITE BLOOD CELL CASTS, pyuria (free WBC cells)	**AIN (Acute interstitial nephritis) or Pyelonephritis**
WAXY CASTS: acellular with sharp edges	Narrow waxy casts: **CHRONIC** ATN/ Glomerulonephritis **Broad waxy casts**: End stage renal disease (tubal dilation).
FATTY CASTS: "Maltese crosses", oval fat bodies	**Nephrotic syndrome** (due to hyperlipidemia).
HYALINE CASTS	**Nonspecific (may be seen in normal urine).** Tamm- Horsfall proteins are secreted by tubular epithelial cells.
Normal or Near Normal UA: few cells with little or no casts	<u>Acute Kidney injury:</u> **Prerenal or Postrenal.** Hypercalcemia, Multiple myeloma.
Hematuria & pyuria (excluding red cell casts)	**UTI,** acute interstitial nephritis (AIN), glomerular disease, vasculitis.
Pyuria alone	**Most common due to infection** Sterile pyuria in tubulointerstitial disease.

$$FENA\% = \frac{Urinary\ conc\ Na}{Plasma\ Na} \times \frac{Plasma\ creatinine}{Urine\ creatinine} \times 100$$

ACUTE TUBULAR NECROSIS (ATN)
- **Epithelial cell, granular or muddy brown casts**

ACUTE INTERSTITIAL NEPHRITIS (AIN)
- **White blood cell casts**

ACUTE GLOMERULONEPHRITIS (AGN)
- **Red blood cell casts, red cells**
- **Dysmorphic RBCs**
    (glomerular origin of RBCs)

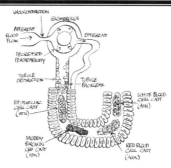

ACUTE INTERSTITIAL NEPHRITIS (AIN)

- **Tubulointerstitial nephritis: A type of intrinsic AKI characterized by an inflammatory or allergic tubulointerstitial injury** with sparing of the glomeruli & blood vessels. 10-15% of AKI.

ETIOLOGIES:

- **Drug hypersensitivity most common (70%)** — especially **NSAIDs** & selective COX-2 inhibitors, **Penicillins, sulfa drugs** (Sulfonamides, Furosemide, Thiazides), **Cephalosporins, Ciprofloxacin, Rifampin, Allopurinol, Proton pump inhibitors,** Immune checkpoint inhibitors.
- Infections (15%) — eg, Streptococcus, Legionella, CMV, EBV, HIV, RMSF, etc. Idiopathic 8%.
- Autoimmune (6%) — eg, SLE, Sjögren syndrome, Cryoglobulinemia. Sarcoidosis, GPA.

CLINICAL MANIFESTATIONS

- **Classic triad: [1] fever, [2] transient maculopapular rash,** & [3] arthralgias (all 3 only seen in 10%).

DIAGNOSIS

- **Urinalysis — white cells (sterile pyuria with positive leukocyte esterase), white cell casts, eosinophiluria, red cells, & proteinuria** [usually subnephrotic range (<3.5 g/day).
- Serum studies: **Increased creatinine, peripheral blood eosinophilia, & ↑serum IgE.**

MANAGEMENT

- **Supportive treatment: Identification & discontinuation of the offending medication mainstay of treatment** (allows for spontaneous recovery). Urgent dialytic therapy if severe.
- **Biopsy proven AIN: Corticosteroids** may be considered in select patients without improvement in renal function within 3-7 days after withdrawal of the offending drug or in severe disease.

VASCULAR

Microvascular: TTP, HELLP syndrome, DIC.

Macrovascular: Aortic aneurysm, renal artery dissection, renal artery or vein thrombosis, malignant hypertension, atheroembolic disease (associated with **ischemic digits/blue toe syndrome** or **livedo reticularis** especially post catheterization, CABG, AAA repair).

POSTRENAL AZOTEMIA (OBSTRUCTIVE UROPATHY)

- **Characterized by obstruction of the passage of urine.** Least common cause of AKI (5-10%).
- **Rare cause of Acute kidney injury because both kidneys need to be obstructed.**

ETIOLOGIES

- Etiologies vary depending on population. Postrenal causes typically result from obstruction of urinary flow. Prostatic hypertrophy is the most common cause of obstruction in older men.
- Kidney stones (eg, ureteral). External compression from tumors. Bladder outlet obstruction (Benign prostatic hypertrophy, Bladder or Prostate cancer). Sloughed off renal papillae.

DIAGNOSIS

- **Increased serum creatinine usually associated with bilateral kidney involvement.**
- Urinalysis May be relatively normal or reveal only a few white cells or red cells.
- **Renal Ultrasound: often initial imaging test to look for signs of obstruction, urinary retention, hydroureter, & Hydronephrosis** (dilatation of the collecting system in one or both kidneys).
- **Postvoid residual: postvoid residual urine >100 mL (determined by a bladder scan or via urethral catheterization if bladder scan is unavailable)** suggests postrenal Acute kidney injury and requires Renal ultrasonography to detect hydronephrosis or outlet obstruction.

MANAGEMENT

- **Removal of the obstruction (eg, catheterization) — readily reversible if corrected quickly.**
- If not corrected, it may lead to Urinary tract infections and End-stage renal disease.

HYDRONEPHROSIS

- Urinary tract obstruction leading to **dilatation of the collecting system in one or both kidneys.**
- <u>Pathophysiology:</u> characterized by **obstruction of the passage of urine.**

ETIOLOGIES:
- Kidney stones (eg, ureteral), tumors, bladder outlet obstruction (Benign prostatic hypertrophy or Prostate cancer) & sloughed off renal papillae.

CLINICAL MANIFESTATIONS
- Usually asymptomatic. Change in urine output, Hypertension, hematuria, and rarely pain.

DIAGNOSIS
- <u>UA:</u> often benign but may show hematuria. <u>Labs:</u> may have increased serum creatinine.
- <u>Ultrasound:</u> **initial imaging of choice — dilatation of the collecting system in one or both kidneys.**
- <u>CT scan:</u> indicated with those with flank pain and suspected Nephrolithiasis or in patients whom visualization of the ureters is needed.

MANAGEMENT
- **Removal of the obstruction** (readily reversible if corrected quickly). May lead to urinary tract infections and possible End-stage renal disease if not corrected.
- Patients often experience post-obstructive diuresis after relief of the obstruction.

HORSESHOE KIDNEY

- **Fusion of one pole of each kidney — most commonly fused at the lower poles.**
- **If kidney ascent into the abdomen is restricted by the inferior mesenteric artery (IMA),** which hooks over the isthmus Horseshoe kidney may develop (they are low lying). The fusion may be associated with entrapment of the inferior renal artery.

RISK FACTORS
- May be associated with other congenital urologic abnormalities (eg, **ureteropelvic junction obstruction most common,** vesicourethral reflux) or genital abnormalities (eg, bicornuate or septate uterus in girls as well as Cryptorchidism & Hypospadias in boys).
- May also be seen in Turner syndrome and Trisomy 13, 18, & 21.

COMPLICATIONS
- **Urine stasis** leads to [1] increased risk for Pyelonephritis & [2] kidney stone formation.
- **Increased risk of renal malignancies** — **Renal cell carcinoma most common** (45% of tumors), Transitional cell cancer, Wilms tumor.

CLINICAL MANIFESTATIONS
- **Majority are asymptomatic and seen as an incidental finding** (eg, antenatal ultrasound).
- **Hematuria or pain** due to urinary infection or obstruction. Renal calculi (20%).
- <u>Hydronephrosis:</u> due to vesicourethral reflux or ureteropelvic junction obstruction.

DIAGNOSIS
- **Ultrasound to detect horseshoe kidneys & evaluate for Hydronephrosis.** Serum creatinine.
- **CT urography best initial imaging to evaluate anatomy and relative renal function.**
- <u>Voiding cystourethrogram</u> to detect vesicourethral reflux (VUR).
- <u>Renal radionuclide scan</u> can differentiate true obstruction from passively dilated systems.

MANAGEMENT
- **Majority of cases require no treatment. UTI or Hydronephrosis treated with antibiotics.**
- Patients with obstruction should be referred to a urologist.

CHRONIC KIDNEY DISEASE (CKD) & END STAGE RENAL DISEASE (ESRD)

Chronic kidney disease: progressive functional decline **≥3 months** to years as evidenced by:

1. Proteinuria
2. Abnormal urine sediment
3. Abnormal serum/urine chemistries
4. Abnormal imaging studies
5. Inability to buffer pH
6. Inability to make urine
7. Inability to excrete nitrogenous waste
8. ↓ synthesis of Vitamin D/Erythropoietin

CHRONIC KIDNEY DISEASE STAGING

Stage 0: At risk patients: DM, HTN, chronic NSAID use, African American/Hispanic/Asian), age >60, SLE, s/p kidney transplant, family history of kidney disease. **Normal GFR, normal urine.**

Stage 1: Kidney damage with normal GFR (or >90)
    Kidney damage = proteinuria, Abnormal UA, serum, imaging

Stage 2: GFR 89-60

Stage 3: GFR 59-30   (3a 59-45) (3b 44-30)

Stage 4: GFR 29-15

Albuminuria
A1 = ACR <30mg/g
A2 = ACR 30-300mg/g
A3 = ACR ≥300mg/g

Stage 5: GFR <15   **End Stage Renal Disease (ESRD) = uremia requiring dialysis and/or transplant.**

Normal Glomerular filtration rate (GFR) is 120-130 ml/min/1.73 m^2

ETIOLOGIES

- **Diabetes mellitus most common cause of End-stage renal disease.**
- **Hypertension second most common cause of End-stage renal disease.**
- Glomerulonephritis, Polycystic kidney disease, Rapidly progressive glomerulonephritis, etc.

CLINICAL MANIFESTATIONS

- Most patients with stages I-IV CKD have no symptoms.
- Uremia: nausea, vomiting, fatigue, malaise, metallic taste, hiccups, altered mentation, irritability, muscle cramps, restless legs, easy bruising, fluid overload, encephalopathy, pericarditis.
- **Hypertension is the most common finding. May develop volume overload (edema).**

DIAGNOSIS

Proteinuria: **single best predictor of disease progression.**

- **Spot Urine Albumin/UCreatinine Ratio (ACR) preferred over 24-hour urine collection.** Spot test estimates grams of protein loss/day.
- Labs in advanced CKD: Increased BUN and creatinine. Hyperphosphatemia, Hypocalcemia, Hyperkalemia, and Metabolic acidosis are commonly seen as a result of advanced CKD.
- Urinalysis: abnormal sediment: may have RBC casts, WBC casts etc. **Broad waxy casts seen in ESRD** (the casts take the shape of dilated & damaged tubules). Urine dipstick
- Estimated GFR: CKD-Epi most accurate; MDRD. Cockcroft-Gault used for Creatinine clearance (eg, "renally" dosing medications excreted by the kidney).
- **Renal ultrasound: bilateral small, echogenic kidneys** (<9-10 cm) **classic in advanced CKD.** Large kidneys may be seen in diabetic nephropathy & Polycystic kidney disease.

MANAGEMENT

- Hypertension: blood pressure control reduces cardiovascular disease risk.
- **Proteinuria: ACE inhibitors or Angiotensin receptor blockers (ARBs) in early disease. SGLT2i.**
- Diabetes control: **Hemoglobin A1C goal <7.0%** if predialysis & not at risk for hypoglycemia.
- Hyperlipidemia: LDL <100 mg/dL, triglycerides <150 mg/dL, HDL >50 mg/dL.
- **Renal osteodystrophy: low serum calcium + high phosphate.** Managed by active vitamin D (Calcitriol) + phosphate binders (eg, Calcium Acetate, Calcium carbonate); Lanthanum or Sevelamer used if both calcium & phosphate levels are elevated.
- Hypocalcemia & Osteomalacia: replace vitamin D and calcium.
- Dialysis: end stage disease (stage 5), acidosis, electrolyte imbalances, ingestion, overload (volume) and uremia. Renal transplant for some end-stage renal disease.
  Dialysis indicated if GFR ≤10 mL/min and/or serum creatinine ≥8mg/dL.
  (In diabetics, if GFR ≤15ml/min and/or serum creatinine ≥6 mg/dL).

CARDIOVASCULAR COMPLICATIONS OF CHRONIC KIDNEY DISEASE

- CKD is an independent risk factor for Cardiovascular disease (CVD), especially if proteinuria is present. Of patients on dialysis, 45% will die of a cardiovascular etiology.
- **80% of patients with earlier stages of CKD will die of underlying CVD prior to progression to End stage kidney disease.**
- Modifiable risk factor management: Traditional modifiable risk factors for CVD, such as Hypertension, tobacco use, and dyslipidemia, should be aggressively treated.

HYPERTENSION

- **Hypertension is the most common complication of Chronic kidney disease (CKD);** The Hypertension tends to be progressive and salt sensitive.
- Hyperreninemic states and exogenous erythropoietin administration may worsen Hypertension.

MANAGEMENT

- **Both pharmacologic and nonpharmacologic therapy:** eg, diet, exercise, weight loss, treatment of obstructive sleep apnea. Low-salt diet (2 g/day) to reduce BP & prevent volume overload.
- **Patients with CKD and volume overload generally respond to the combination of dietary sodium restriction & diuretic therapy, often with a Loop diuretic.**

Blood pressure goals: guidelines differ in terms of goals:
- The American Heart Association recommends <130/80 mm Hg. The Kidney Diseases Improving Global Outcomes (KDIGO) committee recommends <120/80 mm Hg.
- Many advocate for standard office BP goals for higher-risk patients to be 120 to 125/<80 mmHg.

Proteinuric CKD (with or without Diabetes):

- **ACE inhibitors or Angiotensin receptor blockers (ARBs) should be included in the management of proteinuria.** Serum creatinine and potassium should be checked 7–14 days after starting these drugs or with dose adjustment. A rise of creatine ≤30% is expected & tolerable. A rise in serum creatinine >30% from baseline warrants consideration of dose reduction or drug cessation. Hyperkalemia from these medications may also warrant drug cessation, except in patients who can reliably follow a low-potassium diet, adhere to a potassium-binding resin, and be closely monitored.
- **ACE inhibitors, ARBs, & SGLT2 inhibitors help reduce hyperfiltration, which may delay progression of CKD.** SGLT2 inhibitors can slow CKD progression, even in those without diabetes or proteinuria. An initial eGFR decline is often seen several weeks after initiation of SGLT2 inhibitors, & rarely results in the need for therapy cessation because the eGFR commonly stabilizes thereafter.

ANEMIA OF CHRONIC KIDNEY DISEASE

- **Normochromic normocytic anemia due to decreased renal erythropoietin production & Anemia of chronic disease (increased Hepcidin** blocks GI absorption of iron).
- Anemia of chronic disease: low serum iron and low TIBC; Normal or high serum ferritin.
- Initial workup: thyroid function tests, serum vitamin B12 levels, reticulocyte count, and iron stores (ferritin and iron saturation).

Iron supplementation:

- **Iron supplementation: Indicated if serum ferritin is ≤100 ng/mL &/or transferrin saturation (TSAT) <20-30%.** Iron not given if serum ferritin >700 ng/mL or TSAT >30%.
- In patients with TSAT ≤20% & ferritin ≤500 ng/mL, iron is often administered prior to giving an ESA since they may respond with an increase in Hb. Iron withheld if serum ferritin >700 ng/mL.
    An ESA may not be needed if there is adequate response to iron.

Erythrocyte stimulating agents: eg, Erythropoietin, Darbepoetin

- **Erythrocyte stimulating agents: ESAs administered to most patients with CKD who have a hemoglobin (Hb) <10 g/dL, as long as the transferrin saturation (TSAT) is >20% and ferritin >200 ng/mL.** Adverse effects of ESAs: increased risk for Stroke, cardiovascular events, Hypertension, & acceleration of underlying tumor growth (if present).
- Important exceptions to ESA use include patients with active malignancy or history of Stroke.

CHRONIC KIDNEY DISEASE-MINERAL & BONE DISORDER (CKD-MBD)

- Bone disorders **(Osteitis fibrosa cystica** & **Osteomalacia)** associated with **Chronic kidney disease.**

PATHOPHYSIOLOGY
- Mineral bone disorders of CKD occur to disruptions in homeostasis of calcium & phosphorus metabolism, parathyroid hormone (PTH), active vitamin D, & fibroblast growth factor-23 (FGF-23).
- **The failing kidneys do not eliminate phosphate properly (increased phosphate) & simultaneously poorly synthesize active vitamin D [Calcitriol, 1,25(OH) vitamin D].**
- **Secondary hyperparathyroidism**: Increased phosphate and low active vitamin D [1,25(OH) vitamin D] production by the kidney lead to Hypocalcemia and compensatory increase in parathyroid hormone/PTH (secondary Hyperparathyroidism) and decreased bone mineralization by osteoclast activity (PTH pulls the calcium from the bones). This causes high bone turnover.
- Because 1,25(OH) vitamin D normally suppresses PTH production, Vitamin D deficiency leads to Secondary hyperparathyroidism due to lack of inhibition of PTH production.

CLINICAL MANIFESTATIONS
- **Osteitis fibrosis cystica: bone & proximal muscle pain in the context of uremia from high bone turnover due to Secondary hyperparathyroidism** and the effects of PTH on osteoclast activity.
- Pathologic fractures & chondrocalcinosis (calcified cartilage).
- Osteomalacia lack of bone mineralization + low bone turnover that may be seen with Vitamin D deficiency (active form), often associated with decreased serum calcium and phosphate.
- Adynamic bone disease with low bone turnover is a common bone disorder in patients on Dialysis.

DIAGNOSIS
- **Secondary hyperparathyroidism: classic triad — [1] Hypocalcemia + [2] increased phosphate + [3] increased intact PTH.** Calcium levels may be normal early on.
- Increased alkaline phosphatase. Vitamin D levels vary but are often low.
- Radiograph: **Osteitis Fibrosa Cystica: subperiosteal erosions, bony cysts** with thin trabeculum & cortex, **"salt & pepper" appearance of the skull** (punctate trabecular bone resorption in the skull).
- Biopsy: **cystic brown tumors** — describes the appearance of hemosiderin (not an actual tumor).

MANAGEMENT
- Prevention and/or treatment of Osteitis fibrosis & Renal osteodystrophy with predialysis CKD are primarily based on directly suppressing the secretion of PTH (Secondary hyperparathyroidism) via **[1] dietary phosphate restriction** (800–1,000 mg/day), followed by **[2] oral phosphate binders for persistent Hyperphosphatemia** (>5.5 mg/dL) **despite dietary restriction, &**
[3] administration of Calcitriol (or vitamin D analogs) to suppress PTH secretion.
Phosphate binders:
- **If hypocalcemic: calcium-containing binders (eg, Calcium acetate, Calcium Carbonate)** bind phosphate while supplementing calcium. Phosphate goal of <5.5 mg/dL Adverse effects: May result in a positive calcium balance, Hypercalcemia, and subsequent vascular calcification.
- **If calcium is normal: non-calcium binders (eg, Sevelamer carbonate, Lanthanum carbonate).**
- Replenish vitamin D (eg, Cholecalciferol or Ergocalciferol) unless Hyperphosphatemia or Hypercalcemia is present.
- Calcitriol in select patients: active forms of vitamin D (eg, Calcitriol/1,25[OH] vitamin D) if PTH values are persistently >150-200 pg/mL despite treatment of Hyperphosphatemia & repleted vitamin D stores.
Calcimimetics:
- Cinacalcet lowers PTH because it allosterically increases the sensitivity of the calcium-sensing receptor in the parathyroid gland to calcium, suppressing PTH secretion from a different receptor than the vitamin D receptor (can therefore act synergistically with vitamin D analogs).
- Indicated in predialysis CKD if elevated Ca^{+2} or phosphate limits the use of Vitamin D.

HYPERTENSIVE NEPHROSCLEROSIS

- **Chronic systemic HTN** increases capillary hydrostatic pressure in the glomeruli, leading to benign or malignant sclerosis (ischemia resulting from arterial and arteriolar thickening).
- **Hypertensive nephrosclerosis is the second most common cause of End-stage renal disease.**
  Diabetes is the most common of ESRD

RISK FACTORS
- African descent (due to increased presence of the *APOL1* gene mutations), longstanding Hypertension, and underlying kidney disease.

PATHOPHYSIOLOGY
- Hypertensive nephrosclerosis is seen with normal aging but is accelerated due to Hypertension.
- **In CKD, intraglomerular hypertension and glomerular hypertrophy results in compensatory adaptive hyperfiltration (overwork injury) of the remaining nephrons, which over time, results in glomerular scarring (sclerosis and interstitial fibrosis).**
- Nephrosclerosis — hypertrophic thickening of the glomerular afferent arterioles and glomeruli themselves (global or focal segmental) develops in patients with long-standing HTN.
- Results in mild to moderate increase in creatinine levels, microscopic hematuria, and mild proteinuria.

CLINICAL MANIFESTATIONS
- Patients present with a long history of Hypertension often accompanied by retinopathy and left ventricular hypertrophy and which precedes the development of either proteinuria or kidney function impairment.

Renal manifestations:
- Mild elevations in blood urea nitrogen (BUN) and serum creatinine concentrations.
- **Hyperuricemia** may be observed independent of diuretic therapy. Due to decreased renal blood flow.

Urinalysis (UA):
- **Usually benign (bland), with the sediment revealing few cells or casts.**
- **Mild proteinuria (protein excretion usually <1g/day),** hematuria, RBC and WBC casts in urine sediment. May result in Nephrotic syndrome.

Malignant:
- Markedly elevated BP (papilledema, cardiac decompensation, CNS findings).

DIAGNOSIS
- **Usually a clinical diagnosis** (often inferred from the clinical picture and exclusion of other diseases). **Biopsy is rarely required.**
- Renal ultrasound: often normal but may show small atrophic echogenic kidneys in advanced CKD.

Renal biopsy
Usually indicated in unexplained chronic kidney disease, rapid progressive decline in GFR:
- (1) Vascular: **afferent arteriolar & intimal thickening with deposition of homogeneous eosinophilic collagenous material (hyaline arteriolosclerosis)** associated with narrowing of vascular lumina of the large and small renal arteries and glomerular arterioles. (2) **glomerular: focal segmental glomerulosclerosis** or more diffuse sclerosis (sclerotic glomerulus). (3) tubulointerstitial disease: ischemia may have tubular atrophy and dilatation and interstitial fibrosis.

MANAGEMENT
- **Effective treatment of the Hypertension usually slows progression of kidney injury.**
  Nonpharmacologic: Lifestyle modification (eg, diet, sodium restriction, reduction of risk factors).
- It is not clear whether ACE inhibitors and ARBs, which are first line agents for their renoprotective effects in patients with proteinuric Chronic kidney disease, are also protective in patients with benign nephrosclerosis without proteinuria. They may not be more beneficial than other antihypertensive patients with nonproteinuric CKD.
- In advanced disease, Dialysis may be required.

AUTOSOMAL DOMINANT POLYCYSTIC KIDNEY DISEASE (ADPKD)

- **Autosomal dominant disorder** due to mutations of either genes encoding polycystin *PKD1* (85-90%) or *PKD2* (10-15%). Causes 10% of End stage renal disease (ESRD most common cause of death).
- Multisystemic progressive disorder characterized by **formation & enlargement of kidney cysts & cysts in other organs [eg, <u>liver</u> most common (50%), spleen, & pancreas].**

PATHOPHYSIOLOGY
- Vasopressin stimulates cystogenesis and eventually End stage renal disease (ESRD) over time.

CLINICAL MANIFESTATIONS
- **Most are asymptomatic; may present with Hypertension**; patients usually present in their 30s-40s.
- Renal: **intermittent abdominal, back, or flank pain**, Nephrolithiasis, UTIs, & **hematuria.**
  The pain may result from renal cyst infection, hemorrhage, or Nephrolithiasis. Renal dysfunction.
- Extrarenal manifestations: **cerebral "berry" aneurysms** can cause Subarachnoid hemorrhages in 10-15%, hepatic cysts, **<u>Mitral valve prolapse</u> (≤25%), LVH, & colonic diverticula (<u>Diverticulosis</u>).**
- Physical examination: **palpable flank masses or large palpable kidneys. Hypertension.**

DIAGNOSIS
- Urinalysis: hematuria, decreased urine concentrating ability, & subnephrotic proteinuria.
- **Renal ultrasound most commonly used diagnostic imaging test in a patient with a family history of PCKD.** Ultrasound is also used for screening family members with known PCKD.
- **CT scan (or MRI) more sensitive than Ultrasound if there is no history of PCKD.**
- Genetic testing for *PKD1* and *PKD2* mutations may be performed once diagnosed in some cases.

MANAGEMENT
- Simple cyst: observation, periodic reevaluation. **Blood pressure control: ACE inhibitors, or Angiotensin receptor blockers (ARBs) are renoprotective.**
- **Multiple cysts: supportive: increase fluid intake** at least 2 L of water daily (fluids suppress vasopressin production, reducing vasopressin-induced cystogenesis). Limited caffeine consumption. **Dietary sodium restriction:** ≤2 grams intake per day (~5 grams). **Protein reduction**: dietary protein restriction of ≤0.8 grams per kilogram of ideal body weight.
- **High-risk patients: Tolvaptan is a Vasopressin 2 receptor antagonist.** Has the most benefit on the rate of eGFR decline if high-risk; it is expensive & commonly associated with adverse effects.

	HYPOphosphatemia	HYPERphosphatemia
ETIOLOGIES	• **↑ <u>Urinary PO$_4$ excretion:</u>** **Primary Hyperparathyroidism** **Vitamin D deficiency** • **Internal PO$_4$ redistribution:** respiratory alkalosis, excessive IV Glucose, treatment for DKA, refeeding syndrome in ETOHics (insulin shifts phosphate intracellularly). • **Decreased intestinal absorption:** antacids, phosphate binders	• **Renal failure most common** **2^{ry} Hyperparathyroidism** - ↓Ca^{+2}, ↑**Phosphate**, ↑iPTH • **1^{ry} Hypoparathyroidism** - ↓Ca^{+2}, ↑**Phosphate**, ↓iPTH • Vitamin D intoxication - ↑Ca^{+2}, ↑**Phosphate**, ↓iPTH • Iatrogenic, DKA • Rhabdomyolysis, Tumor lysis
CLINICAL MANIFESTATIONS	• **Diffuse muscle weakness, flaccid paralysis (due to ↓ATP)**	• **Soft tissue calcifications** • Most asymptomatic, heart block
MANAGEMENT	Treat the underlying cause. **Phosphate repletion:** if symptomatic or serum PO$_4$ <2.0mg/dL • Potassium phosphate • Sodium phosphate	• **Renal failure: phosphate binders: Calcium acetate (PhosLo), Calcium carbonate, Sevelamer (Renagel)** • Decrease dietary phosphate: dairy products, dark colas. • Hydration, Acetazolamide

RENOVASCULAR HYPERTENSION (RENAL ARTERY STENOSIS)

- **Hypertension secondary to Renal artery stenosis** & decreased blood supply to 1 or both kidneys.
- **Most common cause of <u>secondary</u> Hypertension** and is among the most common potentially correctable causes of secondary Hypertension.

ETIOLOGIES
- **<u>Atherosclerosis</u> most common in the elderly (>65y).** >80% of cases of Renovascular hypertension.
- **<u>Fibromuscular dysplasia</u> most common cause in women <50 years** (10-20%).

PATHOPHYSIOLOGY
- **<u>Renal artery occlusive disease</u>: Decreased renal blood flow leads to activation of the renin angiotensin aldosterone system (RAAS).**
- Activation of RAAS and the subsequent increase in Angiotensin II leads to increase blood pressure via vasoconstriction, sympathetic nervous system stimulation, sodium retention (via aldosterone), and fibroblast activation-related thickening of the vascular walls.

CLINICAL MANIFESTATIONS
- **Suspect if headache & Hypertension <20-30 years (often due to Fibromuscular dysplasia) or >50-55 years (often due to atherosclerosis),** severe HTN, HTN resistant to 3 or more drugs, **<u>abdominal or flank bruit</u> or if Acute kidney injury develops after the ACE inhibitor initiation.**
- <u>Physical examination:</u> **<u>abdominal bruit</u>** seen in ~50% of patients with Renovascular hypertension.

DIAGNOSIS
- Diagnostic testing <u>only</u> indicated if a corrective measure is to be performed if clinically relevant disease is discovered (high likelihood of benefit from an invasive procedure).
- **<u>Hypokalemia</u> may be seen secondary to renal potassium wasting & stimulation of the renin–angiotensin system with secondary hyperaldosteronism.** The hyperaldosteronism results in urinary sodium retention & kaliuresis, which may manifest as Hypokalemia & slight Hypernatremia.
- **<u>Noninvasive options</u> include CT angiography, MR angiography,** & Duplex Doppler ultrasound. CT and MR angiography have better sensitivity, specificity, and anatomic detail than Ultrasonography.
- **<u>Renal catheter arteriography</u>: definitive (criterion standard).** Because it is invasive, **arteriography is reserved if imaging is equivocal, high suspicion with negative imaging findings, and patients anticipated to benefit from an intervention** (revascularization can be performed during the same procedure if stenosis is present). Not used in patients with renal failure.
  - <u>Findings</u> **may show renal artery stenosis** (significant if >70% angiographic stenosis or 50–70% angiographic stenosis associated with a resting mean pressure gradient >10 mm Hg); **"String of beads" appearance if due to Fibromuscular dysplasia.**

MEDICAL MANAGEMENT
Medical therapy is the preferred first-line treatment for Renal artery stenosis.
- **<u>ACE inhibitors or Angiotensin II receptor blockers (ARBs)</u>:** inhibits aldosterone II–mediated vasoconstriction. **However, ACE inhibitors & ARBs are used with caution if bilateral stenosis or in patients with a solitary kidney, with close monitoring of serum electrolytes and serum creatinine** because they can cause Acute kidney injury in these patients (markedly reduced renal blood flow & GFR).
- <u>Add-on hypertensive therapy</u> to ACE or ARBs include long-acting Calcium channel blockers, Thiazide diuretics (eg, Indapamide, Chlorthalidone), Beta blockers, Mineralocorticoid receptor antagonists.

SURGICAL MANAGEMENT
- **<u>Revascularization</u> definitive management** (eg, angioplasty or bypass). May be indicated if severe or inadequate response to medical therapy, recurrent unexplained CHF or pulmonary edema, creatinine >4.0, increased creatinine with ACE inhibitor treatment, >80% stenosis, bilateral disease.
- **<u>Angioplasty</u> with or without stent preferred revascularization technique in atherosclerosis & FMD.** Bypass may be performed if angioplasty is unsuccessful.

HYPERKALEMIA

ETIOLOGIES

- **Decreased renal K+ excretion** — **Kidney injury**, especially End stage renal disease. **Acute or chronic renal failure is by far the most common cause or major contributor to Hyperkalemia.**
- **Hypoaldosteronism** — Primary adrenal insufficiency (Addison disease). Drugs that block aldosterone (eg, **ACE inhibitors, Angiotensin receptor blockers, Spironolactone, Eplerenone).**
- Medications: K+ supplementation, NSAIDs, Cyclosporine, Tacrolimus, **Heparin**, Trimethoprim, other K+-sparing diuretics (Amiloride & Triamterene), Beta-blockers, **Digoxin toxicity**, Succinylcholine.
- **Tissue destruction: (releases K+ from cells)** — **Rhabdomyolysis, Tumor lysis syndrome**, severe burns, massive hemolysis, severe crush injuries.
- K+ extracellular redistribution (shift): **Metabolic acidosis** (eg, DKA), **Insulin deficiency**, catabolic states, Hyperglycemia, Mannitol, **Beta blockers**. Hyperkalemia periodic paralysis.
- **Pseudohyperkalemia: due to hemolysis** — **venipuncture** especially if the patient clenches fist during venipuncture or the tourniquette is left on too long, lab error (lysis of the cells). Patients are often asymptomatic, **thrombocytosis or leukocytosis,** & no ECG changes.

CLINICAL MANIFESTATIONS

Hyperkalemia affects muscle contraction and cardiac conduction; it does not cause seizures.
- **Neuromuscular: muscle weakness (progressive ascending),** fatigue, paresthesias, **paralysis.**
- **Cardiovascular: palpitations, cardiac arrhythmias (potentially life-threatening).**
- Gastrointestinal: abdominal distention, **ileus** (paralyzes intestinal muscles).

DIAGNOSIS

- **Rule out pseudohyperkalemia** & extracellular potassium shift from cells by confirming with **repeat laboratory testing** to rule out spurious Hyperkalemia, **especially without typical ECG changes.**
- **Serum potassium >5.0 mEq/L.** Check labs for potential causes — glucose (hyperglycemia), bicarbonate (acidosis), CBC (hemolysis), Creatine kinase (Rhabdomyolysis).
- ECG: **tall peaked T waves earliest manifestations**, QT interval shortening, **wide QRS**, prolonged PR interval, ST-segment depression, P wave flattening, **sine wave, followed by arrhythmias.**

MANAGEMENT (MILD & MODERATE):

- Most patients with chronic mild Hyperkalemia (≤5.5 mEq/L) or moderate (5.5-6.5) due to chronic kidney disease &/or the use of medications that inhibit the renin-angiotensin-aldosterone system can be managed with **dietary modifications,** diuretics (if applicable), bicarbonate therapy (if metabolic acidosis is present), **& reversal of factors that may cause Hyperkalemia** (eg, NSAIDs).

MANAGEMENT IF SIGNIFICANTLY ELEVATED (>6.5 mEq/L) or ECG changes

[1] IV Calcium gluconate to stabilize the myocardium, followed by [2] intracellular potassium shifting (eg, Insulin with glucose, Beta agonists), followed by [3] K+ elimination (diuretics, GI cation exchangers).
- **[1] IV Calcium gluconate** (or Calcium chloride) **to stabilize the myocardium — does not lower K+ levels but protects against arrhythmias** while other medications take effect. Address causes.
- **[2] Intracellular potassium shifters:**
  - **Parenteral insulin (with glucose):** IV insulin shifts extracellular potassium into cells to **rapidly lowering serum potassium. Insulin is usually given with IV Dextrose to (1) facilitate glucose entry into the cells, which also brings potassium with it and (2) to prevent Hypoglycemia from Insulin therapy** (unless glucose levels >250 mg/dL).
  - **High-dose Beta-2 agonists** are quick-acting to shift potassium intracellularly.
- **[3] K+ elimination (diuretics, GI cation exchangers):**
  - **Loop or thiazide diuretics** with IV saline may be useful to enhance renal potassium excretion.
  - **GI cation exchangers** bind potassium in the GI tract — **Sodium zirconium cyclosilicate** (works within 1 hour) **or Patiromer calcium.** Sodium polystyrene sulfonate (may cause bowel necrosis).
- **Dialysis** [preferably hemodialysis] if kidney function is severely impaired.

HYPOKALEMIA

- **Serum potassium level <3.5 mEq/L.**

ETIOLOGIES
- Hypokalemia is usually caused by [1] **Increased renal and extrarenal loss of K+ (most common),** [2] redistribution (shifting) of K+ between tissues and the ECF (increased intracellular potassium uptake), or [3] insufficient dietary potassium intake.
- **Urinary or GI potassium losses: diarrhea, vomiting,** laxative abuse, NG suction, **diuretic therapy** (including **loop diuretics, thiazides, & carbonic anhydrase inhibitors**). **Increased mineralocorticoid activity (eg, Hyperaldosteronism,** Hyperreninism, Hypercortisolism).
- **Increased intracellular K+ shift: Beta adrenergic activity (Beta-2 agonists), thyroid hormone, Insulin, & alkalosis promote Na+/K+-ATPase mediated cellular uptake of K+, leading to Hypokalemia.** Metabolic alkalosis (hydrogen ions leaves cells in exchange for potassium entering the cells), Medications: Chloroquine, Amphotericin B. Hypothermia. **Vitamin B12 and Folate treatment** (increased blood cell production results in increased K+ uptake by the new cells).
- **Hypomagnesemia** low magnesium opens magnesium-dependent potassium channels, spilling potassium into the urine. Hyperthyroidism (hypokalemic thyrotoxic periodic paralysis).
- Type I (classic distal) & type II (proximal) Renal tubular acidosis. Hyperthyroidism. Licorice.

CLINICAL MANIFESTATIONS
- Hypokalemia is usually asymptomatic but can lead to muscle weakness and cardiac arrhythmias.
- Hypokalemia affects muscle contraction and cardiac conduction; it does not cause seizures.
- **Neuromuscular — severe muscle weakness, paralysis, decreased deep tendon reflexes, ileus, constipation,** nausea & vomiting. Severe Hypokalemia may induce arrhythmias & Rhabdomyolysis.
- **Cardiovascular:** palpitations, arrhythmias (ventricular and atrial), and cardiac arrest.
- **Polyuria & polydipsia: Persistent severe Hypokalemia (eg, <3 mEq/L) induces Nephrogenic Diabetes insipidus** by impairing urinary concentrating ability of the kidney (decreased collecting tubule responsiveness to ADH). Rhabdomyolysis or myoglobinuria with Acute kidney injury.

DIAGNOSIS
- Serum electrolytes (including Magnesium levels). Mild: serum potassium level is 3-3.4 mEq/L; Moderate serum potassium level 2.5-3 mEq/L; Severe: <2.5 mEq/L.
- **ECG: T wave flattening (earliest change), followed by prominent U wave** development. PVCs & ST depressions. **QRS prolongation, prolongation of the PR and QT interval. Torsades de pointes.**

MANAGEMENT
Mild to moderate Hypokalemia:
- **Oral potassium mainstay of treatment** — eg, Potassium chloride if they have Metabolic alkalosis or normal serum bicarbonate; Potassium citrate or acetate in the presence of Metabolic acidosis.
- In patients with potassium loss due to diuretics, Amiloride (potassium-sparing diuretic) may be added. Spironolactone or Eplerenone helpful if due to Primary hyperaldosteronism.
Severe Hypokalemia:
- **Slow IV Potassium chloride given with caution & careful monitoring; reserved if [1] unable to use the enteral route, [2] if severe (K+ <2.5-3.0), or [3] symptomatic (arrhythmias, marked muscle weakness).** Potassium chloride may be given through a peripheral intravenous line at rates up to 10–15 mEq/h diluted in 0.5% or 0.9% normal saline, but higher rates (up to 20 mEq/h) require central access due to increased risk of peripheral vein irritation (burning, sclerosis, phlebitis).
- Intravenous potassium requires frequent monitoring of the plasma K+ concentration due to avoid transient overrepletion and transient Hyperkalemia.
- A saline rather than a Dextrose solution should be used for initial therapy since (Dextrose administration stimulates the release of insulin, which shifts potassium into the cells).
- **Magnesium deficiency should be corrected. It may be difficult to replete potassium in patients with concurrent Hypomagnesemia without magnesium repletion.**

HYPERMAGNESEMIA

ETIOLOGIES
- **Impaired renal Mg^{+2} excretion:** **Renal insufficiency** Chronic kidney disease (CKD) or Acute kidney injury (AKI). **Hypermagnesemia is rare in the absence of kidney failure.**
- **Lithium therapy**; Adrenal insufficiency, Primary hyperparathyroidism, DKA, Tumor lysis syndrome.

Administration of a large magnesium:
- **Excessive magnesium intake: Iatrogenic excess IV magnesium administration (eg, in the management of asthma, preeclampsia, eclampsia, Torsades de pointes, & arrhythmias.**
- **Oral ingestion** — Massive oral ingestion (eg, vitamin supplementation, antacids, laxatives, cathartics, Epsom salts, enemas). Patients with milk-alkali syndrome due to the ingestion of large amounts of calcium and absorbable alkali are more susceptible to develop Hypermagnesemia.

CLINICAL MANIFESTATIONS
- **Decreased deep tendon reflex first sign, muscle weakness,** nausea, vomiting, skin flushing, lightheadedness, ileus (GI hypomotility), somnolence, AMS, dysrhythmia, & **respiratory depression.**
- Increased magnesium levels have **calcium channel blocker-like effects: conduction defects, bradycardia, hypotension, and vasodilation** that may be refractory to fluids & pressors.

DIAGNOSIS
- Serum electrolyte levels. mild (>2.2 but <3 mEq/L); **most are symptomatic when Mg >4 mEq/L.**
- ECG: may be similar to Hypomagnesemia: prolonged QT &/or PR intervals; wide QRS complex.

MANAGEMENT
- **Mild: Discontinue excess sources of Magnesium:** If normal renal function, cessation of Mg+2-containing sources will often normalize Magnesium levels.
- **Severe: IV Calcium gluconate stabilizes the cardiac membranes** in patients with ECG changes. **IV fluids + Furosemide enhance renal Mg^{+2} excretion.** Dialysis for severe or refractory cases.

HYPOMAGNESEMIA

ETIOLOGIES
- **GI losses: intestinal malabsorption** — eg, **chronic alcoholism,** Celiac disease, small bowel bypass. Increased GI (intestinal) losses — **prolonged diarrhea or vomiting, & laxatives.** Anorexia.
- **Renal losses: thiazide & loop diuretics.** Uncontrolled Diabetes mellitus, Renal tubular acidosis.
- Endocrine: Hypoparathyroidism, Hyperaldosteronism, Hypercalcemia, pregnancy.
- Medications: **Proton pump inhibitors (>5 years use),** Amphotericin B, Cisplatin, Cyclosporine, Aminoglycosides. Patiromer (binds to magnesium in the gut).

CLINICAL MANIFESTATIONS
- **Neuromuscular hyperexcitability similar to Hypocalcemia — tetany, increased deep tendon reflexes (one of the first clinical signs), Trousseau & Chvostek signs, tremor,** muscle cramps, muscle twitching, weakness. Altered mental status, confusion, lethargy, vertigo, seizures.
- **Cardiovascular:** Hypertension, arrhythmias, palpitations. **Psychiatric: dementia or psychosis.**

DIAGNOSIS
- **Serum magnesium <1.5 mg/dL.** Hypomagnesemia can cause Hypocalcemia or Hypokalemia.
- ECG: prolonged QT interval, prolonged PR, QRS widening, atrial or ventricular fibrillation, **ventricular tachycardia, Torsades de pointes.**

MANAGEMENT
- **Mild: oral Magnesium oxide.** Diet rich in magnesium (eg, dairy products, seafood, nuts, & cereals).
- **Severe or Torsades: IV Magnesium sulfate** or chloride. Magnesium sulfate preferred in Torsades.
- **Hypocalcemia or Hypokalemia may be induced by Hypomagnesemia & may be refractory to correction until magnesium is repleted.** Hypomagnesemia suppresses PTH release.

HYPERNATREMIA

- **Increased serum sodium (>145 mEq/L)** due to **intracellular free water loss, hypotonic fluid loss** (water deficit relative to total body sodium), or less commonly, hypertonic sodium gain (iatrogenic).
- Hyponatremia does not usually occur if there is [1] an intact thirst mechanism and [2] access to water (ability to intake water); increasing osmolality stimulates thirst, water intake, & ADH secretion.
- Sustained **Hypernatremia seen when appropriate water intake is not possible or impaired (eg, infants, elderly, debilitated patients), impaired thirst mechanism,** or impaired mental status.

ETIOLOGIES: **assess volume status because volume status reflects total body sodium content:**
HYPOvolemic Hypernatremia: (loss of total body water [TBW] > sodium store depletion)
- **renal water loss:** eg, diuretics, osmotic [glycosuria (Diabetes mellitus), Mannitol, urea], renal failure.
- **extrarenal water loss**: eg, **GI loss** — **diarrhea, vomiting;** Skin loss — excessive sweating, burns; respiratory loss: — eg, mechanical ventilation, heat exposure. Vigorous exercise, fever.
ISOvolemic Hypernatremia: (free water loss + decreased water intake + normal sodium stores)
- **AVP/ADH deficiency or resistance (Diabetes insipidus).** No access to water. Vigorous exercise.
- Insensible loss: lungs (tachypnea), sweat (fever, exercise). Other: reset osmostat, Primary hypodipsia.
HYPERvolemic Hypernatremia: (sodium excess or hypertonic sodium gain) — rare.
- **Iatrogenic**: hypertonic fluid administration (eg, sodium bicarbonate, TPN, hypertonic saline). **Excess glucocorticoids**: exogenous glucocorticoids or Cushing syndrome. **Primary hyperaldosteronism.**

CLINICAL MANIFESTATIONS symptoms vary with degree and rapidity of Hypernatremia:
- **Neurological symptoms** due to **shrinkage of brain cells from dehydration (loss of cell volume)** — **thirst most common initial symptom,** confusion, lethargy, disorientation, fatigue, nausea, vomiting, weakness, hypertonia. Severe: Seizures, coma, brain damage, & respiratory arrest.
- **Findings of hypertonicity > hypovolemia: altered mentation, thirst, dry mucous membranes, Hypernatremia, increased serum osmolality.** Findings of hypovolemia > dehydration: orthostasis, elevated BUN & creatinine, **diminished urine sodium.** Both hypervolemia & dehydration (many findings overlap the two): ↓ skin turgor, oliguria, elevated urine osmolality.

DIAGNOSIS
Laboratory studies: serum osmolarity, & assess volume status; serum sodium, urine osmolarity.
- **Increased serum osmolality: Hypernatremia nearly always associated with hyperosmolality.**
- Urine sodium (UNa+): **renal loss: elevated UNa+ (>20 mEq/L); extrarenal loss: decreased UNa+ (<20, often <10).** UNa+ well above 100 mEq/L — ingestion of salt or infusion of hypertonic solution.
- **Urine osmolality:**
  - **Extrarenal water loss: high urine osmolality >600 mOsm/kg (concentrated urine).** The appropriate response to Hypernatremia & serum osmolality >295 mOsm/kg is an increase in ADH & excretion of low volumes (<500 mL/d) of concentrated urine (>600 mOsm/kg).
  - Renal water loss: UNa+ >20 & intermediate Uosm 300-600 — osmotic diuresis or AVP disorder.
  - **Hypernatremia in the setting of dilute urine (decreased urine osmolality <300 mOsm/kg) is characteristic of AVP/ADH deficiency or resistance (formerly Diabetes insipidus).**

MANAGEMENT
Correct sodium ≤0.5 mEq/L/h. **Rapid correction (>0.5 mEq/L/hr) can result in cerebral edema.**
- **Hypotonic fluids: oral pure water preferred route** or feeding tube if present. **D5W (5% Dextrose in water) is the preferred IV solution to replace water deficit.** Other: 0.45% saline, 0.2% saline.
- **Severe hypovolemia: Isotonic fluids Normal saline (0.9%) or Lactated ringers** (eg, tachycardia, low blood pressure, delayed capillary refill), **then switch to hypotonic fluids to correct Hyponatremia & fluid deficit once volume is repleted.** Mild volume depletion (eg, diarrhea or vomiting) — Hypotonic solutions containing sodium (eg, 0.45% sodium chloride with 5% Dextrose).
- Asymptomatic hypovolemic: Hypotonic solution — oral pure water or D5W (5% Dextrose in water).
- Hypervolemic Hypernatremia: [1] Diuretics (eg, Furosemide) to correct volume status PLUS [2] D5W to achieve normal sodium concentration.

HYPONATREMIA

- **Serum sodium <135 mEq/L** due to **increased free water (excess of total body water when compared to total body sodium content) due to inability of kidneys to excrete excess water.**
- Type is determined by **serum osmolality & volume status.** Symptoms vary with rapidity & degree.
- Clinically significant Hyponatremia is **hypotonic Hyponatremia.** Most common electrolyte disorder.

HYPERTONIC HYPONATREMIA:
- **Due to Hyperglycemia or Mannitol infusion.** There is a formula to correct sodium for Hyperglycemia.

ISOTONIC HYPONATREMIA:
- **Lab artifact due to hyperproteinemia or hypertriglyceridemia.** This not true Hyponatremia.

HYPOTONIC hyponatremia: clinically significant Hyponatremia. 3 types determined by volume status:
- **Hypovolemic** renal volume loss: **diuretics,** hypoaldosteronism (ACE inhibitors, Adrenal insufficiency); extrarenal volume loss — **GI loss diarrhea, vomiting,** osmotic laxatives. Burns, fever, Pancreatitis.
- **Isovolemic SIADH,** hypothyroidism, Adrenal insufficiency, reset hypothalamic osmostat, water intoxication (1^{ry} polydipsia), **MDMA (ecstasy),** low solute intake: tea & toast syndrome, beer potomania.
- **Hypervolemic edematous states — Decompensated heart failure, Cirrhosis, Nephrotic syndrome, Acute or chronic renal failure.**

CLINICAL MANIFESTATIONS
- **Neurologic symptoms: primarily due to cerebral edema** — confusion, lethargy, disorientation, fatigue, nausea, vomiting, headache, & muscle cramps. Seizures, coma, or respiratory arrest if severe.

DIAGNOSIS: 3 steps: after a low serum sodium, determine the cause & the effective treatment.
- **Step 1: measure serum (plasma) osmolality.** If true (hypotonic, low osmolality), go to step 2.
- **Step 2: assess volume status** if hypotonic/decreased serum osmolality, assess volume status to determine if hypovolemic vs euvolemic vs hypervolemic. If hypovolemic, check urine sodium.
- **Urine sodium concentration: Urine sodium <20 mEq/L indicates extrarenal loss of volume** [GI (vomiting, diarrhea), blood, or third-spacing volume loss] with preserved renal ability to hold onto sodium (water and electrolyte conservation). **Urine sodium >20 mEq/L suggests renal loss of volume** (diuretics, cortisol deficiency, and salt wasting nephropathies).
- **Urine osmolality:** Urine osmolality & Urine sodium can help distinguish between SIADH and Primary polydipsia. **Primary polydipsia or reset osmostat: low urine sodium <20 mEq/L and low urine osmolality** (<100 mOsm/L), reflecting suppressed ADH secretion. **SIADH: high urine sodium & osmolality** — urine sodium >40 mEq/L & urine osmolality >300 mOsm/L (due to ↑ADH).

MANAGEMENT
- In general, with the exception of severe cases, **correction of serum sodium >0.5 mEq/L/hour can lead to central pontine myelinolysis (demyelination),** leading to permanent neurologic damage.
- When treating Hyponatremia, it is important to consider **volume status,** degree and severity of symptoms, and duration & magnitude of the Hyponatremia. There are main 4 treatments to know:
- **[1] Isovolemic** hypotonic Hyponatremia: **water restriction** (<1L/d). Treat the underlying cause. Water (fluid) restriction is not used if the cause is secondary to Subarachnoid hemorrhage.
- **[2] Hypovolemic** hypotonic Hyponatremia: **volume repletion** — Isotonic fluids [eg, Normal **(0.9%) saline, Lactated ringers].** Treat the underlying cause.
- **[3] Hypervolemic** hypotonic Hyponatremia: **volume removal — sodium restriction ± water restriction ± diuretics if appropriate, depending on cause.** Treat the underlying cause.

[4] Hypertonic (3%) saline if intracranial pathology (eg, Subarachnoid hemorrhage) or if:
- **Severe Hyponatremia (eg, obtunded, coma, seizures, respiratory arrest): IV hypertonic saline regardless of etiology or volume status** — eg, sodium chloride 3% 100 mL IV bolus; repeated up to twice if persistent. Each bolus may raise the serum sodium 1–2 mEq/L.
- **Serum Na+ <120 mEq/L** due to ↑seizure risk — IV 3% saline beginning at a rate of 0.25 mL/kg/hour.
- **Acute Hyponatremia (<48 hours) even if asymptomatic** — 50 mL bolus of 3% saline to prevent the serum sodium from falling further.

APPROACH TO HYPONATREMIA

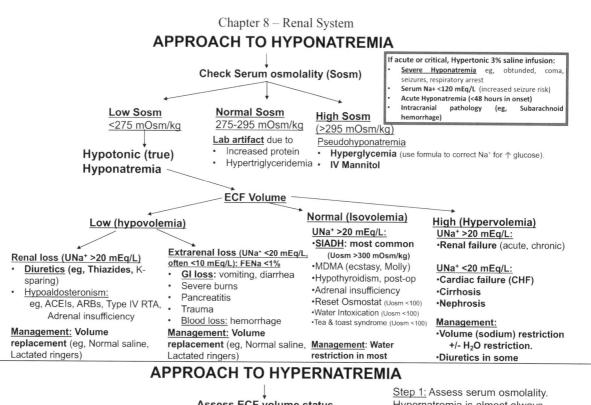

↓
Check Serum osmolality (Sosm)

If acute or critical, Hypertonic 3% saline infusion:
• <u>Severe Hyponatremia</u> eg, obtunded, coma, seizures, respiratory arrest
• <u>Serum Na+ <120 mEq/L</u> (increased seizure risk)
• <u>Acute Hyponatremia</u> (<48 hours in onset)
• <u>Intracranial pathology</u> (eg, Subarachnoid hemorrhage)

Low Sosm <u>**<275 mOsm/kg**</u>

Hypotonic (true) Hyponatremia

Normal Sosm <u>275-295 mOsm/kg</u>
Lab artifact due to
• Increased protein
• Hypertriglyceridemia

High Sosm (>295 mOsm/kg)
Pseudohyponatremia
• **Hyperglycemia** (use formula to correct Na⁺ for ↑ glucose).
• **IV Mannitol**

ECF Volume

Low (hypovolemia)

Renal loss (UNa⁺ >20 mEq/L)
• **Diuretics** (eg, Thiazides, K-sparing)
• Hypoaldosteronism: eg, ACEIs, ARBs, Type IV RTA, Adrenal insufficiency
Management: Volume replacement (eg, Normal saline, Lactated ringers)

Extrarenal loss (UNa⁺ <20 mEq/L, often <10 mEq/L): FENa <1%
• GI loss: vomiting, diarrhea
• Severe burns
• Pancreatitis
• Trauma
• Blood loss: hemorrhage
Management: Volume replacement (eg, Normal saline, Lactated ringers)

Normal (Isovolemia)
UNa⁺ >20 mEq/L:
• <u>SIADH</u>: most common (Uosm >300 mOsm/kg)
• MDMA (ecstasy, Molly)
• Hypothyroidism, post-op
• Adrenal insufficiency
• Reset Osmostat (Uosm <100)
• Water Intoxication (Uosm <100)
• Tea & toast syndrome (Uosm <100)
Management: Water restriction in most

High (Hypervolemia)
UNa⁺ >20 mEq/L:
• Renal failure (acute, chronic)

UNa⁺ <20 mEq/L:
• Cardiac failure (CHF)
• Cirrhosis
• Nephrosis

Management:
• Volume (sodium) restriction +/- H₂O restriction.
• Diuretics in some

APPROACH TO HYPERNATREMIA

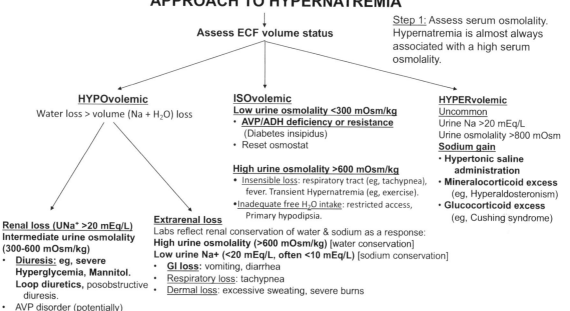

↓
Assess ECF volume status

Step 1: Assess serum osmolality. Hypernatremia is almost always associated with a high serum osmolality.

HYPOvolemic
Water loss > volume (Na + H₂O) loss

ISOvolemic
<u>Low urine osmolality <300 mOsm/kg</u>
• **AVP/ADH deficiency or resistance** (Diabetes insipidus)
• Reset osmostat

<u>High urine osmolality >600 mOsm/kg</u>
• Insensible loss: respiratory tract (eg, tachypnea), fever. Transient Hypernatremia (eg, exercise).
• Inadequate free H₂O intake: restricted access, Primary hypodipsia.

HYPERvolemic
Uncommon
Urine Na >20 mEq/L
Urine osmolality >800 mOsm
Sodium gain
• **Hypertonic saline administration**
• **Mineralocorticoid excess** (eg, Hyperaldosteronism)
• **Glucocorticoid excess** (eg, Cushing syndrome)

Renal loss (UNa⁺ >20 mEq/L)
Intermediate urine osmolality (300-600 mOsm/kg)
• **Diuresis:** eg, severe Hyperglycemia, Mannitol. **Loop diuretics,** posobstructive diuresis.
• AVP disorder (potentially)

Extrarenal loss
Labs reflect renal conservation of water & sodium as a response:
High urine osmolality (>600 mOsm/kg) [water conservation]
Low urine Na+ (<20 mEq/L, often <10 mEq/L) [sodium conservation]
• GI loss: vomiting, diarrhea
• Respiratory loss: tachypnea
• Dermal loss: excessive sweating, severe burns

HYPERVOLEMIA	HYPOVOLEMIA	ISOVOLEMIA
Jugular venous distention (↑JVP)	**Flat neck veins (↓JVP)**	Moist mucous Membranes
Hypertension	**Hypotension, delayed capillary refill**	
Peripheral and presacral edema	**Increased BUN: creatinine >20:1**	
Pulmonary edema	**UNa <20 mEq/L;** increased creatinine	Absence of signs of hyper- or hypovolemia
Decreased hematocrit & protein	Increased hematocrit & protein	
Decreased BUN: creatinine	Dry mucous membranes	
	Decreased skin turgor	

<u>**Findings of Hypovolemia:**</u>

Diminished skin turgor and dry oral mucous membranes are less than ideal markers of a decreased ECFV (hypovolemia) in adult patients because both can also be seen with dehydration (decreased cell volume).

More reliable signs of hypovolemia include decreased jugular venous pressure (JVP), orthostatic tachycardia (increase of >15–20 beats/min upon standing), and orthostatic hypotension (a >10–20 mm Hg drop in blood pressure on standing). More severe fluid loss leads to hypovolemic shock, with hypotension, tachycardia, peripheral vasoconstriction (reduced capillary refill), peripheral hypoperfusion,

	HYPOnatremia	HYPERnatremia
ETIOLOGY	• Due to ❶ impaired kidney free water excretion (*increased ADH secretion*) where the kidney is unable to make dilute urine in the setting of ❷ ↑'ed water intake. • Remember Na disorders are a problem with water handling (not total body sodium)!!	• *MC caused by net water loss* (free water loss, hypotonic fluid loss) or *hypertonic sodium gain (iatrogenic)*. • *Sustained hypernatremia seen when appropriate water intake is not possible/impaired* (ex. infants, elderly, debilitated patients) or impaired thirst mechanism.

CLINICAL MANIFESTATIONS	• Symptoms vary with degree & rapidity of hyponatremia.
	• *CNS dysfunction due to cerebral edema:* hypotonicity shifts water intracellularly ⇨ cerebral edema.
	   – Nonspecific neuro sx: fatigue, headache, nausea, vomiting, muscle cramps, lethargy, AMS, ↓DTR.
	   – Neuro Complications: seizures, coma, permanent brain damage, death, respiratory arrest.
		• Symptoms vary with degree and rapidity of hypernatremia.
		• *CNS dysfunction:* hypertonicity shifts water out of cells ⇨ *shrinkage of brain cells.*
		   – Confusion, lethargy, coma, muscle weakness, lethargy, seizures

LAB FINDINGS	• *Serum Na <135.* May order urine Na & urine osmolality.	• *Serum Na >145.* May order urine Na & urine osmolality.

MANAGEMENT	• **Hypotonic Hyponatremia:**
	   – ISOvolemic: H₂O restriction.* (<1.5L/d). Tx cause.
	   – HYPERvolemic: H₂O + Na restriction.*
	   – HYPOvolemic: normal saline (volume expansion decreases hypovolemic stimulus for ADH secretion).
	• **Hypertonic Hyponatremia: normal saline until hemodynamically stable ⇨ switch to ½ normal saline**
	• **Severe (Iso or Hyper) volemic Hyponatremia: Hypertonic saline + Furosemide*** (rapidly ↑'es Na).
		• *HYPOTONIC FLUIDS:*
		   – *Preferred route is oral* (or feeding tube if present).
		   – *Only hypotonic fluids are appropriate:* Ex. pure water orally, D5W, 0.45%NS, 0.2% saline.
		   – except for cases of frank circulatory compromise, 0.9% normal saline is unsuitable for hypernatremia!

CORRECTION	• *Correct ≤0.5mEq/L/h to PREVENT DEMYELINATION.*	• *Correct ≤0.5mEq/L/h to PREVENT CEREBRAL EDEMA.*

HYPONATREMIA

Critical hyponatremia:
Tx c̄ hypertonic saline
+ Loop diuretic

Serum ↓osm (STEP 1)

Low → HYPOTONIC HYPONATREMIA (TRUE)

Normal → Lab Error (↑Protein, ↑Triglycerides)

High → Hyperglycemia Mannitol

ECF Volume (STEP 2)

Low [HYPOVOLEMIA]

RENAL LOSS (UNa >20)
Diuretics
- Thiazides
- K-sparing
- ACE-I, ARBs
- IV RTA, Hypoaldosteronism
Mgmt: Normal Saline (correct the volume)

EXTRA-RENAL LOSS
[UNa <10], FeNa <1)
- Bleeding
- Burns
- GI (N/V, diarrhea)
Mgmt: Water restriction

Normal (ISOVOLEMIA)
• SIADH, post op
• Hypothyroidism
• Adrenal Insufficiency
• Reset Osmostat
• Water Intoxication
• 1° Polydipsia
Mgmt: Water Restriction

Una <20

High (HYPERVOLEMIA)
Una <20
• CHF, Cirrhosis
• Nephrosis

UNA >20
• Acute/Chronic Renal failure
Mgmt: H₂O/salt restriction

*Note: all will have ↑ADH
• SIADH: inappropriate
• The rest: appropriate

REVIEW OF HYPERNATREMIA

ECF Volume

❶ HYPOvolemic

Renal loss (U_Na > 20
U_osm 300–600
• Severe Hyperglycemia
• Osmotic Diuretics

Extra-renal loss (U_Na <10)
U_osm >400
• Sweating
• Resp Loss
• GI loss (N/V/D)
• Dehydration

❷ ISOvolemic
U_osm <250
• Diabetes insipidus
• Reset Osmostat

❸ HYPERvolemic
• Hypertonic Saline
• Mineralocorticoid Excess

	HYPOmagnesemia	HYPERmagnesemia
ETIOLOGIES	• **GI losses:** *Malabsorption: ETOHics,* Celiac disease, small bowel bypass, diarrhea, vomiting, laxatives. • **Renal losses:** - *Diuretics:* thiazides, loop diuretics. - Diabetes mellitus, renal tubular acidosis. - **Meds:** *proton pump inhibitors (omeprazole),* Amphotericin B, Cisplatin, Cyclosporine, Aminoglycosides.	• RARE. 2 MC causes ❶ *renal insufficiency* or ❷ *increased Mg intake* (ex. overcorrection of hypomagnesemia). ↓Mg excretion. - ***Acute or chronic renal failure:*** ↓Mg excretion. - **Iatrogenic:** excess IV Mg administration in the treatment of asthma, eclampsia, torsades de pointes. - Excess ingestion of Magnesium: vitamins, antacids, milk alkali syndrome. - Lithium toxicity, Adrenal sufficiency.
CLINICAL MANIFESTATIONS	• **Neurovascular:** AMS, lethargy, weakness, muscle cramps, vertigo, seizures, ↑DTR, tetany.* • **Hypocalcemia*:** Trousseau's & Chvostek's signs are due to impaired PTH secretion/release because magnesium is needed to make parathyroid hormone. • **Cardiovascular:** arrhythmias, palpitations (due to hypomagnesemia & associated hypokalemia).	• Nausea, vomiting, skin flushing, dizziness, muscle weakness, AMS, ↓DTR (hyporeflexive).* • Severe: hypotension, bradyarrhythmias, AV conduction blocks, respiratory depression, tachyarrhythmias.
LAB FINDINGS	• Hypomagnesemia. ± hypokalemia & hypocalcemia	• Hypermagnesemia. ± hyperkalemia & hypercalcemia
ECG FINDINGS	• *Prolonged PR & QT interval,* wide QRS, A-fib, V-fib, Ventricular tachycardia (R on T), *Torsades** R ON T PHENOMENON TORSADES DE POINTES	• Similar to hypomagnesemia Prolonged PR & QT interval, wide QRS • May show ECG signs of hyperkalemia • Arrhythmias
MANAGEMENT	**MILD** • Oral Magnesium: ex. Magnesium oxide. **SEVERE** • *IV Magnesium Sulfate.* Also used in *Torsades de pointes** Also used in hypokalemia associated with hypomagnesemia are often refractory to treatment until magnesium is repleted.*	**MILD TO MODERATE:** • *IV fluids + Furosemide* (Lasix): enhances renal magnesium excretion. Also used if severe **SEVERE:** • *Calcium Gluconate:** antagonizes the toxic effects of magnesium & stabilizes the cardiac membrane. • Dialysis in severe cases.

	HYPO kalemia	HYPER kalemia
ETIOLOGIES	• Increased urinary/GI losses: *MC causes - diuretic therapy,* *vomiting, diarrhea.* RTA: classic distal (Type I), proximal (II) • Increased intracellular shifts: *metabolic alkalosis,* β-2 agonists, hypothermia, Chloroquine use, vitamin B12 tx, insulin. • Hypomagnesemia. • Decreased potassium intake: very rare unless superimposed with another cause.	• ↓Renal excretion: *acute or chronic renal failure* (especially if on dialysis & coupled with increased K⁺ intake (ex bananas). ↓aldosterone: *hypoaldosteronism, adrenal insufficiency.* • *Meds: K⁺ supplements, K⁺-sparing diuretics, ACEI/ARB's, digoxin, β-blockers, NSAIDs,* Cyclosporine. • *Cell lysis:* rhabdomyolysis, burns, hypovolemia, thrombocytosis, tumor lysis syndrome, leukocytosis (intracellular release of K⁺ from cell lysis). • K⁺ redistribution: *metabolic acidosis** (DKA), catabolic states • *Pseudohyperkalemia: venipuncture MC,* lab error.
CLINICAL MANIFESTATIONS	• **Neuromuscular:** severe muscle weakness (including respiratory), rhabdomyolysis, *nephrogenic DI: POLYURIA** (affects renal concentrating ability) myoglobinuria, cramps, nausea/vomiting, ileus, ↓*DTR.* • **Cardiovascular:** palpitations, arrhythmias.	Serum levels & symptoms not consistent. Rapidity in serum K⁺ change influences symptoms more than levels. • **Neuromuscular:** weakness (progressive ascending), fatigue, paresthesias, flaccid paralysis. • **Cardiovascular:** palpitations, cardiac arrhythmias. • **GI:** abdominal distention, diarrhea.
LAB FINDINGS	• BMP: potassium < 3.5 mEq/L. Magnesium, glucose, bicarbonate ordered in the workup.	• *Potassium >5.0* mEq/L. Glucose, bicarbonate part of the workup. • ±CBC (hemolysis), ±CK (rhabdomyolysis).
ECG FINDINGS	• *T wave flattening (earliest change)* ⇨ *prominent U wave** ±Hypomagnesemia changes Prominent U wave	• *Tall peaked T waves** ⇨ *QR interval shortening, wide QRS,* prolonged PRI ⇨ *P wave flattening* ⇨sine wave ⇨ arrhythmias. Peaked T waves
MANAGEMENT	• *Potassium replacement:* KCl oral if possible IV KCl given for rapid treatment/severe sx. • High dose KCl given in central line. *Hypokalemia associated with ↑risk of digoxin toxicity.** • Potassium sparing diuretics: *Spironolactone, Amiloride* • *If hypomagnesemia present, it may be hard to replenish potassium (so tx hypomagnesemia)* • Use nondextrose IV solutions (because dextrose induced insulin release will shift K⁺ into cells).	Repeat blood draw to verify not from hemolysis during blood draw (since venipuncture may cause cell lysis). • *IV Calcium gluconate:* stabilizes the cardiac membrane* used for *severe symptoms, K⁺ > 6.5,* ⊕ *significant ECG findings.* Given over 30-60min. Given simultaneously with other tx for hyperkalemia. • *Insulin (with glucose): insulin shifts K⁺ intracellularly* glucose given to prevent hypoglycemia from insulin. • Sodium polystyrene sulfonate (*Kayexalate*): *enhances GI potassium excretion. Lowers total body K⁺* • *Beta₂ agonists:* 4-8 times dosing use for asthma. 12-20mg via nebulizer. • Bicarbonate: not usually given unless metabolic acidosis also present • Loop diuretics, Fludrocortisone (synthetic mineralocorticoid). • Dialysis if severe.

RENAL CELL CARCINOMA [HYPERNEPHROMA, RENAL ADENOCARCINOMA]

- **Tumor of the proximal convoluted renal tubule cells** (they are very metabolically active cells, so they are the most prone to dysplasia). Median age at diagnosis is 64 years (peak 50-70 years).
- **95% of primary tumors originating in the kidney (Clear cell most common** histological pattern).

RISK FACTORS
- **Cigarette smoking most important environmental risk factor.** Native American & Alaskan men.
- **Hypertension, obesity, dialysis;** cadmium exposure, **men,** Von Hippel-Lindau, Sickle cell disease.

CLINICAL MANIFESTATIONS
Characterized by lack of warning signs, variable presentations, and resistance to chemo & radiation.
- **Classic triad** of **[1] hematuria, [2] flank or abdominal pain, & [3] palpable abdominal or flank mass** — classically seen in locally advanced disease but only 10% of cases present with all 3.
- **Paraneoplastic syndromes: Hypertension** (↑ renin) **& Hypercalcemia common** (↑ production of PTHrP). Hypercortisolism (↑ ectopic ACTH production), **Erythrocytosis, hepatic dysfunction.**
- **Left-sided varicocele** if the tumor blocks left testicular vein drainage. Fever, malaise, weight loss.
- METS: **cannon ball metastases to the lungs** (most common site of metastasis) or bone.

DIAGNOSIS: **Abdominal CT scan** initial test. Renal ultrasound, MRI. Anemia > polycythemia.

MANAGEMENT
- **Stage I-III: Radical nephrectomy.** Immune-mediated therapy (eg, interleukin-2 and monoclonal antibody molecular targeted treatment). **Usually resistant to chemotherapy & radiation therapy.**
- In patients with localized Renal cell carcinoma (RCC) treated with nephrectomy, adjuvant immunotherapy with 1 year of adjuvant Pembrolizumab improved disease-free survival.
- Partial nephrectomy patients with bilateral involvement of solitary kidney or an option in early disease.
- **Advanced disease: molecularly targeted agents & debulking nephrectomy** — eg, Nivolumab plus Ipilimumab; Pembrolizumab plus Axtinib; Nivolumab plus Cabozantinib.

NEPHROBLASTOMA (WILMS' TUMOR)

- **Most common in children within the first 5 years of life** (almost all diagnosed by 10 years of age).
- **Most common solid renal malignancy in children (most common abdominal mass in children).**

RISK FACTORS
- May be associated with other GU abnormalities (eg, cryptorchidism, hypospadias, horseshoe kidney). **WAGR (W**ilms tumor, **A**niridia, **G**enitourinary malformations, & mental **R**etardation) due to chromosome 11 abnormalities. Denys-Drash syndrome; Loss of function mutation of tumor suppressor genes WT1 or WT2.
- Beckwith-Wiedemann syndrome: Wilms tumor, adrenal cytomegaly, hemihypertrophy.

CLINICAL MANIFESTATIONS
- **Palpable abdominal mass most common manifestation** with or without other signs or symptoms. **The mass rarely crosses the midline (unlike Neuroblastoma).**
- **Hematuria, constipation,** abdominal pain, nausea, vomiting, hypertension, anemia, anorexia, fever.

DIAGNOSIS
- **Abdominal ultrasound best initial imaging test to evaluate an abdominal mass in children.**
- CT with contrast or MRI most accurate imaging tests. Chest CT: lung is the common site for METS.
- The diagnosis of Wilms tumor is made by histologic confirmation, either at surgical excision or biopsy.

MANAGEMENT
- **Total nephrectomy with lymph node sampling, followed by chemotherapy** (eg, Dactinomycin, Vincristine, & Doxorubicin) — **80-90% cure rate.** Bilateral involvement: Partial nephrectomy.
- Post-surgery radiation therapy if it extends beyond renal capsule, pulmonary METS, or large tumor.

LUNGS: CO_2 regulation via respiratory rate (min-hours). Acidosis stimulates ↑respiration (to blow off excess CO_2). Alkalosis depresses respiration (to retain CO_2).

KIDNEYS:
- **generates new HCO_3^-** by eliminating H^+ from body (adds one HCO_3^- for every H^+ secreted).
- **reabsorbs virtually all filtered HCO_3^- at the proximal tubule.**
  ↑HCO_3^- reabsorption seen with ↑PCO_2, hypovolemia, hypokalemia.

Anion Gap Metabolic Acidosis	Non-Gap Metabolic Acidosis	Acute Respiratory Acidosis	Metabolic Alkalosis	Respiratory Alkalosis
"MUDPILERS"	**"HARDUPS"**	anything that causes hypoventilation, i.e.: "CHAMPP"	**"CLEVER PD"**	**"CHAMPS"**
Methanol	Hyperalimentation		Contraction	anything that causes hyperventilation, i.e.:
Uremia	**Acetazolamide**		Licorice*	
DKA/Alcoholic KA	Renal Tubular Acidosis		Endo* (Conn's, Cushing's)	
Propylene glycol	**Diarrhea**	CNS depression (drugs/CVA)	Vomiting	CNS disease
Isoniazid, Infection	Uretero-Pelvic Shunt	Hemo/Pneumothorax	Excess Alkali*	Hypoxia
Lactic Acidosis	Post-Hypocapnia	Airway Obstruction	Refeeding Alkalosis*	Anxiety
Ethylene Glycol	Spironolactone	Myopathy	Post-hypercapnia	Mech Ventilators
Rhabdo/Renal Failure		Pneumonia	Diuretics*	Progesterone
Salicylates		Pulmonary Edema		Salicylates/Sepsis
Too much acid or little Bicarbonate	**Too much acid or little Bicarbonate**	**Anything that decreases respiration**	**Little acid or too much bicarbonate**	**Anything that causes hyperventilation**

HIGH ANION GAP METABOLIC ACIDOSIS

- **Anion gap >12** due to accumulation of unmeasured anions. $AG = Na^+ — [HCO_3^- + Cl^-]$.
  Metabolic Acidosis: pH <7.35; bicarbonate <22 mEq/L
- ↑**Anion Gap acidosis:** the acid in blood dissociates into H^+ & an anion not routinely measured (the H^+ is buffered by HCO_3^- leaving the unmeasured anion (Ua) to accumulate in serum, creating the AG.

$$HUa + NaHCO_3 \Rightarrow NaUa + H_2CO_3 \Rightarrow CO_2 + H_2O$$

Delta ratio: If High anion gap Metabolic Acidosis is present, calculate the Delta Ratio to assess for additional disorders. Delta ratio = (Measured anion gap [AG] – 12)/(24 – measured bicarbonate)
- Delta ratio 1-2: pure elevated (high) anion gap metabolic acidosis only.
- Delta ratio <1: Normal anion gap acidosis is also present in addition to the high gap acidosis.
- Delta ratio >2: Metabolic alkalosis or compensated chronic respiratory acidosis also present.

ETIOLOGIES
"MUDPILES"
- **Methanol — visual blurring, central scotomata, and blindness common with poisoning.**
- **Uremia** (Chronic kidney disease when the GFR drops below 15–30 mL/min/1.73 m²).
- **Diabetic ketoacidosis,** fasting ketosis (relative hypoinsulinemia), alcoholic ketosis
- **Propylene glycol, Paracetamol**
- **Isoniazid, Infections**
- **Lactic acidosis: eg, sepsis, Metformin, Aspirin intoxication.**

- **Ethylene glycol (antifreeze,** windshield wiper fluid, deicing solutions, solvents). **Triad of [1] flank pain, [2] gross hematuria, and [3] oliguria (Acute kidney injury due to tubular damage** from toxic metabolites); nausea, vomiting, ataxia, AMS, nystagmus, Kussmaul respirations.
  Urinalysis (UA): **envelope- or dumbbell-shaped Ca+ oxalate crystals.** Fluorescent urine under Wood lamp. Acute kidney injury &/or Hypocalcemia may be seen.
  Ethylene glycol or Methanol: very high osmolal gap (>25 mOsm), & profound metabolic acidosis (serum bicarbonate <8 meq/L) with Ethylene glycol & Methanol.
  Management: **Fomepizole** or Ethanol. Severe (pH <7.25): sodium bicarbonate; consider dialysis.

- **Salicylates (Aspirin): may cause a mixed respiratory alkalosis (hyperventilation) + high anion gap metabolic acidosis.** Other signs of toxicity may include tinnitus, nausea, vomiting, AMS.

NORMAL (NON) ANION GAP METABOLIC ACIDOSIS (HYPERCHLOREMIC)

Anion gap <12. AG = Na$^+$ — [HCO$_3^-$ + Cl$^-$].
- **Normal Gap Acidosis:** lost HCO$_3^-$ is replaced by chloride (Cl$^-$), a measured anion, so there is no change in the anion gap formula but there is an **accumulation of Cl$^-$ concentration**. In other cases (diarrhea, type II RTA) there is loss of NaHCO$_3$ and the kidney tries to preserve volume by retaining NaCl (same overall sequelae).

$$HCl + NaHCO_3 \Rightarrow NaCl + H_2CO_3 \Rightarrow CO_2 + H_2O$$

ETIOLOGIES: "HARDUPS"
- **H**yperalimentation
- **A**cetazolamide causes renal loss of both sodium and bicarbonate via inhibition of carbonic anhydrase. Acetazolamide can be used to alkalanize the urine, which acidifies the blood.
- **R**enal Tubular Acidosis: common — type 1 (distal H$^+$ secretion issue; hypokalemia) Type 2 (proximal, loss of bicarbonate; hypokalemia), & Type 4 (hyporeninemic hypoaldosteronism & hyperkalemia). Management: **Type 1** alkali therapy (potassium bicarbonate, potassium citrate, sodium bicarbonate). **Type 2** alkali therapy (like type 1); Thiazide; **Type 4**: Fludrocortisone, dietary K$^+$ restriction.
- **D**iarrhea (acute) common cause — loss of bicarbonate-rich fluid from the small intestine.
- **U**retero-Pelvic Shunt (fistula) or Ureteral diversion (eg, ileal loop).
- **P**ost-Hypocapnia or Pancreatic fistula (due to pancreas releasing bicarbonate-rich fluid).
- **S**pironolactone inhibits the aldosterone receptor, which results in retention of hydrogen ions and potassium at the expense of renal sodium excretion (normally, aldosterone causes sodium retention & renal potassium & hydrogen ion excretion). **Saline (0.9%) in large amounts** (dilutional acidosis).

METABOLIC ALKALOSIS

- **Metabolic alkalosis:** ↑ serum HCO$_3^-$ (>26) & ↑ pH >7.45; requires generating & maintenance factors.
- [1] "Generation" due to loss of acid or gain of alkali; [2] "maintenance" from the kidney's inability to excrete the excess bicarbonate.
- Calculation of expected CO2 compensation: Expected PCO$_2$ = (0.7 × HCO3$^-$) + 20 ± 2.

ETIOLOGIES (GENERATING FACTORS) "CLEVER PD"
- **[1] Loss of H$^+$ from GI tract/kidneys: vomiting or NG suction (loss of gastric HCl$^-$** perpetuated by EFCV depletion), chronic diarrhea (perpetuated by EFCV depletion), **Loop & thiazide diuretics.**
- **[2] Exogenous alkali or contraction alkalosis:** diuresis ⇨ excretion of HCO$_3^-$-poor fluid ⇨extracellular fluid volume (EFCV) "contracts" around a stable level of HCO$_3^-$ ⇨ ↑HCO$_3^-$ concentration.
- **[3] Post hypercapnia:** rapid correction of respiratory hypercapnia (eg, mechanical ventilation) ⇨ transient excess HCO$_3^-$ until the kidney can excrete it.
- **C**ontraction
- **L**icorice (glycyrrhizic acid activates mineralocorticoid receptor: hypokalemia & metabolic alkalosis).
- **E**ndocrine: **Hyperaldosteronism** [eg, Conn syndrome (adrenal adenoma), Cushing syndrome]
- **V**omiting: due to loss of hydrochloric acid produced in the stomach in the vomitus.
- **E**xcess Alkali (eg, Milk-alkali syndrome)
- **R**efeeding Alkalosis (addition of bicarbonate in alimentation therapy)
- **P**ost-hypercapnia
- **D**iuretics — eg, **Loop diuretics, Thiazide diuretics**

Urinary chloride concentration differentiates saline responsive vs. saline unresponsive alkalosis:
- **Decreased urine chloride (<20 mEq/L) Metabolic alkalosis in the setting of hypovolemia: Saline responsive: vomiting & NG aspiration (low end); Diuretics (thiazides, loops) higher end. Treat the hypovolemia with volume expansion (eg, Normal saline [sodium chloride]).**
- **Increased urine chloride (>20 mEq/L** [often >40]): patients who are ECFV-expanded: **Saline unresponsive: excess mineralocorticoids** (eg, Hyperaldosteronism, Cushing syndrome) — often associated with Hypertension, Hypokalemia, Metabolic alkalosis, & mild Hypernatremia.

RESPIRATORY ACIDOSIS (HYPERCAPNIA)

Hypoventilation causes the lungs retain CO_2 (hypercapnia), resulting in a lowering of the pH.
- **Respiratory Acidosis: pH <7.35; $PaCO_2$ >45 mmHg.**

Compensation: complete metabolic compensation by the kidney usually takes a few days. In
Acute respiratory acidosis: HCO_3^- increases by 1 mEq/L for every 10 mm Hg increase in PCO_2.
Chronic respiratory acidosis commonly occurs with underlying pulmonary disease (eg, COPD).
Renal excretion of acid as NH_4Cl results in compensatory metabolic alkalosis:
HCO_3^- increases by 3 mEq/L for every 10 mm Hg increase in PCO_2.

ETIOLOGIES
Any condition that decreases the respiratory rate (hypoventilation).
- **Acute Respiratory failure: CNS depression** (opioids, sedatives, trauma), cardiopulmonary arrest, pneumonia.
- **Chronic respiratory failure:** COPD, obesity, neuromuscular disorders (eg, Myasthenia gravis, Guillain-Barré syndrome, etc.).

Any condition that decreases the respiratory rate:
- "CHAMPP"
- **CNS depression — eg, medications, stroke, opioid intoxication**
- **H**emo/Pneumothorax
- **A**irway Obstruction
- **M**yopathy
- **P**neumonia
- **P**ulmonary Edema

CLINICAL MANIFESTATIONS
- **Acute-onset respiratory acidosis:** fatigue, somnolence, confusion, mental status changes, asterixis, and myoclonus.
- **Severe hypercapnia increases cerebral blood flow & increases intracranial & CSF pressure. Papilledema and seizures may occur as a result.**

MANAGEMENT
- Treat the underlying cause; Severe or refractory: may require noninvasive or mechanical ventilation.
- **Opioid overdose:** if opioid overdose is known or suspected with no other etiology for hypoventilation, **IV Naloxone** may be administered for diagnosis & or therapy.

RESPIRATORY ALKALOSIS (HYPOCAPNIA)

Respiratory Alkalosis: pH >7.45 & $PaCO_2$ <35 mm Hg, often with an **increased respiratory rate.**
- **With hyperventilation, the lungs blow off excess CO_2, resulting in an increased pH.**
- **Acute hyperventilation symptoms: anxiety, perioral numbness, paresthesias.** Tetany results from a low ionized calcium because severe alkalosis increases albumin and calcium binding.

ETIOLOGIES
CHAMPS
- **C**NS disease
- Hypoxia, **H**epatic failure
- Anxiety, **A**sthma
- **M**echanical ventilation
- **P**rogesterone during pregnancy stimulates the respiratory center. **P**neumonia, **P**E
- **S**alicylates/Sepsis. **Salicylates directly stimulate respiration (can present with a mixed respiratory alkalosis + high anion gap metabolic acidosis), especially with alkalemia.**

MANAGEMENT
- Treat the underlying cause. Hyperventilation is usually self-limited since muscle weakness caused by respiratory alkalemia will suppress ventilation.

SIMPLIFIED 3-STEP APPROACH TO ACID BASE DISORDERS

Normal Values: Na: 135-145; Cl: 105, HCO_3^- : 24 (22-26); P_{CO2} = 40 (35-45); AG 10-12; pH: 7.35-7.45, PO_2: 80-100

Step 1: **Identify the most _apparent_ disorder** ✓pH

pH normally 7.35–7.45. If in normal range, still check PCO_2 & HCO_3. If abnormal, a disorder may be present.

> ➤ **If pH >7.45** ⇨ **Alkalosis**
> ➤ **If pH <7.35** ⇨ **Acidosis**
> ➤ If pH is within normal range (high normal or low normal) in the setting of abnormal PCO2 &/or Bicarbonate levels, a fully compensated disorder may be present.

Step 2: **Look at PCO_2 is it normal, low, or high??**
Normal PCO_2 35-45

- **If PCO_2 is in going in the opposite direction as the pH, then the 1ʳʸ disorder is respiratory.**
- Think **RO**ME (In primary **R**espiratory disorders, PCO_2 & pH are in **O**pposite directions).
- Respiratory compensation: in primary metabolic disorders, if the PCO_2 is going in the same direction as the pH, then there is partial respiratory compensation (full compensation if the pH is normal).

Step 3: **Look at [HCO_3^-] it normal, low, or high?**
Normal [HCO_3^-] is 22-26

- **If [HCO_3^-] is in going in the same direction as the pH, then the 1ʳʸ disorder is metabolic.**
- Think RO**ME** (In primary **M**etabolic disorders, HCO_3 & pH are in the same/**E**qual direction).
- Metabolic compensation: in primary respiratory disorders, if the [HCO_3^-] is going in the opposite direction as the pH, then there is a partial metabolic compensation (full compensation if the pH is normal).

Perform step 4 & 5 ONLY if the primary disorder is metabolic acidosis.

Step 4: If Metabolic acidosis is present, calculate the anion gap.
Anion gap (AG) = Na - (Cl⁻ + HCO3⁻). Normal anion gap 10-12

Step 5: **If a high anion gap is present in step 4, perform step 5 — calculate the Delta ratio to look for the presence of additional disorders.**

Delta ratio: (Measured AG – 12)/(24 – measured bicarbonate)

[Measured anion gap – Normal AG (use 12)]

Normal bicarbonate [HCO_3^-] use 24 – measured bicarbonate [HCO_3^-]

- If 1-2 ⇨ a pure elevated anion gap metabolic acidosis only is present.
- <1 ⇨ normal anion gap metabolic acidosis is also present.
- >2 ⇨ metabolic alkalosis or compensated chronic respiratory acidosis is also present.

EXAMPLE 1: 21-year-old with Type I DM presents with nausea vomiting, and fruity breath.

pH: 7.29   paCO2: 22   HCO3: 13   Na: 134 Cl: 91 HCO3: 12

CASE 1: pH: 7.45   paCO2: 56   HCO3: 37

CASE 2: pH: 7.29   paCO2: 58   HCO3: 22

CASE 3: pH: 7.32   paCO2: 34   HCO3: 14   Na: 135 Cl: 109 HCO3: 14

CASE 4: pH: 7.49   paCO2: 42   HCO3: 36

CASE 5: pH: 7.36   paCO2: 58   HCO3: 29

CASE 6: pH: 7.25   paCO2: 25   HCO3: 10   Na: 140 Cl: 77 HCO3: 10

CASE 7: pH: 7.48   paCO2: 28   HCO3: 18

CASE 8: pH: 7.28   paCO2: 26   HCO3: 11   Na: 129 Cl: 100 HCO3: 10

EXAMPLE 1 explained: 21-year-old with Type I DM presents with nausea vomiting, and fruity breath.

Na: 134   Cl: 91   BUN: 29   pH: 7.29   pCO2: 22
K: 5.8   HCO3: 13   Cr: 1.6   HCO3: 12   glucose: 780

Step 1: **Identify the most *apparent* disorder** ✓pH

pH normally 7.35 – 7.45. **pH = 7.29** ↓⇨*Acidosis*

Step 2: **Look at P$_{CO2}$ is it normal, low, or high??**

Normal P$_{CO2}$ 35–45. **pCO2: 22**↓   Normal [HCO$_3^-$] 22-26. **HCO3: 12**↓

- Think RO**ME** (In primary **M**etabolic disorders, HCO3 & pH are in the same/**E**qual direction)
  = ***primary metabolic acidosis.***
- In primary metabolic disorders, if the P$_{CO2}$ is going in the same direction as pH (which it is in this example), then there is partial respiratory compensation.

Perform step 4 & 5 ONLY if a metabolic acidosis is the primary disorder (which it is in this example)

Step 4: If metabolic acidosis is present, calculate the anion gap.

AG = Na - (Cl⁻ + HCO3⁻) Normal anion gap 10 – 12. 134 – (91 + 13) = 30 = ↑*AG acidosis*

Step 5: If high anion gap is present, calculate the **Delta Ratio** to look for the presence of additional disorders.

(Measured AG – 12)/(24 – measured bicarbonate) (30-12)/(24-13) = **1.64**

- If 1-2 = **pure elevated anion gap metabolic acidosis = final answer** (probably DKA in this case).

ANSWERS

Case 1: Primary Metabolic Alkalosis with full respiratory compensation (normal pH)

Case 2: Primary Respiratory Acidosis uncompensated (since HCO3 is normal)

Case 3: Normal Gap Metabolic Acidosis with partial respiratory compensation.

Case 4: Primary Metabolic Alkalosis uncompensated (since PCO2 is normal)

Case 5: Primary Respiratory Acidosis with full metabolic compensation (normal pH)

Case 6: Mixed disorder: Primary elevated anion gap acidosis + metabolic alkalosis (delta >2).

Case 7: Primary Respiratory Alkalosis with partial metabolic compensation.

Case 8: Primary high anion gap metabolic acidosis with partial respiratory compensation + concurrent non anion gap acidosis (since delta <1)

RENAL TUBULAR ACIDOSIS (RTA)

- Renal tubular dysfunction that results in a hyperchloremic normal anion gap metabolic acidosis in otherwise well-functioning kidneys (relatively normal glomerular filtration rate).
- **Proximal (Type 2) failure to reabsorb bicarbonate in the proximal tubule (bicarbonate wasting):** **Multiple myeloma (light chain gammopathy),** Fanconi syndrome, Carbonic anhydrase II deficiency, <u>Meds:</u> **Acetazolamide, Topiramate,** Ifosfamide. Heavy metals (mercury, cadmium, copper, lead), Wilson disease.
- <u>Distal (Type 1)</u> **impaired acid secretion (urine acidification) into distal tubule: Sjögren syndrome, Rheumatoid arthritis, hypercalciuria,** Toluene (glue sniffing); <u>Meds:</u> Lithium, Ifosfamide, Amphotericin B.
- <u>Type 4 (hyporeninemic hypoaldosteronism)</u> inability to remove enough potassium, interfering with kidney's ability to remove acid: **Diabetic nephropathy resulting in Chronic kidney disease,** Mineralocorticoid deficiency, **Sickle cell disease, Systemic lupus erythematosus,** Medications (eg, Heparin, ACE inhibitors, ARBs), Cyclosporine, TMP-SMX, Potassium sparing diuretics.

TYPE	PATHOGENESIS	SERUM K⁺	Serum Ca	URINE PH	Nephrolithiasis
2: Proximal	↓ bicarbonate reabsorption in the proximal tubule	Low	Normal	≤5.3 Variable	No
1: Distal (distal tubule)	**Defective hydrogen secretion** (H+/K+ antiporter)	Low	**High**	**≥5.5** UNa >25	**Yes**
4: hyporeninemic hypoaldosteronism	**Hyperkalemia** results in ↓ ammonia (NH3) synthesis in the proximal tubule.	**High**	Normal	<5.5 Variable	No

- <u>Management:</u> **Type 1** alkali therapy (potassium bicarbonate, potassium citrate, or sodium bicarbonate). **Type 2** alkali therapy (similar to type 1); Thiazide; **Type 4**: Fludrocortisone, dietary K⁺ restriction.

CLASSIC BONE DISEASES				
RESULT	CALCIUM	PHOSPHATE	PTH	ALKALINE PHOSPHATASE
HYPOPARATHYROIDISM	• Decreased	• Increased	• Decreased	• Increased
PRIMARY HYPERPARATHYROIDISM	• Increased	• Decreased	• Increased	• Increased
SECONDARY HYPERPARATHYROIDISM Associated with RENAL OSTEODYSTROPHY	• Decreased	• Increased	• Increased	• Increased
OSTEOMALACIA Due to Vitamin D deficiency	• Decreased or normal	• Decreased or normal	• Increased	• Increased
OSTEOPOROSIS	• Normal	• Normal	• Normal	• **Normal** • May increase with an acute fracture
PAGET DISEASE OF THE BONE	• Normal	• Normal	• Normal	• **Markedly elevated**

RENAL PHOTO CREDITS

Membranous nephropathy:
Nephron, CC BY-SA 3.0 <https://creativecommons.org/licenses/by-sa/3.0>, via Wikimedia Commons

Focal segmental glomerulosclerosis
Nephron, CC BY-SA 3.0 <https://creativecommons.org/licenses/by-sa/3.0>, via Wikimedia Commons

Postinfectious glomerulonephritis:
Nephron, CC BY-SA 3.0 <https://creativecommons.org/licenses/by-sa/3.0>, via Wikimedia Commons

Goodpasture syndrome:
Nephron, CC BY-SA 3.0 <https://creativecommons.org/licenses/by-sa/3.0>, via Wikimedia Commons

CHAPTER 9 – GENITOURINARY SYSTEM (MALE AND FEMALE)

URGE INCONTINENCE (OVERACTIVE BLADDER)

- Involuntary urine leakage preceded by or accompanied by a sudden urge to urinate due to uninhibited bladder contractions.
- **Most common cause of established incontinence in older adults** (two-thirds of cases).
- <u>Risk factors</u>: Increased age, idiopathic, & bladder infection (eg, cystitis).

PATHOPHYSIOLOGY
- **Detrusor muscle overactivity:** detrusor muscle is stimulated by muscarinic acetylcholine receptors. **Detrusor overactivity leads to uninhibited (involuntary) detrusor muscle contractions during bladder filling.**

CLINICAL MANIFESTATIONS
- **Increased urgency with no warning, frequency, small volume voids, & nocturia.**
- **Urgency: Sudden strong urge to void with an inability to make it to the bathroom in time** (urinary leakage after the onset of an intense urge to urinate that cannot be forestalled).
- Men have similar symptoms, but detrusor overactivity & urethral obstruction from BPH often seen.

WORKUP
- <u>Urinalysis & microscopy:</u> Because urinary tract infection is a common reversible cause, Urinalysis with Urine culture is appropriate for most patients. Urine cytology & cystoscopy if tumor is suspected.

MANAGEMENT
Conservative:
- **Bladder training cornerstone of treatment** (75% improvement). Patients start by voiding on a schedule based on the shortest interval recorded on a bladder record; gradual lengthening of the interval between voids by 30 minutes each week using relaxation techniques to postpone the void urge.
- **Lifestyle modifications & Kegel exercises: Trial of pelvic floor muscle strengthening (Kegel exercises)** can decrease the frequency of incontinence, **lifestyle therapy & behavioral changes** (eg, decreased fluid intake; avoidance of spicy foods, citrus fruit, chocolate, alcohol, & caffeine).
- Adjunctive medication if initial treatments do not provide sufficient symptom relief or if patients prefer pharmacotherapy.
- **Beta-3 adrenergic agonists & antimuscarinic agents are the primary medical options.**

Beta-3 agonists (Mirabegron, Vibegron)
- <u>Mechanism of action</u>: detrusor muscle relaxation with similar efficacy but less incidence of adverse effects compared to the antimuscarinics.
- <u>Adverse events:</u> headache, GI effects (nausea, diarrhea, constipation), rhinorrhea, nasopharyngitis. Urinary retention. Hypertension with Mirabegron (avoid in if uncontrolled Hypertension).

Antimuscarinic (anticholinergic) agents:
- **Trospium or Darifenacin. Tolterodine (short- & long-acting), Fesoterodine, Oxybutynin, Solifenacin, Propiverine.**
- <u>Mechanism of action:</u> Anticholinergics block muscarinic receptor stimulation by acetylcholine, reducing smooth muscle contraction of the bladder. This leads to increased bladder capacity.
- <u>Common adverse effects:</u> dry mouth, dry eyes, constipation, blurred vision for near objects, tachycardia, drowsiness, & decreased cognitive function. Older adults are at increased susceptibility to adverse drug reactions. Avoid anticholinergics in patients with Myasthenia gravis or Glaucoma.

Third-line therapies:
- Noninvasive office-based acupuncture-like nerve stimulation.
- **Botulinum toxin A** office-based injections of **Onabotulinum toxin A (Botox)** into the detrusor muscle. Effective and associated with increased resolution of symptoms compared to medications but may lead to urinary retention and the need for self-catheterization and urinary tract infections.
- Surgically implanted nerve stimulation devices (SNM), including electrical stimulation (percutaneous tibial nerve stimulation).
- <u>Surgical</u>: bladder augmentation increases bladder compliance, sling procedures, or urethropexy.

OVERFLOW INCONTINENCE

- **Urinary retention & incomplete bladder emptying** leads to involuntary urine leakage once the bladder is full (it overflows).

PATHOPHYSIOLOGY
- Overflow urinary incontinence is caused by [1] bladder detrusor muscle underactivity (impaired contractility) or [2] bladder outlet or urethral obstruction, resulting in leakage from a full bladder.

ETIOLOGIES
[1] Bladder detrusor muscle underactivity (bladder atony):
- **Neurological disorders or autonomic dysfunction** — **peripheral neuropathy** (eg, Diabetic neuropathy, vitamin B12 deficiency, alcoholism), **damage to spinal detrusor efferent nerves** (eg, Multiple Sclerosis, spinal injuries, spinal stenosis), low estrogen state (vaginal atrophy). Stroke.
- **Anticholinergics** (eg, tricyclic antidepressants, antihistamines, antimuscarinics) relax the detrusor muscle, increase bladder capacity, and cause urinary retention.

[2] Bladder outlet or urethral obstruction:
- **Benign prostatic hypertrophy;** external compression of the urethra (eg, Uterine fibroids, pelvic organ prolapse, urethral stricture, or overcorrection of the urethra from prior pelvic floor surgery). Prostate cancer, fecal impaction.

CLINICAL MANIFESTATIONS
- **Loss of urine with no warning** (as in urge) **or no triggers** (as in stress). May be continuous.
- **(1) continuous urinary leakage: continuous urinary leakage or constant dribbling of small volumes of urine.** Leakage often occurs with changes in position, especially if the bladder is full.
- **(2) incomplete bladder emptying, weak or intermittent urinary stream, hesitancy, frequency, & nocturia.**

Physical examination:
- **Neuropathy (if due to bladder underactivity):** may have **decreased perineal sensation.**
- Urinary retention: palpable lower abdominal mass (due to persistently full bladder).
- **Increased post void residual (PVR) >150-200 ml** or >1/3 total volume.

DIAGNOSIS:
- Clinical. Increased post void residual (PVR) >150-200 ml or >1/3 total volume.
- Bladder ultrasound: enlarged bladder. Urodynamic testing in selected patients (not usually needed).

MANAGEMENT
- Management focuses on addressing the underlying cause (eg, medication changes, lifestyle modifications, correction of prolapse).

MANAGEMENT OF BLADDER ATONY
- **Intermittent or indwelling catheterization first-line treatment.**
- **Cholinergics** (eg, **Bethanechol**) — increase detrusor muscle activity.

MANAGEMENT OF BPH:
- **Alpha adrenergic blockers for rapid symptom relief** (eg, **Terazosin, Prazosin, Tamsulosin**). Frequent toileting, double voiding, and suprapubic pressure may be helpful.
- **5-alpha reductase inhibitors** (eg, **Finasteride**) may provide additional benefit in men with prostate enlargement.
- Decompression: If medical therapy fails to allow for adequate bladder emptying, surgical decompression is an alternative. For the nonoperative candidate with urinary retention, intermittent or indwelling catheterization may be an option.
- For the patient with a poorly contractile bladder, augmented voiding techniques (eg, double voiding, suprapubic pressure) may be beneficial.

STRESS INCONTINENCE

Outlet incompetence:
- Involuntary leakage of urine that occurs once **increased abdominal pressure** (eg, exertion, coughing, laughing, sneezing) **> than urethral pressure** & resistance to urine flow.
- **Most common type of incontinence in younger women (highest incidence 45–49 years).**

ETIOLOGIES
- **Laxity of the pelvic floor muscles (eg, childbirth, surgery, postmenopausal estrogen loss, urologic procedures).** Although rare in men, post prostatectomy may be associated with Stress incontinence.
- **Urethral hypermobility** — insufficient support from the pelvic floor musculature and the vaginal connective tissue to the urethra & the bladder neck. Dysfunction of the urethral sphincter.

CLINICAL MANIFESTATIONS
- **Urine leakage during times of increased intra-abdominal pressure** — eg, coughing, laughing, sneezing, straining, lifting heavy objects, or exercising.
- There is no urge to urinate prior to leakage (as in Urge incontinence) or constant dribbling of urine (as in Overflow incontinence).
- Testing can be performed by asking patient to cough firmly while he or she has a full bladder. Instantaneous leakage of urine is highly suggestive of Stress incontinence.

MANAGEMENT
The initial management of Stress incontinence includes:
- **Pelvic floor muscle strengthening (Kegel) exercises: initial treatment of choice for mild to moderate Stress incontinence.** Instruct the patient to pull in the pelvic floor muscles and hold for 6–10 seconds and to perform three sets of 8–12 contractions daily.
- Kegel exercise can be supported with biofeedback, electrical stimulation, bladder training (eg, timed voidings).
- **Lifestyle modifications: used in conjunction with pelvic floor exercises** — protective garments & pads, weight loss, smoking cessation, & decreased intake of caffeine, alcohol, & fluid.
Other management:
- Genitourinary syndrome of Menopause: Topical vaginal estrogen if due to Vaginal atrophy.
- Pessaries or vaginal weighted cones may be helpful in some women (eg, incomplete efficacy with lifestyle changes & muscle strengthening or situational stress incontinence) but should be prescribed only by providers with experience using them and with patient education.
- **Surgery: (eg, midurethral sling) — higher success rates** (96%) **than conservative therapy but often reserved for individuals not responsive to conservative and nonsurgical therapy.** More rapid & definitive treatment.
Medications not usually helpful:
- No medications are approved for the treatment of Stress incontinence, and a clinical practice guidelines from the American College of Physicians recommends against pharmacologic treatment.
- Alpha-agonists (eg, Midodrine & Pseudoephedrine) are only mildly efficacious.

UTERINE PROLAPSE

- Uterine herniation into or beyond the vagina.
- Risk factors: **weakness of pelvic support structures: most common after childbirth** (especially traumatic), increased pelvic floor pressure: multiple vaginal births, obesity, repeated heavy lifting, increased age, constipation.

CLINICAL MANIFESTATIONS

- Pelvic or vaginal fullness, pressure, heaviness, bulging, or "falling out" sensation (eg, protrusion of tissue from the vagina). Low back pain, abdominal pain.
- Symptoms may be worse with prolonged standing and relieved with lying down.
- Urinary urgency, frequency, or stress incontinence. Sexual dysfunction.

PHYSICAL EXAMINATION

Bulging mass especially with increased intrabdominal pressure (eg Valsalva).
- Grades: 0 (no descent) to 4 (through the hymen).
- **Grade 0: no descent**
- Grade 1: uterus descent into the upper 2/3 of the vagina
- Grade 2: the cervix approaches the introitus
- Grade 3: the cervix is outside the introitus
- **Grade 4: entire uterus is outside of the vagina – complete rupture**

May be accompanied by
- **Cystocele:** posterior bladder herniating into the **anterior vagina,**
- **Enterocele:** pouch of Douglas – small bowel herniating into the **upper vagina,** or
- **Rectocele:** distal sigmoid colon or rectum herniating into the **posterior distal vagina.**

MANAGEMENT

- **Kegel exercises (pelvic floor muscle exercises),** behavioral modifications, weight control.
- Vaginal pessaries elevate & support the uterus. Estrogen treatment may improve atrophy.
- Treatment is generally not indicated for women with asymptomatic prolapse.

Surgical management:
- Hysterectomy or uterus-sparing techniques including uterosacral or sacrospinous ligament fixation.
- Vaginal and abdominal approaches (open, laparoscopic, or robotic) and with and without graft materials.

PEYRONIE DISEASE

- **Acquired localized fibrotic changes of the tunica albuginea leading to abnormal penile curvature.**

PATHOPHYSIOLOGY

- The cause of excessive collagen (fibrous tissue) is unknown but contributing factors include penile trauma (eg, sexual activity with a semi rigid phallus), tissue ischemia, & genetic susceptibility.

CLINICAL MANIFESTATIONS

- **Penile pain** especially with erections, **curvature, induration, shortening &/or sexual dysfunction.**
- Palpable fibrous scar tissue plaques along the dorsum penile shaft. Affects up to 10% of men.

MANAGEMENT

- Observation: **urologist referral. Observation is an option for mild curvature (≤30 degrees)** in men with satisfactory erectile function. Medical and/or surgical management may be needed if worsening of mild curvature or if sexual dysfunction occurs.
- **Medical or surgical management:** if curvature ≥30 degrees or associated with sexual dysfunction.
  Within 3 months of onset: Oral Pentoxifylline is a nonspecific phosphodiesterase inhibitor that decreases transforming growth factor beta-1-mediated fibrosis, prevents deposition of collagen type I, and reduces calcification. Surgery is an alternative for severe or refractory disease.
  >3 months: Intralesional injection with collagenase _Clostridium histolyticum,_ followed by penile traction therapy. Surgery is an alternative for severe or refractory disease.

VESICOURETERAL REFLUX (VUR) & REFLUX NEPHROPATHY

- **Retrograde passage of urine from the bladder into the upper urinary tract, increasing infection risk.**
- Normally, the ureterovesical junction (UVJ) allows urine to enter the bladder but prevents retrograde flow of urine into the ureter, especially during voiding. This protects the kidney from high pressure in the bladder and from contamination by bacteria in the urine from the bladder.

TYPES
- **Primary VUR: anatomic deficiencies of the ureterovesical junction (UVJ)** [eg, inadequate closure of or incompetent UVJ] that contains a segment of the ureter within the bladder wall. Low-grade reflux (grades I, II) associated with high rate of spontaneous resolution. **Most common type of VUR.**
- Secondary VUR: due to abnormally high voiding pressure in the bladder that leads to failure of the closure of the UVJ during bladder contraction or altered voiding habits (inhibiting the urge to void).

CLINICAL MANIFESTATIONS
- **Prenatal presentation** — antenatal Hydronephrosis seen on **prenatal ultrasound**.
- **Postnatal presentation** — **febrile illness or UTI.** Children with VUR are at risk for recurrent febrile or symptomatic UTIs, (the risk increases with the severity of VUR). Many are asymptomatic. In older children, symptoms may include chills, high fever, flank pain, nausea and vomiting, and/or lower urinary tract symptoms (eg, dysuria, hematuria, urgency, or incontinence).

DIAGNOSIS
Prenatal presentation:
- **Initial postnatal renal Ultrasound is performed in all patients with prenatal Hydronephrosis.**
- VCUG is performed in infants with persistent postnatal abnormal ultrasound findings (eg, urinary tract dilation) or who develop a UTI.

Postnatal presentation:
- **Renal & bladder Ultrasound often the initial imaging ordered to evaluate the urinary tract in children** (but may miss significant VUR). Also performed in children <2y of age with a febrile UTI. **Renal scarring and/or Hydronephrosis may be suggestive of VUR.**
- **Contrast voiding cystourethrogram** (VCUG) **obtained in children after a first febrile or symptomatic UTI who have an anomaly on kidney Ultrasound**, have Hypertension or poor growth, or have combination of temperature ≥39°C (102.2°F) & a pathogen other than *Escherichia coli.*
- **The diagnosis of VUR is based on demonstration of reflux of urine from the bladder to the upper urinary tract by** either [1] **Contrast voiding cystourethrogram (criterion standard)** or [2] Radionuclide cystogram (RNC) as an alternative; they determine the degree & severity of VUR.

MANAGEMENT
Low grades (grades I and II):
- **Observation or continuous antibiotic prophylaxis** since there is a chance of spontaneous resolution. Prophylactic antibiotic therapy are also used for individuals who are not toilet trained. Antibiotic options include **Trimethoprim-sulfamethoxazole, Trimethoprim, or Nitrofurantoin; age ≤2 months: Cephalexin, Ampicillin, Amoxicillin.** Continuous antibiotic prophylaxis reduces the risk of recurrent UTI, Pyelonephritis, and subsequent renal scarring.
- Grade I to II reflux have the lowest risk for renal scarring but are still at risk for recurrent UTIs.
- Surgical correction is not usually indicated in individuals with low-grade reflux due to a high likelihood of spontaneous resolution unless there is breakthrough UTI on medical therapy.

Intermediate- or high-grade (grades III & IV):
- **Prophylactic antibiotic therapy initially.**
- Surgical correction (definitive management) is reserved for all patients with grades III to IV with breakthrough infection on medical therapy (eg, recurrent UTI or Pyelonephritis) or who have serious adverse effects from prophylactic antibiotic therapy.
- Surgical correction is also indicated in patients with persistent grade IV and V beyond 2-3 years of age.

Complications of VUR: Pyelonephritis, UTIs, Hypertension, renal scarring, Chronic kidney disease.

ACUTE CYSTITIS

- <u>Pathophysiology:</u> usually an ascending infection of the lower urinary tract from the urethra.

ETIOLOGIES
- ***Escherichia coli* most common (>80%),** Other gram-negative uropathogens — *Klebsiella, Proteus, Enterobacter, & Pseudomonas.* **Staphylococcus saprophyticus** second most common cause in sexually active women. *Enterococcus* species with indwelling catheters.

RISK FACTORS
- <u>Women:</u> sexual intercourse "honeymoon cystitis", spermicidal use (especially with diaphragm).
- <u>Pregnancy:</u> progesterone & estrogen cause ureter dilation & inhibition of bladder peristalsis.
- Elderly & Postmenopausal, Diabetes mellitus, & presence of an indwelling catheter. In children, UTIs may indicate Vesicourethral reflux.
- Infants should receive a bladder and renal ultrasound to rule out congenital abnormalities.
- **Complicated: underlying condition with risk of therapeutic failure**: symptoms >7 days, pregnancy, diabetics, immunosuppression, indwelling catheter, anatomic abnormality, elderly, males.
- Uncomplicated cystitis in men is rare and often denotes underlying pathologies (eg, infected stones, prostatitis, or chronic urinary retention). May need further work to assess for cause.

CLINICAL MANIFESTATIONS
- **<u>Irritative symptoms:</u> dysuria** (burning), **frequency, urgency, hematuria, suprapubic discomfort.**
- <u>Physical examination</u> **may elicit suprapubic tenderness, but examination is often unremarkable.** Systemic toxicity (eg, fever >99.9°F/37.7°C, chills, rigor) is usually absent in lower tract infections.

DIAGNOSIS
- For most women with suspected Acute simple cystitis, especially classic symptoms, no additional testing is necessary to make the diagnosis. Urine culture & susceptibility testing are usually not needed in women with acute simple Cystitis unless at risk for infection with a resistant organism.
- **<u>Urinalysis & dipstick:</u> pyuria (≥10 WBCs/hpf),** hematuria, ⊕ leukocyte esterase (pyuria); ⊕ nitrites, cloudy urine, bacteriuria. Increased pH with Proteus.
- **<u>Urine culture on clean-catch mid-stream specimen:</u> definitive diagnosis.** Women: ≥1,000 CFU/ml of uropathogens. Epithelial (squamous cells) = contaminated urine specimen.
  - <u>Indications:</u> complicated or recurrent UTI, infants or children, elderly ≥65 years, males, urologic abnormalities, refractory to treatment, Diabetics, catheterized patients, symptoms ≥7 days.

MANAGEMENT OF UNCOMPLICATED
- **<u>1st-line:</u> Nitrofurantoin or Trimethoprim-sulfamethoxazole or Fosfomycin** (if resistance < 20%).
- **<u>2nd-line:</u> Fluoroquinolones** (eg, Ciprofloxacin, Levofloxacin) first line if sulfa allergies or increased resistance patterns (otherwise, reserved use). **Cephalosporins (eg, Cephalexin, Cefpodoxime).**
<u>Adjunctive therapy:</u>
- Increase fluid intake, void after intercourse; hot Sitz baths may provide relief of discomfort.
- **<u>Phenazopyridine</u> is a bladder analgesic. Inform the patient Phenazopyridine turns the urine an orange color.** Not used >48 hours due to adverse effects (eg, methemoglobinemia, hemolytic anemia).

COMPLICATED
- **Fluoroquinolones PO or IV, Aminoglycosides** x 7-10 or 14 days (depending on the severity).
CYSTITIS DURING PREGNANCY
- **Amoxicillin, Amoxicillin-clavulanate, Cephalexin, Cefpodoxime, Nitrofurantoin, Fosfomycin.** Sulfisoxazole is safe except in last days of pregnancy (can lead to kernicterus).
- **Avoid Aminoglycosides, Fluoroquinolones, and Doxycycline.**
- **Avoid Trimethoprim-sulfamethoxazole in the first trimester.**

ASYMPTOMATIC BACTERIURIA OR COLONIZATION

Asymptomatic patient with incidental bacteriuria on Urinalysis or on ≥2 urine cultures.

- **No treatment needed:** general population, elderly, diabetics, nonpregnant premenopausal women, spinal cord injury patients or patients with chronic indwelling urinary catheters.
- **Treatment needed: pregnancy**, patients undergoing urologic intervention or hip arthroplasty.
- Pregnancy requires screening & treatment for bacteriuria because its presence may be associated with increased risk of pre-term birth, perinatal death, & maternal Pyelonephritis.

ACUTE PYELONEPHRITIS

- **Infection of the upper genitourinary tract (kidney parenchyma & renal pelvis).**
- Usually an ascending infection from the lower urinary tract.

ETIOLOGIES

- ***Escherichia coli* most common (>80%)**; other gram-negative uropathogens (eg, *Proteus, Enterobacter, Klebsiella* & *Pseudomonas*). *Enterococcus* species with indwelling catheters.

RISK FACTORS

- Diabetes mellitus, history of recurrent UTIs or kidney stones, pregnancy, congenital urinary tract malformations.
- Diabetics may develop emphysematous Pyelonephritis due to gas-producing bacteria.

CLINICAL MANIFESTATIONS

- **Upper tract symptoms: fever, shaking chills, back or flank pain. Nausea & vomiting not common but suggestive of Pyelonephritis.** Bacteremia develops in 20-30% of individuals.
- Lower tract (irritative) symptoms: dysuria, urgency, & frequency.

PHYSICAL EXAMINATION

- ⊕ **costovertebral angle tenderness, fever, & tachycardia.**

DIAGNOSIS

- In suspected acute complicated UTI or Acute pyelonephritis, obtain urine for both Urinalysis (either by microscopy or by dipstick) and culture with susceptibility testing.
- UA: **Pyuria [≥10 WBCs/hpf]**, ⊕leukocyte esterase, ⊕ Nitrites (90% bacteria causing UTIs), hematuria, cloudy urine, bacteriuria. **WBC casts hallmark of Pyelonephritis. Increased pH with Proteus.**
- **Urine culture definitive diagnosis.**
- CBC: leukocytosis with left shift.

OUTPATIENT MANAGEMENT

- **Fluoroquinolones first-line** (if resistance rate <10%) — **eg, Ciprofloxacin, Levofloxacin.**
- If resistance >10%, initiate with a long-acting parenteral agent (eg, IV or IM Ceftriaxone, Gentamicin, Tobramycin, Ertapenem) followed by an oral Fluoroquinolone. Alternatives for oral follow-up after LA parenteral agents include TMP-SMX, Ampicillin-sulbactam, Cefpodoxime, Cefdinir, or Cefadroxil.

INPATIENT MANAGEMENT

- **Third- or fourth generation Cephalosporins (eg, Ceftriaxone), extended-spectrum Penicillins (Piperacillin-tazobactam), Ampicillin, Fluoroquinolones, or Aminoglycosides** for a total duration 2 weeks.
    - Indications for admission include older age, signs of obstruction, comorbid conditions, inability to tolerate oral antibiotics, persistently high fever (eg, >38.4°C/>101°F) or pain.

PREGNANCY

- **IV Ceftriaxone first-line;** Piperacillin-tazobactam. Aztreonam if Penicillin-allergic.
- Avoid Trimethoprim-Sulfamethoxazole, Aminoglycosides, Fluoroquinolones, & Tetracyclines.

URETHRITIS

- **Urethritis (inflammation of the urethra)** is a common manifestation of Sexually transmitted infections (STIs) among males.

TYPES
- **Nongonococcal urethritis (NGU):**
    - *Chlamydia trachomatis* **is the most common cause of nongonococcal urethritis.** *Chlamydia trachomatis* **is the most common bacterial STI in the US.** 5–14-day incubation period followed by purulent or mucopurulent discharge. May be associated with pruritus, hematuria, or dyspareunia. Up to 40% asymptomatic. **Coinfection with *N. gonorrhoeae* common.**
    - Other agents include *Mycoplasma genitalium* **(second most common cause of NGU)**, *Ureaplasma urealyticum, Trichomonas vaginalis,* & viruses.

- **Gonococcal urethritis**
    - *Neisseria gonorrhoeae:* abrupt onset of symptoms (especially within 4-7 days). Opaque, yellow, white or clear thick discharge, pruritus. Many patients are asymptomatic.

CLINICAL MANIFESTATIONS
- **Asymptomatic infection**: **The majority of affected persons are asymptomatic.** 5-10% of cases of laboratory-documented gonococcal urethritis and up to 42% of males with NGU are asymptomatic.
- **Dysuria (painful urination) most common symptom)** in both gonococcal & NGU.
- **Urethral discharge, penile or vaginal pruritus;** discharge at the urethral meatus in males.
- Abdominal pain or abnormal vaginal bleeding.

Physical examination:
- On exam, discharge may be grossly evident or may only be detectable after gentle milking of the penis.
- The meatus may appear inflamed or edematous.

DIAGNOSIS
- **In general, the diagnosis and treatment of Urethritis should occur at the time of the presenting visit.** Send NAAT for *N. gonorrhoeae* and *C. trachomatis* (preferably first-void/catch).

Point-of-care stain available: (gram stain, methylene blue, gentian violet) available:
- **Nongonococcal: ≥2 WBCs/hpf in high-prevalence settings (≥5 in lower-prevalence settings) + no intracellular diplococci, treat for Nongonococcal infection** (eg, Doxycycline) if low suspicion for gonococcal infection. If there is a high suspicion for gonococcal infection, treat with regimen that provides gonococcal and chlamydial coverage. Urethral swab performed in some men.
- **Gonococcal: if gram-negative intracellular diplococci present** — **treat for Gonococcal urethritis** (eg, Ceftriaxone).
- Urinalysis or dipstick: ⊕ leukocyte esterase on dipstick or ≥10 WBCs/hpf (pyuria) on microscopy in men.
- If none of these findings are present, a presumptive or suspected diagnosis of Urethritis can be made in sexually active males with suggestive symptoms. NAAT should still be performed when possible.

Point-of-care stain NOT available:
- **Treat with regimen that provides both gonococcal AND chlamydial coverage** if any of the following is present: 1) mucopurulent discharge, 2) ⊕ leukocyte esterase on first-void urine, 3) ≥10 WBCs/hpf on microscopy of spun sediment from first void/catch urine.

Nucleic acid amplification (NAAT):
- **Most sensitive & specific for *C. trachomatis, N. gonorrhoeae,* & *M. genitalium*** (recommended over culture).
- First-void or first-catch urine is ideal as NAAT of a first-catch urine is highly sensitive & specific (test of choice for identification of pathogens most commonly associated with urethritis).

INITIAL THERAPY
- **Initial therapy is often empiric at the point-of-care** and should be offered to males with suspected or confirmed urethritis based on evidence for gonococcal versus nongonococcal urethritis (NGU).

Nongonococcal urethritis (NGU):
- Empiric treatment of nongonococcal urethritis (NGU), in which Gram stain shows no gram-negative diplococci in WBC and clinical suspicion for *N. gonorrhoeae* is low, should be targeted against *C. trachomatis* as the most likely pathogen.
- **Doxycycline 100 mg orally twice daily for 7 days is the first-line treatment for Chlamydia and is also the empiric treatment of nongonococcal urethritis (NGU),** in which Gram stain shows no gram-negative diplococci in WBC and clinical suspicion for *N. gonorrhoeae* is low. There is greater microbial efficacy with Doxycycline compared with Azithromycin for *C. trachomatis* and there is concern that the single-dose Azithromycin regimen could increase resistance in *M. genitalium.*
- **Azithromycin (either as 500 mg orally on day 1 then 250 mg orally daily for 4 days; or as a single 1-gram dose), although the single-dose regimen is associated with lower *C. trachomatis* microbiologic cure rates than Doxycycline** and may promote emergent Macrolide resistance in *M. genitalium.* The single observed 1-gram oral dose is an alternative if adherence to a multi-day regimen is a concern.

N. gonorrhoeae (Gonococcal Urethritis):
- **Ceftriaxone: single intramuscular dose of Ceftriaxone (500 mg for individuals <150 kg or 1 g for individuals ≥150 kg)** is recommended in males with symptoms of urethritis who have microscopic evidence of gonococcal urethritis (eg, gram-negative intracellular diplococci in the urethral exudate) or high clinical suspicion of gonococcal infection based on the revised CDC guidelines.
- **If testing results for *C. trachomatis* are not available or has not been ruled out at the time of treatment, presumptive therapy for Chlamydia coinfection is also indicated (eg, Doxycycline 100 mg twice daily for 7 days).** Azithromycin (1-gram single oral dose) is an alternative.

Directed therapy of *M. genitalium*:
- **Moxifloxacin** 400 mg orally for 7 days is the preferred treatment of patients with **proven *M. genitalium* infection.**
- **High-dose Azithromycin** (1 g once followed by 500 mg daily for the next 3 days) is a reasonable alternative as long as the patient had not previously received it for the current infection.

FOLLOW UP
Sexual activity:
- To reduce transmission risk, males with infectious Urethritis should be instructed to refrain from sexual activity for at minimum 7 days following the initiation of therapy (including single-dose therapy) AND until their symptoms have completely resolved.
- Recurrent and persistent symptoms should prompt reevaluation for possible reinfection, antimicrobial resistance, or the possible involvement of pathogens that were not covered by the empiric regimen.

Repeat testing:
- In males with confirmed gonorrhea, chlamydia, and trichomonas, repeat testing for these pathogens with nucleic acid amplification testing (NAAT) is warranted 3 months after treatment because there is a high rate of reinfection. Repeat testing should be performed regardless of whether sexual partners were treated.

Test of cure:
- A test of cure is a microbial diagnostic test (eg, culture or NAAT) that is performed 1-3 weeks following treatment, regardless of symptom resolution, to document eradication of the pathogen.
- In general, a test of cure is not necessary for males with urethritis treated with first-line regimens for *N. gonorrhoeae* or *C. trachomatis.*

PROSTATITIS

- Prostate gland inflammation secondary to an ascending infection.

ETIOLOGIES OF ACUTE PROSTATITIS

- **>35 years:** *Escherichia coli* **most common,** other gram-negatives — *Proteus*, Enterobacteriaceae (*Klebsiella, Enterobacter & Serratia* species), *Pseudomonas.*
- **<35 years (or older men engaging in high-risk sexual behavior): Chlamydia & Gonorrhea most common,** *E. coli, Treponema, Trichomonas, Gardnerella.*
- Children: viral (Mumps most common cause).

ETIOLOGIES OF CHRONIC PROSTATITIS

- *Escherichia coli* **most common (~80%),** *Proteus, Enterococci, Trichomonas*, HIV, inflammatory.
- Structural or functional abnormality, recurrent UTIs.
- Acute prostatitis may progress to chronic (>3 months).

CLINICAL MANIFESTATIONS

- **Irritative voiding symptoms: frequency, urgency, & dysuria.** Cloudy urine.
- Obstructive symptoms: hesitancy, poor or interrupted stream, dribbling, straining to void, & incomplete emptying.
- **Acute: Flu-like symptoms** — eg, **spiking fever, chills,** malaise, arthralgias, myalgias [eg, **lower (sacral) back or abdominal pain]. Perineal or suprapubic pain** (often dull and poorly localized).
- **Chronic prostatitis: usually presents as recurrent UTIs or intermittent dysfunction.** Malaise, arthralgias. Symptoms are milder. Fever not common.

Physical examination:
Boggy (firm, edematous) prostate = Prostatitis
- Acute: **exquisitely tender,** normal or hot, **boggy (firm, edematous) prostate.**
- Chronic: **usually nontender, boggy (firm, edematous) prostate.**

DIAGNOSIS

- **Urinalysis & Urine culture: pyuria, bacteriuria, & hematuria in Acute prostatitis.** UA & culture often negative in Chronic prostatitis, so prostatic massage is often done in Chronic prostatitis to increase bacterial yield on UA/culture. **Avoid prostatic massage in Acute prostatitis** (may cause bacteremia). Gram stain & culture should be obtained.
- Transrectal Ultrasound or CT of the pelvis with IV contrast helpful for suspected Prostatic abscess.

MANAGEMENT

- **Acute >35 years: Fluoroquinolones or Trimethoprim-sulfamethoxazole** x 4-6 weeks (outpatient); both achieve high levels in prostatic tissue. If hospitalized: [1] IV fluoroquinolones with or without Aminoglycoside OR [2] Ampicillin with or without Gentamicin.
- **Acute <35 years or STI likely:** cover for Gonorrhea & Chlamydia — **Ceftriaxone plus Doxycycline** (Azithromycin is an alternative to Doxycycline).
- Hospitalized: Ampicillin (2 gram every 6 hours) PLUS Gentamicin (1.5 mg/kg every 8 hours).
- Chronic: Fluoroquinolones or Trimethoprim-sulfamethoxazole for 6-12 weeks.
  Alpha blockers (eg, Tamsulosin), hot sitz baths, & NSAIDs can help with chronic pain syndrome.
- Refractory chronic: **Transurethral resection of the prostate (TURP).**

EXAM TIP

- Acute Prostatitis: **exquisitely tender,** normal or hot, **boggy (edematous) prostate.**
- Chronic Prostatitis: **usually nontender** (or minimally tender), **boggy (edematous) prostate.**
- Benign prostatic hypertrophy: symmetrically enlarged, firm, nontender prostate.
- Prostate cancer: rock hard prostate.

EPIDIDYMITIS & EPIDIDYMO-ORCHITIS

- Epididymal pain & swelling thought to be secondary to retrograde infection or reflux of urine. Bacterial infection most common cause.

ETIOLOGIES
- **Men 14-35 years:** *Chlamydia trachomatis* **(most common) &** *Neisseria gonorrhoeae*. *Ureaplasma, E. coli, Treponema, Trichomonas,* & *Gardnerella*. Enterobacteriaceae (insertive anal intercourse).
- **Men >35 years:** enteric organisms — (*E. coli* most common), *Klebsiella, Pseudomonas,* & *Proteus*.
- Prepubertal: viruses, bacterial (*E. coli, Mycoplasma pneumoniae*).

CLINICAL MANIFESTATIONS
- **Gradual onset (over a few hours to days) of localized testicular pain and swelling** (orchitis), usually unilateral pain, swelling, & tenderness of the epididymis. Groin, flank, or abdominal pain.
- May be associated with fever, chills, irritative symptoms (dysuria, urgency, frequency), or urethritis.

PHYSICAL EXAMINATION
- Scrotal swelling and tenderness. **Epididymal tenderness & induration (posterior & superior to the testicle).** The affected testis is usually in normal (vertical) position.
- **Positive Prehn sign — relief of pain with scrotal elevation** (classic but not reliable).
- **Positive (normal) cremasteric reflex** — elevation of the testicle after stroking the inner thigh.

DIAGNOSIS
- **Scrotal ultrasound best initial test — enlarged epididymis & increased testicular blood flow.** Scrotal ultrasound also performed to rule out Testicular torsion.
- UA: pyuria [≥10 WBCs/hpf], ⊕ leukocyte esterase, &/or bacteriuria.
- Nucleic acid amplification testing (NAAT) for *N. Gonorrhoeae* & *Chlamydia*.

MANAGEMENT
- **Supportive management: scrotal elevation, NSAIDs, cool compresses.**
- **<35 years or STI likely:** [no insertive anal intercourse] **cover** *Chlamydia* **&** *N. Gonorrhoeae* — **Doxycycline** (100 mg bid x 10 days) **PLUS single dose IM Ceftriaxone 500 mg for individuals <150 kg or 1 g for individuals ≥150 kg.** Azithromycin 1g x 1 dose is an alternative to Doxycycline.
- **Individuals who practice insertive anal intercourse:** coverage for *N. gonorrhoeae, C. trachomatis,* & enteric pathogen infections: **Ceftriaxone** (500 mg for individuals <150 kg or 1 g for individuals ≥150 kg) **PLUS a Fluoroquinolone (eg, Levofloxacin** 500 mg orally once daily for 10 days).
- **>35 years, low risk for STIs: cover enteric organisms (eg,** *E. coli*) — **Fluoroquinolones** (eg, **Levofloxacin**, Ciprofloxacin, Ofloxacin). **Trimethoprim-sulfamethoxazole is an alternative.**
- Bacterial in children: Cephalexin or Amoxicillin.

ORCHITIS
ETIOLOGIES
- **Viral most common** — eg, **Mumps virus (Paramyxovirus),** Echovirus, coxsackie, rubella. Orchitis is the most common complication of Mumps in postpubertal men 1-2 weeks after (20-30% of cases).

CLINICAL MANIFESTATIONS
- **Scrotal pain, swelling, and tenderness (unilateral 70%;** bilateral in 10-30%).
- Physical examination: The overlying scrotal skin can be edematous and erythematous; scrotal tenderness and swelling sparing the epididymis.

MANAGEMENT
- **Symptomatic management first-line** — NSAIDs, bed rest, scrotal support, & warm or cool packs.

TESTICULAR TORSION

- **Spermatic cord twists & cuts off testicular blood supply** due to congenital malformation.
- **Adolescents (10-20 years of age) & neonates at highest risk. True urologic emergency.**
- Pathophysiology: insufficient fixation of the lower pole of the testis to the tunica vaginalis (**bell-clapper deformity**), leading to increased mobility of the testicle, which can cause it to twist.

CLINICAL MANIFESTATIONS
- **Abrupt (sudden) onset of moderate to severe unilateral scrotal, inguinal, or lower abdominal pain (usually <6 hours).** Testicular torsion may occur after an inciting event (eg, trauma, vigorous physical activity), spontaneously, or often, may wake the patient out of sleep (due to cremasteric contraction with nocturnal erections). May have a prior, less severe episodes that self-resolved.
- If **nausea or vomiting** is present, **suspect torsion** (both are usually absent in Epididymitis).

PHYSICAL EXAMINATION
- **Firm (hard), tender, swollen testicle; retracted testicle (high-riding) most specific finding** — may have a horizontal [transverse] lie in an anterior position.
- **Negative Prehn sign** — **no pain relief with scrotal elevation.**
- **Negative (absent) cremasteric reflex** on affected side — no elevation of the testicle after stroking the inner thigh **(most sensitive finding).**

DIAGNOSIS
- **Clinical diagnosis** — in patients with a history & physical examination suggestive of Torsion, imaging studies should not be performed (confirmatory imaging should not delay surgical management), rather, these individuals should undergo immediate urologic consultation for surgical exploration.
- **Emergency surgical exploration (definitive diagnosis); preferred over US if torsion is very likely.**
- **Testicular Doppler ultrasound** most commonly used imaging modality in equivocal cases — decreased or absent testicular blood flow. **Imaging should not delay surgical exploration.**
- Radionuclide scan — most specific imaging study (rarely used).

MANAGEMENT
- **Surgical exploration with urgent detorsion & orchiopexy (fixation of the testes) ideally within 6 hours of pain onset** (extended periods of ischemia >8 hours associated may cause necrosis).
- Manual detorsion should be performed if surgical intervention is not immediately available.
- Orchiectomy if the testicle is not salvageable.

TORSION OF APPENDIX TESTIS

- Most cases are seen in children 7-14 years.

CLINICAL MANIFESTATIONS
- Abrupt testicular pain (usually more gradual compared to Testicular torsion).
Physical examination:
- **Torsed appendage "blue dot" sign** — **bluish discoloration in the scrotal area directly over the torsed appendage (infarction and necrosis).**
- May also be associated with a reactive hydrocele.

DIAGNOSIS
- Primary a clinical diagnosis.
- Color doppler US: low echogenicity of the torsed appendage with a central hypoechogenic area.

MANAGEMENT
- **Local application of ice, analgesics (eg, NSAIDs), supportive underwear, and reassurance.**
- Surgical excision of the appendix testis is usually only performed with persistent pain after initial management.

CRYPTORCHIDISM [UNDESCENDED TESTES]

- **Failure of spontaneous testicular descent into the scrotum by 4 months of age (or corrected age for preterm infants).**
- 2-5% of full-term & ~30% of preterm infants are born with an undescended testis; however, most undescended testes at birth descend spontaneously within the first 3-4 months of life (~70%).
- **Most commonly found just outside the external ring (suprascrotal) 60%,** followed by the inguinal canal (25%), and less commonly in the abdomen (15%).

INCREASED RISK
- **Preterm delivery** (30% of preterm vs. 5% in full-term infants)
- **Low birth weight** <2.5 kg or small for gestational age at birth
- Maternal obesity or Diabetes.

CLINICAL MANIFESTATIONS
- Empty, small, or poorly rugated scrotum or hemiscrotum. Absence of a palpable testicle in the scrotum.
- Most common on the right side. 10% bilateral.
- May have inguinal fullness (if located in the inguinal canal).

DIAGNOSIS
- Clinical diagnosis based on physical examination in a majority of cases.
- Imaging is not routinely necessary to locate nonpalpable testes. When imaging is needed, scrotal ultrasound or MRI may be indicated.

MANAGEMENT
- **Orchiopexy is recommended as soon as possible after 4-6 months of age for congenitally undescended testicles and definitely should be done before 2 years of age (ideally before 1 year of age).** If testes have not descended by 4 months of age, they are unlikely to descend and generally require surgical manipulation into and attachment to the scrotum (orchiopexy, orchidopexy).
- **Observation can be done only if <6 months of age.** Most descend by 3 months of age (rarely spontaneously descend after 4-6 months of age).
- hCG or gonadotropin releasing hormone: human chorionic gonadotropin stimulates testosterone & hormonal testicular descension. Rarely used due to low response rates and lack of long-term efficacy. Hormone therapy may be used for Cryptorchidism associated with Prader-Willi syndrome.
- If performed early, surgical correction also may reduce the risk of infertility and Testicular cancer.
- Orchiectomy recommended if detected at puberty to reduce Testicular cancer risk.

COMPLICATIONS
Increased risk of
- **Testicular cancer** (reduced with early orchiopexy)
- **decreased fertility**
- **Testicular torsion, &**
- **Inguinal hernia.**

TESTICULAR CANCER

- **Most common solid tumor in young men 15–35 years (average age 32 years).**
- Prognosis: generally excellent — one of the most curable solid cancers (5-year survival rate ~95%).

RISK FACTORS:
- **Cryptorchidism (most significant)** — 4-10 x risk in both the undescended & normal testicle.
- Caucasians, Klinefelter's syndrome, Hypospadias. Slightly more common on the right than the left.

MAJOR TYPES
- **Germinal cell tumors (GCT) most common (95%).**
  - **Nonseminomas:** embryonal cell carcinoma, teratoma, yolk sac (most common in boys ≤10 years), Choriocarcinoma (worst prognosis). Mixed tumors (seminomatous + nonseminomatous components). Mixed tumors are treated like Nonseminomas. **Nonseminomas are associated with increased serum alpha-fetoprotein & beta-hCG and resistance to radiation.**
  - **Seminoma (pure):** The 4 S of Seminoma — **Simple (lacks the tumor marker alpha-fetoprotein), Sensitive (sensitive to radiation), Slower growing**, & associated with **Stepwise spread.**

- NonGerminal cell tumors most common (3%).
  - Leydig cell tumors: may be benign. May secrete hormones (eg, androgens or estrogens), which may lead precocious puberty in 6- to 10-year-old boys or gynecomastia, erectile dysfunction, or loss of libido in adults (26 to 35-year-old males).
  - Sertoli cell tumors: often benign. May secrete hormones (eg, estrogens, androgens).
  - Gonadoblastoma, Testicular lymphoma.

CLINICAL MANIFESTATIONS
- **Testicular mass most common (usually painless);** painless testicular swelling or firmness.
- May have dull pain or testicular heaviness. Acute pain in only 10%. Gynecomastia rare.
- Patients may have cough, shortness of breath, or hemoptysis as a result of lung metastases.

Physical examination:
- **Firm, hard, nontender fixed mass that does not transilluminate.** Secondary Hydrocele seen in 10%.

DIAGNOSIS
- **Scrotal ultrasound initial test of choice** — Seminoma (hypoechoic mass). Nonseminoma (cystic, nonhomogeneous mass).
- Tumor markers: **Alpha-fetoprotein is elevated in Nonseminomas (80-85%) & not elevated in pure Seminomas.** Increased beta-hCG in Nonseminomas (especially Choriocarcinoma) & <25% of Seminomas. Lactate dehydrogenase (LDH) helpful in assessing metastatic disease.
- Staging: High-resolution CT of the abdomen, pelvis, and chest.

MANAGEMENT
- **Low-grade (Stage I) Nonseminoma (limited to testes):** radical orchiectomy; this can be followed by [1] active surveillance if no risk factors or [2] followed by active surveillance, chemotherapy (eg, single-agent Carboplatin), or nerve-sparing retroperitoneal lymph node dissection if ≥1 risk factors.
- **Stage II Nonseminoma: radical orchiectomy; can be followed by nerve-sparing retroperitoneal lymph node dissection (IIA) or chemotherapy (IIB or IIC)** [eg, Etoposide + Cisplatin; Cisplatin, Etoposide & Bleomycin].
- **Low-grade Seminoma: radical orchiectomy is curative.** May be followed by active surveillance or may need radiation therapy to paraaortic lymph nodes or single-agent Carboplatin chemotherapy.
- Stage II seminoma: radical orchiectomy; usually followed by either radiation therapy or Cisplatin-based combination chemotherapy, depending on the extent of retroperitoneal disease.
- Persistent tumor markers after orchiectomy: BEP (Bleomycin, Etoposide, Cisplatin) x 3 cycles or EP x 4 cycles.

HYDROCELE

- Serous fluid collection within the parietal and visceral layers of the tunica vaginalis, which directly surrounds the testis and the spermatic cord. **Most common cause of painless scrotal swelling.**

ETIOLOGIES
- Idiopathic most common.
- Inflammatory: acute reactive Hydrocele can occur with inflammatory conditions (eg, Epididymitis, Orchitis, Torsion, Testicular tumor).

TYPES
- **Communicating: peritoneal/abdominal fluid enters the scrotum via a patent processus vaginalis that failed to close.**
- Noncommunicating: derived from fluid from the mesothelial lining of the tunica vaginalis (no connection to the peritoneum).

CLINICAL MANIFESTATIONS
- **Painless scrotal swelling;** may increase throughout the day. Often anterior and lateral to the testes.
- May complain of dull ache or heavy sensation with increasing size.
Physical examination:
- **Translucency (scrotal sac transilluminates well).** Fluid located anterior and lateral to the testis.
- **Communicating hydrocele: swelling worse (may change in size) with Valsalva or standing and improves with recumbency;** Noncommunicating hydroceles do not change in size.

DIAGNOSIS
- **Testicular ultrasound initial test of choice** — used to rule out associated testicular tumor, other masses, or inflammatory scrotal conditions (eg, Epididymitis, Orchitis).

MANAGEMENT
- **Watchful waiting: usually no treatment needed;** most do not require intervention — often resolves within the first 12 months of life in infants. In adults, Hydroceles are often self-limited.
- Surgical excision of the Hydrocele sac may be needed if it persists beyond 1 year of age in infants, older patients with communicating hydroceles (elective) to reduce the risk of hernia, Hydroceles associated with complications, or persistent pain or pressure sensation.

SPERMATOCELE & EPIDIDYMAL CYST

- **Retention epididymal cyst** (scrotal mass) of a tubule of the rete testis or the epididymal head that contains sperm. It is considered a spermatocele if ≥2 cm.

CLINICAL MANIFESTATIONS
- Painless, cystic testicular mass.

PHYSICAL EXAMINATION
- **Round, soft mass in the head of the epididymis superior, posterior, & separate from the testicle,** freely movable mass above the testicle that **transilluminates.** Does not change in size with Valsalva.

DIAGNOSIS
- Scrotal ultrasound.

MANAGEMENT
- **No treatment is usually necessary** unless the mass is bothersome.
- Surgical excision for chronic pain (rarely needed).

VARICOCELE

- **Cystic testicular mass of <u>varicose veins:</u> pampiniform venous plexus & internal spermatic vein.**
- **Most common surgically correctable cause of male infertility** (seen in ~30% of infertile men because the increased temperature from the increased venous blood flow inhibits spermatogenesis).
- **<u>Most are left-sided</u>** [increased left renal vein pressure transmitted to left gonadal (internal spermatic) vein because it enters the left renal vein at a perpendicular angle "nutcracker effect"].

CLINICAL MANIFESTATIONS

- Asymptomatic Varicoceles found in 10% of the population. May cause testicular atrophy.
- Usually painless but may cause a dull ache or heavy sensation. May be associated with infertility.

<u>Physical examination:</u>
- **Soft scrotal mass with a "bag of worms" feel superior to the testicle.**
- **Dilation worsens when patient is upright or with Valsalva.**
- Less apparent when the patient is supine (recumbency) or with testicular elevation.

DIAGNOSIS

- Clinical diagnosis.
- **<u>Ultrasound:</u> initial test of choice** — dilation of the pampiniform plexus >2 mm.

MANAGEMENT

- **<u>Observation in most</u> — most Varicoceles do not require surgical intervention.**
- **<u>Surgery</u> may be used in some cases for pain, infertility**, or delayed testicular growth — spermatic vein ligation, varicocelectomy, or percutaneous venous embolization.

ASSOCIATIONS

- **Right-sided Varicocele may be due to retroperitoneal or abdominal malignancy** (unilateral right-sided Varicoceles are otherwise uncommon).
- Sudden onset of **left-sided varicocele in an older man** may be possibly due to **Renal cell carcinoma.**

URETHRAL STRICTURE

- Narrowing of the urethral lumen.

ETIOLOGIES

- Infection (eg, STI or UTI), trauma or instrumentation of the urethra (eg, catheterization), idiopathic.

CLINICAL MANIFESTATIONS

- **<u>Chronic obstructive voiding symptoms</u>: weak urinary stream** & incomplete bladder emptying, recurrent UTIs, urinary spraying; <u>Irritative symptoms:</u> frequency or dysuria. Ejaculatory dysfunction.

DIAGNOSIS

- **[1] <u>Noninvasive studies:</u> uroflowmetry & ultrasound postvoid residual [PVR] measurement: poor bladder emptying (increased PVR) & low peak rate of urine flow** (<15 ml/s).
- [2] <u>Testing if abnormal noninvasive studies:</u> **Patients with symptoms and poor bladder emptying (increased postvoid residual) should undergo retrograde urethrogram**, cystourethroscopy, voiding cystourethrogram, or ultrasound urethrography.

MANAGEMENT

- Options include Endoscopic treatment (dilation, cold knife incision, incision with electrocautery or laser), intermittent catheter dilation, or surgical reconstruction of the urethra (eg, Urethroplasty).
- Prophylactic antibiotics recommended prior to cystourethroscopy & surgery.
- <u>Complications:</u> urinary fistula.

BLADDER CARCINOMA

- **Most common urinary tract malignancy.**
- **Urothelial (transitional cell) carcinoma most common type of Bladder cancer in the US** (90%). Other types: Squamous cell carcinoma, adenocarcinoma, Sarcoma, & Small cell.

RISK FACTORS
- **Tobacco smoking most common (>60%).** Age >40y, **Caucasian,** Male gender (3x more common).
- **Occupational exposure to aniline dyes in paint/pigment, leather, & rubber** (20%): eg, auto or metal workers, beauticians, textile & electrical, carpets, paints, plastics, & industrial chemicals.
- **Medications: Cyclophosphamide,** Pioglitazone.
- Long-term indwelling catheter use. Squamous cell carcinoma: infected bladder stones, Schistosomiasis.

CLINICAL MANIFESTATIONS
- **Hematuria — most common presenting symptom, typically intermittent, gross, painless, and present throughout micturition (may be microscopic).** Hydronephrosis with flank pain.
- Irritative voiding symptoms — **dysuria** (second most common symptom), urgency, & frequency.

DIAGNOSIS
- **UA with microscopy & cultures to rule out benign causes** (eg, hematuria from BPH, urinary tract infection, pyelonephritis, cystitis, prostatitis, and passage of renal calculi). The presence of otherwise unexplained hematuria after an initial workup may represent urothelial cancer in individuals >35 years until proven otherwise, although many causes are benign.
- **Workup for Bladder cancer: initial evaluation with cystoscopy, renal function testing, and upper urinary tract imaging (CT urography preferred imaging of the GU tract). Cytology may be an adjunctive to cystoscopy,** especially in patients with high pretest probability of disease.
- **Cystoscopy with biopsy criterion standard for diagnosis & staging of Bladder cancer & management of Bladder cancer** [can be both diagnostic & curative (can be resected on initial Cystoscopy)]. All patients with gross hematuria & many with significant microscopic hematuria should undergo a Cystoscopy and Urinary cytology.
- **Imaging of GU tract:** initial evaluation for Bladder cancer should include imaging of the upper urinary tract to determine the location and extent of tumor as well as to detect sites of multifocal disease. **CT urography with contrast is preferred to assess local extent of the disease** [has largely replaced Intravenous pyelography (IVP) for upper tract imaging]. MRI imaging is an alternative.
- **Urine cytology: commonly used as an adjunct to Cystoscopy to detect carcinoma in situ (CIS) and upper-tract malignancies.** If not, suggestive urine cytology or negative cytology in high-risk patients should be followed by Cystoscopy & possibly bladder biopsy. Urinary cytology is most helpful in diagnosing high-grade tumors & carcinoma in situ. Low-grade, noninvasive tumors may be missed by routine cytologic analysis (relatively poor sensitivity, especially if low-grade).

MANAGEMENT
- **Localized or superficial (non-muscle-invasive): complete transurethral resection of the bladder tumor [TURBT or electrocautery] mainstay of therapy** + follow-up every 3 months.
- **Muscle-invasive: Neoadjuvant Cisplatin-based chemotherapy followed by Radical cystectomy with urinary diversion is the standard of care for muscle-invasive Bladder cancer** (improves overall survival). Cisplatin-based chemotherapy & immunotherapy may be used as adjuvant therapy.
- **Metastatic disease: Platinum-based chemotherapy** — MVAC (Methotrexate, Vinblastine, Doxorubicin, & **Cisplatin**), dose-dense MVAC, or Gemcitabine plus Cisplatin. Checkpoint inhibitor Immunotherapy is an option for those ineligible for chemotherapy: Anti-PDL-1 inhibitors: eg, Atezolizumab, Durvalumab, Avelumab; Anti-PD-1 inhibitors: eg, Pembrolizumab, Nivolumab.
- **Recurrent Intravesicular immunotherapy with Bacillus Calmette-Guérin (BCG) vaccine if electrocautery is unsuccessful** — immune reaction stimulates cross reaction with tumor antigens. Do not use BCG if immunosuppressed or if gross hematuria is present (may cause BCG-related sepsis). Alternative intravesicular chemotherapeutic agents include Mitomycin, Gemcitabine, Epirubicin, and Docetaxel.

PARAPHIMOSIS

- **Retracted foreskin in an uncircumcised male that cannot be returned to its normal anatomic position covering the glans penis** — the foreskin cannot be pulled forward.
- **Urological emergency that requires urgent manual reduction of the foreskin.**

PATHOPHYSIOLOGY:
- Retracted foreskin becomes trapped behind the corona of the glans & forms a tight band, constricting penile tissues.
- Resultant venous congestion can lead to arterial compression, penile necrosis, and gangrene.

ETIOLOGIES
- Forceful retraction of phimotic foreskin (Phimosis).
- Triggers include infection, trauma, or hair tourniquets.
- Infants and young boys: usually physiologic or iatrogenic (retraction by the caretaker).
- Adolescents & adults: can occur after balanoposthitis or penile inflammation (eg, Diabetes mellitus) or after sexual activity.

CLINICAL MANIFESTATIONS
- **Severe penile pain & swelling of the shaft and glans of the penis distal to the constricting ring.**
- Erythema and engorgement of the penis distal to the obstruction and proximal flaccidity.

PHYSICAL EXAMINATION
- **Enlarged, painful glans & distal foreskin with a constricting band of foreskin behind the glans at the coronal sulcus.**

MANAGEMENT
- **Manual reduction:** restore original position of the foreskin combined with pain control. If time permits, edema reduction with cool compresses or pressure dressings can be used prior to gentle pressure on the glans with both thumbs while holding the shaft straight to restore the foreskin to its normal position. **If manual reduction is unsuccessful, urology consult for possible reduction with a dorsal slit procedure should be done.**
- Methods to reduce swelling: ice, compression bandages, granulated sugar (may be time consuming).
- **Definitive management: incision (eg, dorsal slit) or circumcision.**

PHIMOSIS

- **Inability to retract the foreskin proximally over the glans penis.**
- Phimosis is not a urological emergency (unlike Paraphimosis).
- Physiologic phimosis occurs naturally in uncircumcised newborns.

PATHOPHYSIOLOGY
- Distal scarring of the foreskin (eg, after trauma, inflammation or infection).

MANAGEMENT
Nonsurgical management:
- **Proper hygiene & stretching exercises of the foreskin (many spontaneously resolve).**
- **Topical Corticosteroids** for 4-8 weeks can increase foreskin retractility (may be an adjunct to stretching). Betamethasone 0.05% to 0.10% twice daily applied from the tip of the foreskin to the glandis corona, along with daily manual preputial retraction.
Surgical management:
- **Circumcision definitive management.**

BENIGN PROSTATIC HYPERPLASIA (BPH)

- **Prostate hyperplasia (periurethral or transitional zone)** in which prostatic enlargement (BPE) can result in compressive Benign prostatic obstruction & bladder outflow obstruction, with lower urinary tract symptoms (LUTS) due to obstruction at the level of the bladder neck.
- Common in older men (discrete nodules in the periurethral zone). Hyperplasia is part of the normal aging process & is hormonally dependent on increased dihydrotestosterone production.

CLINICAL MANIFESTATIONS
- **Irritative (storage) symptoms:** daytime urinary frequency, urgency, nocturia, overflow incontinence.
- **Obstructive symptoms:** weak, slow, splitting, spraying, or intermittent stream force; hesitancy, incomplete emptying, terminal dribbling, straining to void. BPH may also be asymptomatic.
- **Digital rectal exam: uniformly (symmetrically) enlarged, smooth, firm, non-tender, rubbery (elastic) prostate supports the diagnosis of BPH.**

WORKUP
- No further evaluation is recommended if no significant symptoms or if not impacting health.
- **UA: to look for hematuria or other causes of symptoms & Post-void residual (PVR) volume** used with LUTS/BPH symptoms to evaluate for retention. A bedside bladder scanner may be used.
- Prostate Specific Antigen: most useful to assess prostate volume for 5ARI therapy (PSA >1.5 ng/dL).
- Urine cytology: if increased risk of Bladder cancer (history of tobacco use, irritative bladder symptoms or hematuria) or in the setting of abnormal UA if indicated.

MANAGEMENT
- **Observation (watchful waiting): if asymptomatic or mild symptoms** (monitored annually). **Lifestyle changes**; eg, avoiding fluids prior to bedtime or before going out, decreased consumption of mild diuretics (eg, caffeine, alcohol), and double voiding to further empty the bladder.
- **Alpha-1 blockers: best initial therapy to rapidly relieve symptoms** but they do not change prostate size.
- **5-alpha reductase inhibitors: if BPE to reduce the size of the prostate over time (6-12 months).**
- Phosphodiesterase 5 inhibitor (Tadalafil): alternative in men with both BPH & Erectile dysfunction.
- In men with <u>low</u> post-void residual urine volumes and irritative symptoms, anticholinergics or beta-3 agonists are a reasonable alternative or adjunct to Alpha-1 adrenergic antagonists.

Surgical management:
- Option if persistent, progressive, or refractory despite combination therapy for 12-24 months.
- **Transurethral resection of prostate (TURP)** — removes excess prostate tissue, relieving the obstruction; however, it may cause sexual dysfunction, urinary incontinence. Laser prostatectomy.

ALPHA-1 BLOCKERS: Tamsulosin (most uroselective), Alfuzosin. Doxazosin, Terazosin
- Mechanism of action: **smooth muscle relaxation of prostate & bladder neck, leading to decreased urethral resistance, obstruction relief, & increased urinary outflow.** Alpha-1a activation in the prostate & urethra normally causes bladder neck contraction & decreases urinary flow.
- Indications: **provide rapid symptom relief (in days) but no effect on the clinical course of BPH.**
- Adverse effects: nonselective — **dizziness & orthostatic hypotension (due to alpha-1b antagonism) most common.** Retrograde ejaculation or anejaculation.

5-ALPHA REDUCTASE INHIBITORS (Finasteride, Dutasteride)
- Mechanism of action: **androgen inhibitor** — inhibits the conversion of testosterone to dihydrotestosterone, **suppressing prostate growth; reduces bladder outlet obstruction.** Doesn't provide immediate relief but **has positive effect on clinical course of BPH (size reduction of the prostate & decreases need for surgery)** unlike Alpha blockers. **Reduces size in 6-12 months.**
- Indications: BPH & male pattern baldness.
- Adverse effects: sexual or ejaculatory dysfunction. Decreased libido, breast tenderness & enlargement — increased peripheral testosterone conversion to estrogen by aromatase. Potential increased risk of high-grade Prostate cancer.

PROSTATE CANCER

- After skin cancer, Prostate cancer is the most common cancer in men in the US.
- Prostate cancer is the second most common cause of cancer deaths in men (behind Lung cancer). However, most men die with Prostate cancer than from it (usually slow-growing).
- **Adenocarcinoma most common type** (95%).
- **Prostate cancer arises most commonly in the posterior lobe (peripheral zone).**

RISK FACTORS
- **Increasing age >40 years (strongest risk factor), genetics, Black race, diet (eg, high in animal fat,** decreased vegetable intake), family history of Prostatic cancer.
- The risk for Prostate cancer increases as PSA level rises, but no specific numerical threshold accurately determines the presence of Prostate cancer. Changes of PSA over time is more helpful.

CLINICAL MANIFESTATIONS
- **Most are asymptomatic** and are diagnosed either via an abnormal digital rectal exam or via workup after an abnormal PSA or until invasion of bladder, urethral obstruction, or bone involvement.
- **Urethral obstruction**: urinary frequency, urgency, retention, decreased urinary stream, hematuria.
- **Systemic symptoms: back or bone pain: increased incidence of METS to the bone.** Weight loss.
- **Digital rectal exam (DRE): hard, indurated, discrete nodular, enlarged, asymmetrical prostate.**

DIAGNOSIS
- **Prostate Specific Antigen (PSA):** PSA elevation is often seen with Prostate cancer & the likelihood of cancer increases with higher PSA values; However, PSA is not specific for malignancy (can be seen in other prostate disorders). Abnormal values may be based on general number (>4 ng/mL) or based on age-related normal values. Prior to further evaluation, repeat the PSA test in a few weeks to confirm that the PSA level remains elevated. Elevated alkaline phosphatase level if bony METS.
- **Transrectal Ultrasound-guided needle biopsy: most accurate test.** Indications include [1] life expectancy is at least 10 years (some biopsy if life expectancy is >5 years) and [2] PSA is higher than the range for the patient's age cohort, or PSA has increased >0.75 ng/mL over one year, or abnormal abnormality on DRE (palpable mass). Multiparametric MRI can be used to characterize the tumor.
- Bone scan may be indicated to rule out metastasis If PSA >10 ng/dL.
- **Gleason grading system determines aggressiveness or malignant potential of Prostate cancer.** Higher grade suggests more benefit from surgical removal.

MANAGEMENT
- Appropriate management is controversial because many cases are latent and do not progress while others metastasize. Active surveillance is a preferred option for most with very low-risk disease.
- Local disease: options [1] include observation/active surveillance (eg, low risk, clinically localized, or life expectancy <10 years) or [2] definitive local therapy (eg, external beam radiation therapy, brachytherapy, or radical prostatectomy). **Adverse effects of prostatectomy include incontinence & erectile dysfunction** (more likely compared to radiation).
- **Locally advanced & very high-risk Prostate cancer**: Treatment options include External beam radiation therapy (RT) with or without brachytherapy, long-term androgen deprivation therapy (ADT), or radical prostatectomy. External beam RT plus brachytherapy and ADT are often preferred rather than radical prostatectomy for patients with biopsy grade group 5 disease.
- **Lymph node involvement** — usually treated with definitive RT plus ADT. However, for young males with minimal regional lymphatic spread suspected, radical prostatectomy as part of a combination strategy that includes postoperative ADT and/or RT is an option.
- **Disseminated metastases**: ADT, which may be combined with Docetaxel.
- **Hormonal therapy: androgen deprivation therapy (ADT)** — GnRH agonist (Leuprolide, Goserelin) or GnRH antagonist (Degarelix, Relugolix) for medical castration without surgery. Abiraterone is a 17-hydroxylase (CYP17) inhibitor, a key enzyme in androgen synthesis, that blocks both testicular and adrenal androgen production. It decreases progression of metastatic Prostate cancer.

SCREENING FOR PROSTATE CANCER

Decision to screen is not routinely recommended but should be individualized based on shared decision making:
- Discussion of risk/benefit of screening is important prior to initiating PSA testing.
- In 2018, the USPSTF issued a revised (Grade C) recommendation for men 55–69 years that the decision to undergo periodic PSA-based screening should be an individual one. This acknowledges while screening offers some men a small potential benefit of reducing the chance of dying from prostate cancer, many other men will experience potential harms from screening
- For men aged ≥70 years, the USPSTF recommends against PSA-based screening (Grade D recommendation).

Initiation of screening:
- **Average risk:** if indicated, screening should start at age 50 with PSA.
- **High-risk:** If at high risk for development of prostate cancer (African American men, family history of prostate cancer, known to have the BRCA-1 or BRCA-2 gene mutation), **screen should start between 40-45 years.**

ENURESIS

- **Distinct episodes of urinary incontinence (bedwetting) while sleeping in children ≥5 years of age in a person who usually has voluntary control.**
- **Monosymptomatic:** Enuresis in the absence of lower urinary tract infection symptoms & without bladder dysfunction. Associated with a high rate of spontaneous resolution.

PRIMARY ENURESIS
- **Absence of any period of nighttime dryness. Most common type.** May have a family history.

SECONDARY ENURESIS
- **Enuresis after a dry period of ≥6 months.** Usually due to a psychological stressor (eg, birth of a sibling, parental divorce) or a medical condition (eg, UTI).
- Less common organic etiologies of Enuresis include spinal cord abnormalities, Diabetes insipidus, seizures, obstructive sleep apnea, Chronic kidney disease, and Psychogenic polydipsia.

WORKUP
Evaluation: complete history, physical examination, voiding diary, & Urinalysis (UA):
- **Urinalysis (UA): all patients with Enuresis should be evaluated with UA** even if Urinary tract infection is not highly suspected.

MANAGEMENT
- **Behavioral therapy: first-line therapy** — motivational therapy (especially in children 5-7 years), education & reassurance. Use of washable products & room deodorizers. Bladder training: regular voiding schedule, deliberate voiding prior to sleeping, waking the child up to urinate intermittently. Avoidance of caffeine-based & drinks with high sugar content. Fluid restriction.
- **Enuresis alarm: most effective long-term therapy for Primary enuresis. Usually used if children fail to respond to behavioral therapy.** Often attempted before medical therapy. A sensor is placed on a bed pad or in the undergarments and goes off when wet. Usually continued until there is a minimum of 2 weeks of consecutive dry nights.
- **Desmopressin (DDAVP): used in patients with Primary enuresis in nocturnal polyuria with normal bladder function capacity refractory to behavioral intervention.** Better for short-term use. Mechanism of action: **synthetic antidiuretic hormone (ADH),** which reduces urination. May cause Hyponatremia so patients may use liberal amounts of salt to reduce the incidence.
- **Imipramine: a Tricyclic antidepressant (TCA) that may be used in select refractory cases.** Mechanism of action: stimulates ADH secretion, detrusor muscle relaxation, & decreases time spent in REM sleep.

NEPHROLITHIASIS [KIDNEY STONE DISEASE (RENAL CALCULI)]

TYPES
- **Calcium: calcium oxalate most common type of stone (~75%). Calcium phosphate** (~15%). Low urine citrate increases risk Calcium oxalate stones (envelope- or dumbbell-shaped on UA).
- **Uric acid:** 5-8%. Increased uric acid due to high protein foods, gout, chemotherapy (tumor lysis). **Acidic urine promotes uric acid stone formation.**
- **Struvite: composed of Magnesium ammonium phosphate. May form staghorn calculi in the renal pelvis due to urea-splitting organisms (eg, Proteus,** Klebsiella, Pseudomonas, Serratia, & Enterobacter) which **increase urine pH** (>8.0) or be a complication of a UTI with these organisms.
- **Cystine:** Rare (1-3%). Congenital defect in reabsorption of the amino acid cysteine.

CLINICAL MANIFESTATIONS
- **Acute Nephrolithiasis usually presents with [1] renal colic &/or [2] painless gross hematuria (less common).** May be an asymptomatic incidental finding.
- **Renal colic: sudden, constant upper lateral back or flank pain over the costovertebral angle, often waxing and waning pain,** that may radiate to the groin or anteriorly (testicle in men, labia in women). **May be difficult to find a comfortable position (no alleviating factors).**
- Nausea, vomiting, frequency, **hematuria.** Distal ureter stones may cause dysuria & urinary urgency.
- **Costovertebral angle tenderness** if upper ureteral or kidney pelvic obstruction. Usually afebrile.

Location of pain: pain varies with stone location:
- **proximal ureteral stones — flank pain, CVA tenderness**
- midureteral stones — midabdominal pain
- **distal ureteral stones — groin pain (ipsilateral testicle in men & ipsilateral labium in women).**

DIAGNOSIS
- **UA:** initial test — **microscopic or gross hematuria** (85%). ⊕ Nitrites if infectious. Ca phosphate: wedge-shaped prisms. Ca oxalate: envelope- or dumbbell-shaped. **Acidic urine (pH < 5.0): uric acid & cystine. Alkaline urine (pH >7.2) & coffin lid stone shape associated with struvite stones.**
- **Noncontrast CT abdomen & pelvis: imaging test of choice for suspected Nephrolithiasis** to confirm the presence of a stone and assess for signs of urinary obstruction (eg, Hydronephrosis).
- **Renal & bladder Ultrasound: detects stones or complications (eg, Hydronephrosis), first-line if pregnant or in young children** (US sometimes in combination with abdominopelvic radiography).
- KUB radiographs: **only calcium & struvite stones are radiopaque** (visible on radiographs). May miss small stones even if radiopaque. Cystine & uric acid are radiolucent (hard to see).
- Intravenous pyelography — not used as often. Less sensitive & specific than CT scan.

MANAGEMENT
Stones <5-mm in diameter: 80% chance of spontaneous passage. Strain urine for stone analysis.
- **IV or oral fluids & analgesics: NSAIDs (eg, Ketorolac, Ibuprofen)** provide pain relief & have ureteral-relaxing effects; preferred over opioids. Antiemetics if nauseous (eg, Metoclopramide).
- **Stones at the ureterovesicular junction (UVJ), which is the narrowest point of the urinary tract,** & ureteropelvic junction (UPJ) may make the passage of small stones difficult.

Stones 5 to ≤10 mm in diameter: 20% chance of spontaneous passage.
- **Alpha blocker: (eg, Tamsulosin)** 10-14 days (no more than 4 weeks) may facilitate stone passage. Alpha blockers relax the musculature of the ureter and lower urinary tract. Nifedipine alternative.
- **Elective extracorporeal shock wave lithotripsy:** may be used to break up larger stones that are less likely to pass spontaneously. May need multiple treatments to reduce the size of the stones.
- **Ureteroscopy with/without stent: provides immediate relief to an obstructed or at-risk kidney.**
- **Percutaneous nephrolithotomy:** most invasive. **Used for large stones (>10 mm), struvite,** or if other less invasive modalities fail. Incision is made in the back & the stone is removed via a tube.
- If uric acid stones presents, alkalinization of the urine to pH >6.5 helps to dissolve uric acid stones.

Stones >10 mm should be referred to urology for further management & intervention.

RISK FACTORS FOR NEPHROLITHIASIS

[1] Dietary Risk Factors

- Dietary factors that are associated with an increased risk of Nephrolithiasis include animal protein, oxalate, sodium, sucrose, and fructose. Vitamin C (Calcium oxalate stones in men).
- **Dietary factors associated with a lower risk include calcium, potassium, and phytate intake.**

[2] Nondietary risk factors:

- Age, race, body size, and environment are important risk factors for Nephrolithiasis.
- The prevalence of stone disease is highest in middle-aged white men, but stones can form at any age.
- Weight gain increases the risk of stone formation.
- Working in a hot environment or lack of ready access to water or a bathroom, increases stone risk.

[3] Urinary risk factors:

- **Lower urinary volume leads to higher risk of lithogenic factors (supersaturation).**
- **Urine calcium:** higher urine calcium increases the likelihood of formation of calcium oxalate and calcium phosphate stones.
- Higher urine oxalate increase the risk of calcium oxalate stones.
- **Lower urine citrate excretion increases the risk of stone formation because urine citrate is a natural inhibitor of calcium-containing stones.**
- **Urine pH:** Uric acid stones form only when the urine pH is consistently ≤5.5, whereas calcium phosphate stones are more likely to form when the urine pH is ≥6.5. Cystine is more soluble at higher urine pH. Calcium oxalate stones are not influenced by urine pH. Struvite stones form with high pH.

NEPHROLITHIASIS PREVENTION

- **For all stone types, consistently increased fluid (diluted urine) reduces the likelihood of crystal formation.** The urine volume should be at least 2 liters daily.

Calcium:

- **Calcium oxalate most common. Calcium phosphate.** Calcium stones make up ~90% of all stones.
- **Risk factors: decreased fluid intake most common,** alkaline urinary pH, **higher urinary calcium,** high urine oxalate, **lower urine citrate.** Males, **medications (loop diuretics, acetazolamide, antacids, chemotherapeutic drugs, Indinavir & Topiramate),** high animal protein intake, hypercalcemia, polycystic kidney disease, & increased vitamin C intake in men.
- **Prevention: increased fluid intake, Thiazide diuretics (lowers urinary calcium excretion), low sodium diet,** decreased animal protein diet, foods rich in alkali (eg, fruits and vegetables) can increase urine citrate (urine citrate is a natural inhibitor of calcium-containing stones). **Avoid high-dose Vitamin C supplements for patients with Calcium oxalate stones.**

Uric acid:

- 5-8%. Increased uric acid due to high protein foods, gout, chemotherapy (tumor lysis). **The 2 main risk factors for uric acid stone formation are [1] persistently low urine pH (acidic urine) & [2] higher uric acid excretion** (Gout & increased cell turnover). Not usually visualized on a KUB.
- Prevention: **increased fluids,** decreased purine-containing foods. **Urine alkalinization** can be achieved by increasing foods rich in alkali (eg, fruits, vegetables) & reducing the intake of foods that produce acid (eg, animal flesh), potassium citrate. **Allopurinol or Febuxostat.**

Struvite:

- **Composed of Magnesium ammonium phosphate. May form staghorn calculi** in the renal pelvis due to **urea-splitting organisms (eg, *Proteus,* *Klebsiella, Pseudomonas, Serratia* & Enterobacter)** or be a complication of a UTI with these organisms. Prevention: control the source of infection.

Cystine:

- Rare (1-3%). Congenital defect in reabsorption of the amino acid cysteine from the urine. Not usually visualized on a KUB.
- Prevention: **dietary modification, low sodium, urine alkalinization.**
  Chelating agents in refractory cases.

HEMATURIA

ETIOLOGIES
- Hematuria not explained by an obvious underlying condition (eg, cystitis, ureteral stone) is relatively common (eg, trauma, vigorous exercise, idiopathic, menses). In many of these patients, especially in young adult patients, the hematuria is often transient with no sequelae.
- **Causes vary with age, with the most common cause in individuals <35 years of age being [1] inflammation or [2] infection of the prostate or bladder, or [3] Nephrolithiasis**.
- If >35 years, a kidney or urinary tract malignancy or Benign prostatic hyperplasia may be the cause.
- **Upper GU tract (eg, kidneys & ureter): Nephrolithiasis (40%),** Kidney disease (20%), Renal cell carcinoma, trauma (10%), Diabetes mellitus, Sickle cell trait or disease.
- **Lower GU tract: BPH (most common cause of microscopic hematuria in men),** Urothelial cell cancer (in the absence of infection) 5%. Sexual or physical activity & illness.
- Pseudo hematuria: Rhabdomyolysis, beets, rhubarb, myoglobinuria (contains heme), hemoglobinuria.
- Medications: Ibuprofen, Phenazopyridine, Rifampin. **Cyclophosphamide (hemorrhagic cystitis).**

TIMING OF HEMATURIA
- **Terminal: bladder irritation (eg, stone or infection) or prostate.**
- Throughout micturition: bladder, ureter, or kidneys. **Initial urethral in origin.**

DIAGNOSIS
- **Urinalysis: usually initial test of choice to assess for hematuria (≥3 RBCs/hpf)** to rule out benign causes (eg, UTI or Pyelonephritis). Repeat UA after 6 weeks to assess for resolution of hematuria.
- Urine culture may be performed if UA is suggestive for UTI (eg, ⊕ leukocyte esterase &/or nitrite, increased WBCs, UTI symptoms).
- Measurement of BUN and creatinine should also be performed.

Symptoms suggestive of Nephrolithiasis:
- **Noncontrast computed tomography [CT] or Ultrasound initial imaging in the evaluation of patients who present with hematuria and unilateral flank pain suggestive of obstructive Nephrolithiasis.** Ultrasound may be the initial test of choice for Nephrolithiasis after UA in pregnant patients, in children, or if CT scan cannot be performed. Abdominal radiographs in some.

Noninfectious urine on UA + gross hematuria with visible blood clots in the urine:
- **CT urography (upper tract imaging) & urgent urology referral for evaluation, cystoscopy (± adjunctive urine Cytology),** especially if >35 years, smoking history, or Bladder cancer risk factors. **CT urography is the workup of choice after noninfectious UA in patients >35 years old, especially if initial imaging is negative.** Intravenous pyelogram is an alternative to CT urography to evaluate the kidney, ureters etc.

Gross hematuria without visible blood clots in the urine:
- **Patients with Acute kidney injury or glomerular bleeding should be referred to nephrology.**
- **Nonpregnant patients** without Acute kidney injury or findings suggestive of glomerular bleeding **should have CT urography & urology referral for Cystoscopy.** Pregnant patients should have Kidney & bladder ultrasound rather than CT, mainly to rule out ureteral obstruction or urolithiasis.

Microscopic hematuria:
- Patients with Acute kidney injury or findings suggestive of glomerular bleeding should be referred to nephrology.
- Nonpregnant patients with risk factors for malignancy of the kidney or bladder, or have a prior history of a urologic disorder (eg, Benign prostatic hypertrophy, nephrolithiasis), should undergo CT urography and urology referral for Cystoscopy.
- Nonpregnant patients who have no findings suggestive of glomerular bleeding, no risk factors for malignancy, and no history of urologic disease do not require imaging studies or cystoscopy. However, nephrology evaluation and imaging may be indicated for persistent, unexplained microscopic hematuria.
- Pregnant patients should be evaluated with a Kidney and bladder ultrasound; further evaluation should be avoided, if possible, until after delivery.

PENILE CANCER

- Rare in the US, Europe, & other industrialized countries. <u>Older men</u>: mean age at diagnosis is 60 years.
- **<u>Squamous cell carcinoma</u>: most common type. Commonly associated with Human papillomavirus [HPV 16,** 18, 6], **tobacco exposure, lack of circumcision [eg, lack of hygiene (smegma,** phimosis; circumcision &/or good hygiene reduces risk)], HIV, urethral stricture, penile trauma (eg, penile tear, chronic penile rash), obesity.
- <u>Bowen's disease:</u> leukoplakia on the shaft of the penis or scrotum. Peak incidence >50 years. Associated with HPV 16. Minority progresses to Squamous cell carcinoma.

CLINICAL PRESENTATION

- **Penile skin abnormality, mass, palpable lesion, or penile ulcer (often painless) & common on the glans > coronal sulcus > prepuce.** Rare presentations include rash, bleeding, & balanitis.
- **May have inguinal lymphadenopathy** (30-60%); may be inflammatory or metastatic.
- Squamous cell carcinoma in situ involving the penis (erythroplasia of Queyrat).

DIAGNOSIS

- Biopsy. May seed to inguinal lymph nodes, followed by pelvic and retroperitoneal lymph nodes.

MANAGEMENT

- <u>Early disease:</u> limited excision with organ-preserving strategies.
- <u>Bulky stage T2 to T4 tumors, high risk</u>: penile amputation with therapeutic lymph node dissection.

ERECTILE DYSFUNCTION

- Consistent or recurrent inability to generate or maintain a sufficiently rigid penile erection.

ETIOLOGIES

- **<u>Vascular</u> most common due to decrease arterial inflow (eg, atherosclerosis, diabetes).**
- Neurologic, psychogenic (eg, normal nocturnal, morning, or masturbatory erections and situational erectile dysfunction); prolactinoma, trauma, surgery.
- <u>Medications</u>: beta-blockers, thiazide diuretics, spironolactone, calcium channel blockers, SSRIs, TCAs.
- Abrupt onset most likely psychological whereas gradual worsening indicates systemic causes.

DIAGNOSIS

- History & physical exam, lipid level, glucose level, testosterone level, other hormone testing.
- Nocturnal penile tumescence used to evaluate sleep erections.
- <u>Duplex Doppler ultrasound</u> to evaluate penile blood flow and characterize penile anatomy.

MANAGEMENT

Phosphodiesterase-5 inhibitors: Sildenafil, Tadalafil, Vardenafil, Avanafil
- <u>Indications</u>: **first-line therapy for Erectile dysfunction.**
- <u>Mechanism of action</u>: **phosphodiesterase-5 inhibition increases cyclic GMP & potentiates nitric oxide-mediated penile smooth muscle relaxation,** improving ability to generate & maintain an erection.
- <u>Adverse effects</u>: **headache, flushing, rhinitis, visual disturbances (blue vision), hearing loss.**
- **Alpha blocker concomitant use may drop blood pressure.** Initiate and titrate in stepwise fashion.
- <u>Contraindications</u>: **PDE5Is not used with Nitrates or patients with cardiovascular disease** (may cause severe hypotension — synergistic nitric oxide).

Second-line therapies:
- <u>Vacuum erection device</u> (eg, vacuum pump), often followed by band constriction to maintain erection.
- <u>Intracavernosal injection therapy</u>: Intraurethral prostaglandin E1 (Alprostadil) injection or suppository in combination with Papaverine (causes vasodilation — increased arterial inflow).
- <u>Third-line therapies:</u> Penile prosthesis or corrective penile revascularization.
- Psychotherapy if due to psychogenic reasons.

Testosterone:
- Hormone replacement if documented hypogonadism [testosterone is low (eg, androgen deficiency)].

PRIAPISM

- Prolonged, painful penile erections in the absence of sexual stimulation.
- **Ischemic (low-flow):** decreased <u>venous</u> outflow may lead to a compartment syndrome, increasing acidosis, & hypoxia in the cavernous tissues. Painful & rigid erection. **Most common type.**
- **Nonischemic (high-flow):** increased <u>arterial</u> inflow due to a fistula between the cavernosal artery & corpus cavernosum. Commonly related to **perineal or penile trauma.** Less painful & not fully rigid compared to ischemic. **The penis may be semierect &/or painless if Nonischemic.**

ETIOLOGIES
- **Idiopathic most common** (50%), **Sickle cell disease** (10%), injection of erectile agent for erectile dysfunction (eg, Papaverine, Prostaglandin E1), drugs (eg, cocaine, marijuana), alcohol.
- <u>Medications:</u> **PDE-5 inhibitors, Trazodone**, Antipsychotics, Anticonvulsants, Alpha blockers.
- <u>Neurologic:</u> head trauma, meningitis, Subarachnoid hemorrhage, & postoperative.
- <u>Trauma</u> may cause high flow Priapism and may cause rupture of the cavernosal artery.

DIAGNOSIS
- Primarily based on history and physical examination. Cavernous blood gas analysis or Doppler ultrasound can be performed to distinguish between ischemic and nonischemic Priapism.
- **<u>Cavernosal blood gas</u>: high flow results similar to ABG & normal glucose.**
  Low flow shows hypoglycemia, hypoxemia, hypercarbia, & acidemia.
- <u>Doppler ultrasound:</u> May be performed as an alternative to cavernosal blood gas to differentiate between ischemic and nonischemic types of Priapism — <u>Nonischemic:</u> normal or high blood flow. <u>Ischemic:</u> minimal or absent blood flow.

MANAGEMENT OF ISCHEMIC (LOW-FLOW)
- Ischemic Priapism requires rapid detumescence to avoid long-term sequelae, and urgent urologic consultation should be obtained.

<u>Corporal aspiration, irrigation, & α-adrenergic agonist (eg, Phenylephrine) first line if Ischemic:</u>
- **<u>Intracavernosal injection with a sympathomimetic:</u> eg, <u>Phenylephrine</u>: first-line medication (if <4 hours duration.** <u>Mechanism of action:</u> **Alpha agonists** cause contraction of the cavernous smooth muscle, which increases venous outflow. <u>Adverse effects</u> include acute Hypertension, headache, and cardiac arrhythmia. <u>Contraindications:</u> cardiac or cerebrovascular history.
- **<u>Needle aspiration</u> of corpus cavernosum & irrigation to remove blood especially if >4 hours duration with or without Phenylephrine** (combination therapy is more effective). Ice packs. Fluid and oxygenation added to combination therapy in patients with Sickle cell disease.
- <u>Shunt surgery</u> may be performed if not responsive to repeated medical & aspiration therapy.

MANAGEMENT OF NONISCHEMIC (HIGH-FLOW)
- **<u>Observation</u> — most resolve within hours to days. Once ischemic Priapism has been ruled out, observation alone is appropriate for initial management of nonischemic Priapism.**
- <u>Refractory:</u> nonpermanent arterial embolization or surgical ligation may be used if refractory or in patients who prefer an intervention rather than observation.

PREMATURE EJACULATION (PE)

- Rapid or early ejaculation and is defined according to three essential criteria: (1) brief ejaculatory latency; (2) loss of control; and (3) psychological distress in the patient and/or partner.

MANAGEMENT
- **Mainstays of therapy include <u>Selective serotonin reuptake inhibitors (SSRIs)</u> [eg, Paroxetine), topical anesthetics, & Psychotherapy** when psychogenic and/or relationship factors are present.
- <u>Second line:</u> Clomipramine (a serotonergic Tricyclic) if SSRIs are ineffective or not tolerated.

HYPOSPADIAS

- Congenital anomaly of the male urethra that results in **abnormal <u>ventral</u> placement of the urethral opening,** penile curvature, and abnormal foreskin development.
- The urethral opening can be glandular or coronal (85%), on the shaft, the scrotum, or perineum.
- Second most common congenital in males after Cryptorchidism.

PATHOPHYSIOLOGY:
- **<u>Failure of the urogenital folds to fuse during development</u>** — abnormal development of the urethral fold & the ventral foreskin of the penis. **Proximal Hypospadias associated with Cryptorchidism** (8-10%); **Inguinal hernia** (9-15%) or other GU abnormalities (eg, VUR).

CLINICAL MANIFESTATIONS
- Increased risk of UTIs, deflection of the urinary stream, erectile dysfunction.
Physical examination:
- **Ventral placement of the urethral meatus** (representing the remnant urethral groove).
- **<u>Dorsal hooded foreskin</u>:** Abnormal foreskin with incomplete closure around the glans (dorsal hooded prepuce). **Abnormal ventral penile curvature (chordee) when proximally displaced.**
- May have underdeveloped penis or Cryptorchidism.

DIAGNOSIS
- Urologic evaluation for surgical repair to be performed at 6 months. No further workup if isolated.
Severe Hypospadias or Undescended testes:
- <u>Karyotyping analysis</u>: In some cases, severe Hypospadias can be indicative of a disorder of sex development (eg, androgen receptor mutation). Hypospadias may represent either virilization of a genotypic female (XX) or undervirilization of a genotypic male (XY).
- <u>Pelvic ultrasound</u> may also be indicated to assess for internal genitalia (eg, uterus).

MANAGEMENT
- **<u>Defer early neonatal circumcision</u>: these patients should NOT be circumcised in the neonatal period because the foreskin may be used to repair the defect.**
- <u>Elective surgical correction</u> (arthroplasty) may include penile straightening. **Hypospadias repair usually performed in healthy full-term infants most commonly 6 months-1 year of age.**

EPISPADIAS

- Congenital anomaly of the male urethra — **abnormal <u>dorsal</u> placement of the urethral opening.**
- **Often associated with bladder exstrophy** (protrusion of the bladder wall through a defect in the abdominal wall).

PATHOPHYSIOLOGY
- <u>Epispadias:</u> **failure of midline penile fusion.**
- <u>Bladder exstrophy:</u> in utero rupture of an overdeveloped cloacal membrane, leading to herniation of the lower abdominal contents.

CLINICAL MANIFESTATIONS
- <u>Males:</u> **opening of the urethral meatus on the dorsal (top) surface of the penis, dorsal (upward) curvature of the penis, absent dorsal foreskin.** Dorsiflexion of the penis.
- <u>Females:</u> bifid clitoris and small, laterally displaced labia minora.

DIAGNOSIS
- The diagnosis of bladder exstrophy is often made via prenatal Ultrasound.

MANAGEMENT
- <u>Surgical correction</u> of curvature, urethral reconstruction; bladder neck reconstruction if incontinent.

SCROTAL INJURIES

CLINICAL MANIFESTATIONS
- Clinical findings that suggest significant scrotal trauma include marked testicular pain, scrotal swelling, laceration into or through the dartos fascia, or a large scrotal hematoma.
- Blood at the meatus or ecchymosis of the penis, perineum or scrotum suggest urethral injury.

DIAGNOSIS
Urinalysis & Scrotal Ultrasound:
- Urinalysis and Doppler ultrasound of the scrotum are often obtained in patients who experienced scrotal trauma, especially with significant pain and swelling after blunt scrotal trauma.

Suspected urethral injury:
- **Retrograde urethrography** is indicated for patients with suspected urethral injury.

MANAGEMENT
Minor trauma:
- **For most patients, pain or scrotal swelling is minimal and the testes appear normal.**
  - **Supportive treatment** consists of rest, ice packs as tolerated, supportive underwear (briefs instead of boxers), & Nonsteroidal anti-inflammatory medications (eg, Ibuprofen) for pain.
  - Initial management of scrotal trauma includes analgesia and, in patients with penetrating scrotal trauma including human or animal bites to the scrotum, antibiotic prophylaxis, tetanus prophylaxis, and if indicated, rabies and other viral prophylaxis.

More serious injuries require Urology consultation and further management depending on the injury.

URETHRAL PROLAPSE

- Rare; most commonly occurs in prepubertal females 2-10 years of age & postmenopausal women.

CLINICAL MANIFESTATIONS
- Urethral prolapse may present with vaginal bleeding, dysuria, and/or difficulty with urination in postmenopausal women. May be asymptomatic in children.
- Rarely, a large prolapse may become strangulated and result in pain, bleeding, and urinary symptoms.

Physical examination:
- **The urethral mucosa protrudes through the meatus & presents as a dusky red or purplish annular (donut-shaped) mass at the urethral location or anterior vaginal wall;** sensitive vulvar mass separated from the vagina. The tissue may be friable and become infected.
- Diagnosis is confirmed on identification of the urethral meatus as the central opening in the prolapsed tissues. Urethral catheterization may be required if direct observation during voiding is not possible
- Rule out urinary tract infection, which is frequently associated with urethral prolapse.

MANAGEMENT
Refer all patients with confirmed or suspected urethral prolapse for follow-up with a urologist.
Consult urology emergently for signs of urethral strangulation.
- **Medical therapy** consists of warm sitz baths twice daily and a short course of topical estrogen cream applied two to three times to the urethra after the sitz bath for 2 weeks. Then, the urethra is reassessed, and treatment is continued if the prolapse has not resolved and is still present. The prolapse will usually resolve within a few weeks of topical estrogen treatment.
- Surgical therapy is reserved for strangulation or failed medical therapy. Indwelling catheter inserted for 24 hours after surgery.

Pediatric urologist referral:
- A necrotic distal urethra, which may require excision under general anesthesia.
- Persistence of the prolapse, which may require assessment for a urethral polyp and reduction under general anesthesia.

URETHRAL INJURIES

- More common in men. Long-term complications include Urethral stricture.

ETIOLOGIES

- Anterior urethral injuries: **direct perineal trauma most common (80%) blunt or penetrating — straddle-type injuries or falls most common,** direct blows to the perineum, penile fracture. Penetrating trauma (eg penile urethra). Pelvic fractures; traumatic catheterization. Sexual assault.
- Posterior urethral injury (prostatic or membranous portions) — eg, pelvic fractures, motor vehicle collisions, fall from heights, **traumatic childbirth during vaginal deliveries in women.**

CLINICAL MANIFESTATIONS

- **Gross hematuria,** difficulty urinating, urinary retention, inability to void, lower abdominal pain.

Physical examination:

- **Blood at the urethral meatus (anterior urethral injury). Vaginal bleeding in females.**
- **Swelling or ecchymosis (hematoma) of the scrotum, penis, labia, or perineum.**
- **Hallmark triad of urethral injury:** [1] blood at the urethral meatus, [2] inability to void, & [3] distended bladder.
- High-riding prostate in males (rare).
- May have difficulty (resistance) to gentle passage of Foley catheter. May need suprapubic catheterization for bladder drainage in these patients. **Foley catheters should not be inserted if there is a suspicion of Urethral injury until it has been ruled out (eg, via Retrograde urethrogram).**

DIAGNOSIS

- Assess for injuries & fractures (eg, pelvic fractures). Urinalysis (UA).
- **Retrograde urethrogram diagnostic imaging of choice for anterior urethral injury — may demonstrate extravasation of contrast from the urethra; must be done prior to transurethral catheterization** & may interfere with completion of CT abdomen and pelvis assessment for other injuries. Urethroscopy is an alternative and is more helpful in assessment of women.
- CT cystography can assess for coexisting bladder injury. Trauma surgeon &/or urology consult.

MANAGEMENT

- **Non-operative management:** bladder drainage (eg, suprapubic catheter placement); monitoring for healing.
- Surgical repair: indicated in severe injuries. May involve **temporary suprapubic catheter placement for bladder drainage prior to delayed repair.**

TUMOR MARKER	MAIN ASSOCIATIONS
ALPHA FETOPROTEIN	• **Hepatocellular carcinoma** • **Nonseminomatous germ cell testicular cancer** • Decreased in Down syndrome (Trisomy 21) "AFP is down in Down syndrome"
hCG	• **Nonseminomatous germ cell testicular cancer** • **Choriocarcinomas,** Teratomas • **Trophoblastic tumors** (eg, hydatidiform molar pregnancy)
CA-125	• **Ovarian cancer**
CA 19-9	• **Pancreatic cancer** • GI – Colorectal, Esophageal & Hepatocellular cancers
CALCITONIN	• **Medullary thyroid cancer**
CEA	• **Colorectal cancer** • Medullary thyroid, pancreatic, gastric, lung & breast cancers
PROSTATE SPECIFIC ANTIGEN (PSA)	• **Prostate cancer** • Can also be elevated in BPH & Prostatitis

FOURNIER GANGRENE

- **Necrotizing fasciitis (soft tissue) infection with <u>involvement of the perineal, genital (scrotal), or perianal areas.</u>** May rapidly spread to involve the thighs, abdominal wall, and chest.
- **Considered a urological emergency;** High fatality rate >40%.

MICROBIOLOGY

- **<u>Fournier gangrene is usually a polymicrobial infection</u>** (aerobes and anaerobes) — facultative organisms (*E. coli, Klebsiella,* enterococci), *Group A Streptococci, Staphylococcus aureus,* & anaerobes (*Bacteroides, Fusobacterium, Clostridium,* anaerobic or microaerophilic streptococci).

RISK FACTORS

- **<u>Immunocompromised states</u>: Diabetes mellitus &/or alcohol abuse seen in most patients. Most common in Diabetic males [20-79 years of age (esp. >50y)];** smoking, Cirrhosis, HIV.
- **Males 10 times more affected** than women. Cancer, chemotherapy. SGLT-2 inhibitors. Obesity.

PATHOPHYSIOLOGY

- **The most common causes are infection and trauma** — eg, breach in the integrity of the skin or mucosa (GI, urethral) or traumatic wounds. Often begins as a benign infection (eg, localized cellulitis, UTI) or simple abscess, with rapid spread of inflammation & infection along the fascial planes of adjacent soft tissue. Results in microthrombosis of the small subcutaneous vessels & development of gangrene of the overlying skin.

CLINICAL MANIFESTATIONS

- **<u>Early symptoms:</u> severe genital or peritoneal pain (may be out of proportion to examination findings early on), pruritus, cellulitis with edema, & patchy erythema of the genital or scrotal area.** The pain may be poorly localized & spread rapidly to the anterior abdominal wall & gluteal muscles. **Involvement in men may include the scrotum, perineum, and penis**; involvement in women may involve the labia. Prodromal symptoms of lethargy & fever may occur.
- **The early symptoms are often followed by rapid progression of erythema, edema extending past the visible erythema, fever, dusky-appearing skin.** Purulent draining may be seen. Systemic toxicity (eg, hypotension, tachycardia, fever, tachypnea, sepsis, shock, and organ dysfunction).

Physical examination:
- **Fever, erythema of the scrotum and perineum, marked edema extending past the visible erythema, subcutaneous crepitus, skin bullae & blisters, ecchymosis, gangrenous changes (eg, necrosis, patchy dusky or black skin discoloration).**

DIAGNOSIS

- Prompt recognition of Fournier gangrene in its early stages may prevent extensive tissue loss that occurs when the diagnosis and intervention are delayed. **Imaging should not delay urologic or surgical consultation or intervention. Definitive diagnosis made during surgical exploration.**
- <u>CT scan</u> **best initial imaging** & may reveal disease extent (often shows spread of infection beyond what is seen on the skin). Fat stranding; gas in the tissues is highly specific for Necrotizing fasciitis.
- <u>Bedside US</u> may show scrotal wall thickening, & "dirty shadowing"; hazy look due to air in the tissues.

MANAGEMENT

- **Treat with aggressive fluid resuscitation, broad spectrum antibiotics** (gram-positive, gram-negative, and anaerobic coverage); **early, extensive, and aggressive surgical debridement of necrotic tissue; hemodynamic support, and ICU admission.** Hyperbaric oxygen used in some.
- <u>Empiric regimen</u>: **A Carbapenem (eg, Imipenem or Meropenem) or Piperacillin-tazobactam PLUS an agent with activity against Methicillin-resistant *Staphylococcus aureus* (eg, Vancomycin) PLUS Clindamycin** (for its antitoxin effects against toxin-elaborating strains of beta-hemolytic streptococci and *S. aureus*). Daptomycin or Linezolid are alternatives to Vancomycin.

CHAPTER 10 – NEUROLOGIC SYSTEM

SEVERE NONEXERTIONAL HYPERTHERMIA (HEAT STROKE)

- Occurs during strenuous activity in hot humid weather.

CLINICAL MANIFESTATIONS
- **Elevated core body temperature (generally >40.5°C [105°F]), central nervous system dysfunction (eg, altered mental status, SEIZURES),** exposure to severe environmental heat, and the absence of another explanation for hyperthermia.

MANAGEMENT
- Ensuring adequate airway protection, breathing, and circulation; rapid cooling; and treatment of complications. Tracheal intubation and mechanical ventilation are often necessary.
- **Hypotension or volume depletion is treated with IV isotonic crystalloid.**
- **Rapid cooling using <u>evaporative and convective techniques</u> (eg, naked patient is sprayed with a mist of lukewarm water while fans are used to blow air over the moist skin, ice-wet towel rotation)** rather than other noninvasive (eg, cold water immersion) or invasive (eg, peritoneal lavage) techniques. There is no role for antipyretic agents. Continuous core temperature monitoring with a rectal or esophageal probe is necessary in all patients being treated for heat stroke.
Complications:
- **<u>Organ or tissue damage</u>:** renal or hepatic failure, Disseminated intravascular coagulation, acute respiratory distress syndrome, Rhabdomyolysis.

TRAUMATIC BRAIN (INTRACRANIAL) INJURY

- Sequelae from an external force injuring the brain (head trauma).
- Can result in cognitive, physical, social, emotional, and behavioral symptoms.

ETIOLOGIES
- **Falls (especially in the elderly) most common,** motor vehicle collisions.

CLASSIFICATION OF SEVERITY
- The Glasgow coma scale (GCS) is scored between 3-15, 3 being the worst and 15 the best.
- It is composed of 3 parameters: [1] best eye response (E), [2] best verbal response (V), and [3] best motor response (M). The components of the GCS should be recorded individually; for example, E4V2M2 results in a GCS score of 8.
  - Mild: score of ≥13
  - Moderate: score of 9-12
  - Severe: score of ≤8

	SCORE
Eye opening	4
Spontaneous	4
Response to verbal commands	3
Response to pain	2
No eye opening	1
Best Verbal Response	5
Oriented	5
Confused	4
Inappropriate words	3
Incomprehensible sounds	2
No verbal response	1
Best Motor Response	6
Obeys commands	6
Localizing response to pain	5
Withdrawal response to pain	4
Flexion to pain	3
Extension to pain	2
No motor response	1

PATHOPHYSIOLOGY
- Primary: intra- and extraparenchymal hemorrhages and diffuse axonal injury.
- Secondary: molecular damage, which can be worsened by fever, seizures, hypoxia, and hypotension.

MANAGEMENT OF SEVERE TRAUMATIC BRAIN INJURY (TBI)
- Managed in a neurosurgical ICU with frequent clinical & neurological assessments.
- Prevention of hypoxia (PaO$_2$ <60 mm Hg), hypotension (SBP <100 mm Hg). Endotracheal intubation.
- Surgical evaluation of hematomas based on hematoma size, mass effect, and neurological status.
- **Reduction of intracranial pressure: options include elevate the head of bed, hyperventilation, IV Mannitol or Hypertonic saline.**
  - Hyperventilation should be avoided in the first 24 to 48 hours and should not exceed PaCO$_2$ <30 mmHg except as a temporizing measure in a patient with impending cerebral herniation.
  - Positive end-expiratory pressure (PEEP) up to 15-20 cm H$_2$O may be utilized to manage acute respiratory distress syndrome (ARDS) following TBI while ICP is monitored.
- For patients with severe TBI and an abnormal CT scan revealing evidence of mass effect from lesions such as contusions, hematomas, or swelling, ventriculostomy and ICP monitoring along with treatment of elevated ICP to target pressures <22 mm Hg is recommended.
- Short-term (one-week) use of antiseizure drugs for the prevention of early seizures (eg, Levetiracetam), Fosphenytoin.
- Fever and hyperglycemia should be avoided (may exacerbate secondary injury).

ACUTE MILD TRAUMATIC BRAIN INJURY [TBI] (CONCUSSION SYNDROME)

- **Reversible mild traumatic brain injury leading to alteration in mental status**, with or without loss of consciousness.
- May result after blunt force or an acceleration/deceleration head injury. Indirect or direct injury.

CLINICAL MANIFESTATIONS
- Headache, dizziness, nausea, psychological symptoms, unsteady gait, and cognitive impairment.
- Change in personality, brief loss of consciousness, overt confusion, brief amnesia, blurring of vision.
- **Confusion**: confused or blank expression, blunted affect.
- **Amnesia**: pretraumatic (retrograde) or posttraumatic (antegrade) amnesia. The duration of retrograde amnesia is usually brief.
- Delayed responses & emotional changes: emotional instability.
- Signs of increased intracranial pressure: persistent vomiting, worsening headache, increasing disorientation, changing levels of consciousness.

DIAGNOSIS
- Patients who have suffered loss of consciousness or have persistent symptoms should be referred to an emergency department.
- **Noncontrast CT head is the study of choice for evaluating most acute head injuries.**
- MRI study of choice if prolonged symptoms >7-14 days or with worsening of symptoms not explained by concussion syndrome.
- CT angiography of the head or neck with IV contrast if vascular injury is suspected.

MANAGEMENT
- **Cognitive & physical rest is the mainstay of management of patients with a concussion.**
- **Some form of observation** is recommended for a minimum of 24 hours (outpatient or inpatient).
- **Patients may resume strenuous activity after resolution of symptoms & recovery of memory as well as cognitive functions.**
- Neurosurgical or neurologic consult if CT scan shows mass effect, substantial hematomas (epidural, subdural, cerebral), subarachnoid hemorrhage, pneumocephalus, depressed skull fracture, cerebral edema.
- Current guidelines state that after an athlete's third concussion, he or she should terminate the current season but may return to play the subsequent season if asymptomatic.

PANCE PREP PEARL OF THE WEEK

LOWER MOTOR NEURON
Muscles are **FLABBY**
- **F**asciculations in advanced stage
- **F**laccid paralysis (flabby muscle)
- **L**oss of muscle tone & strength
- **A**reflexia (decreased DTR)
- **B**abinski towards the **B**asement downwards
- **Y**oung (infantile poliomyelitis known as infantile paralysis)

Conditions: Bs:
- Guillain-**B**arré Syndrome,
- **B**otulism,
- Poliomyelitis (**B**aby),
- Cauda Equina Syndrome (**B**ack)
- **B**ell palsy

UPPER MOTOR NEURON
Muscles are **SPASTIC**
- **S**light muscle loss **(no atrophy)**
- **P**ositive Babinski (toe up), Posturing
- **A**bsence of fasciculations
- **S**trong **T**one (Spastic paralysis)
- **T**one increased (Spastic paralysis)
- **I**ncreased deep tendon reflexes
- **C**lonus

- **Conditions:** S: **S**troke (CVA), Multiple **S**clerosis, Cerebral pal**S**y **S**pinal cord or brain damage (ex traumatic brain injury)

CRANIAL NERVES

EYELID
- CN III opens the eyelid (damage causes ptosis)
- CN VII closes the eyelid

PUPILLARY REFLEX
- CN II afferent (sensory)
- CN III efferent (motor)

CORNEAL REFLEX
- CN V (afferent) sensory
- CN VII (efferent) motor

CRANIAL NERVE		FUNCTIONS & ASSESSMENTS	DISEASE ASSOCIATION
I. OLFACTORY	S	Smell	Anosmia
II. OPTIC	S	Visual acuity: tests Snellen chart & accommodation Visual fields Pupillary light reflex: swinging flashlight test to assess afferent pupillary response (CN III efferent; CN II afferent).	Optic neuritis Marcus Gunn pupil (pupil appears to dilate when light is shone in the affected eye).
III. OCULOMOTOR	M	(1) Eye movement: most of the ocular muscles, except the lateral rectus (CN 6) [LR6] and superior oblique muscles CN4 [SO4]. (2) Opens the eyelid: supplies the levator palpebrae. (3) Pupil constriction and accommodation efferent pupillary response (CN III efferent; CN II afferent).	Eye is "down and out". Ptosis Blown pupil: fixed and dilated pupil. Diabetes can cause CN III palsy with pupil sparing.
IV. TROCHLEAR	M	Superior oblique muscle [SO4]: depresses the eye when adducted in isolation (down and out).	Diplopia is usually worse on downgaze & gaze away from side of affected muscle (difficulty looking down). Head tilt away from the side of the lesion (towards unaffected side) to reduce their diplopia.
V. TRIGEMINAL	B	(1) Motor function: muscles of mastication, closing the jaw, moves chin from side to side. (2) Sensory function: facial sensation 3 branches: ophthalmic, maxillary, and mandibular branches. (3) Corneal reflex involuntary blinking of the eyelids elicited by stimulation of the cornea. CN V only carries sensory information (afferent). [CN VII - motor function (efferent)]. Sensory: light touch with cotton wisp to test the 3 division of the nerve.	Trigeminal neuralgia Cluster headache Herpes Zoster Ophthalmicus Loss of blink reflex Jaw deviation towards the side of the lesion
VI. ABDUCENS	M	Lateral eye motion: Lateral rectus muscle functions to abduct the ipsilateral eye (look away from the nose) [LR6].	Abducens nerve palsy causes esotropia & horizontal diplopia. Idiopathic intracranial hypertension.

VII. FACIAL	B	[1] <u>Motor</u>: muscles of facial expression [eg, blinking of the eyelid, raising eyebrows, smile, closing the eyelid (orbicularis oculi), puffing cheeks], stapedius muscle, tear glands, corneal reflex [motor function (efferent)]. [2] <u>Sensory</u>: taste anterior 2/3 of tongue; Somatic fibers to the external ear. [3] <u>Parasympathetic</u>: salivation & lacrimation.	Bell palsy CN 7 palsy Ramsay Hunt syndrome Loss of blink reflex
VIII. ACOUSTIC	S	<u>Hearing</u>: assess with Weber & Rinne test & speech. <u>Vestibular function</u>: balance & proprioception	Vestibular Neuritis Labyrinthitis Acoustic Neuroma
IX. GLOSSO PHARYNGEAL	B	<u>Motor</u>: swallowing (raises part of the throat). Check gag reflex & soft palate elevation. <u>Sensory</u>: taste involving the posterior 1/3 of tongue.	Difficulty swallowing Absent gag reflex Dysfunction of the parotid gland.
X. VAGUS	B	<u>Motor</u>: voice, soft palate, gag reflex <u>Sensory</u>: relays to the brain sensory information about organs. Gag, swallow, and cough. Check uvula <u>Visceral sensory</u>: cardiovascular (including Aortic arch and bodies), respiratory, & GI systems.	<u>Cranial nerve X (10) palsies:</u> palate droop Dysphagia <u>Deviation of the uvula</u> away from the side of the lesion (towards the strong side). <u>Loss of gag reflex</u> (the sensory component of this reflex is mostly via CN IX). <u>A hoarse voice</u> can indicate Vagus nerve injury (the recurrent laryngeal nerve branches off of the Vagus nerve).
XI. ACCESSORY	M	<u>Sternocleidomastoid & Trapezius</u> (motor) Have the patient <u>shrug their shoulders against resistance</u> (both together and one at a time). Have the patient turn their head.	Shoulder droop
XII. HYPOGLOSSAL	M	<u>Tongue</u>: inspect for fasciculations & asymmetry. Have the patient stick out their tongue, and then move it from side to side. Push out their cheek from the inside of their mouth and oppose their movements.	<u>Lesions (palsies)</u>: The tongue will deviate toward the side of lesion with CN XII damage. Muscle atrophy can also be visible on exam so symmetry can be assessed.

M = motor; S = sensory; B = both

CERVICAL RADICULOPATHY

	C5	**C6**	**C7**	**C8**
	C5	C6	C7	C8
MOTOR	Shoulder abduction (deltoid) Elbow flexion (palm up)	**Elbow flexion (thumb up)** Forearm Wrist extension	Elbow extension Wrist flexion	Finger flexion
MUSCLES	**Deltoid, Biceps**	**Biceps, Brachioradialis** Extensor carpi radialis	Triceps Flexor carpi radialis	**Finger flexors**: Flexor digitorum superficialis
SENSORY	**Lateral upper arm** (below deltoid & above elbow), axillary nerve	**Lateral forearm:** **Radial side of hand &** **forearm (including <u>thumb</u>** **& index finger)**	**Radial side of fingers** 2,3,4 (**middle finger**) Posterior forearm	**Ulnar side:** **Little finger** **Ulnar side of 4th finger**
REFLEXES	**Loss of bicep jerk reflex**	**Brachioradialis & biceps**	**Triceps jerk reflex**	

HEADACHES

PRIMARY HEADACHE

- **Multiple entities that cause episodic and chronic head pain in the absence of disease, traumatic injury, or underlying pathological processes.**
- The most common of these are Tension-type headache, Migraine, and the Trigeminal autonomic cephalalgias, including Cluster headache; Rebound (medication overuse) headache: chronic or nearly daily headaches associated with frequent use of medication for acute head pain.

SECONDARY HEADACHE

- Head pain in the presence of disease, traumatic injury, or underlying pathological processes.
- Examples include Meningitis, Subarachnoid hemorrhage, Intracranial hypertension, Hypertensive crisis, Acute glaucoma, brain tumor.
- Suspect secondary if abrupt or progression of severity.

Secondary headache disorders may be suspected if

- <u>Systemic symptoms</u>: eg, fevers, chills, myalgias, weight loss.

- Neurological symptoms, especially if focal neurologic deficits.

- Older onset ≥50 years of age.

- Sudden onset headache (eg, Subarachnoid hemorrhage).

- Progressive headache or substantial pattern change in usual pattern.

- Positional

- Papilledema

- Precipitated by the Valsalva maneuver or exertion.

TENSION-TYPE HEADACHE (TTH)

- **Most common overall cause of Primary headache.** Mean age of onset ~30 years of age.
- Risk factors: mental stress, sleep deprivation, eye strain, poor posture, hunger.

CLINICAL MANIFESTATIONS

- **[1] Bilateral, [2] pressing, tightening "bandlike, viselike, tight cap" nonthrobbing (nonpulsatile) steady or aching, occipitonuchal or bifrontal headache, usually [3] mild to moderate in intensity.** Often described as "dull", "pressure", "head fullness" or "heavy weight on their head or shoulders". The pain often builds gradually & vary from 30 minutes-7 days in duration.
- Exacerbating factors: **worse with stress, fatigue, noise, or glare.** May have poor concentration.
- **[4] Not worsened with routine activity** such as walking or climbing stairs (as in Migraine).
- **Usually not pulsatile & not associated with nausea, vomiting, photophobia & phonophobia (one may be present but not both), or focal neurological symptoms** (auras).

Physical examination:

- **No focal neuro deficits; may have increased pericranial muscle tenderness** (head, neck, shoulders).

DIAGNOSIS: Clinical — diagnosis of exclusion of other causes of headache; there are no specific tests. Imaging usually not usually needed unless atypical or suspicious for a secondary cause of headache.

MANAGEMENT

- **Simple analgesics** — **NSAIDs mainstay of abortive treatment (eg, Ibuprofen or Naproxen) or Aspirin, Acetaminophen, caffeine.** Local heat. Behavioral (eg, relaxation).
- Severe: Ketorolac, Metoclopramide; Chlorpromazine (Diphenhydramine added to prevent dystonia).
- **Chronic management: Tricyclic antidepressants (eg, Amitriptyline). Amitriptyline is the most studied and has the strongest evidence of efficacy.** Nortriptyline. Mirtazapine, Venlafaxine. Anticonvulsants: Topiramate, Gabapentin. **Electromyographic (EMG) biofeedback & relaxation.**

TRIGEMINAL NEURALGIA [TN] (TIC DOULOUREUX)

- Pathophysiology: **compression of the trigeminal nerve (cranial nerve 5) root by the superior cerebellar artery or on occasion a tortuous vein (90%).** Idiopathic (10%).
- **Most common in middle-aged women (60%).** Affects maxillary (V2) & mandibular (V3) divisions.
- **In younger patients (<40 years) or bilateral TN, consider Multiple sclerosis as a cause.**

CLINICAL MANIFESTATIONS

- Headache: **[1] sudden, unilateral, brief, episodic, severe, stabbing, sharp, lancinating, electric shock-like pain** along 2nd/3rd division of CN5, maximal in onset, **[2] lasts seconds up to 2 minutes.**
- Radiation: **pain starts near the mouth & shoots to the eye, ear, or nostril on the ipsilateral side;** Often occurs many times throughout the day. May be associated with facial spasm.
- **[3] trigger zones may generate severe pain:** innocuous stimuli — eg, washing the face, brushing the teeth, touching those areas, shaving, talking, chewing, grimacing, exposure to a draft of air.

Physical examination:

- Usually normal but light palpation of "trigger zones" of the affected CN5 division may trigger attack.

DIAGNOSIS

- Usually a clinical diagnosis in the absence of history or physical findings suggestive of other cause.
- **MRI of the brain with and without contrast is recommended, especially in patients <40 years or bilateral TN (to rule out Multiple sclerosis)** or if structural brain lesions are suspected.

MANAGEMENT

- **Carbamazepine or Oxcarbazepine first-line therapy for Trigeminal neuralgia.** Monitor CBC & LFTs (Carbamazepine can cause Hepatoxicity, agranulocytosis, aplastic anemia, & low platelets). Oxcarbazepine is an active metabolite of Carbamazepine with fewer adverse effects.
- **Alternative agents: Gabapentin, Baclofen, Lamotrigine,** and Pimozide. Valproic acid. Botox.
- Severe or recalcitrant cases: surgical decompression, rhizotomy, gamma knife surgery may be used.

MIGRAINE HEADACHE

- **~75% of all persons who experience Migraines are women.** Strong family history (80%).
- Although unknown, Migraines are thought to be likely secondary to numerous intra- and extracranial changes, such as **activation of the trigeminovascular system** (eg, trigeminal nerve afferent activation and firing), alteration of blood-brain permeability, **cranial vasodilation via vasogenic peptide release (eg, CGRP)**, & neurogenic inflammatory changes in the pain sensitive meninges.
- <u>Migraine without aura</u> — **most common type (75%).** <u>Migraine with aura</u> **classic (25%).**

CLINICAL MANIFESTATIONS

- **<u>Prodrome affective or vegetative symptoms</u>** appearing 24-48 hours prior to the onset of headache — increased yawning, euphoria, depression, irritability, food cravings, constipation, neck stiffness.
- **<u>Headache:</u> [1] episodic <u>lateralized (unilateral), throbbing (pulsatile) headache</u> localized in the frontotemporal & ocular area, moderate to severe in intensity, [2] usually <u>4-72 hours in duration</u>. [3] Often associated with <u>nausea, vomiting, photophobia, &/or phonophobia</u>.**
- **<u>Worsened with routine physical activity</u>** (eg, walking climbing stairs), stress, lack or excessive sleep, alcohol, specific foods, hormonal (eg, oral contraception, menstruation), odors, skipped meals.
- **<u>Auras (25%):</u> focal neurologic symptoms that accompany (within 60 minutes) or follow headache, often lasting <60 minutes** (5-20 minutes). **<u>Visual most common</u>: flashing or zigzags of light, scintillating scotomas),** auditory, somatosensory, function loss (eg, aphasia, hearing).
- <u>Physical examination:</u> Usually normal. May have aphasia, dysarthria, paresthesias, or weakness.

DIAGNOSIS:

- <u>Clinical diagnosis:</u> <u>at least 2</u>: unilateral pain, throbbing (pulsatile) pain, aggravated by movement, moderate or severe intensity; <u>plus at least 1</u>: nausea, vomiting, photophobia, or phonophobia.
- Neuroimaging is not necessary in most unless unexplained abnormal findings on neuro examination.

ABORTIVE (SYMPTOMATIC) MANAGEMENT

Migraine therapy must be individualized; a standard approach for all patients is not possible.

- IV fluids & placing the patient in a dark & quiet room are helpful in severe cases.
- **<u>Mild to moderate:</u> <u>Simple analgesics</u>** (eg, NSAIDs, Acetaminophen, or Aspirin) **first line alone or in combination with other compounds (eg, Acetaminophen, Aspirin, and/or caffeine).** If unresponsive to analgesics, the **combined use of an NSAID with a triptan may be effective.**
- **<u>Moderate to severe:</u> <u>Migraine-specific agents</u>** for moderate to severe Migraine attacks and in those who respond poorly to NSAIDs or combination analgesics — **5-hydroxytryptamine–1 (5-HT 1b/1D) receptor agonists — (Triptans, Sumatriptan-Naproxen, Ergotamines) either alone or in combination with Dopamine receptor antagonists** (eg, Metoclopramide, Prochlorperazine, Chlorpromazine); **CGRP antagonists (eg, Ubrogepant), 5-HT1F receptor agonists (Lasmiditan).**
- <u>Severe Migraine with nausea/vomiting attacks in an emergency department</u> — initial treatment with either subcutaneous Sumatriptan or a parenteral antiemetic agent rather than other migraine-specific drugs. **When using intravenous (IV) Metoclopramide or Prochlorperazine (dopamine antagonists) for nausea/vomiting during a Migraine, adjunctive use of Diphenhydramine is recommended to prevent extrapyramidal symptoms (eg, dystonic reactions, akathisia).**
- <u>Adjunctive Dexamethasone</u> to reduce recurrence of early headaches but doesn't provide immediate relief.
- <u>Pregnancy:</u> Acetaminophen → Antiemetics (eg, Promethazine) → NSAIDs → Opioids (eg, Oxycodone).

PROPHYLACTIC (PREVENTATIVE) eg, ≥15 headache days per month for >3 months:

- **<u>First-line:</u> <u>Antihypertensives</u>: Beta-blockers (Propranolol, Metoprolol), <u>Antidepressants</u>: Tricyclic antidepressant (Amitriptyline), Venlafaxine, or <u>Anticonvulsants</u>: Topiramate, Valproate.**
- <u>Alternatives:</u> Calcium channel blockers (eg, Verapamil, Flunarizine), ARB (Candesartan), NSAIDs, **CGRP antagonists (Rimegepant, Ubrogepant),** <u>Monoclonal antibodies</u>: to the CGRP receptor (eg, Erenumab) or the peptide (eg, Eptinezumab, Framnezumab, Galcanezumab).
- <u>OnabotulinumtoxinA</u> may be beneficial in patients with intractable, chronic Migraine that have failed to respond to at least 3 conventional preventive medications. Occipital nerve block, Nortriptyline.

SEROTONIN [5-HT 1B/1D] RECEPTOR AGONISTS (TRIPTANS)

Oral: **Rizatriptan & Eletriptan tend to be the most effective**, Almotriptan.
Sumatriptan (oral, subcutaneous, or nasal spray); **Zolmitriptan** (nasal, oral).

- Mechanism of action: **serotonin (5HT-1b/d) agonists** can stop Migraine attacks via vasoconstriction & blockage of nociceptive (pain) pathways in the brainstem & trigeminovascular system.
- Indications: **moderate to severe Migraines or no response to analgesics in mild disease.**
- Adverse effects: **often mild and transient — chest tightness from vasoconstriction,** nausea, vomiting, abdominal cramps, flushing, malaise.
- Contraindications: Because of their vasoconstricting properties, Triptans are contraindicated in individuals with a history, symptoms, or signs of ischemic cardiac, cerebrovascular, or peripheral vascular syndromes (Ischemic stroke or ischemic heart disease, uncontrolled Hypertension, angina, pregnancy; hemiplegic or basilar migraines). Not used within 24 hours of the use of Ergotamines.

SEROTONIN [5-HT 1B/1D] RECEPTOR AGONISTS (ERGOTAMINES)

Ergotamine (oral), **Dihydroergotamine** (IM, IV, SQ, and intranasal)

- Mechanism of action: Nonselective serotonin (5HT-1) receptor agonists that stop Migraines via cranial vasoconstriction & blockage of nociceptive (pain) pathways in the brainstem & trigeminovascular system (eg, trigeminal nucleus caudalis and trigeminal sensory thalamus).
- Indications: **Reserved use due to its adverse effects & contraindications (Triptans are associated with lower occurrence of adverse effects compared to Ergotamines).**
- Adverse effects: Rebound headache. **Excessive use can cause** Ergotism: **eg, seizures, spasticity, irritability, numbness, psychiatric changes (including psychosis).**
- Contraindications: Because of their vasoconstricting properties, they are contraindicated in individuals with a history, symptoms, or signs of ischemic cardiac, cerebrovascular, or peripheral vascular syndromes (eg, Ischemic stroke or ischemic heart disease, uncontrolled hypertension, angina, pregnancy; hemiplegic or basilar migraines). Hepatic or renal disease.

ABORTIVE MIGRAINE THERAPY – ANTIEMETICS

- **Metoclopramide** (IV), **Chlorpromazine** (IV or IM), **Prochlorperazine** (IV or IM).
- Mechanism of action: **Dopamine receptor antagonists.** May also reduce headache pain intensity.
- Indications: **nausea &/or vomiting** in patients with Migraine.
- Adverse effects: **Extrapyramidal symptoms** – **acute dystonic reactions** (dyskinesias characterized by intermittent spasmodic or sustained contractions of muscles in the face, neck, trunk, etc.). **IV Diphenhydramine can be given to prevent or treat dystonic reactions.** QT prolongation.

CGRP RECEPTOR ANTAGONISTS [oral gepants: Rimegepant, Ubrogepant]

- Mechanism of action: **Calcitonin gene-related peptide receptor antagonists** inhibit pain transmission, reduce neurogenic inflammation, and minimize artery dilatation without active vasoconstriction.
- Indications: Effective in the acute treatment of Migraine with relief from pain, other symptoms, and functional disability (associated with pain- and symptom-free state at 2 hours). **Oral options for the acute treatment of Migraine in patients with either insufficient response or contraindication to treatment with Triptans (eg, Coronary artery disease).**
- Adverse effects: Gepants are extremely well tolerated with only a small number of patients reporting troublesome adverse effects, such as mild nausea. Rare adverse effects include rash, dyspnea, and hypersensitivity.

5-HT 1F RECEPTOR AGONISTS (DITANS) Lasmiditan (oral)

- Mechanism of action: **Highly selective 5-HT 1F receptor agonist that aborts Migraine attacks via inhibition of neuropeptide and neurotransmitter release and inhibition of PNS trigeminovascular and CNS pain signaling pathways.**
- Indications: Acute management of Migraine attacks. **Safe in patients with cardiovascular or cerebrovascular disease — Ditans have no vascular effects because the 5-HT 1F receptor is located in the central and peripheral nervous system but not vasculature.**
- Adverse effects: The major side effect is dizziness. Other adverse effects include somnolence, paresthesia, fatigue, and nausea. Patients are advised not to drive for 8 hours after treatment.

CLUSTER HEADACHE

- Cluster headache is characterized by hypothalamic activation with secondary activation of the trigeminal-autonomic reflex, probably via a trigeminal-hypothalamic pathway.
- Cluster headache is one of the trigeminal autonomic cephalalgias (TACs).

RISK FACTORS
- **Male gender**: men are 3-4 times more affected than women.
- **Young & middle-aged males (onset 20-40 years of age)** but can occur at any age.
- **Consumption of alcohol, tobacco use,** Prior brain surgery or trauma, family history.

TRIGGERS
- **Worse at night** (onset of attacks is nocturnal in ~50% of patients), **alcohol,** stress, or ingestion of specific foods, hot weather, watching TV, use of Nitroglycerin, sexual activity, glare.

CLINICAL MANIFESTATIONS
- Headache: **[1] recurrent episodes of severe (excruciating), unilateral, periorbital, deep (retroorbital), or temporal pain that is sharp & lancinating. Headaches usually last 15 minutes to 3 hours, with spontaneous remission; [2] a sense of restlessness &/or agitation.**
- Bouts occur several times a day often in the same location and may be around the same time of day.
- Episodic form: a bout may last 6-12 weeks while remissions last ≥3 months, up to 12 months or longer.
- Chronic form attacks occur without significant periods of remission.

PHYSICAL EXAMINATION
[3] Ipsilateral cranial autonomic symptoms/signs:
- **Partial Horner's syndrome: ptosis &/or miosis.**
- **Nasal congestion or rhinorrhea, conjunctival injection or lacrimation, and eyelid edema or forehead/facial sweating, occurring only during the pain attack.**
- Autonomic symptoms are indicative of both parasympathetic hyperactivity and sympathetic impairment. Sweating and cutaneous blood flow may also increase on the painful side.

DIAGNOSIS
- Clinical diagnosis.
Neuroimaging often obtained to exclude cranial lesions if suspected Cluster headache.
- MRI performed with and without contrast or a noncontrast Computed tomography (CT) scan to exclude abnormalities of the brain and pituitary gland in patients without a previous diagnosis.

ACUTE MANAGEMENT
- **100% Oxygen first-line (6-12L for 15-20 minutes).** Most patients respond to oxygen therapy, it is often effective in <10 minutes, & carries no risks or adverse effects. **Triptans alternative therapy.**
- **Triptans (fast-acting): SQ Sumatriptan (preferred) or Zolmitriptan intranasal spray.**
- For patients with acute Cluster headache who do not respond to or tolerate initial therapy with oxygen &/or triptans, alternatives include intranasal Lidocaine, oral Ergotamine, or IV Dihydroergotamine.
- Noninvasive vagus nerve stimulation FDA approved for acute treatment of attacks in episodic Cluster headache using three 2-min stimulation cycles applied at the onset of headache on the side of pain.
- For patients with relatively short bouts, limited courses of oral glucocorticoids (eg, 10-day course of Prednisone, beginning at 60 mg daily for 7 days and followed by a rapid taper), may interrupt pain.

PROPHYLAXIS (PREVENTATIVE THERAPY) FOR CHRONIC CLUSTER HEADACHE:
- **Verapamil first-line medical therapy for Cluster headache prophylaxis.** A short course of glucocorticoids to provide rapid benefit during the initial titration of Verapamil. Glucocorticoids alone (eg, **Prednisone**) can be used for episodic infrequent active cluster periods lasting <4 weeks.
- **Alternatives:** Galcanezumab (CGRP ligand monoclonal antibody), **Lithium, Topiramate. Valproate**.
- **Suboccipital greater occipital nerve block.** Class A recommendation. Adverse events are nonserious, including transient injection site pain and low-level headache.

IDIOPATHIC INTRACRANIAL HYPERTENSION (PSEUDOTUMOR CEREBRI)

- **[1] Idiopathic increased intracranial (CSF) pressure** on CSF examination via LP with
- **[2] no clear identifiable cause evident on neuroimaging** (eg, MRI or CT).

PATHOPHYSIOLOGY
- Symptoms of increased intracranial pressure occur due to an imbalance between the production and reabsorption of cerebrospinal fluid (CSF). The exact pathophysiology is not well understood.

ETIOLOGIES
- **Idiopathic no specific cause found in most cases.**
- **Most commonly seen in overweight women of childbearing age (20–44 years).**
- Medications: **withdrawal from long-term corticosteroid use,** growth hormone, thyroid replacement, oral contraceptives, **long-term Tetracycline use, & vitamin A toxicity.**
- Thrombosis of the transverse venous sinus as a complication of otitis media or chronic mastoiditis.
- Endocrine disturbances: hypoparathyroidism, hypothyroidism, thyroid replacement therapy, Addison disease, uremia. Chronic pulmonary disease, Systemic lupus erythematosus.

CLINICAL MANIFESTATIONS
Signs & symptoms of **increased intracranial pressure (↑ ICP):**
- **Headache: most common presenting symptom — often lateralized, pulsatile (throbbing), worse with straining,** Valsalva, or changes in posture (eg, bending forward). Often occurs daily.
- **Retrobulbar pain that may be worse with eye movements or globe compression.** Back pain.
- **Nausea, vomiting. Pulsatile tinnitus** (patients often describe hearing rushing water or wind).
- **Visual changes** eg, **transient visual obscurations** that may last seconds at a time, photopsia, horizontal diplopia. **May lead to blindness if not treated** in up to 32%.

Ocular examination:
- Funduscopic exam: **papilledema hallmark (usually bilateral & symmetric** but may be unilateral and/or asymmetric) — blurred optic discs and engorged retinal veins. **Visual field loss** may be seen.
- **Cranial nerve VI/6 (abducens nerve) palsy** may cause **diplopia** & esotropia.

DIAGNOSIS
- **CT scan: performed prior to Lumbar puncture (LP) to rule out intracranial mass.**
- **Lumbar puncture: increased CSF pressure (≥250 mm H$_2$O) with otherwise normal CSF.**
- **MRI + MR venography ideal neuroimaging to rule out secondary causes.** Usually normal; may show posterior sclera flattening, vertical tortuosity of the orbital optic nerve, or empty sella.

MANAGEMENT
- **Acetazolamide first-line (carbonic anhydrase inhibitors decrease CSF production). Weight loss recommended in obese patients.**
- Furosemide or other diuretics may be adjunctive if symptoms worsen while on Acetazolamide.
- Topiramate is another carbonic anhydrase inhibitor that may also result in weight loss.
- Short course of systemic corticosteroids if acute visual loss as a temporizing measure to rapidly reduce ICP prior to surgical intervention. Repeat lumbar puncture reduces intracranial pressure.
- **Refractory: CSF shunting (Optic nerve sheath fenestration or Ventriculoperitoneal shunt).**

CLASSIC CSF FINDINGS

1. MULTIPLE SCLEROSIS	High IgG and discrete IgG oligoclonal bands
2. GUILLAIN BARRÉ SYNDROME	High protein with normal white blood cell (WBC) count
3. BACTERIAL MENINGITIS	High protein with increased WBC (primarily polymorphonuclear neutrophils), decreased glucose
4. VIRAL (ASEPTIC) MENINGITIS	Normal glucose, increased WBCs (lymphocytes)
5. FUNGAL or TUBERCULOSIS MENGITIS	Decreased glucose, increased WBCs (lymphocytes)
6. IDIOPATHIC INTRACRANIAL HTN	Increased CSF pressure with otherwise normal CSF
7. SUBARACHNOID HEMORRHAGE	Xanthochromia, blood in the CSF

ACUTE BACTERIAL MENINGITIS

- Bacterial infection of the meninges.
- 25% have a recent history of concomitant Otitis or Sinusitis that could predispose to *S pneumoniae.*

ETIOLOGIES

Streptococcus pneumoniae:
- **Most common cause bacterial in adults of all ages** & children ages >3 months–10 years.

Neisseria menigitidis:
- **Most common in older children** (10 years–19 years of age).
- **Second most common bacterial cause in adults.**
- May be associated with a **petechial (purpuric) rash** (eg, trunk, legs, conjunctivae).

Group B *Streptococcus* (*S. agalactiae*):
- **Most common cause in neonates <1 month** (part of the vaginal flora) & infants <3 months.

Listeria monocytogenes:
- **Increased incidence in neonates, >50 years, & immunocompromised states** (eg, history of glucocorticoid use, alcoholism, pregnant, AIDS or HIV, chemotherapy).

Neonates:
- Group B *Streptococcus, Escherichia coli,* & gram-negative rods are common causes of neonatal meningitis. *Listeria monocytogenes* is also an important pathogen.
- *Haemophilus influenzae* (reduced incidence due to Hib vaccine)

CLINICAL MANIFESTATIONS

The classic clinical triad of Meningitis is [1] fever, [2] headache, and [3] nuchal rigidity.
- Meningeal symptoms: **headache, fever, neck stiffness, photosensitivity,** chills, nausea, vomiting.
- May develop confusion, **altered mental status changes**, and seizures. Back pain or stiffness.
- **Petechial rash on the skin &/or mucous membranes is suggestive of *Neisseria meningitidis*.**

PHYSICAL EXAMINATION

Meningeal signs:
- **Nuchal rigidity (neck stiffness)**
- **Positive Brudzinski** attempted passive neck flexion produces knee and/or hip flexion.
- **Positive Kernig sign** inability to extend the knee &/or leg with the hip at 90° flexion.

Focal neurologic findings seen in 30% — eg, hemiparesis, sensory deficits, cranial nerve palsies.

DIAGNOSIS

- **Lumbar puncture + CSF examination** best initial test & definitive diagnosis — decreased glucose <45, increased polymorphonuclear neutrophils, increased protein, increased pressure. Gram stain: **gram-negative diplococci (*N. meningitidis*); gram-positive diplococci (*S. pneumoniae*).**
- **Head CT scan** best initial test prior to LP ONLY if mass effect must be ruled out (if any of these are present) — **papilledema, seizures, confusion, focal neurologic findings,** >60 years, immunocompromised, or history of CNS disease.

	NORMAL	BACTERIAL	VIRAL (ASEPTIC)	FUNGAL/TB
Opening pressure (cm H$_2$0)	5-20 cm	Increased	Normal or mildly increased	Normal or Mildly increased
Appearance	Normal	Turbid	Clear	Fibrin web
Protein (g/L)	0.18 – 0.45	Increased	Normal or mildly increased	Increased
Glucose (mg/100mL)	50-80	**Decreased (<45)**	**Normal**	**Decreased**
WBC Count	0-5 (no RBC's)	100-100,000 (pleocytosis) **>80% Neutrophils (PMN's)**	10-300 **Lymphocytes**	10-200 **Lymphocytes**
Gram Stain	Normal	60-90% positive	Normal	

MANAGEMENT
- **Antibiotics should be started immediately after Lumbar puncture is performed**, or immediately after blood cultures are obtained if a CT scan is going to be performed before the LP (eg, contraindications to LP). **Antibiotics given immediately if septic shock is present.**
- <u>Adjunctive Dexamethasone</u> should be given shortly before or at the same time as the first dose of antibiotics, when indicated. In adults, **Dexamethasone has been shown to reduce mortality and sequelae of *S. pneumo*.** Also recommended in children if *H. influenzae* type B is suspected (reduces incidence of CN VIII-related hearing loss). Not used in neonates <1 month.

Empiric treatment for >1 month-50 years of age:
- **Vancomycin + Ceftriaxone** (or Cefotaxime or Cefepime) + adjunctive Dexamethasone.

Empiric treatment for >50 years of age:
- **Vancomycin + Ceftriaxone + Ampicillin** (for Listeria) + adjunctive Dexamethasone.

Empiric treatment for neonates (up to 1 month):
- **Ampicillin + either Gentamicin and/or Cefotaxime.** Dexamethasone is <u>not</u> given in this group.

Empiric treatment for head trauma or post-neurosurgical procedure:
- Vancomycin + EITHER Ceftazidime or Cefepime (to cover aerobic gram-negative organisms, eg, *Pseudomonas*).

Additional management for *N. meningitidis*:
- **<u>Droplet precautions:</u>** continued for 24 hours after antibiotic initiation with suspected or confirmed *N. meningitidis* infection. Switch to IV aqueous Penicillin G once confirmed sensitivity to Penicillin.
- **<u>Post-exposure prophylaxis</u>: Ciprofloxacin** (500 mg oral x 1 dose) or **Rifampin** (600 mg orally every 12 hours for 2 days). **Prophylaxis only needed for "close contacts" with prolonged exposure (>8 hours) or direct exposure to respiratory secretions** (eg, household contacts, roommates, kissing, sharing utensils, performing mouth to mouth resuscitation etc.).
- Prophylaxis is <u>not</u> recommended for healthcare workers who have not had direct exposure to respiratory secretions.

NORMAL PRESSURE HYDROCEPHALUS [NPH]

- **[1] Dilation of the cerebral ventricles with [2] normal opening pressures on lumbar puncture.**

PATHOPHYSIOLOGY
- Unknown but thought to be a local pressure effect due to impaired CSF absorption after a CNS injury (eg, Subarachnoid hemorrhage, chronic meningitis, tumors, inflammatory disease, head injury etc.).

CLINICAL MANIFESTATIONS
- **<u>Triad</u> ❶ gait disturbance, ❷ urinary incontinence, & ❸ dementia/cognitive dysfunction** — "wobbly, wet, & wacky". NPH is more common in elderly patients.
- **<u>Gait disturbances:</u> wide-based, shuffling gait** — a *"magnetic"* gait **(as if the feet are stuck to the floor) with gait apraxia (freezing).** May be associated with postural instability, especially when attempting to turn. Gait disturbance is the most prominent & often the earliest feature.
- **<u>Urinary incontinence;</u>** may present as **urinary urgency early in the disease or frequency.**
- **<u>Dementia</u>** subcortical — impaired executive function, psychomotor depression, forgetfulness, apathy.
- <u>Other:</u> weakness, lethargy, malaise, rigidity, hyperreflexia, & spasticity.

DIAGNOSIS
- **<u>Neuroimaging:</u> <u>Ventriculomegaly</u> (ventricular enlargement)** in the absence of or out of proportion to sulcal dilation. MRI is superior to CT scan.
- Lumbar puncture (LP): **CSF pressure is usually normal** (<200 mm H_2O). <u>Positive lumbar tap test:</u> **Large fluid volume LP (35-50 mL) may be therapeutic, with improvement of symptoms.**

MANAGEMENT
- **<u>Ventriculoperitoneal shunt</u> treatment of choice.** Gait abnormalities usually the most improved.

ASEPTIC MENINGITIS

- Clinical and laboratory evidence of **Meningitis with <u>negative routine bacterial cultures.</u>**

<u>ETIOLOGIES</u>
- **<u>Enteroviruses</u> most common cause of viral Meningitis** (eg, **Coxsackieviruses & Echoviruses**).
- Other viruses (eg, HSV-2, VZV), mycobacteria, fungi, Syphilis, Lyme disease, medications, malignancy.

<u>CLINICAL MANIFESTATIONS</u>
- **Classic symptoms of Meningitis (eg, headache, fever, neck stiffness) but may be milder.**
- <u>Preceding systemic symptoms</u> may include myalgias, fatigue, anorexia, abdominal pain, diarrhea.
- <u>Meningeal symptoms:</u> **headache, neck stiffness, photosensitivity, fever,** chills, nausea, vomiting.
<u>Physical examination:</u>
- **Meningeal signs: nuchal rigidity, positive Brudzinski sign** (neck flexion produces knee and/or hip flexion), **positive Kernig sign** (inability to straighten the knee with hip flexion).
- **No focal neurological deficits in Aseptic meningitis helps to distinguish it from Encephalitis.**

<u>DIAGNOSIS</u>
- **Diagnosis of exclusion** after ruling out bacterial meningitis. PCR testing of the CSF fluid.
- **<u>Lumbar puncture</u> best initial test and most accurate** if no symptoms or signs of mass effect. <u>CSF</u> classic findings: **<u>normal glucose, lymphocyte predominance</u>,** ↑ protein count (usually <200).

<u>MANAGEMENT</u>
- **<u>Supportive:</u> eg, antipyretics, IV fluids, analgesics, and antiemetics.** Most have a benign & self-limited course with resolution even without specific therapy. Treat any underlying causes.

ENCEPHALITIS

- **Inflammation of the <u>brain parenchyma</u>,** most commonly due to infection or autoimmune process.

<u>ETIOLOGIES</u>
- **<u>Herpes simplex virus-1</u> most common identified virus.** Associated with a poor prognosis.
- Varicella zoster virus, Epstein-Barr virus, measles, mumps, rubella, HIV, St. Louis & West Nile viruses.

<u>CLINICAL MANIFESTATIONS</u>
- <u>Meningeal symptoms:</u> **headache, neck stiffness, photosensitivity, fever,** chills, nausea, vomiting, **seizures.** May range from minor deficits, behavioral changes, to complete unresponsiveness.
- **<u>Focal neurological deficits</u>: The presence of <u>altered mental status</u>, changes in personality, speech, & movement distinguishes Encephalitis from Aseptic meningitis.**

<u>PHYSICAL EXAMINATION</u>
- **<u>Focal neurological deficits</u> hallmark of Encephalitis** — eg, hemiparesis, sensory deficits, cranial nerve palsies, exaggerated deep tendon reflexes, pathologic reflexes, myoclonus, tremor, ataxia.

<u>DIAGNOSIS</u>
- **<u>CT scan of the head</u> must be performed first to rule out space-occupying lesions** (these patients often have altered mental status, requiring imaging before LP).
- **<u>Lumbar puncture</u>** criterion standard & performed after CT — **normal glucose, increased lymphocytes (lymphocytic pleocytosis), similar to Aseptic meningitis.** ↑ CSF RBCs with HSV.
- **<u>MRI:</u>** preferred modality— **temporal lobe involvement characteristic of HSV** (or frontal lobe).
- **<u>PCR testing</u> of CSF fluid is the most accurate test for Herpes encephalitis.**

<u>MANAGEMENT</u>
- **<u>IV Acyclovir</u>: early empiric treatment for HSV Encephalitis should be initiated as soon as possible** in Encephalitis with no obvious cause. Supportive management (antipyretics, antiemetics).

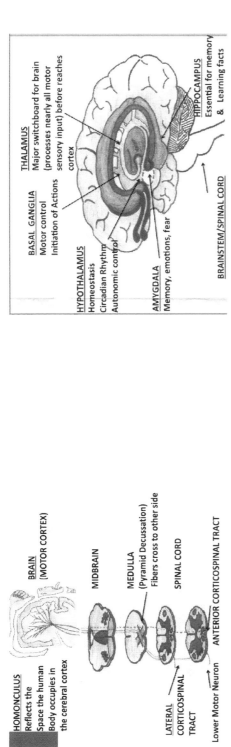

BASAL GANGLIA DISORDERS: since the basal ganglia is involved in coordinated movement, emotion & cognition, problems can lead to movement disorders (*dyskinesias, dystonias, Parkinsonism, Huntington's disease*) or behavior control (*Tourette's, obsessive compulsive*).

"EXTRAPYRAMIDAL SYMPTOMS"	
DYSKINESIA	*Involuntary spasms, repetitive motions or abnormal voluntary movement.*
DYSTONIA	*Sustained contraction* (muscle spasm) especially of antagonistic muscles (ex simultaneous biceps & triceps contraction) ⇨ *twisting of the body, abnormal posturing* (ex. torticollis, writer's cramp).
MYOCLONUS	Sudden *brief, sporadic involuntary jerking/twitching* of 1 muscle or muscle group (not suppressible).
TICS	Sudden, *repetitive nonrhythmic movements or vocals* using specific muscle groups. Tics are *suppressible* (unlike myoclonus which is not suppressible). Ex. Tourette syndrome.
CHOREA	*Rapid involuntary jerky, uncontrolled, purposeless movements.* Ex. *Huntington chorea* (due to caudate nucleus atrophy in the basal ganglia). Sydenham's chorea (rheumatic fever)
MUSCLE SPASMS	Muscle contractions. **Tonic:** *prolonged sustained contraction/rigidity;* **Clonic:** *repetitive rapid movements*
TREMORS	Rhythmic movement of a body part. - **Resting tremor:** tremor at rest (ex Parkinson disease) - **Postural tremor:** tremor occurs while holding position against gravity. - **Intentional tremor:** tremor occurs during movement or when approaching nearer to a target.

PARKINSONISM: disorders associated with tremor, bradykinesia, rigidity, and postural instability. Includes:

❶ *Parkinson disease:* loss of the dopamine producing cells of the substantia nigra (in the basal ganglia).

❷ *Dopamine antagonists: medications that block dopamine include the typical antipsychotics (Haloperidol, Droperidol, Fluphenazine, Chlorpromazine) > atypical antipsychotics (ex. Olanzapine, Clozapine, Risperidone).* Antiemetics: *Prochlorperazine, Promethazine, Metoclopramide.*

❸ *Lewy body disease:* loss of dopaminergic neurons leads to motor features similar to Parkinson disease. Loss of anticholinergic neurons lead to dementia (similar to Alzheimer's), visuospatial dysfunction & recurrent visual hallucinations.

❹ Other: head trauma, HIV, carbon monoxide or mercury poisoning, CNS dysfunction (ex stroke, meningitis).

663

MOVEMENT DISORDERS

HUNTINGTON DISEASE

- **Autosomal dominant neurodegenerative disorder characterized by involuntary choreatic movements with cognitive and behavioral disturbances.**

PATHOPHYSIOLOGY
- **Inheritance of trinucleotide repeats of cytosine, adenine, and guanine (CAG/glutamine) on the Huntingtin [HTT] gene on chromosome 4** (4p16.3).
- This leads to neurotoxicity (loss of GABA-producing neurons in the striatum) as well as cerebral, putamen, & caudate nucleus atrophy. **The disease <u>predominantly affects the striatum</u> (<u>caudate nucleus & putamen)</u>** but progresses to involve the cerebral cortex and other brain regions.

EPIDEMIOLOGY
- Both sexes are affected equally.
- **Symptoms usually begins between ages 30-50 years of age** but may begin as early as infancy, juvenile HD if onset < 20 years of age, or in older individuals.

CLINICAL MANIFESTATIONS
Symptoms usually appear 30-50 years of age.
- **3 hallmark manifestations: 3 Ms: M**ood, **M**ovement, & **M**emory — **behavioral & mood changes → chorea** (rapid involuntary movements), → **dementia.**
- **Behavioral changes:** personality, cognitive, intellectual, & psychiatric changes including irritability, moodiness, antisocial behavior, or psychiatric disturbances.
- **Chorea: brief, abrupt, involuntary, or arrhythmic movements of the face, neck, trunk, & limbs initially.** Chorea worsens with voluntary movements & stress (may disappear with sleep). Fidgetiness or restlessness may be the early symptoms. Tics, grimacing, ataxia, & falls may occur.
- **Dementia:** most develop dementia before 50 years of age with primarily executive dysfunction.
- Gait abnormalities, ataxia (often irregular & unsteady), incontinence.
- Psychiatric dysfunction: depression, suicidal ideation, anxiety. Psychosis, sleep disturbances.
Physical examination:
- Restlessness, fragility.
- Quick, involuntary hand movements. Unsteady or irregular gait. Brisk deep tendon reflexes.

DIAGNOSIS
- **Clinical symptoms + family history (if known) + neuroimaging + genetic confirmation.**
Neuroimaging:
- **CT or MRI: cerebral & <u>striatal (caudate nucleus & putamen) atrophy</u> with subsequent widening in the frontal horns of the lateral ventricle (boxcar ventricle sign).**
- PET scan: decreased glucose metabolism (↓ metabolic rate) in the caudate nucleus & putamen.
Genetic DNA testing (confirmatory) criterion standard:
- **Trinucleotide CAG expansion repeats** on the short arm of chromosome 4 in the Huntingtin gene – **the number of CAG expansion repeats determine how early the onset of symptoms will occur.**

MANAGEMENT
- **No cure. Usually fatal within 15-20 years after presentation (due to disease progression).**
No medication stops the disease progression or is curative:
- **Vesicular monoamine transporter type 2 (VMAT2) inhibitor — eg, Deutetrabenazine, Valbenazine, or Tetrabenazine for dyskinesia or chorea.** They are dopamine depleters.
- **Antidopaminergics: alternatives to VMAT2 inhibitors** — atypical antipsychotics (eg, Risperidone, Olanzapine, Aripiprazole, Quetiapine) > typical antipsychotics (eg, Haloperidol).
- Benzodiazepine use intermittently may help with chorea & sleep, especially during stressful situations. SSRIs or Tricyclic antidepressants for mood symptoms.

ESSENTIAL TREMOR (ET)

- Autosomal dominant inherited disorder (30-70%) or sporadic. Incidence increases with age.

CLINICAL MANIFESTATIONS
- **Intentional action tremor** — **postural bilateral (symmetrical) action tremor,** most commonly **affecting the upper extremities & head** (hands, forearms, head, neck, &/or voice). Face, trunk, & legs less common.
- **Tremor worsened** with **action & intentional movement,** postural eg, **holding affected body part against gravity** (eg, arms held outstretched), **adrenergic activity** (eg, **emotional stress, anxiety**).
- **Tremor improved** with alcohol ingestion, when the body part is supported, and with rest.

PHYSICAL EXAMINATION
- Tremor is more pronounced with [1] the arms suspended against gravity in a fixed posture (eg, outstretched arms) and [2] during goal-directed activity (eg, on finger to nose testing, the tremor increases at the end of approaching the target or holding a position against gravity). 6-12 Hz tremor.
- Besides the tremor, no other significant neurologic findings seen, other than cogwheel phenomenon.

DIAGNOSIS
- Diagnosis of exclusion based on history, **family history**, physical after ruling out other causes.

MANAGEMENT
- **Medical treatment not usually needed if mild.** Less impaired patients may opt not to be treated. Reduction of tremors with weighting the limb (adaptive devices), non-medical relaxation techniques, and biofeedback. Avoidance of stimulants (eg, caffeine) or medications known to exacerbate tremors.

Medical:
- <u>First-line:</u> **Propranolol &/or Primidone (barbiturate) if no relief with Propranolol. Propranolol is often the first-line therapy of choice in most cases, unless contraindicated** [eg, heart block, Asthma, or type 1 Diabetes mellitus, CHF, bradycardia]. **Primidone used if contraindications to Beta blockers.** <u>Adverse effects of Primidone:</u> sedation, drowsiness, fatigue, depression, nausea, vomiting, ataxia, malaise, dizziness, unsteadiness, confusion, vertigo.
- <u>Second line:</u> Topiramate, Benzodiazepine if intermittent (eg, Alprazolam), Gabapentin, Pregabalin.

Interventional therapy:
- For patients who fail or tolerate adverse effects of medication treatment, surgical options include Deep brain stimulation, focused Ultrasound, Thalamotomy, or Botulinum toxin injections.

ESSENTIAL TREMOR	PARKINSON DISEASE
• Mainly tremor affects **upper extremities, head, neck, & voice**	
INTENTIONAL POSTURAL • **Worse with** (1) goal-directed activity, (2) fixed postures against gravity, (3) increased beta-adrenergic activity (stress, excitement, anxiety)	**RESTING tremor** • Worse at rest & stress
• **Improved with** rest, alcohol, **Propranolol,** affected body part is fully relaxed and supported.	• **Improved with** voluntary activity, intentional movement, & sleep.
• Usually **BILATERAL & SYMMETRICAL**	• **Usually starts on ONE SIDE of the body**

665

PARKINSON DISEASE

- Neurodegenerative movement disorder due to **deceased dopamine resulting from idiopathic loss of dopaminergic neurons in the striatum & substantia nigra & the presence of Lewy bodies.**
- Onset of symptoms 45-65 years most common. Usually a clinical diagnosis.

PATHOPHYSIOLOGY
- **Idiopathic degeneration of dopamine-producing neurons within the pars compacta of the substantia nigra** and Norepinephrine-producing cells of the locus coeruleus in the brainstem.
- **Decreased dopamine leads to imbalance of dopamine & acetylcholine, resulting in improper movement due to failure of acetylcholine inhibition in the basal ganglia** (acetylcholine is an excitatory CNS neurotransmitter; dopamine is inhibitory).
- It also affects dopamine's ability to initiate movement.
- **The pathologic hallmark of PD seen on post-mortem histology is eosinophilic cytoplasmic inclusions (Lewy bodies)** & loss of pigment cells seen in the substantia nigra.

CLINICAL MANIFESTATIONS
Motor triad: resting tremor, bradykinesia, & muscle rigidity (cardinal motor symptoms of PD).
- **Resting tremor:** often the first symptom. **"Pill-rolling" resting tremor of the hand.**
  Lips & mouth may be involved. Frequency 4-6 Hz.
  - **Tremor is worse at rest, emotional stress, excitement, and walking.**
  - **Tremor improves with voluntary activity, intentional movement, and sleep.** Typically, the tremor disappears with action of the involved limb & reemerges with maintained posture.
  - Usually confined to one limb or one side for years before it becomes generalized.
- **Bradykinesia: slowness of voluntary movement & decreased automatic movements** (eg, lack of swinging of the arms while walking & a gait with small shuffling steps).
- **Rigidity: sustained increased resistance to passive movement — cogwheel rigidity** ratchety pattern of resistance and relaxation as the examiner moves the limb through its full range of motion. Festination: increasing speed while walking. Freezing: inability to initiate stepping.
- **Postural instability, including a flexed (stooped) posture, and loss of postural reflexes is a sign of more advanced disease.** Unsteadiness when turning, difficulty stopping, & falls. Postural instability may significantly impact the quality of life. Early in the disease, postural reflexes are preserved.
- Nonmotor symptoms: **include the loss of smell (anosmia),** constipation, excess salivation or drooling (sialorrhea), & sleep dysfunction.
- Behavioral symptoms include personality changes, anxiety, **depression occurs in up to 40% of patients with PD and is the most prevalent neurobehavioral change in PD.**
- Dementia in 50% (usually a late finding).
Physical examination:
- Normal deep tendon reflexes. Usually no muscle weakness.
- **Face involvement: relatively immobile face (fixed facial expressions),** widened palpebral fissure, **Myerson's sign:** tapping the bridge of nose repetitively causes a sustained blink.
  Decreased blinking. **Seborrheic dermatitis of the scalp & face common.** Olfactory dysfunction.
- **Postural instability:** usually a late finding. Pull test — standing behind the patient & pulling the shoulders causes the patient to fall or take steps backwards. **Micrographia.**

MANAGEMENT
- **Levodopa-carbidopa — most effective treatment** & best tolerated, especially in older adults.
- **Dopamine agonists** (eg, Bromocriptine, Pramipexole, Ropinirole) may be used as initial treatment.
- **Deep brain stimulation is extremely effective for rigidity and tremors in select patients.**
- Anticholinergics (eg, Trihexyphenidyl, Benztropine)
- Amantadine — increases dopamine. MAO-B inhibitors (eg, Selegiline, Rasagiline)
- COMT inhibitors (eg, Entacapone, Tolcapone).

LEVODOPA

Mechanism of action:
- Levodopa is converted to dopamine once it crosses the blood brain barrier.
- **Carbidopa reduces amount of Levodopa needed** & also reduces the peripheral conversion of levodopa into dopamine, reducing the adverse effects of Levodopa.

Indications:
- **Most effective treatment for the cardinal motor symptoms of PD.**

Adverse effects:
- Gastrointestinal: **anorexia, nausea, & vomiting** (can be reduced by taking in divided doses).
- Orthostatic (postural) hypotension common. CNS: **somnolence, headache,** confusion.
- Behavioral: anxiety, agitation, confusion, depression. **Psychosis & hallucinations upon initiation.**
- Dyskinesia (involuntary movements especially the lower extremities) & akinesia.
- **On-off phenomena:** off periods of akinesia may alternate over a few hours with on periods of improved mobility. In some cases, off periods may respond to Apomorphine or Istradefylline.
- Levodopa should be used at the minimum dose of clinical efficacy to reduce wearing off effect. If Levodopa is stopped abruptly, a syndrome similar to Neuroleptic malignant syndrome can occur.

DOPAMINE AGONISTS: PRAMIPEXOLE, ROPINIROLE, ROTIGOTINE

Mechanism of action:
- Directly stimulates dopamine receptors, increasing dopamine levels (less motor adverse effects).
- Less motor adverse effects than Levodopa but not as effective as Levodopa. Rotigotine transdermal.

Indications:
- **Can be used as first-line agents in younger patients (<65 years) to delay the use of Levodopa.** If patient is not sensitive to Levodopa, they will often be insensitive to dopamine agonists.

Adverse effects:
- Similar to Levodopa: orthostatic hypotension, headache, dizziness, hallucinations, confusion, anorexia, nausea, vomiting, sleepiness. Peripheral edema. Weight gain.
- More frequent nonmotor side effects compared to Levodopa (eg, sleep disturbances, somnolence, dizziness, impulse control such as compulsive shopping or gambling, hypersexuality from dopamine reward effect). Pramipexole is contraindicated in patients with active Peptic ulcer disease.

ANTICHOLINERGICS — TRIHEXYPHENIDYL, BENZTROPINE, BIPERIDEN, ORPHENADRINE

Mechanism of action:
- Anticholinergic (antimuscarinic) that blocks the excitatory effects of acetylcholine.

Indications:
- **Most useful as monotherapy in younger patients (<70 years) with tremor as the predominant symptom without significant bradykinesia or gait disturbance.**
- **Does not improve bradykinesia.** Not used in patients with cognitive impairment due to adverse effects.
- Adjunctive treatment for severe tremor despite Levodopa or dopamine agonists.

Adverse effects:
- Anticholinergic: constipation, dry mouth, blurred vision, tachycardia, urinary retention, ↓ sweating.
- **May worsen Glaucoma & Benign prostatic hypertrophy.** CNS toxicity confusion, hallucinations.

AMANTADINE

Mechanism of action:
- Increases presynaptic dopamine release & inhibits dopamine reuptake.

Indications:
- **Low-potency** antiparkinsonian therapy that can help early on with **mild symptoms who are at risk for dyskinesia** (improves long-term Levodopa-induced dyskinesia).

Adverse effects:
- Livedo reticularis and ankle edema.
- Rare — restlessness, agitation, confusion, psychosis, & hallucinations (more likely in older patients).

SELECTIVE MAO-B INHIBITORS — SELEGILINE, RASAGILINE, SAFINAMIDE

Mechanism of action:
- **Increases dopamine in the striatum** (MAO-B normally breaks down dopamine).

Indications:
- Can be used as early therapy in patients with very mild sign and symptoms.
- May have neuroprotective properties in PD.

Adverse effects:
- Nausea & headache most common; confusion, hallucinations. Falls, insomnia.

COMT INHIBITORS — ENTACAPONE, TOLCAPONE

- Mechanism of action: Catechol-O-methyltransferase inhibition prevents dopamine breakdown.

Indications:
- **Adjunctive treatment with Levodopa** (prolongs the therapeutic dose of Levodopa) in patients experiencing wearing "off" periods. Not used as monotherapy.

Adverse effects:
- Nausea, orthostatic hypotension, hallucination, orthostatic hypotension, GI symptoms, brown discoloration of the urine.
- **Tolcapone associated with hepatotoxicity** (avoided in patients with liver disease).

AMYOTROPHIC LATERAL SCLEROSIS (ALS) [LOU GEHRIG'S DISEASE]

- **Neurodegenerative disorder due to necrosis of BOTH upper & lower motor neurons**, leading to **progressive motor degeneration**. Idiopathic etiology. Upper motor neuron findings result from degeneration of frontal lobe motor neurons & corticospinal tract. The lower motor neuron findings occur due to degeneration of lower motor neurons in the brainstem and spinal cord.
- **Degeneration & gliosis of axons within the anterior & lateral columns of the spinal cord.**

CLINICAL MANIFESTATIONS
- **Asymmetric limb weakness is the most common presenting symptom,** muscle weakness, loss of ability to initiate & control motor movements. Progressive muscular atrophy
- Bulbar palsy: dysphagia, dysarthria, speech problems, **difficulty in chewing, aspiration**.
- Cognitive impairment (frontotemporal dysfunction).
- **Mixed upper & lower motor neuron** signs & symptoms are hallmark.
- Upper motor neuron: spasticity, stiffness, hyperreflexia, weakness, slowness of movement, incoordination, weakness, dysarthria, dysphagia.
- Lower motor neuron: progressive bilateral fasciculations, muscle atrophy, hyporeflexia, weakness.
- **Sensation, voluntary eye movement, sphincter function (bowel & bladder), and sexual function are usually spared** (sensory examination is usually normal).
- Motor impairment may involve limb, bulbar, axial, and respiratory function.

DIAGNOSIS
- **Electromyography (EMG) & nerve conduction studies: active denervation** (fibrillations and positive sharp waves with reduced amplitudes of motor nerve conductions & reinnervation in muscle groups). Elevated creatine phosphokinase (CPK) levels.

MANAGEMENT
- **Riluzole only drug known to impact ALS (reduces the progression for up to 6 months). Decreases excitotoxic damage to neurons by reducing glutamate buildup in neurons.**
- Edaravone. Sodium phenylbutyrate-Taurursodiol.
- Dextromethorphan/Quinidine for pseudobulbar affect; Baclofen & Tizanidine for spasticity.
- CPAP, BiPAP, & ventilator may be needed as the disease advances.

PROGNOSIS
- Usually fatal within 3-5 years after onset — **Respiratory failure most common cause of death.**

TOURETTE DISORDER (SYNDROME)

- Idiopathic movement disorder characterized by vocal tics, motor tics, & Obsessive-compulsive disorder.
- **Associated with Attention deficit hyperactivity disorder (30-60%); Obsessive-compulsive disorder (30%)** & other behavioral and psychosocial problems.
- **Onset usually in childhood** (onset 2-6 years) with peak severity 10-12 years of age with decreased symptoms in adolescence & significant decrease in adulthood. Most common in boys.

PATHOPHYSIOLOGY
- Idiopathic. May be due to excess dopamine + GABA deficiency in the caudate nucleus.

CLINICAL MANIFESTATIONS
- <u>**Motor tics:**</u> **most common initial symptom — usually involves the face, head, or neck** (eg, **blinking most common initial symptom,** facial grimacing, shrugging, head thrusting, sniffling).
- <u>**Verbal or phonetic tics:**</u> eg, grunts, throat-clearing, sniffing, barking, moaning, coughing, obscene words (coprolalia), repetitive phrases, repeating the phrases of others (echolalia).
- <u>Self-mutilating tics</u>: hair pulling, nail biting, biting of the lips etc. May have complex motor tics.

DIAGNOSTIC CRITERIA
- **Multiple motor & ≥1 vocal tics** (not required to occur concurrently) **for >1 year** since the first tic (frequency may wax and wane).
- **Onset prior to age 18 years.** Not caused by a substance or medical condition.

MANAGEMENT
- <u>**Habit reversal therapy**</u> **first-line — tic awareness & response training (most don't need medications).** Education, counseling, and supportive care.

<u>Medical management:</u>
- **Alpha-2 adrenergic agonists: Guanfacine or Clonidine first-line agents**, especially in those who also have ADHD or predominant behavioral symptoms (eg, impulse control). Sedation is the most common adverse effect (especially Clonidine), orthostatic hypotension, bradycardia, irritability.
- <u>Dopamine blocking agents:</u> <u>VMAT2 inhibitors</u> **Deutetrabenazine, Valbenazine (dopamine depleters via VMAT2 inhibition).** Antipsychotics not used as often (eg, Haloperidol, Pimozide, Aripiprazole).
- Topiramate can be used; Clonazepam may also be used as adjunct.

CEREBRAL PALSY

- **CNS disorder associated with muscle tone, movement, & postural abnormalities** due to brain injury during the perinatal or prenatal period. Types include spastic, dyskinetic, & ataxic.

CLINICAL MANIFESTATIONS
- **Spasticity is hallmark.**
- Varying degrees of motor deficits. May develop seizures.
- Often associated with intellectual or learning disabilities & development abnormalities.

<u>Physical examination:</u>
- Hyperreflexia, limb-length discrepancies, congenital defects, & persistent primitive reflexes.

DIAGNOSIS
- Primarily clinical but MRI is often performed in patients.
- Workup includes screening for commonly associated conditions.

MANAGEMENT
- Multidisciplinary approach. Pain management.
- <u>Spasticity</u>: Baclofen, Diazepam. Antiepileptics for seizures.

RESTLESS LEGS SYNDROME [RLS] (WILLIS-EKBOM DISEASE)

- **Disorder characterized by [1] an unpleasant sensation in the legs + [2] an irresistible urge to move, emerging during inactivity, <u>most prominent in the evening, transiently relieved by movement</u>.**
- <u>Etiologies:</u> usually primary (idiopathic) but may occur secondary to **reduced iron stores in the CNS,** pregnancy, peripheral neuropathy, uremia, & chronic alcohol use. ⊕ Family history in 40-60%.

CLINICAL MANIFESTATIONS

- **Uncomfortable or unpleasant sensation** (eg, itching, burning, paresthesias, crawling, creeping, pulling, drawing, or stretching) **in the legs** (occasionally the arms) **with inactivity (eg, lying in bed, sitting) that creates an urge to move the legs. Symptoms improve with leg movement.**
- **Symptoms worsen in the evening & with prolonged periods of rest or inactivity.**
- During sleep, periodic limb movements may disturb sleep or cause the patient to awake from sleep.

DIAGNOSIS

- Clinical diagnosis. <u>Iron store workup</u> usually performed as part of workup for underlying causes.

MANAGEMENT

- **<u>Oral iron supplementation</u> recommended in patients with a serum ferritin levels <75 mcg/L** because of the association with Iron deficiency in the central nervous system.
- <u>On-demand therapy (intermittent symptoms):</u> Carbidopa-Levodopa on an as-needed basis.
- **First-line daily medication: Gabapentoid (Pregabalin, Gabapentin).** A dopamine agonist (eg, Pramipexole, Ropinirole, Rotigotine) is an alternative to Gabapentoids but may augment symptoms.
- <u>Refractory:</u> Benzodiazepines as adjunctive treatment. (eg Clonazepam), low-dose Opioids.

BELL PALSY

- **Idiopathic, unilateral lower motor neuron CN VII (facial nerve) palsy leading to hemifacial weakness & paralysis due to inflammation or compression.** Maximal weakness attained by 48h.
- **Although idiopathic, reactivation of this virus Herpes simplex virus (HSV) type 1 DNA** in the geniculate ganglion may be responsible for most cases. House-Brackmann grading system for severity.
- <u>Risk factors:</u> Diabetes mellitus, pregnancy (especially the 3rd trimester), post URI, dental nerve block.

CLINICAL MANIFESTATIONS

- <u>Prodrome:</u> **ipsilateral hyperacusis (ear pain)** 24-48 hours, followed by sudden onset of weakness.
- **<u>Motor dysfunction:</u> <u>Unilateral hemifacial weakness or paralysis</u> (forehead included) — unable to lift affected eyebrow,** wrinkle forehead, smile; loss of the nasolabial fold, drooping of the corner of mouth, biting the inner cheek, eye irritation (decreased lacrimation & **inability to fully close eyelid**). <u>Bell phenomenon:</u> eye on the affected side moves laterally & superiorly when eye closure is attempted. The **weakness & paralysis ONLY affects the face** (no other neurological deficits).
- **<u>Sensory dysfunction:</u> Taste disturbance involving the anterior 2/3 of the tongue.**

DIAGNOSIS

- **Clinical diagnosis of exclusion.** Electromyography and nerve excitability or conduction studies.

MANAGEMENT

- **<u>No specific treatment is required</u>** (>85% of cases resolve within 1 month) — **<u>supportive:</u> artificial tears** (replaces lacrimation, reduces vision problems). Eye lubricant, paper tape, &/or patches worn during sleep if eye closure not possible to prevent corneal ulceration. Massage weakened muscles.
- **<u>Prednisone,</u> especially if started within the first 72 hours of symptom onset, reduces the time to full recovery & increases the likelihood of complete recuperation** at 9–12 months (12–15%).
- Acyclovir in combination with glucocorticoids in severe cases has been shown to improve symptoms & recovery timing. The presence of incomplete paralysis in week 1 most favorable prognostic sign.
- The presence of incomplete paralysis in week 1 most favorable prognostic sign.

GUILLAIN BARRÉ SYNDROME (ACUTE IDIOPATHIC POLYNEUROPATHY)

- Group of conditions due to **acquired autoimmune-mediated demyelinating polyradiculopathy of the _peripheral_ nervous system,** characterized by rapidly evolving muscular weakness.

ETIOLOGIES
- **Increased incidence with _Campylobacter jejuni_ (most common antecedent infection) or other antecedent GI or respiratory infection.** Influenza A and B.
- CMV, Epstein-Barr virus, HIV, Mycoplasma infections, immunizations, & postsurgical.

PATHOPHYSIOLOGY:
- **_Molecular mimicry_: Inflammatory neuropathy triggered by an immune response to an antecedent event producing antibodies that cross react with shared epitopes on peripheral nerve (neural antigens).** _C. jejuni_ has lipooligosaccharides in the bacterial wall similar to gangliosides on peripheral nerves. This creates antiganglioside autoantibodies that attack nerves.
- _Demyelination_: **The autoantibodies and macrophages attack the myelin sheath of the peripheral nerves (Schwann cells);** breakdown of the blood-nerve barrier at the dural attachment allows transudation of plasma proteins into the cerebrospinal fluid (high CSF protein with normal cell count). **Demyelination causes conduction slowing, resulting in muscle weakness.**

CLINICAL MANIFESTATIONS
- **_Symmetric, ascending, progressive, flaccid muscle weakness & sensory changes_ (paresthesias, pain)** hours to days — **distal lower extremities first.** Often 2-4 weeks after antecedent infection.
- **_Cranial nerve & bulbar symptoms_** — Cranial nerves III, IV, & VI may lead to ophthalmoplegia (oculomotor weakness); involvement of the glossopharyngeal, vagus, & hypoglossal cranial nerves may lead to bulbar symptoms (oropharyngeal weakness with swallowing difficulties).
- **May develop _weakness of the respiratory muscles_,** necessitating ventilatory support.
- **_Sensory deficits_ paresthesias/numbness (hands & feet), pain, cramps. _Autonomic dysfunction_:** eg, ileus, wide fluctuations in blood pressure, fever, tachycardia or bradycardia, urinary retention.

Physical examination:
- **_Lower motor neuron signs_: _decreased or absent deep tendon reflexes_,** flaccid muscle weakness.
- **Sensory deficits** & cranial nerve palsies (eg, CN VII, III, IV, and VI).
- **_Autonomic dysfunction_:** tachycardia, arrhythmias, hypotension, hypertension, breathing difficulties.
- _Miller Fisher syndrome_: subvariant characterized by the clinical triad of ophthalmoplegia, ataxia, and areflexia. Associated with anti-GQ1b antibodies.

DIAGNOSIS
- **_Electrophysiologic studies:_ Nerve conduction studies [NCS] (most specific test)** & needle Electromyography — decreased motor nerve conduction velocities & amplitude. NCS reveals demyelination (absent or prolonged H reflexes &/or F wave latencies) with sural sparing pattern.
- **LP (CSF analysis): high protein** (45-200 mg/dL) **+ normal WBC count** (seen 1-3 weeks after onset).
- _Autoantibody testing_ — Antiganglioside antibody testing may be useful to help identify patients with atypical symptoms (eg, anti-GM1, anti-GD1A, anti-GT1A, and anti-GQ1B).
- **_Pulmonary function test:_** assesses forced vital capacity & negative inspiratory force — **decline in FVC (≤20 mL/kg) or NIF (<30 cm H_2O) denote respiratory failure & often warrants intubation.**

MANAGEMENT
- **IV immune globulin (IVIG) or Plasmapheresis first line for antibody removal and neutralization.** They are equally effective for typical GBS & best within 4 weeks of symptom onset. IVIG may be preferred in children & adults with cardiovascular instability; IVIG is better tolerated.
- Mechanical ventilation if respiratory failure or decreased FVC on PFTs.
- **Prednisone _not_ indicated** as steroids show no benefit in GBS & may even delay long-term recovery.
- _Prognosis:_ by 4 weeks after onset, >90% of patients have reached the nadir of the disease. >80% achieve independent ambulation after 6 months.

MYASTHENIA GRAVIS (MG)

- **Autoimmune peripheral nerve disorder of the neuromuscular junction due to autoantibodies against the acetylcholine receptor on the muscles, leading to <u>fluctuating muscle weakness</u>.**

EPIDEMIOLOGY
- <u>Bimodal distribution</u>: **most common in young women <40 years and older men >50 years.**
- **Strong association with an abnormal thymus gland (hyperplasia or thymoma),** HLA B8 & DR3.

PATHOPHYSIOLOGY
- **<u>Type II hypersensitivity</u>: Autoantibodies against acetylcholine (nicotinic) postsynaptic receptor at the neuromuscular junction** prevent ACh from exciting the postsynaptic muscle. This decreases skeletal muscle neuromuscular transmission, leading to weakness. Autoantibodies against receptor-associated protein, muscle-specific tyrosine kinase (MuSK), or LRP4 may be seen.
- <u>T cell-dependent</u> T cells stimulate B-cell autoantibody production.
- Transient worsening of myasthenic symptoms can be precipitated by concurrent infection, surgery, pregnancy, childbirth, & medications (eg, Fluoroquinolones, Aminoglycosides, Beta blockers).

CLINICAL MANIFESTATIONS
2 main manifestations: ❶ ocular weakness & ❷ generalized weakness **<u>worsened with repeated use</u>.**
- **<u>Ocular weakness</u>: diplopia, ptosis,** or blurred vision usually initial symptoms. **Pupils are spared.**
- **<u>Skeletal muscle weakness</u>: fluctuating skeletal muscle weakness <u>worsened with repeated muscle use</u> & throughout the day, often with true muscle fatigue, is the hallmark cardinal feature of Myasthenia gravis.** Fatigue is manifest by contractile force of the muscle, not tiredness. **Fluctuating weakness improves after a brief period of rest & is often mild earlier in the day.**
- **<u>Bulbar (oropharyngeal) weakness</u>:** fatigue with prolonged chewing, dysphagia, dysphonia, & dysarthria. **<u>Respiratory muscle weakness</u>** may lead to **respiratory failure = Myasthenic crisis.**
- **<u>Bedside ice pack test</u>:** can be used to support the diagnosis of Myasthenia gravis in patients with ptosis, but it is **not** helpful for those with extraocular muscle weakness. **Application of ice for 10 minutes improve ocular symptoms of MG.**
Sensation, deep tendon reflexes, & pupil reaction are usually preserved. No autonomic symptoms.

DIAGNOSIS
- **<u>Serologic antibody testing</u>: <u>Acetylcholine receptor antibodies</u> initial test of choice for MG (positive in 85%).** Thymic hyperplasia is frequent in AChR-Ab positive MG.
- **<u>MuSK antibodies</u> obtained if ACR antibodies negative** (often negative in isolated ocular MG).
- <u>Anti-striated muscle antibodies</u>: useful marker for Thymoma in early onset MG. LRP4 antibodies.
- **<u>Electrophysiology testing</u>: Repetitive nerve stimulation (RNS) and single-fiber Electromyography (SFEMG) are the most accurate tests for MG. <u>Repetitive nerve stimulation</u> — most frequently used electrodiagnostic test for MG. RNS positive for MG if the decrement is >10%** (not specific). RNS is usually performed first, followed by SFEMG, if the diagnosis is still uncertain. SFEMG — positive for MG if there is increased jitter due to decreased neuromuscular junction transmission (nonspecific). The variability in time of the second action potential relative to the first is called "jitter".
- **<u>Chest imaging</u>: (eg, chest CT or MRI) should be done in all patients diagnosed with MG to detect thymus gland abnormalities (eg, hyperplasia, thymoma).**

MANAGEMENT
- **<u>Long-term</u>: Acetylcholinesterase inhibitors (eg, Pyridostigmine or Neostigmine) first-line treatment** of symptoms. Glucocorticoids. Azathioprine, or Mycophenolate are steroid alternatives.
- **<u>Myasthenic crisis or severe</u>: Plasmapheresis or IV immunoglobulin (IVIG).**
- **Thymectomy,** even if thymus gland is normal, can improve symptoms and removes the source of antibodies. Useful if no improvement with medical management. Glucocorticoids if >60 years.
- **Avoid medications known to worsen MG (eg, Fluoroquinolones, Aminoglycosides, Beta blockers).**

ACETYLCHOLINESTERASE INHIBITORS Pyridostigmine, Neostigmine

- <u>Mechanism:</u> Acetylcholinesterase inhibitors prevent acetylcholine breakdown in the synapse.

<u>Indications:</u>
- **First-line medical management of Myasthenia gravis.**
- **Pyridostigmine usually preferred over Neostigmine** due to a longer duration of action.

<u>Adverse effects:</u>
- <u>Cholinergic adverse effects:</u> **muscarinic — abdominal cramping, diarrhea**, increased salivation and bronchial secretions, nausea, vomiting, sweating, and bradycardia. Acetylcholine causes SLUDD-C (salivation, lacrimation, urination, digestion, defecation, and pupillary constriction).
- <u>Nicotinic adverse effects</u> — fasciculations and muscle cramping.
- Glycopyrrolate & Hyoscyamine are anticholinergic drugs with little to no effect on the nicotinic receptors. They are used to help control some adverse effects of acetylcholinesterase inhibitors.
- **Cholinergic crisis** — excessive anticholinesterase medication, leading to paradoxical weakness, nausea, vomiting, pallor, sweating, salivation, diarrhea, miosis, bradycardia, & respiratory failure.

LAMBERT-EATON MYASTHENIC SYNDROME (LEMS)

- **Autoimmune disease due to antibodies against the <u>presynaptic</u> terminal voltage-gated calcium channels lead to decreased acetylcholine release from the presynaptic nerve terminals at the neuromuscular junction, leading to muscle weakness.**
- **<u>Malignancy:</u> >50% associated with malignancy — Most commonly & strongly associated with Small cell lung cancer** & less often with other malignancies (eg, lymphoproliferative disorders).

PATHOPHYSIOLOGY
- <u>Paraneoplastic phenomenon:</u> The expression of voltage-gated calcium channel (VGCC) antigens on surface membrane of SCLC tumor cells & other neural antigens induce autoantibody production.
- <u>Proximal muscle weakness:</u> These autoantibodies cross-react with presynaptic VGCC antigens and interfere with the normal calcium flux required for the release of ACh. **Decreased acetylcholine release decreases muscle contraction and results in subsequent weakness.**
- <u>Autonomic symptoms:</u> certain VGCC subtypes on autonomic presynaptic fibers are also targeted.

CLINICAL MANIFESTATIONS
- **<u>Typical LEMS triad</u>: [1] proximal muscle weakness, [2] areflexia, & [3] autonomic dysfunction.**
- **Proximal muscle weakness that <u>improves with repeated muscle use</u>** (unlike Myasthenia gravis). The weakness may cause difficulty arising from a chair, gait alteration, or managing stairs.
- **<u>Autonomic symptoms:</u> dry mouth most common,** postural hypotension, & erectile dysfunction.

<u>Physical examination:</u>
- **<u>Hyporeflexia:</u> decreased or absent deep tendon reflexes** & sluggish pupillary response.
- **Recovery of lost deep tendon reflexes or improvement in muscle strength with vigorous, brief muscle activation is a unique feature of LEMS.** No significant muscle atrophy.

DIAGNOSIS
- <u>Serological testing</u>: **P/Q-type voltage-gated calcium channel antibody assay** (85%-95%).
- **<u>Electrophysiology</u>:** <u>Repetitive nerve stimulation</u> (RNS) testing — **low CMAP (compound muscle action potential) amplitude at rest, reproducible post-exercise increase in CMAP** of at least 100% compared with pre-exercise baseline value, a decremental response at low rates of RNS, and an incremental response at high-rate stimulation.
- **<u>Chest imaging:</u>** CT or MRI of the chest to assess for underlying malignancy.

MANAGEMENT
- **Treat the underlying malignancy.**
- <u>Initial symptomatic management:</u> Amifampridine (3,4-diaminopyridine). Pyridostigmine.
- <u>Second-line:</u> Plasmapheresis, IVIG, oral immunosuppressants.

MULTIPLE SCLEROSIS (MS)

- **Autoimmune, inflammatory <u>demyelinating disease of the CNS</u>** of idiopathic origin associated with **axon degeneration of white matter (brain &/or spinal cord). Affects the <u>oligodendrocytes</u>.**
- Most common in **women & young adults 20-40 years.** Associated with HLA DRB*15:01 & HLA-DR2.
- <u>Risk factors</u>: reduced sunlight exposure (colder climates), vitamin D deficiency, Epstein-Barr virus.

<u>3 MAIN TYPES OF MS:</u>
- **[1] <u>Relapsing-remitting disease</u> most common — episodic exacerbations.**
- [2] <u>Progressive disease</u>: progressive decline without acute exacerbations.
- [3] <u>Secondary progressive</u>: relapsing-remitting pattern that becomes progressive.

<u>CLINICAL MANIFESTATIONS</u>
- **Sensory disturbances followed by weakness, fatigue, & visual disturbances most common presenting symptoms.** Sensory deficits (pain, paresthesias, numbness, tingling), motor deficits (weakness, gait/balance problems, limb unsteadiness). Visual disturbances (**diplopia, Optic neuritis). Trigeminal neuralgia.** Dysarthria. CNS lesions occur at different times & locations.
- **<u>Uhthoff's phenomenon</u>:** worsening of symptoms with heat (eg, exercise, fever, hot tubs, weather).
- <u>Spinal cord symptoms</u>: bladder or bowel dysfunction (eg, Overflow incontinence). Spastic paraparesis.

<u>PHYSICAL EXAMINATION</u>
- **<u>Upper motor neuron signs</u>: spasticity, upward Babinski, hyperreflexia,** muscle rigidity.
- **<u>Lhermitte's sign</u>:** neck flexion causes lightning-shock type pain radiating from the spine down the leg.
- **<u>Marcus-Gunn pupil</u> with Optic neuritis — during swinging-flashlight test from the unaffected eye into the affected eye, the pupils appear to dilate** (due to less than normal pupillary constriction). Due to delayed conduction through the affected optic nerve.
- <u>Internuclear ophthalmoplegia</u> — inability to adduct the eye on the side of the lesion with nystagmus in the other eye.
- <u>Cerebellar</u>: Charcot's neurologic triad (nystagmus, staccato speech, and intentional tremor).
- <u>Spinal cord symptoms</u>: bladder, bowel, or sexual dysfunction. Vertigo, ataxia.

<u>DIAGNOSIS</u>
Mainly clinical: at least 2 distinct episodes of CNS deficits at different CNS locations.
- **<u>MRI with gadolinium</u> best initial & most accurate test — hyperintense white matter plaques** hallmark finding. There should be proof ≥2 areas of white matter involvement before the diagnosis is made (eg, periventricular, infratentorial, cortical/juxtacortical, and spinal cord).
- **<u>Lumbar puncture</u> indicated if negative MRI: <u>increased IgG & IgG oligoclonal bands</u>** — small discrete bands in the gamma globulin region seen on electrophoresis, which reflects inflammatory cells penetrating the blood brain barrier. Increased IgG index.

<u>MANAGEMENT — ACUTE EXACERBATION</u>
- **<u>IV high-dose Glucocorticoids</u> first line treatment of acute exacerbations of MS.**
- **<u>Plasmapheresis</u> (Plasma exchange therapy) if not responsive to glucocorticoids.**

<u>PREVENTION OF RELAPSE & PROGRESSION:</u>
- **<u>Escalation therapy</u>: Interferon beta or Glatiramer first line agents.**
- **<u>Monoclonal antibody disease-modifying therapies (DMTs)</u>** if initial therapy is ineffective or partially effective, second-line drugs are used for escalation of therapy — eg, **Natalizumab,** anti-CD20 agents (eg, **Ocrelizumab,** Ofatumumab, Ublituximab, Rituximab), Fingolimod, Alemtuzumab, Teriflunomide. Dimethyl fumarate. Natalizumab associated with PML (test for JC virus antibodies).
- Amantadine helpful for fatigue symptoms. **<u>Spasticity</u>: Baclofen,** Tizanidine, & Diazepam.
- **<u>Induction therapy</u> used in aggressive MS** — more potent immunosuppressant agents early in the course of the disease (eg, Ocrelizumab, Mitoxantrone, Fingolimod, Natalizumab, Alemtuzumab).

ASTROCYTOMA

- **Tumors derived from astrocytes.** Astrocytes are star-shaped glial cells of the brain & spinal cord that support the endothelial cells of the blood-brain barrier, provide nutrients for cells, maintain extracellular ion balance, and also repair the brain after injury.
- Can appear in any part of the brain. **Most often infratentorial in children (supratentorial in adults).**

TYPES OF ASTROCYTOMAS
- PILOCYTIC ASTROCYTOMA (GRADE I): (Juvenile Astrocytoma) — typically localized. Considered the **"most benign" of all the Astrocytomas. Most common in children & young adults.** Other grade I Astrocytomas include cerebellar Astrocytoma & desmoplastic infantile.

- DIFFUSE ASTROCYTOMA (**Grade II** or Low-grade) Types: Fibrillary, Gemistocytic, & Protoplasmic. They tend to invade surrounding tissues but grow at a relatively slow pace. May present with seizures.

- ANAPLASTIC ASTROCYTOMA: **(Grade III).** Rare but aggressive.

- GRADE IV: **Glioblastoma multiforme is the most common primary CNS tumors in adults.**

- Subependymal Giant cell Astrocytoma — ventricular tumors associated with tuberculous sclerosis.

CLINICAL MANIFESTATIONS
1. **Focal deficits: most common.** Depends on the location of the lesion. Most common in the frontal & temporal areas of the cerebral hemisphere.
   - General symptoms: **headaches (may be worse in the morning, may wake patients up at night, may be positional), cranial nerve deficits, seizures,** altered mental status changes, neurological deficits, ataxia, vision changes, weakness.
2. **Increased intracranial pressure:** due to mass effect ⇨ headache, nausea, vomiting, papilledema, ataxia, drowsiness, lethargy, stupor, coma.

DIAGNOSIS
1. **CT scan or MRI with contrast:** Grade I & II non-enhancing. Grade III & IV are enhancing.
2. Brain biopsy: usually guided by imaging studies. Histologic appearance includes:
   - **Pilocytic Astrocytomas (Grade I)** generally form sacs of fluid (**cystic**), or may be enclosed within a cyst. Although they are usually slow-growing, these tumors can become very large. **Rosenthal fibers eosinophilic corkscrew fibers.** Compact areas of bipolar cells.

   - **Diffuse Astrocytomas** tend to contain microcysts and mucus-like fluid. They are grouped by the appearance and behavior of the cells for which they are named.

   - **Anaplastic Astrocytomas** tend to have tentacle-like projections that grow into surrounding tissue, making them difficult to completely remove during surgery.

   - **Astrocytoma Grade IV (Glioblastoma)** may contain cystic material, calcium deposits, blood vessels, and/or a mixed grade of cells.

MANAGEMENT
- Pilocytic Astrocytoma: Surgical excision. In adults and older children, radiation may follow surgery if the tumor cannot be completely removed.
- Diffuse Astrocytoma: Surgery if the tumor is accessible & can be completely removed. Radiation therapy (RT) may be adjunctive to surgery or for unresectable tumors.
- Anaplastic Astrocytoma: Surgical resection ⇨ RT. ±Chemotherapy after radiation or if recurrent.
- Astrocytoma Grade IV: Surgical resection ⇨ Radiation therapy (RT) + Chemotherapy.

GLIOBLASTOMA MUTLIFORME [GRADE 4 ASTROCYTOMA]

- **Most common & most aggressive primary malignant CNS tumors in adults.**
- **Glioblastoma (Grade IV Astrocytoma):** heterogenous mixture of poorly differentiated astrocytes.

TYPES
- **PRIMARY: most common** (60%). **Seen in adults >50 years.** Arises de novo (new). **Most common type & most aggressive.**
- **SECONDARY:** (40%). Most common <45y. Due to malignant progression from a low-grade Astrocytoma (grade II) or anaplastic Astrocytoma (grade III). May transform as early as 1 year or >10 years.

RISK FACTORS
- Males, >50 years, HHV-6, Cytomegalovirus (CMV) infection, history of ionizing radiation.

VARIANTS
- "Classic": 97%. Presence of extra copies of the epidermal growth factor receptor gene (EGFR). TP53 is rarely mutated in this type (note that other tumors are associated with TP53 mutation).
- Mesenchymal: high rates of mutations & alterations including the gene encoding for neurofibromatosis type I. TP53 often mutated. An alteration of MGMT (a DNA repair enzyme).

CLINICAL MANIFESTATIONS
- Focal deficits depend on the location of the tumor. Most common in the frontal & temporal areas of the cerebral hemisphere.
- **Patients usually present in the sixth and seventh decades of life with headache, seizures, or focal neurologic deficits.**
- General: **headache (may be worse in the morning, may wake patients up at night, may be positional),** cranial nerve deficits (eg, fixed, dilated pupil from a CN III palsy), altered mental status, neurological deficits, ataxia, vision changes, weakness, seizures.

DIAGNOSIS
- **Brain MRI with contrast initial study of choice** — classic finding is heterogenous lesion with **variable ring of enhancement with central necrosis, surrounded by edema & irregular (serpiginous) margins.** Mass effect may cause Hydrocephalus. **May cross the corpus callosum ("butterfly" glioma).**
- Histology (usually post-surgical): malignant astrocytes + necrotizing, hemorrhagic center surrounded by pleomorphic cells in a **pseudopalisading pattern (tumor cells lining the area of necrosis).**

MANAGEMENT
- Treatment involves maximal surgical excision when possible, followed by adjuvant partial-field external-beam radiotherapy (6000 cGy in thirty 200-cGy fractions) with concomitant chemotherapy with Temozolomide (alkylating agent), followed by 6 months of adjuvant Temozolomide.
- Implantation of biodegradable polymers containing Carmustine chemotherapy into the tumor bed after resection of the tumor or addition of tumor treating fields (scalp electrodes delivering low-intensity electric currents) may also be used in some.

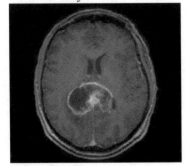 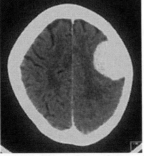 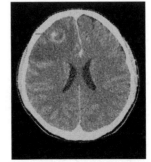

Butterfly glioma   Meningioma (dural attachment)   CNS lymphoma (ring-enhancing)

MENINGIOMA

- **Usually benign, slow-growing tumors arising from arachnoid meningothelial cells of the meninges (covering the brain & spinal cord). Most common primary CNS tumor.**
- **Most commonly arises from the dura** or sites of dura reflection (eg, venous sinuses, falx cerebri).
- Meningiomas are classified by the WHO into 3 histologic grades of increasing aggressiveness: grade I (benign), grade II (atypical), and grade III (malignant). They rarely invade brain tissue.

RISK FACTORS
- Females (estrogen receptors on tumor cells), radiation exposure, Neurofibromatosis type 2 (NF2), and history of cranial irradiation. Their incidence increases with age. Most are located supratentorial.

CLINICAL MANIFESTATIONS
- Often asymptomatic (incidental finding) or causes **symptoms due to compression & displacement of the brain** (usually does not invade the brain parenchyma). **Headaches, seizures, or focal neurologic signs** (depending on the location of the tumor). Fixed dilated pupil (CN III) common.

DIAGNOSIS
- **MRI with contrast** preferred: **uniform extra-axial intensely enhancing, well-defined lesion often attached to the dura** (resembling a snowball). May have **increased calcifications**.
- Histology: **spindle-cells concentrically arranged in a whorled pattern.**
  Psammoma bodies: concentric round calcifications.

MANAGEMENT
- **Asymptomatic: observation if small;** can be observed with serial MRI studies annually or biennially.
- **Symptomatic or large: surgical excision when possible** (transarterial embolization may be performed prior to surgery). External beam Radiation therapy may be used if not a surgical candidate or as adjuvant in some (eg, partially resected tumors). Stereotactic radiosurgery.

CNS LYMPHOMA

- Primary seen without evidence of systemic disease. **Variant of extranodal Non-Hodgkin lymphoma (NHL).** Secondary is more common.
- **Secondary: METS from another site** (eg, NHL in the neck, chest, groin, abdomen) **especially Diffuse large B cell lymphoma (90%).** Burkitt's lymphoma (10%), T-cell, or low-grade lymphomas.

RISK FACTORS:
- **Epstein-Barr virus (EBV) positive in 90% of patients,** immunosuppression — eg, AIDS, post-transplant, receiving immunosuppressant treatment (eg, high-dose steroids, chemotherapy). Males.

CLINICAL MANIFESTATIONS
- Focal deficits: depends on the location. Visual changes, steroid-refractory posterior uveitis.

DIAGNOSIS
- **CT scan or MRI with contrast:** hypointense **ring-enhancing lesion** in the deep white matter on CT.
- Biopsy: usually guided by imaging study. Systemic staging is performed prior to treatment.
- Staging includes CT of abdomen/pelvis, PET scan, bone marrow biopsy, slit lamp examination.

MANAGEMENT
- **Primary: Methotrexate most effective chemotherapy (given with Folinic acid/Leucovorin)** may be used with other chemotherapeutics (eg, Rituximab). Chemotherapy not usually given at the same time as radiation (increased risk of leukoencephalopathy). Radiation therapy, corticosteroids.
- **Secondary:** when an aggressive approach is feasible, **induction therapy (eg, R-CHOP) plus high-dose Methotrexate-based regimen,** followed by consideration of consolidative therapy with high-dose chemotherapy and autologous hematopoietic cell transplantation (IICT) in eligible patients.

OLIGODENDROGLIOMA

- Oligodendrocyte — a type of cell that makes up the supportive (glial) tissue of the brain, which are responsible for myelination of CNS axons. These tumors can be found anywhere within the cerebral hemispheres, often in the cortical gray matter (**especially the frontal & temporal lobes**).
- Oligodendrogliomas most often occur in middle-aged adults; more common in women.

CLINICAL MANIFESTATIONS
- May be asymptomatic (incidental finding) as the tumor grows slowly.
- Focal deficits: include headaches, seizures, & personality changes (depends on the tumor location).

DIAGNOSIS
- MRI with contrast (preferred) or CT scan: Hypointense or isodense lesions with coarse calcifications.
- Brain biopsy: guided by imaging studies. **1p/19q codeletion &** *IDH* **mutations (Isocitrate dehydrogenase) associated with better response to Temozolomide & combo chemoradiotherapy.**
- Histologic appearance: soft, grayish-pink *calcified* tumors, areas of hemorrhage &/or cystic. **Chicken-wire capillary pattern** with perinuclear clearing **("fried-egg" appearance)** seen on microscopy.

MANAGEMENT
Surgery ⇨ radiation therapy & chemotherapy: Temozolomide. Procarbazine, Lomustine, & Vincristine (PCV).

EPENDYMOMA

- **Arises from ependymal (radial glial) cells** lining the ventricles & central canal of the spinal cord column.
- **Most common in children 1-5 years of age** (mean age at diagnosis is 5 years of age) & young adults.
- **Most are infratentorial: arising from fourth ventricle (70%), intramedullary spinal cord, & medulla.**

CLINICAL MANIFESTATIONS
- Infants: Hydrocephalus (↑ in head size), irritability, sleeplessness, depressed mental status, & vomiting.
- Older children & adults: nausea, vomiting, headache. May cause Cauda equina in adults.

DIAGNOSIS
- CT scan or MRI with contrast: hypointense T1, hyperintense T2. Enhances with gadolinium.
- Brain biopsy: **perivascular pseudorosettes tumor cells surrounding a blood vessel.**

MANAGEMENT
- **Surgical resection ⇨ adjuvant radiation therapy** or postoperative Chemotherapy.

HEMANGIOMAS

- **Hemangioma:** abnormal buildup of blood vessels in the skin or internal organs. 2% of all 1ry brain tumors. Von Hippel-Lindau syndrome 10% — (Hemangiomas, tumors of the liver, pancreas & kidney).
- **Hemangioblastoma:** arises from the blood vessel lining. Benign, slow growing well-defined tumors. MC found in the posterior fossa (**brainstem & cerebellum**). Often >40 years. May occur in the cerebral hemispheres or spinal cord. **Retinal hemangiomas associated with von Hippel-Lindau syndrome.**
- Hemangiopericytoma: originate from the cells surrounding the blood vessels & the meninges. May spread to the lung & liver.

CLINICAL MANIFESTATIONS
- Hemangioblastoma: headache, nausea, vomiting, gait abnormalities, poor coordination of the limbs. May produce erythropoietin (secondary polycythemia). Hemangiopericytoma: depends on tumor location.

DIAGNOSIS
- CT scan or MRI.
- Biopsy: well-defined borders, usually does not invade surrounding healthy tissue. **Foam cells with high vascularity.**

MANAGEMENT: **surgical resection.** Radiation may be used in tumors attached to the brainstem.

DELIRIUM

- **Acute, abrupt <u>transient</u> change of consciousness or altered cognition due to an identifiable cause** (eg, medication effect, sleep disturbance, medical condition, electrolyte abnormalities, uremia, organ failure, substance intoxication or withdrawal etc.). **No focal neurological findings.**
- **Rapid onset associated with fluctuating mental status changes & marked deficit in short-term memory.** Visual hallucinations, tremulousness, and myoclonus/asterixis may be seen.
- <u>Laboratory workup:</u> serum electrolytes, glucose, BUN, creatinine, calcium, CBC, Vitamin B12, TFTs, urinalysis & urine culture. Drug levels, toxicology screen, liver function testing, & ABG as needed.
- **<u>Management</u>: treat the cause. Rapid onset & full recovery is seen within 1 week in most cases.**
- <u>Prevention:</u> reorientation, sleep facilitation, keep blinds open, noise reduction, family visits, out of bed,

ALZHEIMER DEMENTIA

- **Most common type of dementia.** Usually disease of elderly (>65 years) but may occur earlier.
- <u>Risk factors:</u> Increasing age, genetics, family history.

PATHOPHYSIOLOGY
- Unknown — 3 hypotheses: [1] <u>Amyloid hypothesis:</u> **extracellular amyloid-beta protein deposition (senile plaques)** in the brain are neurotoxic. [2] <u>Tau hypothesis:</u> **neurofibrillary tangles (hyperphosphorylated tau proteins)** are neurotoxic. [3] <u>Cholinergic hypothesis:</u> **acetylcholine deficiency** leads to memory, language, & visuospatial changes.
- <u>Histologic findings:</u> **amyloid-beta protein deposition (senile plaques)** in the brain. Amyloid precursor proteins (APP) are normally degraded by alpha-cleavage. Beta cleavage of APP results in Amyloid-beta accumulation. **Neurofibrillary tangles = intracellular aggregations of tau protein** (an insoluble cytoskeletal microtubule element).

CLINICAL MANIFESTATIONS
- **<u>Short-term memory loss</u> often first symptom; progressive decline to long-term memory loss.**
- **<u>Cognitive deficits</u>:** disorientation, behavioral & personality changes, language difficulties, loss of motor skills, visuospatial function, etc. Impaired executive functioning. Usually gradual in nature.
- **<u>Neuropsychiatric and behavioral symptoms:</u>** common in middle and late stages of AD but may occur early in the course in some patients. Changes in environment may destabilize the patient.
- <u>Noncognitive neurologic deficits:</u> apraxia, myoclonus, and seizures can occur in late stages of AD.

DIAGNOSIS
- **Montreal Cognitive Assessment (≤25 is abnormal) → Mini-Mental State Examination.** If positive MMSE, do lab screening. There are no specific tests.
- Workup to rule out other causes include MRI of the brain, Vitamin B12, TFTs (rule out hypothyroidism), CBC, renal and liver tests, VDRL or RPR to rule out Syphilis,.
- **<u>MRI</u> preferred neuroimaging test — cortex atrophy (eg, medial temporal lobe atrophy),** reduced hippocampal volume, white matter lesions. Aβ positron emission tomography (PET) scan.

MEDICAL MANAGEMENT
- **<u>Acetylcholinesterase inhibitors</u>: increase cholinergic transmission (Donepezil, Rivastigmine, Galantamine).** Used to improve memory function & symptom relief for patients with newly diagnosed Alzheimer disease (AD) dementia (does not slow down the disease progression).
- **<u>NMDA antagonist</u>: Memantine — can be added to Acetylcholinesterase inhibitors or used as monotherapy in moderate to advanced Dementia** (eg, MMSE ≤18).
  <u>Mechanism:</u> **blocks NMDA receptor, slowing calcium influx & nerve damage.** Glutamate is an excitatory neurotransmitter of the NDMA receptor. Excitotoxicity causes cell death. NMDA antagonists reduce glutamate excitotoxicity. May be adjunctive.
- <u>Aducanumab</u> is approved by the US Food and Drug Administration (FDA) for the treatment of mild AD with Aβ PET scan. Reduces brain amyloid levels (although clinical benefit is uncertain).

VASCULAR DEMENTIA

- **Any dementia that is primarily caused by cerebrovascular disease or impaired cerebral blood flow**, or in which **impaired cerebral blood flow is a contributing causative factor.**
- **Hypertension most important risk factor.** Diabetes mellitus, history of CVA, Dyslipidemia.
- **Prevention: strict blood pressure control.**

CLINICAL MANIFESTATIONS
- **Sudden stepwise progression cognitive executive function decline — random infarct then decline traced back to a definitive point in time** ⇨ stable then another infarct ⇨ decline.
- **Cortical findings:** depend on area affected. Medial frontal: executive dysfunction, apathy, abulia. Left parietal: apraxia aphasia, agnosia. Right parietal: hemineglect, confusion, visuospatial abnormalities.
- **Subcortical findings:** focal motor deficits, gait abnormality, urinary difficulties, personality changes.

DIAGNOSIS
- Clinical diagnosis. Workup similar to Alzheimer disease — rule out other causes of symptoms (eg, B12 and folate levels, RPR, etc.). Vascular dementia is the second most common cause of Dementia.
- MRI: white matter lesions, cortical or subcortical infarcts. **CT scan may show lacunar infarcts**.

FRONTOTEMPORAL DEMENTIA (PICK DISEASE)

- **Localized brain degeneration of the frontotemporal lobes.** May progress globally.
- Histology: **Pick bodies** (round or oval aggregates of Tau protein) seen on silver-staining of the cortex.

CLINICAL MANIFESTATIONS
- **Marked changes in social behavior, personality, & language (aphasia) are early signs of FTD (relative sparing of memory);** eventual executive & memory dysfunction when advanced. The onset of dementia is earlier than Alzheimer disease (usually presents in the sixth decade).
- **Behavioral variant: disinhibition or socially inappropriate behaviors, apathy, hyperorality** (binge-eating, changes in food preferences, putting large amounts of food in their mouth), **compulsive ritualistic behaviors,** loss of sympathy & empathy. Deficits in executive control.
- **Language variant:** language difficulty, progressive reduction in speech, nonfluent aphasia (early).
- **Preserved visuospatial.** In advanced disease, they may have positive primitive reflexes (palmomental & palmar grasp). May have Parkinsonism.

MANAGEMENT
- Nonpharmacologic behavior modification; physical, occupational, & speech therapy; supervision.
- **No specific medical management. SSRIs (eg, Citalopram) or Trazodone may be used for neurobehavioral symptoms of FTD despite nonpharmacologic interventions.**

DEMENTIA WITH LEWY BODIES [DIFFUSE LEWY BODY DISEASE]

- Progressive dementia characterized by the diffuse presence of Lewy bodies (abnormal neuronal protein deposits) in comparison to Parkinson disease, where the Lewy bodies are localized.
- Histology: Cortical Lewy bodies (abnormal deposition of alpha-synuclein proteins).

CLINICAL MANIFESTATIONS
- 4 core features may occur early [1] **recurrent well-formed visual hallucinations,** [2] **cognitive fluctuations (episodic delirium),** [3] **Parkinsonism** (bradykinesia, tremor, rigidity, postural instability), **& [4] rapid eye movement (REM) sleep behavioral disorder.** Dream reenactment.
- Supportive: Delusions, **sensitivity to antipsychotics & antiemetic drugs** (may respond with catatonia, cognitive dysfunction, or life-threatening muscle rigidity); **autonomic dysfunction** orthostatic hypotension, constipation, urinary incontinence. Hypersomnia. Dementia late findings.
- **Dementia mainly deficits in attention, executive function, & visuospatial**. Memory loss rare.
- Treatment of the Parkinsonian symptoms may worsen the neuropsychiatric symptoms and vice versa.

FOCAL SEIZURE

Abnormal neuronal discharge from one discrete section of 1 brain hemisphere (eg, temporal or frontal lobe).
- **Focal seizure with retained awareness**: consciousness fully maintained.
- **Focal seizure with impaired awareness**: consciousness impaired.

CLINICAL MANIFESTATIONS
- **Motor:** **tonic (muscular rigidity), clonic (rhythmic jerking), or myoclonic movements.** Additional findings may include **[1] Jacksonian march: starts in one localized area (eg, fingers) and then spread to more parts of the affected limb or body. [2] Todd's paralysis: seizures may be followed by a neurologic deficit (localized paresis) for minutes up to 24 hours.**
- Sensory: paresthesias, numbness, pain, heat, cold, sensation of movement, olfactory, flashing lights.
- Autonomic: abdominal (pain, nausea, vomiting, hunger), cardiovascular (sinus tachycardia), blood pressure changes, flushing, piloerections, sweating, bronchoconstriction.
- Psychologic: fear, déjà vu, hallucinations. Vision (flashing lights or formed hallucinations).
- Auras: (focal seizure with sensory or psychic symptoms) may precede, accompany, or follow seizure onset: vision change, dyspepsia, déjà vu, paresthesias, hearing disturbance, abnormal taste or smell.

Focal sensory, motor, or autonomic symptoms depending on the lobe affected:
- **Temporal lobe focal onset seizures can cause autonomic or psychological symptoms** [eg, dyspepsia, **auditory hallucinations**, olfactory sensations (intense odors), sense of fear (involvement of the amygdala)]. Focal seizures arising from the temporal or frontal cortex may also cause alterations in hearing, olfaction, or emotional state, or an epigastric sensation that rises from the stomach or chest to the head. **Temporal lobe seizures can also have motor symptoms.**
- **Frontal Lobe: prominent motor manifestations (supplementary motor area),** loud vocalizations, shaking, twitching, stiffness of the face or limbs, bicycling movements, Jacksonian march.
- **Occipital Lobe seizures frequently begin with sudden visual changes** (eg, poorly formed colors or lights, scotomas, amaurosis, flashing of lights), illusions (eg, micropsia or metamorphopsia), seeing complex figures, or visual hallucinations.
- **Parietal Lobe sensory deficits:** subjective tingling, paresthesias, or numbness of the contralateral limb or body. Lack of awareness of a body part, vertigo, and language disturbances.

Additional findings in Focal seizures with impaired awareness:
- **Seizure:** behavioral arrest & staring lasting between 30-120 seconds (<3 minutes). The patients are generally unaware & unresponsive during this period. May preceded by an aura.
- **Automatisms: repetitive stereotyped behaviors** — **oral automatisms (lip smacking, chewing, facial grimacing,), manual automatisms (eg, picking at clothes repeatedly, patting, fidgeting),** subtle dystonic limb posturing (sustained contortion of the hand or foot), coordinated movements or repeating words or phrases. Seen with temporal lobe (mesial) seizures.
- **Post ictal phase: symptoms after the seizure include fatigue, somnolence, confusion, difficulty speaking or comprehending, and headache, usually resolving within minutes but may last for up to several hours.** The patient may be amnestic to the event itself.

DIAGNOSIS
- **Initial workup is to rule out reversible causes** — eg, Hypoglycemia, Hyponatremia, uremia.
- **(1) Basic labs:** CBC, electrolytes, calcium, magnesium, liver and renal function tests, UA, RPR.
- **(2) Urine toxicology** to rule out drugs as a cause (eg, Heroin, cocaine).
- **(3)** Neuroimaging: **CT scan:** to rule out intracranial pathology (eg, mass, bleed). **MRI better imaging.**

Electroencephalogram (EEG): EEG is the primary tool for the diagnosis of epilepsy.
- Focal with retained awareness — focal discharge at the onset of the seizure.
- Focal with impaired awareness — interictal spikes or with slow waves in the temporal or frontotemporal area. The interictal EEG may be normal, or it may demonstrate focal slowing and epileptiform discharges.

MEDICAL MANAGEMENT
- **Focal: Carbamazepine and Lamotrigine first line. Valproate,** Oxcarbazepine, Levetiracetam.

ABSENCE (PETIT MAL) SEIZURE

Generalized seizure (involving both hemispheres).
- **Most commonly seen in childhood** — **age at onset usually 4–10 years** (often ceases by early puberty or 20 years of age in most patients).

CLINICAL MANIFESTATIONS
- **Pause/stare: sudden brief lapses of consciousness & loss of awareness <u>without</u> loss of body tone** (patient remains upright), **blank staring episodes with pauses (behavioral arrest) with unresponsiveness. Episodes typically last between 5-10 seconds** (rarely >30 seconds). If prolonged >10 seconds, it can be associated with **eyelid twitching & automatisms (lip smacking).**
- **Prompt return to baseline after the spells** — **no postictal phase or confusion & no auras.**
- May occur up to hundreds of times daily. Because the signs are so subtle, patients are often thought to be "daydreaming" or are often misdiagnosed as having Attention deficit disorder.
- **Triggers: may be provoked by hyperventilation** or by emotions (eg, anger, fear).

DIAGNOSIS
- <u>EEG</u>: **bilaterally synchronous & symmetrical 3 Hertz** (3 cycles per second) **spike-and-slow-wave discharges** (2.5–5 Hz) that start and end abruptly superimposed on a normal EEG background.

MANAGEMENT
- **Ethosuximide first-line medical management.**
- **Second line: Valproic acid alternative to Ethosuximide.** Lamotrigine or Topiramate.
- <u>Medications to avoid</u>: some sodium channel blockers (eg, Carbamazepine, Gabapentin, Phenytoin, Pregabalin) can exacerbate Absence seizures.

ATONIC SEIZURES

- **Sudden partial or complete loss of muscle and postural tone lasting 1-2 seconds.**
- A very brief seizure may result in only a **quick head drop or nodding movement; a longer seizure will cause the patient to collapse (drop attack), which can lead to body or head injury.**
- Consciousness is briefly impaired, but the seizure is not usually associated with postictal confusion.

Electroencephalogram (EEG)
- The EEG shows brief, generalized spike-and-wave discharges followed immediately by diffuse slow waves that correlate with the loss of muscle tone.

MYOCLONIC SEIZURES

- **Myoclonus is a sudden, brief, sporadic, involuntary muscle contraction (twitching/limb jerking) of one muscle or a group of muscles, usually without loss of consciousness.**
- Due to cortical (vs subcortical or spinal) dysfunction.
- **Myoclonic seizures usually coexist with other forms of generalized seizures but are the predominant feature of Juvenile myoclonic epilepsy (JME).**
- **JME is most common in the morning & may be triggered by sleep deprivation.**
- A physiologic form of myoclonus is the sudden jerking movement noted while falling asleep.
- Pathologic myoclonus is most commonly seen in association with metabolic disorders, degenerative CNS diseases, or anoxic brain injury.

ELECTROENCEPHALOGRAM (EEG)
- EEG shows **bilaterally synchronous spike-and-slow-wave discharges immediately prior to the movement** and muscle artifact associated with the myoclonus.

MANAGEMENT
- **Valproate first-line for JME.** Levetiracetam, Lamotrigine, Topiramate, Zonisamide, Clonazepam.

GENERALIZED (GRAND MAL) SEIZURE

- **Simultaneous neuronal discharge of both hemispheres (diffuse brain involvement).**
- Generalized tonic clonic (Grand mal) most common type.

CLINICAL MANIFESTATIONS
- **Tonic-clonic (Grand Mal): sudden loss of consciousness with tonic activity [contraction & rigidity, which may include a loud moan/ictal cry] for 10-20 seconds that may be associated with respiratory arrest, followed by 1-2 minutes of clonic activity** (repetitive, rhythmic, symmetric jerking usually lasting <3 minutes) followed by **postictal phase (eg, confusion, unresponsiveness, muscle flaccidity, headache, fatigue, muscle ache). Cyanosis, tongue-biting, bowel incontinence or urinary incontinence can occur.** Patients may gradually regain consciousness over minutes to hours.
- Clonic: repetitive rhythmic jerking (usually lasting < 2-3 minutes) often associated with postictal state.
- Myoclonic: sudden, brief, sporadic involuntary twitching of one muscle or a group of muscles, usually without loss of consciousness.
- Tonic: loss of consciousness followed by rigidity.
- Atonic: sudden partial or complete loss of muscle and postural tone ("drop attacks") may cause injury.
- Absence: nonconvulsive brief lapse of consciousness with brief staring episodes or without loss of postural tone.

DIAGNOSIS
Workup of first seizure:
- **Initial workup is to rule out reversible causes** — eg, Hypoglycemia, Hyponatremia, uremia, and drug intoxication should be ruled out.
- [1] **Basic lab tests:** CBC, electrolytes including calcium and magnesium, liver and renal function tests, UA, RPR.
- [2] **Urine toxicology** to rule out drugs as a cause (eg, Heroin, cocaine).
- [3] Neuroimaging: **CT scan**: to rule out intracranial pathology (eg, mass, bleed). **MRI better imaging.**
- Serum prolactin assessment has limited utility as a diagnostic test for epileptic seizures (not part of the routine evaluation). In selected cases, an elevated serum prolactin & lactic acid immediately after a seizure may be useful in differentiating generalized tonic-clonic and focal seizures from psychogenic pseudo seizures.

Electroencephalogram (EEG):
- **EEG is the main diagnostic tool for the evaluation and characterization of seizures.**
- Tonic phase: The EEG during the tonic phase of the seizure shows a progressive increase in generalized low-voltage fast activity, followed by generalized high-amplitude, polyspike discharges.
- Clonic phase: the high-amplitude activity is typically interrupted by slow waves to create a spike-and-slow-wave pattern. The postictal EEG shows diffuse suppression of all cerebral activity, then slowing that gradually recovers as the patient awakens.

MANAGEMENT
- Treat the underlying cause if known.
- **Long-term options for Epilepsy include Lamotrigine, Valproic acid, Topiramate, Levetiracetam, Phenytoin, Carbamazepine, Phenobarbital. Levetiracetam & Lamotrigine safest in pregnancy.**
- Absence: Ethosuximide first line; Valproic acid second line.
- Myoclonic: Valproic acid.
- **Simple Febrile seizures are benign and self-limiting; preventive medications are not recommended.** Antipyretic medications do not reduce recurrence risk. Antiepileptic medications may prevent recurrence but have side effects. **Febrile seizures most common in children 6 months–5 years and are associated with fever, especially with viral illnesses.**

STATUS EPILEPTICUS

- A single, continuous epileptic seizure [1] lasting ≥5 minutes, or [2] >1 seizure within a 5-minute period without recovery in between the episodes. Considered a neurologic emergency.

ETIOLOGIES
- Structural abnormalities, infections (eg, meningitis, encephalitis), metabolic abnormalities, medications, toxins.

DIAGNOSIS: Neuroimaging: once stabilized to determine if intracranial mass or hemorrhage is present.

MANAGEMENT
- **Benzodiazepines are the preferred initial agents (Lorazepam** usually preferred). They are associated with rapid control of seizure. Additional doses can be given. Midazolam (IM, nasal, buccal) can be used as initial therapy if an IV access cannot be established. Rectal Diazepam if no IV.
- **Second line: In addition to Benzodiazepines, IV loading with Levetiracetam, Fosphenytoin, Phenytoin, or Valproate if no response to Benzodiazepine &/or to prevent seizure recurrence.** Lacosamide or Phenobarbital are alternatives.
- **Third line: Phenobarbital if no response to Phenytoin or other second-line agent (refractory).** Lacosamide is an alternative.
- General anesthesia: Midazolam or Propofol can be used (also used if no response to above).

COMPLICATIONS
- Hypoxia, aspiration, respiratory failure, cardiac arrhythmias.

PHENYTOIN & FOSPHENYTOIN

Mechanism of action:
- **Stabilizes neuronal membranes and stops seizure propagation by blocking voltage-gated sodium channels (VGNA+).** Fosphenytoin is a prodrug for Phenytoin.

Indications:
- Generalized tonic-clonic & Focal seizures.
- Seizure prophylaxis.
- Status epilepticus after Benzodiazepines.
- Since Phenytoin is **highly protein-bound (~90%)**, dosing adjustments need to be made for patients with **hypoalbuminemia** due to **alcoholism, impaired liver function,** or **severe malnutrition.**

PHENYTOIN

- **Mechanism:** stabilizes neuronal membranes by blocking voltage-gated sodium channels.
- Indications: generalized tonic-clonic & focal seizures (simple & complex), seizure prophylaxis. **Status epilepticus after benzodiazepines**

SIDE EFFECTS

P-450 inducer & induces lupus-like syndrome

H yperplasia of the gums & **H**irsutism

E rythema multiforme, Stevens-Johnson syndrome

N europathies: vertigo, ataxia, headache

Yield: if you don't give it slow, it can cause **hypotension & arrhythmias**

T eratogenicity (cleft lip & palate, microcephaly)

O steopenia

I nhibits folic acid absorption (megaloblastic anemia)

N ystagmus

SLOW·DOWN

YIELD TO

Slow to prevent low BP & arrhythmias

CARBAMAZEPINE

Mechanism of action:
- **Stabilizes neuronal membranes and stops seizure propagation by blocking voltage-gated sodium channels (VGNA⁺).** Decreases seizure spread by increasing the refractory period of the channels, decreases synapse transmission, & inhibits action potentials.
- Exact mechanism in Trigeminal neuralgia & Bipolar disorder is unknown.

Indications:
- **Epilepsy**: Generalized tonic-clonic & Focal seizures
- **Trigeminal neuralgia first-line therapy.** Oxcarbazepine (active metabolite with less adverse effects).
- **Bipolar disorder: [1] Sodium valproate and Carbamazepine are alternative mood stabilizers to Lithium and [2] are useful for rapid cycling or mixed features.**
- AVP/ADH deficiency (Central diabetes insipidus) second line after Desmopressin.

Adverse effects:
- **The most common adverse effects of Carbamazepine are dizziness, drowsiness, ataxia, nausea, & vomiting.**
- Gastrointestinal: nausea, vomiting, anorexia, **hepatotoxicity (increased LFTs, so monitor LFTs).**
- Neurologic: dizziness, ataxia, diplopia, CNS depression (eg, drowsiness, sedation), cognitive dysfunction.
- **Hyponatremia (causes SIADH)** — Hyponatremia is usually mild, transient, and reversible.
- **Stevens-Johnson syndrome (test for HLA-B*1502** — genetic susceptibility marker in Asians associated with an increased risk of developing Stevens-Johnson syndrome).
- Diplopia, arrhythmias.
- Rash, renal toxicity, suicidal ideation.
- **Blood dyscrasias: agranulocytosis, aplastic anemia**, thrombocytopenia — rare occurrence.
- **Teratogenic potential: craniofacial anomalies (eg, cleft lip & palate), spina bifida,** cardiovascular and cutaneous malformation, hypospadias, and developmental delays.
- Cardiac: Arrhythmias. Carbamazepine can exacerbate heart failure patients or even lead to cardiac dysfunction in healthy patients due to its tendency to cause homocysteinemia.

Medication interactions:
- **Inducer of the CP450 system** (CYP450 3A4) — can reduce the levels of other medications.
- **Drug-induced lupus.**
- Carbamazepine is contraindicated in use with Nefazodone (decreases Nefazodone's efficacy).
- Contraindications: **Not used in Absence (Petit mal) seizures** — can worsen absence seizures.

Monitoring:
- Therapeutic blood level 8–12 mcg/mL.
- **Monitor CBC & LFTs** to assess for hepatoxicity, agranulocytosis, aplastic anemia, & low platelets.

ETHOSUXIMIDE

Mechanism of action:
- **Calcium channel blockade: Ethosuximide blocks low-threshold (T-type) calcium channels, especially in the thalamic neurons** that act as pacemakers to generate rhythmic cortical discharge. This leads to motor cortex depression, elevation of the stimulation threshold, and decreased neuronal firing.

Indications:
- **Drug of choice for Absence (Petit mal) seizures** — can only be used in Absence seizures.

Adverse effects:
- **Drowsiness**, sleep disturbance, hyperactivity, ataxia, dizziness, headache, rash (**Stevens-Johnson syndrome), GI upset** (nausea, vomiting, diarrhea), weight gain.
- Caution: renal or hepatic failure.
- Monitoring: UA, CBC, LFTs.

PHENOBARBITAL

Mechanism of action:

- **Barbiturate that <u>binds to GABA receptors</u>** (different site than Benzodiazepines) **& potentiates GABA-mediated CNS inhibition as a result of _increased duration_ of chloride ion channel openings.** Inhibits sodium channels and acts as an antagonist at some glutamate receptors.

Indications:

- Partial (simplex & complex) or generalized (tonic-clonic) seizures.
- **Status epilepticus after Phenytoin administration.** Can be used in pregnant women and children.

Adverse effects:

- Sedation (toxicity), sleep wake cycle alteration, cognitive dysfunction, tolerance, dependence, ataxia.
- **<u>Inducer of P450 system</u>** — induction of hepatic drug metabolism
- <u>Psychological</u>: suicidality, **depression,** hyperactivity in pediatric patients, dependence.
- Permanent neurologic deficit if injected into or near peripheral nerves. Stevens-Johnson syndrome.

BENZODIAZEPINES

- **Lorazepam, Diazepam, Midazolam**

Mechanism of action:

- **<u>Potentiates GABA-mediated CNS inhibition</u>** — Benzodiazepines interact with postsynaptic GABA A receptor–chloride ion channel macromolecular complex at several sites within the CNS. Benzodiazepines _<u>increase the frequency of chloride ion channel openings</u>_, facilitating the inhibitory effects of GABA (decreased rate of neuronal discharge).
- Functions as an anxiolytic, sedative-hypnotic, anticonvulsant, and muscle relaxant.
- **Lorazepam is the most effective Benzodiazepine for seizures & has a shorter half-life (but longer "seizure' half-life) compared to Diazepam.**

Indications:

- Generalized and absence seizures, anxiety, sedation, muscle spasm.
- **First-line for acute generalized (tonic-clonic) seizures & status epilepticus** (usually followed by Phenytoin loading to prevent seizure recurrence), alcohol withdrawal, delirium tremens, & eclampsia (recurrent seizures after magnesium sulfate administration).
- <u>Seizure prevention</u>: during Alcohol withdrawal, Delirium tremens, & Eclampsia (recurrent seizures after IV Magnesium sulfate administration).

Adverse effects:

- **Sedation, tolerance, dependence**, ataxia, paradoxical reaction increased suicide.
- Monitor blood pressure after IV administration.
- <u>Contraindications or caution</u>: suicide risk.
- <u>Overdose</u>: **Flumazenil antagonizes the Benzodiazepine receptors**. It is used for Benzodiazepine sedation reversal and Benzodiazepine overdose.

LAMOTRIGINE

Mechanism of action:

- **Blocks Na+ and Ca²⁺ channels, decreases presynaptic glutamate release.** Inhibits glutamate's effect on the NMDA receptor, reducing neuronal activity.

Indications:

- Generalized tonic-clonic, focal, myoclonic, and absence seizures.

Adverse effects:

- Dizziness, ataxia, nausea, tremor, headache, diplopia, Stevens-Johnson syndrome, drug interactions.

LEVETIRACETAM

Mechanism of action:

- Binds the SV2A protein on glutamate-containing transmitter vesicles & **reduces glutamate release**.

Adverse effects:

- Somnolence, dizziness, agitation, anxiety, irritability, depression.

VALPROIC ACID, DIVALPROEX SODIUM

Mechanism of action:

- Multiple mechanisms — potentiates GABA-mediated CNS inhibition, inhibits glutamate & NMDA receptors, increases refractory period of voltage-gated sodium channels, modulates Ca^{2+} channels.
- Divalproex sodium is the stable, coordinated compound of sodium Valproate and Valproic acid.

Indications:

- **Valproic acid is an anticonvulsive and mood stabilizer medication.**
- Seizures: Partial (simple and complex), generalized (tonic-clonic & absence). **First-line for myoclonic seizures. Valproate has the broadest spectrum of all antiseizure medications. Absence seizures: blocks T-type Ca^{2+} channels, reducing thalamic spike & wave patterns.**
- **Bipolar disorder:** [1] Sodium valproate and Carbamazepine are alternative mood stabilizers to Lithium and [2] are useful for rapid cycling or mixed features. Headaches: Migraine prophylaxis.

Adverse effects:

- **Common adverse effects include drowsiness (sedation), nausea, tremor, hair loss (alopecia), weight gain, hepatotoxicity, and inhibition of hepatic drug metabolism** (CYP2C9, CP450).
- GI: **Pancreatitis, hepatotoxicity,** nausea, vomiting, **weight changes** (anorexia and weight gain).
- **Teratogenic Valproate has the highest risk of birth defects of any of the commonly used antiepileptic drugs** — though multiple fetal malformations are possible, **neural tube defects (eg, spina bifida) are the most common abnormalities seen after Valproate use.** Valproate should be avoided if patient is not already on it prior to pregnancy or only used in very select cases.
- **Inhibitor of the CP450 system** leading to drug-drug interactions. Thrombocytopenia.
- **Neurological: headache, sedation, tremor, ataxia,** tinnitus, blurred vision, nystagmus, photosensitivity. Increased suicidality. Hyponatremia due to SIADH.

Monitoring:

- Therapeutic levels: 80-120 mcg/mL.
- **Liver enzymes should be monitored beginning with baseline and frequently during therapy,** especially during the first 6 months.
- Valproic acid is contraindicated in patients with hepatic disorders or significant hepatic impairment.

TOPIRAMATE

Multiple mechanisms of action:

- Blocks sodium channels (eg, ligand & gated channels), increases GABA receptor activity, glutamate receptor antagonist, & reduces depolarization by AMPA/Kainate receptor antagonism.

Indications:

- Generalized (tonic-clonic) seizures, partial (simple & complex) seizures.
- Migraine prophylaxis. **Obesity and Binge-eating disorders (due to its weight loss effects).**

Adverse effects:

- **Nephrolithiasis:** Treatment with Topiramate causes systemic metabolic acidosis (carbonic anhydrase inhibition), markedly lowers urinary citrate excretion, and increases urinary pH. These changes **increase the propensity to form calcium phosphate kidney stones**.
- **CNS symptoms: paresthesias,** sedation, drowsiness, headache, dizziness, ataxia, psychomotor slowing, memory impairment, fatigue, nausea. Hyperthermia. Acute myopia, glaucoma.
- **Weight loss and decrease appetite; this adverse effect may be a benefit in some conditions.**

GABAPENTIN

Mechanism of action:

- **Blocks presynaptic voltage-gated calcium channels specifically possessing the alpha-2-delta-1 subunit,** inhibiting the release of excitatory neurotransmitter. Although Gabapentin is structurally related to GABA, it does not bind to GABA receptors or affect GABA degradation or uptake.

Indications:

- Partial (simple & complex) seizures.
- **Neuropathy:** Peripheral neuropathy & neuropathic pain, Fibromyalgia, post-herpetic neuralgia.

Adverse effects:

- CNS symptoms: dizziness, sedation (somnolence), ataxia, nystagmus. **Can worsen Absence seizures.**

SEIZURE CLASSIFICATION	MANIFESTATIONS	MISCELLANEOUS
PARTIAL (FOCAL) SEIZURES	*Confined to small area of brain (focal part of one hemisphere).*	May become generalized.
SIMPLE PARTIAL	*CONSCIOUSNESS FULLY MAINTAINED* EEG: focal discharge at the onset of the seizures.	May have focal sensory, autonomic, motor sx^ May be followed by transient neurologic deficit (Todd's paralysis) lasting up to 24 hours.
COMPLEX PARTIAL (TEMPORAL LOBE)	*CONSCIOUSNESS IMPAIRED.* Starts focally. EEG: interictal spikes with slow waves in the temporal area. Aura (seconds – minutes) ⇨ impaired consciousness.	*AURAS:* sensory/autonomic/motor symptoms of which the patient is aware of. May precede/accompany or follow. Complex partial includes: *AUTOMATISMS: ex: lip smacking, manual picking, patting, coordinated motor movement (ex. walking).*
GENERALIZED SEIZURES	*Diffuse brain involvement (both hemispheres)*	
❶ ABSENCE (PETIT MAL) Nonconvulsive	Brief lapse of consciousness; patient usually unaware of attacks. *Brief staring episodes, eyelid twitching.* *NO post-ictal phase.*	May be clonic (jerking), tonic (stiffness) or atonic (loss of postural tone). *MC in childhood ⇨ usually ceases by 20y* EEG: bilateral symmetric 3Hz *spike & wave* action or may be normal.
❷ TONIC-CLONIC (GRAND MAL)	Tonic Phase: **loss of consciousness ⇨ rigidity,** sudden arrest of respiration (usually <60sec) ⇨ clonic phase. Clonic Phase: **repetitive, rhythmic jerking*** *(lasts <2-3 minutes)* ⇨ postictal phase. Postictal phase: *flaccid coma/sleep: variable duration.*	May be accompanied by incontinence, tongue biting or aspiration with postictal confusion. *Auras are prewarnings to seizures* EEG: generalize high-amplitude rapid spiking. May be normal in between seizures.
❸ Myoclonus	*Sudden, brief, sporadic involuntary twitching* *No LOC*	*May be 1 muscle or groups of muscles*
❹ Atonic	*"Drop attacks" – sudden loss of postural tone**	
Status Epilepticus	Repeated, generalized seizures without recovery >30mins	

^motor: jerky, rhythmic, movements one area (focal) or spread to other parts of the affected limb or body (spread = "Jacksonian March"). Tonic or clonic.
^sensory: paresthesias, numbness, pain, heat, cold, sensation of movement, olfactory, flashing lights (photopsia).
^autonomic: abdominal (nausea, vomiting, pain, hunger); cardiovascular (sinus tachycardia).

MANAGEMENT OF SEIZURES
1. **Absence (Petit Mal):** *Ethosuximide 1st line** (only works for absence); *Valproic acid* 2nd line (S/E: hepatitis, pancreatitis); Lamotrigine.
2. **Grand Mal:** *Valproic acid, Phenytoin, Carbamazepine, Lamotrigine,* Topiramate, Primidone, Levetiracetam, Gabapentin, Phenobarbital, Midazolam
3. **Status Epilepticus:** *Lorazepam or Diazepam ⇨ Phenytoin ⇨ Phenobarbital.* Thiamine + Ampule of D50. Place in lateral decubitus position with all possible harmful objects cleared away from the area.
   Myoclonus: Valproic acid, Clonazepam. Febrile: Phenobarbital.
4. **Myoclonus:** Valproic acid, Clonazepam. Febrile: Phenobarbital.

Benzodiazepines (Lorazepam, Diazepam): increases GABA (GABA is an inhibitory neurotransmitter in the CNS).
Phenytoin: blocks Na+ channels in the CNS (takes longer to work). **S/E:** *gingival hyperplasia, Steven Johnson Syndrome, hirsutism*
Barbiturates: (Phenobarbital): binds to GABA receptors to ↑GABA-mediated CNS inhibition.
   • *Prolactin levels are increased in seizures** (helps to differentiate it from pseudoseizures).
   • *EEG helps to establish the diagnosis & localize the lesions**.

ANTICONVULSANT MEDICATIONS

SEIZURE MEDICATION	MECHANISM OF ACTION	INDICATIONS	SIDE EFFECTS
ETHOSUXIMIDE (Zarontin)	Blocks Ca^{+2} channels ⇨ motor cortex depression (elevates stimulation threshold, decreases neuronal firing).	Ind: *drug of choice for absence* *(only used in absence)*	S/E: drowsiness, ataxia, dizziness, headache, rash, GI upset (diarrhea), weight gain. **Caution**: patient with renal or hepatic failure. **Monitoring**: CBC, UA, ↑LFTs
VALPROIC ACID (Depakene) DIVALPROEX SODIUM (Depakote)	Multiple mechanisms of action: - ↑es GABA's effects (↑CNS inhibition) - inhibits glutamate/NMDA receptor-mediated neuronal excitation.	Ind: absence sz, complex-partial sz, epileptic seizures (Grand Mal). Acute mania in bipolar disorders.	S/E: *pancreatitis, hepatotoxicity**, GI problems, thrombocytopenia, monitor levels. CI/Cautions: hepatic disorders
LAMOTRIGINE (Lamictal)	Blocks Na & Ca channels, decreasing presynaptic glutamate & aspartate release. Also inhibits glutamate's effects on NMDA receptor ⇨ decreased neuronal activity.	Ind: absence, grand mal & partial complex seizures.	*Rash, Steven Johnson Syndrome (SJS),* headache, diplopia
PHENYTOIN (Dilantin)	MOA: stabilizes neuronal membranes [limits firing of action potentials by blocking Na-dependent channels] – related to barbiturates. *Does not cause CNS depression*	Ind: generalized tonic-clonic seizures, complex partial seizures, *seizure prophylaxis**, - *status epilepticus: started after benzodiazepine.*	**Monitoring: *drug levels***, CBC, UA, significant drug-drug interactions. S/E: *rash (erythema multiforme/SJS), gingival hyperplasia**, nystagmus, slurred speech, hematologic cx, *hirsutism,* dizziness, teratogenic, *hypotension, arrhythmias (esp with rapid administration >50mcg/min).*
CARBAMAZEPINE (Tegretol)	Blocks Na+ channels, decreases seizure spread. Exact mechanism in trigeminal neuralgia & bipolar disorder is unknown.	Ind: *seizure disorders, bipolar d/o. trigeminal neuralgia (drug of choice),* central diabetes insipidus.*	S/E: *Hyponatremia (causes SIADH)*, SJS* dizziness, drowsiness, N/V, ↑LFT's, arrhythmias *blood dyscrasias (rare).*
TOPIRAMATE (Topamax)	Blocks Na channels, ↑es GABA activity, glutamate receptor antagonist.	Grand Mal, partial seizures	Weight loss, nephrolithiasis, paresthesias, headache, hyperthermia
BENZODIAZEPINES LORAZEPAM (Ativan) DIAZEPAM (Valium)	MOA: *potentiates GABA-mediated CNS inhibition* *Lorazepam most effective* (has shorter ½ life than diazepam).*	Generalized sz, absence sz, anxiety, chemo-related N/V, sedation, muscle spasms. Status epilepticus, *benzodiazepine 1st line for status epilepticus** (usually followed by phenytoin "loading" to prevent seizure recurrence).	S/E: sedation, ataxia, paradoxical reaction. *Flumazenil reverses sedation.** CI/Cautions: Suicide risk, *monitor BP after dose.*
PHENOBARBITAL	Barbiturate: binds to GABA receptor potentiating GABA-mediated CNS inhibition	*Status epilepticus after phenytoin if status epilepticus persistent* Febrile seizures in children	S/E: permanent neurologic deficit if injected into or near peripheral nerves. *Depression, osteoporosis, irritability.*

TRANSIENT ISCHEMIC ATTACK (TIA)

- **<u>Transient acute episode of ischemic neurologic deficits</u>** caused by focal brain, spinal cord, or retinal ischemia **<u>without acute infarction or tissue injury on neuroimaging</u>**. **Usually lasts <1 hour (more commonly minutes);** <24 hours.
- ~30% of patients with stroke have a history of TIAs and 5–10% of patients with TIAs will have a stroke within 90 days. Risk factors: **Hypertension most important,** cardiovascular risk factors.

<u>3 MAIN TYPES</u>
- <u>Embolic:</u> Atrial fibrillation, left ventricular thrombus, Heart failure, Endocarditis, Atrial septal defects.
- <u>Large artery (low flow):</u> ischemia due to atherosclerosis & atherothrombosis.
- <u>Lacunar:</u> involvement of the penetrating small vessels.

<u>CLINICAL MANIFESTATIONS</u>
- **Focal neurologic &/or speech deficits** depending on the artery involved (resembles stroke pattern). **Most last for a few minutes with <u>complete</u> resolution within 1 hour.**
- **Amaurosis fugax:** transient monocular vision loss — "temporary shade down on one eye".
- <u>Physical examination:</u> **a carotid bruit may be heard.**

<u>DIAGNOSIS</u>
[1] Neuroimaging + [2] neurovascular imaging + [3] tests to rule out cardioembolic source.
- <u>Neuroimaging</u> **MRI preferred neuroimaging (more sensitive); in emergent settings, CT scan may be performed initially to rule out hemorrhage (faster results) or if MRI is not available.**
- **Neurovascular imaging CT or MR angiography, carotid Doppler US,** transcranial Doppler US.
- <u>Conventional angiography</u> definitive diagnosis but invasive.
- <u>Ancillary testing:</u> rule out cardioembolic source (ECG, telemetry, & Echocardiogram/TEE). Rule out metabolic or hematologic cause of neurologic symptoms (eg, hypoglycemia, CBC). HIV & Syphilis.

<u>MANAGEMENT</u>
- Place patient in the supine position to increase cerebral perfusion, avoid lowering blood pressure unless >220/120 mm Hg. Thrombolytics contraindicated in TIA.
- Patients presenting within 72 hours of TIA with ABCD^2≥3 admit. If score is <3, obtain basic laboratory tests, ECG, echocardiogram, carotid & brain imaging within 24-48h as an outpatient.

Noncardiogenic TIA:
- **<u>Dual antiplatelet therapy</u>: Aspirin + either Clopidogrel** or Ticagrelor, **followed by Aspirin only** substantially reduces the risk of future TIA or strokes **if high risk (ABCD^2 score ≥4) started while evaluating the ischemic mechanism.** <u>Alternative:</u> Aspirin + extended-release Dipyridamole.
- <u>Aspirin monotherapy</u> — **Aspirin (162-325 mg/daily)** alone for <u>low-risk TIA</u> (ABCD^2 score <4).
- <u>Long-term risk factor reduction</u> (eg, DM, lipid control, hypertension control, smoking cessation, weight reduction, regular exercise); **statin therapy regardless of LDL levels.**
- **<u>Revascularization</u>: Carotid endarterectomy recommended if internal carotid artery stenosis 50-99%** with a life expectancy of at least 5 years + Aspirin. Endovascular intervention & stenting.

Cardiogenic (Nonvalvular Atrial fibrillation):
- **<u>Oral anticoagulation</u>** — Warfarin or a direct oral anticoagulant (eg, Dabigatran, Rivaroxaban, Apixaban, Edoxaban).

ABCD² SCORE ASSESSMENT IN TIA

The risk of stroke after a TIA is significantly increased, and the risk is highest during the days immediately following the TIA. The ABCD^2 tool is designed to predict the risk of stroke in the 3-90 days after a TIA. Patients receive one point each for:
- **A**ge >60 beats/minute
- **B**lood pressure >140/90 mm Hg
- **C**linical symptoms (one point for slurred speech or two points for unilateral weakness)
- **D**uration (one point for > 10 minutes or two points for >60 minutes); **D**iabetes

<u>ABCD² SCORE:</u>
- 0-3 points = 3.1% 90-day stroke risk; 4-5 points = 9.8% 90-day stroke risk; 6-7 points = 17.8% 90-day risk.

LACUNAR (SMALL SUBCORTICAL) INFARCTS

- **Small subcortical infarcts** (<1.5 cm in diameter) **due to small-vessel disease involving a penetrating branch of the cerebral arteries in the pons and basal ganglia.**
- Lacunar infarcts account for 15-30% of Ischemic strokes.

RISK FACTORS:
- **80% have a history of <u>Hypertension</u>.** Longstanding Diabetes mellitus.

5 CLASSIC PRESENTATIONS
- **[1] <u>Pure motor:</u> most common presentation. Hemiparesis or hemiplegia in the absence of sensory or "cortical signs"** (eg, aphasia, agnosia, neglect, apraxia, or hemianopsia). Involves the internal capsule and the corona radiata (branches originating from the middle cerebral artery).
- **[2] <u>Ataxic hemiparesis:</u> ipsilateral weakness and clumsiness in the leg > arm.** Involves the pons (branches from the basilar artery) or the internal capsule (branches from the MCA).
- **[3] <u>Pure sensory deficits</u> — numbness, paresthesias of the arm, face, and leg on one side of the body in the absence of motor or "cortical" signs.** Involves the thalamus (branch from the PCA).
- **[4] <u>Sensorimotor:</u> weakness and numbness of the face, arm, and leg on one side of the body** in the absence of "cortical" signs. Located in the thalamus and internal capsule (arises from middle and cerebral artery penetrators).
- **[5] <u>Dysarthria (clumsy hand syndrome):</u>** dysarthria, facial weakness, dysphagia and slight weakness and clumsiness of one hand in the absence of "cortical" signs.

DIAGNOSIS
- <u>CT scan</u> — **small punched-out hypodense areas (lacunar infarcts) usually in the central & noncortical areas (eg, basal ganglia).**

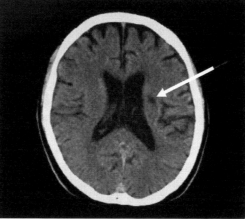

Photo credit: Shutterstock (used with permission)

MANAGEMENT
- **Aspirin; risk factor reduction** (eg, control of Hypertension & Diabetes mellitus; smoking cessation).
- <u>Good prognosis</u> — partial or complete deficit resolution ranging from hours up to 6 weeks.

CEREBRAL EDEMA

- Clinically significant brain edema requiring treatment develops in 10–20% of patients with ischemic stroke and is responsible for 80% of the mortality resulting from large MCA infarcts.

MANAGEMENT
- <u>Surgical management</u>: decompressive hemicraniectomy.
- **<u>Medical management</u> to decrease intracranial pressure includes osmotherapy with Mannitol or hypertonic saline, head elevation, sedation, and a short course of hyperventilation.**
- Corticosteroids are not usually effective & may be potentially harmful.

ISCHEMIC STROKE

- Acute onset of neurological deficits due to death of brain tissue from ischemia.

Ischemic most common type of stroke (80%). Causes include thrombotic and cardioembolic.

- **Thrombotic most common type of Ischemic stroke (2/3) due to Atherosclerosis.**
- **Cardioembolic (1/3)** — from the heart, aortic arch, or large cerebral arteries. **Sources include Atrial fibrillation (most common),** valvular disease, patent foramen ovale (paradoxical venous emboli).

RISK FACTORS

- **Hypertension is the most significant & modifiable risk factor for Stroke.**
- Dyslipidemia, diabetes, Atrial fibrillation, cigarette smoking, & other atherosclerotic risk factors.
- Nonmodifiable risk factors: males, increasing age, ethnicity, and family history.

Anterior circulation symptoms (eg, Anterior cerebral artery, Middle cerebral)

- **Contralateral arm or leg weakness and contralateral sensory deficits.**
- Visual changes: **contralateral homonymous hemianopsia** (on opposite side of the stroke).
- **Middle cerebral artery: unilateral weakness and/or numbness (upper extremity > lower), facial droop (with forehead sparing), forced gaze deviation towards the side of the lesion, visual field cuts, and, if in the dominant hemisphere, speech deficits** (eg, dysarthria, aphasia).
- **Anterior cerebral artery most commonly, patients present with motor deficits characteristically involving the lower extremity contralateral to the infarct site (leg > arm).** Abulia, agitation, motor perseveration, memory impairments, emotional lability, or incontinence, as well as anosognosia, are some of the classic neuropsychologic features associated with ACA.

Posterior circulation symptoms:

- **V's: v**omiting, **v**isual changes (diplopia), **v**ertigo; Nystagmus, nausea, coma, drop attacks, ataxia.
- Contralateral arm/leg weakness and contralateral sensory deficits.

DIAGNOSIS

- **Noncontrast head CT best initial test to rule out hemorrhagic Stroke** (rapid acquisition; in the acute phase, "time is the brain," & MRI brain takes much longer to complete than a CT scan). CT may be normal in the first 6-24 hours; later, CT may show hypodense lesion. MRI more accurate.
- **Neurovascular imaging: CT angiography (most common), MR angiography, carotid Doppler ultrasound,** transcranial US. Performed to [1] diagnose large-vessel occlusion amenable to thrombectomy & [2] asses for atherosclerosis as the etiology. Conventional angiography rarely used.
- Ancillary testing: ECG, echocardiography/TEE, & cardiac monitoring to rule out embolic causes.

IMMEDIATE MANAGEMENT

- **Within 3 hours of symptom onset: thrombolytic (Alteplase/rTPA) if no contraindications.** Contraindications include blood pressure ≥185/110 mm Hg, recent bleeding, bleeding disorder, INR > 1.7, & recent trauma. **Thrombolytics can be used within 4.5 hours in some patients**: <80 years old + <25 on NIH stroke scale (not maximally severe) + not a diabetic with a previous stroke.
- **Mechanical thrombectomy can be performed within 24 hours of symptom onset of large artery occlusion in the anterior circulation.** Compared to Alteplase alone, thrombectomy is associated with improved reperfusion, early neurological recovery, and improved functional outcome.
- **>3-4.5 hours of symptom onset: Conservative — eg, Aspirin + long-term risk factor reduction.**
- Blood pressure should only be lowered IF blood pressure ≥185/110 mm Hg if thrombolytics are to be used or ≥220/120 mm Hg if no plan to use thrombolytics to protect the ischemic penumbra.
- DVT prophylaxis: Low molecular weight heparin during hospitalization.

LONG-TERM (OUTPATIENT) MANAGEMENT

- **Antiplatelet therapy: Aspirin therapy should not be initiated until 24 hours after the time of thrombolytic therapy.** If patient was already on Aspirin prior to stroke, either add Dipyridamole or switch to Clopidogrel. Aspirin when administered within 48 hours of ischemic stroke onset modestly reduces the risk of early stroke recurrence and long-term disability.
  Clopidogrel, Dipyridamole, and other antiplatelet agents are other long-term options.
- **Statin therapy** should be initiated regardless of LDL level (**St**roke = **St**atin)!

MIDDLE CEREBRAL ARTERY (MCA) ISCHEMIC STROKE

- **Most common type of ischemic stroke**. Think **MC**A is the **M**ost **C**ommon **A**rtery involved.

CLINICAL MANIFESTATIONS

- **Neurological deficits:** contralateral sensory & motor deficits <u>greater in face & arm</u> > leg > foot.
- **Facial involvement:** facial droop only involves the lower half of the face (patient will still be able to raise forehead on both sides).
- **Visual:** contralateral homonymous hemianopsia (loss of visual fields on the opposite side of the stroke). This leads to **gaze preference towards the side of the lesion initially.**

Dominant hemisphere (left in 90%):

- **Aphasia** (Broca – expressive or Wernicke's – sensory). Br**o**ca is an **o**utput problem — partial ability to produce language (spoken, manual, or written) with intact comprehension. Wern**i**cke's (sensory) aphasia is an **i**nput problem — they have difficulty understanding incoming language, so they produce large amounts (fluent) speech that lack content & meaning.
- **Math comprehension deficits & agraphia.**

Nondominant hemisphere (usually right in most):

- Spatial deficits, dysarthria, **neglect of the other side**, anosognosia, apraxia, **flat affect, impaired judgment, & impulsivity**.

ANTERIOR CEREBRAL ARTERY (ACA) ISCHEMIC STROKE

CLINICAL MANIFESTATIONS

- **Contralateral sensory &/or motor deficits (hemiparesis, sensory loss, & facial paralysis) <u>greater in the lower extremity</u> > face, arm** (upper extremity & face may be spared).
- <u>Left-sided lesions</u> presented with more transcortical motor aphasia, in which patients have difficulty responding spontaneously with speech, but repetition is preserved.
- <u>Right-sided lesions</u> presented with more acute confusional state and motor hemineglect (unilateral motor function is lost).
- **Urinary incontinence.** Grasp or sucking reflexes and rigidity.
- **Contralateral homonymous hemianopsia** may lead to gaze preference towards the side of the lesion initially.
- **Personality/cognitive deficits**: frontal lobe dysfunction — **confusion, flat affect, impaired judgment, abulia** (slowness & prolong delays to perform acts), **gait apraxia.**

POSTERIOR CEREBRAL ARTERY (PCA) ISCHEMIC STROKE

Vs of **V**ertebral: **v**ertigo (including nystagmus), **v**omiting, **v**isual changes (eg, diplopia).

Posterior cerebral artery:

- **Contralateral homonymous hemianopsia (may spare the macula);** alexia without agraphia (if dominant hemisphere - left PCA); visual hallucinations, sensory loss, coma, limb ataxia, nystagmus, cerebellar signs, nausea, vomiting & drop attacks. Visual perseverations (calcarine cortex).
- <u>Deep segments of the PCA:</u> **hypersomnolence, cognitive deficits,** ocular findings, hypoesthesia, and ataxia. Ocular findings may include **homonymous hemianopsia** (visual field deficits in one half of their visual field) that **may spare the macula**. Paresis of vertical eye movement.
- **Larger infarcts that involve the deep structures can lead to hemisensory loss and hemiparesis due to the involvement of the thalamus and the internal capsule.**
- Superficial infarcts present with visual and somatosensory deficits, impairment of stereognosis, tactile sensation, & proprioception. **Spontaneous pain (thalamus);** cranial III nerve palsy, motor deficits.

Vertebrobasilar artery:

- **"Crossed symptoms":** ipsilateral cranial nerve deficits; contralateral motor/sensory deficits.
- **Diplopia,** dizziness, nausea, **vomiting, vertigo,** limb and gait ataxia, coma, cerebellar dysfunction.
- **Asymmetric but bilateral deficits are the rule in basilar infarcts** (eg, hemiparesis with motor or reflex abnormalities on the nonhemiparetic side). Dysarthria, dysphagia, hiccups.

Cerebellar Infarction

- **Ataxia, nausea, vomiting, headache, dysarthria, and vertigo symptoms.**
- Edema and rapid clinical deterioration may complicate cerebellar infarction.

STROKE TYPE	CLINICAL MANIFESTATIONS	DIAGNOSIS	MANAGEMENT
ISCHEMIC STROKE **LACUNAR INFARCT**	*MC type (80%). Due to* ❶ *thrombotic MC** (49%) ❷ *emboli* (31%) ❸ *cerebrovascular occlusion.* *Small vessel disease* (*penetrating branches* of cerebral arteries in pons, basal ganglia. ❶ PURE MOTOR MC (hemiparesis, hemiplegia) ❷ ATAXIC HEMIPARESIS & clumsiness leg >arm ❸ DYSARTHRIA (CLUMSY HAND SYNDROME) ❹pure sensory loss (numbness, paresthesias). *History of HTN 80%**	**CT scan:** *small punched out hypodense areas.* Lesions usually central & in noncortical areas: ex basal ganglia	Aspirin. Control risk factors (HTN & DM). Good prognosis: partial or complete deficit resolution ranging from hours up to 6 weeks. **ISCHEMIC STROKE MANAGEMENT** •*Thrombolytics within 3 hours* of onset (4.5 hours in some cases). •Tissue plasminogen activator (rTPA) *Alteplase** given if no evidence of hemorrhage. *Alteplase only rTPA effective in ischemic stroke.** CI: BP ≥185/110, recent bleed/trauma, bleeding d/o. •Antiplatelet therapy: Aspirin, Clopidogrel, Dipyridamole. Aspirin used in the acute setting if after 3 hours & thrombolytics aren't given or at least 24h after thrombolytics. •±Anticoagulation tx if cardioembolic •Only lower BP if ≥185/110 for thrombolytics or ≥220/120 if no thrombolytic use or if MAP >130 •**Note:** *strokes with facial involvement involves the lower half of face** (patient will still be able to raise both eyebrows)!
ANTERIOR CIRCULATION **Middle Cerebral Artery** *MC type** (70%)	• Contralateral sensory/motor loss/hemiparesis: GREATER IN FACE, ARM* > leg/foot. • Visual: contralateral homonymous hemianopsia, *gaze preference towards side of lesion* (x1 – 2 days). • *Dominant* (usually L-side): *aphasia: Broca (expressive), Wernicke (sensory)*, math comprehension, agraphia. • *Nondominant* (usually R-side): spatial deficits, dysarthria, left-side neglect, anosognosia, apraxia	**ISCHEMIC STROKE DIAGNOSIS** *Noncontrast CT scan to rule out hemorrhage in suspected stroke.* CT scan may be normal during 1st 6-24 hours.	
Anterior Cerebral Artery 2%	• Contralateral sensory/motor loss/hemiparesis: GREATER IN LEG/FOOT* > upper extremity ⇨ abnormal gait. • *Face spared:** speech preservation. Slow responses • Frontal lobe & mental status impairment; *impaired judgment, confusion. Personality changes* (flat affect)* • *URINARY INCONTINENCE*.* Upper motor neuron weakness. • Gaze preference towards side of the lesion (early on).		
POSTERIOR CIRCULATION **Posterior Cerebral Artery**	• *Visual hallucinations, contralateral homonymous hemianopsia. "crossed sx"** (ipsilateral cranial nerve deficits + contralateral muscle weakness), coma, drop attacks.		
Basilar Artery **Vertebral Artery**	• Cerebellar dysfunction, CN palsies, ↓vision, ↓bilateral sensory • *Vertigo, nystagmus, N/V, diplopia,* ipsilateral ataxia.		
HEMORRHAGIC STROKE *20% of strokes. Headache, vomiting favors ICH or SAH*. Impaired consciousness without focal symptoms favors SAH. ↑mortality*			
Spontaneous ICH	*Commonly caused by HTN** especially in *basal ganglia. LOC*, N/V, hemiplegia, hemiparalysis. Sx usually mins-hrs gradually increasing in intensity.	Noncontrast CT (*Do not perform LP if ICH is suspected).** Mass effect ± cause herniation if LP done).	Supportive vs. hematoma evacuation If ↑ intracranial pressure ⇨ Head elevation, ± IV Mannitol, hyperventilation
Subarachnoid Hemorrhage (SAH)	*Sudden "worst h/a of my life"** ⇨ *brief LOC, N/V, meningeal irritation** signs (nuchal rigidity), seizures. MC 2ry to rupture of berry aneurysm* or AVM. No focal neurologic symptoms*	1. CT scan. 2. If CT negative & high suspicion ⇨ Lumbar puncture: xanthochromia (RBC's)* esp if >12h & ↑CSF pressure*	Bedrest, no exertion/straining, anti-anxiety meds, stool softeners; ± cautious lowering of BP (only if >220/120 or MAP >130)
'Berry' Aneurysm	*MC circle of Willis (asymptomatic until SAH)*	*Angiography gold standard*	±Aneurysm clipping or coiling.

4 TYPES OF INTRACRANIAL HEMORRHAGE

EPIDURAL HEMATOMA (HEMORRHAGE)	SUBDURAL HEMATOMA (HEMORRHAGE)	SUBARACHNOID HEMORRHAGE (SAH)	INTRACEREBRAL HEMORRHAGE (ICH)
LOCATION • *Arterial bleed MC* between skull & dura.*	**LOCATION** • *Venous bleed MC*.* Between dura & arachnoid due to *tearing of cortical bridging veins*. MC in elderly.*	**LOCATION** • *Arterial bleed* between arachnoid & pia	**LOCATION** • *Intraparenchymal*
MECHANISM • *MC after Temporal bone fracture* ⇨ middle meningeal artery* disruption.	**MECHANISM** • *MC blunt trauma* often causes bleeding on other side of injury "contre-coup". Venous bleed.*	**MECHANISM** • *MC Berry aneurysm rupture, AVM*	**MECHANISM** • HTN, AVM, trauma, amyloid ArterioVenous Malformation
CLINICAL MANIFESTATIONS • Varies. brief LOC ⇨ lucid interval ⇨ coma; headache, N/V, focal neuro sx, rhinorrhea (CSF fluid). • CN III palsy if tentorial herniation.	**CLINICAL MANIFESTATIONS** • Varies. May have focal neuro sx.	**CLINICAL MANIFESTATIONS** • *Thunderclap sudden headache "worse h/a of my life"* ±unilateral, occipital area. ± LOC. N/V, Meningeal sx: stiff neck, photophobia, delirium*. • *No focal neurologic deficits* usually. • Terson syndrome: retinal hemorrhages.	**CLINICAL MANIFESTATIONS** • *Headache, N/V, ± LOC,* hemiplegia, hemiparesis. Not associated with lucid intervals
DIAGNOSIS • *CT: convex (lens – shaped)* bleed* • *Does NOT cross suture lines. Usually in temporal area**	**DIAGNOSIS** • CT: concave (crescent-shaped) bleed*. • *Bleeding can cross suture lines*	**DIAGNOSIS** • CT scan performed first. If CT negative ⇨ LP: xanthochromia (RBC's), ↑CSF (ICP) pressure. • *4-vessel angiography* after confirmed SAH.	**DIAGNOSIS** • CT: intraparenchymal bleed. • *Do NOT perform LP if suspected because it may cause brain herniation!*
MANAGEMENT • ± herniate if not evacuated early. Observation if small. If ↑ICP: Mannitol, hyperventilation, head elevation, ± shunt	**MANAGEMENT** • Hematoma evacuation vs. supportive Evacuation if massive or ≥5mm midline shift.	**MANAGEMENT** • Supportive: bed rest, stool softeners, lower ICP. Surgical coiling or clipping. ± lower BP gradually (ex. *Nicardipine*, *Nimodipine*, Labetalol).	**MANAGEMENT** Supportive: gradual BP reduction. ± IV Mannitol if ↑ICP ±Hematoma evacuation if mass effect

EPIDURAL

SUBDURAL

SUBARACHNOID

INTRACEREBRAL

EPIDURAL HEMATOMA

- Bleeding in the potential space between the skull & dura mater. Usually resulting from **blunt trauma.**

PATHOPHYSIOLOGY
- **Most common due to rupture of the <u>middle meningeal artery,</u> often associated with a <u>temporal bone fracture.</u>** May lead to hemorrhagic stroke & brain herniation. Mean age 20-30 years of age.

CLINICAL MANIFESTATIONS
- **3 classic phases — [1] <u>brief loss of consciousness</u> followed by [2] a <u>lucid interval</u>** (patient regains consciousness with complete transient recovery) followed by **[3] <u>subsequent neurologic deterioration</u>** mental status changes to coma as a result of increased intracranial pressure.
- During the deterioration phase, headache, vomiting, aphasia, hemiparesis, seizures, & coma may occur.
- <u>Uncal herniation:</u> **ipsilateral cranial nerve III palsy — fixed, dilated "blown" pupil can be seen on the ipsilateral side of the injury (tentorial herniation compressing CN III).**
  <u>Cushing reflex</u>: triad of hypertension, bradycardia, & respiratory irregularity.

DIAGNOSIS
- **<u>Head CT without contrast</u> initial test of choice: "bulging" <u>biconvex (lens-shaped) hyperdensity</u> usually in the temporal area that does <u>not</u> cross suture lines** because the collection is limited by firm attachments of the dura to the cranial sutures. The margins are usually sharp.

MANAGEMENT
- **<u>Hematoma evacuation & craniotomy</u> treatment of choice in most symptomatic acute EDH,** hematoma volume >30 ml regardless of Glasgow coma score, GCS <9 with pupillary abnormalities.
- May be observed closely with serial imaging every 6-8h if small and the patient is in good condition.
- <u>Increased intracranial pressure:</u> head elevation, short-term hyperventilation, & hyperosmolar therapy (IV Mannitol or hypertonic saline).

SUBDURAL HEMATOMA

- Venous bleeding in the potential space between the dura mater and the arachnoid membranes.
- <u>ETIOLOGY:</u> **most commonly due to <u>tearing of the cortical bridging veins</u> after blunt trauma (acceleration-deceleration injury** of the brain parenchyma). Bleeding may occur with minor trauma.

RISK FACTORS
- **<u>Significant brain atrophy</u> elderly & chronic alcoholic use** (atrophy puts tension on bridging veins).
- Coagulopathy (eg, anticoagulant use, thrombocytopenia).
- **<u>Shaken baby syndrome</u> (abusive head trauma), especially if <u>bilateral retinal hemorrhages</u> seen.**

CLINICAL MANIFESTATIONS
- Because the bleeding is venous, it can develop over a longer period of time compared to Epidural.
- **Varies but usually a gradual increase in generalized neurologic symptoms** (eg, headache, dizziness, nausea, vomiting) or focal neurologic symptoms. Loss of consciousness may occur.

DIAGNOSIS
- **<u>Head CT without contrast</u> — <u>concave (crescent-shaped)</u> bleed that <u>can cross the suture lines</u>.** If severe, midline shift may occur due to increased intracranial pressure.
- CT scan may negative immediately after the injury so serial imaging may be needed.

MANAGEMENT
- **<u>Nonoperative management:</u> if clinically stable with a small hematoma or no CT signs of brain herniation (eg, midline shift <5 mm) or no signs of increased intracranial pressure.**
- Management includes neurosurgical consultation, blood pressure control, reversal of anticoagulation.
- <u>Surgical management:</u> **surgical evacuation may be indicated if≥5 mm or greater midline shift or severe.** Options include burr hole trephination, craniotomy, and decompressive craniectomy.

SUBARACHNOID HEMORRHAGE (SAH)

- Bleeding between the arachnoid membranes & the pia mater. 5-10% of all Strokes.

ETIOLOGIES
- **Most commonly due to a <u>ruptured saccular (berry) aneurysm</u> at the anterior communicating artery (Circle of Willis). Blunt trauma,** Arteriovenous malformation, or stroke.

RISK FACTORS
- **Cigarette smoking and Hypertension most important.**
- **Polycystic kidney disease,** atherosclerotic disease, smoking, excessive alcohol intake, Ehlers-Danlos syndrome, Marfan syndrome, family history. More common in females.

CLINICAL MANIFESTATIONS
- **<u>Headache</u> most common symptom — <u>sudden</u> or rapid onset of an intense thunderclap headache (severe, rapidly progressing with maximal intensity at its onset) that is often unilateral in the occipital area. Often described as "the worst headache of my life".**
- May be associated with delirium, nausea, vomiting, **meningeal symptoms (photophobia, neck stiffness, fever),** decreased level of consciousness, hemiparesis, and occasionally, seizures.
- May have **loss of consciousness** initially.
- Prodromal symptoms: May have a history of a prior, milder headache (sentinel leak).

PHYSICAL EXAMINATION:
- Hypertension is often present on physical examination.
- **Meningeal signs:** may be present — eg, nuchal rigidity, positive Brudzinski and Kernig signs.
- Usually not associated with focal neurologic deficits but may have a CN III palsy (fixed, dilated, "blown" pupil).
- **Terson syndrome: preretinal hemorrhages** may be seen and are associated with a poorer prognosis (higher association with abrupt increase in intracranial pressure).

DIAGNOSIS
- **<u>Noncontrast head CT</u> initial study of choice — subarachnoid bleeding (white hyperdensity) most commonly found in the basal cisterns.** May also be seen in the Sylvian fissures, interhemispheric fissure, & suprasellar, ambient, and quadrigeminal cisterns. Most are picked up on Head CT performed within 6 hours of symptom onset. LP if negative CT + high clinical suspicion.
- **<u>Lumbar puncture:</u> performed if CT is negative + no papilledema** or focal signs — **<u>xanthochromia</u>** (yellow to pink color of the CSF fluid due to breakdown of RBCs in the CSF), elevated red blood cell count that does not diminish from cerebrospinal fluid (CSF) tube 1 to tube 4, increased CSF protein from bilirubin, and increased CSF pressure). Most sensitive ≥12 hours after symptom onset.
- **<u>4-vessel CT or MR angiography</u> usually performed <u>after</u> confirmed SAH** (on neuroimaging or LP) to identify source of bleeding & other aneurysms. Digital subtraction angiography may also be used.

MANAGEMENT
- **<u>Supportive management:</u>** bed rest, analgesia, stool softeners (avoid straining), lower intracranial pressure, and venous thromboembolism prophylaxis. **Nimodipine reduces cerebral vasospasms, improving neurologic outcomes in aneurysmal SAH** (eg, 60 mg orally every 4 hours).
- Blood pressure should be titrated to a target systolic blood pressure (SBP) <160 mm Hg or mean arterial pressure (MAP) <110 mm Hg for most patients with SAH. Lowering blood pressure may decrease the risk of rebleeding but may also increase the risk of infarction. If needed, Labetalol, Nicardipine and Enalapril are preferred antihypertensives. Discontinue antithrombotic agents.
- Ventriculostomy may be needed if SAH is associated with Hydrocephalus.
- **<u>Prevention of rebleeding:</u> endovascular coiling or surgical clipping of aneurysm or AVM used to prevent rebleeding** (coiling is often preferred over clipping).
- Complications: rebleeding, hydrocephalus, cerebral vasospasms. **Hyponatremia (treat with Hypertonic saline).**

INTRACEREBRAL HEMORRHAGE (ICH)

- Bleeding within the brain parenchyma.
- May compress the brain, ventricles, and sulci.

RISK FACTORS
- **Hypertension most common overall cause of spontaneous ICH.**
- **Cerebral amyloid angiopathy is the most common cause of nontraumatic ICH in the elderly.**
- **Arteriovenous malformation** is the most common cause in children.
- Trauma, older age, high alcohol intake, and coagulopathy.

CLINICAL MANIFESTATIONS
- Neurologic symptoms usually increase within minutes to hours — **headache, nausea, vomiting, syncope, focal neurologic symptoms** (hemiplegia, hemiparesis, seizures), **altered mental status** (lethargy, obtundation, etc.).

Physical examination:
- May have focal motor and sensory deficits.

DIAGNOSIS:
- **Noncontrast head CT: initial neuroimaging of choice.** Vascular imaging (eg, CT or MR angiography or digital subtraction angiography) is performed when an underlying vascular lesion is suspected.

MANAGEMENT
- **Supportive:** gradual blood pressure reduction. Blood pressure reduction: IV Labetalol, Nicardipine, Esmolol, Hydralazine, Nitroprusside and Nitroglycerin. Aggressive reduction only if systolic BP (SBP) >220 mmHg to <220, then gradual reduction (over a period of hours) to a target range of 140-160 mmHg if the patient remains stable.
- **Prevention of increased intracranial pressure (ICP)** — raising the head of the bed 30 degrees, limiting IV fluids, blood pressure management, analgesia & sedation. Reduction of ICP if present: IV mannitol of Hypertonic saline, temporary hyperventilation.

BASILAR SKULL FRACTURE

- Most commonly occur after traumatic head injuries. **Most involve the temporal bone.**

CLINICAL MANIFESTATIONS
- Varies. May have no symptoms.
- Headache, altered mental status, **focal cranial nerve (eg, CN VII, VIII),** or neurologic deficit.

PHYSICAL EXAMINATION
- **Periorbital ecchymosis (Raccoon eyes), retroauricular or mastoid ecchymosis (Battle's sign), hemotympanum (blood behind the tympanic membrane [retroauricular]), clear rhinorrhea or otorrhea (CSF leak).**

DIAGNOSIS
- Noncontrast head CT: in addition to the fracture, pneumocephalus may be seen.

MANAGEMENT
- **Nonoperative in most without underlying brain injury.** All patients with Basilar skull fractures require admission for observation. Complications may include CSF leak, cranial nerve injury, and Meningitis. Tetanus if needed and prophylactic antibiotics.
- Surgical management may be indicated if there is mass effect on the brain parenchyma or CSF leak.
- Depressed skull fractures are often considered open fractures and are admitted to neurosurgery.

HANGMAN'S [C2 (AXIS) PEDICLE] FRACTURE

- **Traumatic bilateral fractures (spondylolysis)** of the pedicles or pars interarticularis of the axis cervical vertebra (C2). Second most common C2 fracture (after odontoid fractures).
- May lead to **spondylolisthesis at the C2-C3 level (anterior dislocation/displacement of C2 on C3).**
- **Unstable fracture.** 30% are associated with cervical spinal fractures.

MECHANISM OF INJURY

- **Extreme hyperextension & axial loading**: occurs when the cervicocranium (the skull, atlas, and axis functioning as a unit) is thrown into **sudden extreme hyperextension from extension forces, resulting from abrupt deceleration (eg, forced extension of an already extended neck, such as the chin hitting a steering wheel,** diving injuries, or during contact sports).
- **Usually not associated with spinal cord injury**: despite being unstable, **spinal cord damage is often minimal with a Hangman fracture** because the AP diameter of the neural spinal canal is widest (greatest) at C2, and bilateral pedicle fractures permit spinal canal decompression.
- Higher energy injuries resulting in severe extension forces may result in dislocation of the C2-3 facet complex and damage the C2-3 disc. Vascular imaging should be performed in all C1 to C3 fractures.

CLINICAL MANIFESTATIONS

- Neck pain with palpation in the posterior portion of the neck.
- Neurologic exam is usually intact but may be associated with radiculopathy or myelopathy.

DIAGNOSIS

- **Cervical radiographs:** subluxation of C2 on C3. **CT scan mainstay of imaging;** MRI.

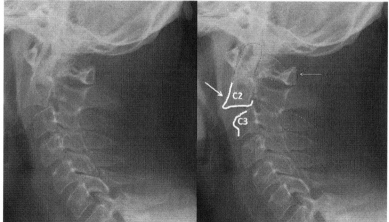

Hangman Fracture
Note slipping of C2 forward compared to C3 (white arrow).

Hangman Fracture
By Lucien Monfils (Own work) [GFDL (http://www.gnu.org/copyleft/fdl.html) or CC BY-SA 3.0 (http://creativecommons.org/licenses/by-sa/3.0)], via Wikimedia Commons

MANAGEMENT

- **Rigid collar** placed for stabilization on immediate evaluation of suspected cervical fractures.
- **Nonoperative:** Type I (<3mm horizontal displacement) stable rigid cervical collar 4-6 weeks. Type II (3-5 mm displacement) closed reduction in axial traction followed by halo-vest orthosis (immobilization) for 8-12 weeks.
- Operative: Type II (>5 mm displacement with severe angulation) may be treated with internal fixation and bone grafting between C2 and C3. Type III facet dislocations often need surgical intervention.

ATLAS FRACTURE & TRANSVERSE LIGAMENTAL INSTABILITY

MECHANISM OF INJURY

- Hyperextension & compression injuries.
- Low risk of neurologic complications. May be associated with an axis fracture.

ATLANTO-OCCIPITAL DISLOCATION

- **Extreme flexion injury** involving the atlas (C1) & the axis (C2) can cause an unstable atlanto-occipital or atlanto-axial joint dislocation, with or without an associated odontoid fracture.
- Highly unstable and severe ligamentous injury at the craniocervical junction with dislocation resulting from damage to ligaments and/or bony structures connecting the skull to the upper cervical spine. **AOD is more common among children than adults (3:1) and young adults.**

MECHANISM OF INJURY

- **High-energy trauma** involving large acceleration & deceleration forces transmit excessive force to the craniocervical junction & lead to ligamentous disruption (high-speed MVAs or falls from heights).

CLINICAL MANIFESTATIONS

- Because of the relatively wide cross-sectional area of the spinal canal at the CCJ, spinal cord injury is uncommon. **However, when present, neurological injury from AOD can be devastating, resulting in sudden death secondary to brainstem injury (often called internal decapitation).**

Survivors of AOD may present with:

- **Isolated severe neck pain** up to 20% may have normal neurological examination at presentation.
- **Neurologic deficits: cruciate paralysis with <u>paralysis of the upper extremities and sparing the lower extremities (classic)</u>,** cranial nerve deficits (eg, abducens, hypoglossal, vagus), unilateral or bilateral weakness, or quadriplegia. Hyperreflexia with clonus, positive Babinski sign.
- **Patients may present with unconsciousness and respiratory arrest.**

DIAGNOSIS

- <u>Plain radiographs</u>: abnormalities in the measurements of the basion-dental interval and the basion-atlantal interval. <u>CT scan</u> preferred imaging.

MANAGEMENT

- **Immediate management:** in the field and the emergency department includes **confirmation of a stable airway, assessment for respiratory instability, hemodynamic stabilization, and application of rigid cervical collar** at the trauma scene for stabilization of the neck.
- **Definitive management: halo immobilization, followed by internal occipitocervical fixation and fusion.** Cervical traction should be avoided (10% risk of neurological deterioration).

ATLANTO-AXIAL DISLOCATION

- Loss of stability between the atlas and axis (C1–C2), resulting in loss of normal articulation.
- An unstable cervical spine injury occurring due to a direct blow to the occiput resulting in transverse ligament rupture. Rare but potentially fatal.
- **Etiologies: most commonly congenital (eg, Down syndrome).** Purely traumatic rare in the absence of predisposing factor. Rotatory atlanto-axial dislocation is an unstable cervical spine injury, caused by a flexion-rotation mechanism. May be seen in inflammatory diseases (eg, Rheumatoid arthritis).

CLINICAL MANIFESTATIONS

- **Most cases appear in adolescents** — eg, **child with minor neck pain &/or neck movement restriction** (eg, inability or unwillingness to turn their head), or chronically progressive spinal canal compression: neurologic & respiratory symptoms (eg, sphincter disturbances, cranial nerve deficits, respiratory depression, and rarely, quadriplegia and death if untreated.
- In adults, usually seen with Rheumatoid arthritis, Osteoarthritis, Inflammatory spondyloarthropathy.

DIAGNOSIS

- Best visualized on open-mouth odontoid radiographs or computed tomography (CT) scan: **increase in the size of the predental space on imaging;** reduced space available for spinal cord (SAC).

MANAGEMENT

- <u>Types I & II</u>: **Posterior fusion procedure.** <u>Type III</u>: transorally released anteriorly → posterior fusion.

ATLANTOAXIAL JOINT INSTABILITY

- **Instability between the atlas (C1) and axis (C2).** Excessive movement may compress spinal cord.

MECHANISM OF INJURY
- <u>Traumatic:</u> extreme flexion-rotation injuries. May compress the spinal cord &/or brainstem.
- **<u>Non traumatic:</u> degenerative changes: Down syndrome, Rheumatoid arthritis,** Os odontoideum.

CLINICAL MANIFESTATIONS
- Neck pain, **restricted neck movements (especially rotation);** neurological symptoms or deficits.
- **<u>Myelopathy:</u>** muscle weakness, hyperreflexia, wide gait, bladder dysfunction. Brainstem signs.

DIAGNOSIS
- **<u>Open-mouth (odontoid) view</u>: may see increase in the atlanto-dens interval (ADI).** ADI >3.5mm considered unstable. **CT scan preferred imaging** or MRI.

MANAGEMENT
- <u>Depends on the cause:</u> **ADI >10 mm in the setting of Rheumatoid arthritis indicates surgery.** Os odontoideum with symptoms of myelopathy & a widened may need a posterior C1-C2 fusion.

CLAY-SHOVELER (CERVICAL SPINOUS PROCESS) FRACTURE

- **Spinous process avulsion fracture most common at the lower cervical vertebrae (C7 most common)** or upper thoracic vertebrae (C6, C7, T1, and T2).

MECHANISM OF INJURY
- **<u>Forced neck flexion</u>: the paraspinal muscle pulls off a piece of the spinous process (avulsion fracture), especially after sudden deceleration injuries** (eg, MVA, from shoveling soil).
- **Usually, a stable injury** resulting from flexion-extension of the spine.

CLINICAL MANIFESTATIONS
- **Neck pain or pain between the shoulder blades or base of the neck.**
- May have localized tenderness or crepitus with reduced range of motion of the neck. Usually no neurologic deficits.

DIAGNOSIS
- **<u>Cervical radiographs</u>: lateral view best view** — oblique fracture line with fragment displaced posteroinferiorly. AP view — double spinous process shadow suggestive of displacement.
- **CT scan preferred over radiographs.**

MANAGEMENT
- **<u>Nonoperative</u> first-line management: NSAIDs, rest, immobilization in hard collar for comfort.**
- Surgical excision only needed if nonunion or persistent pain.

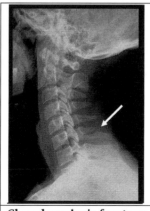
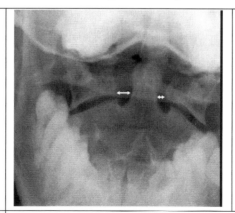
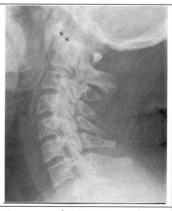

| Clay shoveler's fracture | Atlantoaxial joint instability | increased ADI interval |

BURST (JEFFERSON) FRACTURE OF THE ATLAS ARCH (C1)

- **Bilateral fractures of both the anterior & posterior arches of the atlas (C1).** Type II atlas fracture.
- Stability is determined by the involvement of the transverse ligament **(ligament disruption = highly unstable).** May be associated with a C1/C2 dislocation.

MECHANISM OF INJURY
- **Axial load on the back of the head** **(± extension force) or hyperextension of the neck (eg, caused by diving, football).** 2-part fracture of the anterior ring of the atlas & 2-part fracture of posterior ring.

CLINICAL MANIFESTATIONS
- Upper neck pain, decreased range of motion, usually without neurologic symptoms.
- Physical examination: neurologic exam is usually normal.

DIAGNOSIS
- **Lateral radiographs: increase in the predental space between C1 & the odontoid (dens), atlantodens interval >3 mm in adults & >5 mm in children. CT scan ideal imaging.**
- Open-mouth (odontoid) view: may also show **step-off of the lateral masses of the atlas** (when the transverse diameter of the atlas is 7 mm > that of the axis, suspect transverse ligament rupture).

MANAGEMENT
- Nonoperative management: **external immobilization (hard cervicothoracic orthosis vs. halo ring and vest) for 6-12 weeks for stable fractures (intact transverse ligament).**
- Operative: posterior C1-C2 fusion vs. occipitocervical fusion if unstable or significantly displaced.

ODONTOID PROCESS [AXIS (DENS)] C2 FRACTURES

- **Fracture of the dens (odontoid process) of the axis (C2).**
- Mechanism: head placed in forced flexion or extension in an anterior-posterior orientation (eg, forward fall onto the forehead). Type II from lateral loading forces.
- Type I: oblique fracture at the tip of odontoid above the transverse ligaments. Stable.
- **Type II: fracture at the base of the odontoid process (dens) where it attaches to C2. Most common type. Unstable.** High association with nonunion in >50% of patients treated with halo vest immobilization. Os odontoideum appears like a type II fracture on radiographs.
- Type III: extension of the fracture through the upper portion of the body of C2.

CLINICAL MANIFESTATIONS
- Neck pain worse with motion. May have dysphagia if large retropharyngeal hematoma is present.
- Physical exam: usually no neurologic deficits because the cervical canal is widest at C2 area.

DIAGNOSIS
- **AP odontoid (open mouth) view** radiograph imaging: may show prevertebral soft tissue swelling on lateral images. **Place patient in a rigid cervical collar during evaluation.**
- **CT scan best test to delineate fracture pattern**. MRI if symptoms of spinal cord injury.

MANAGEMENT
- Os odontoideum (aplasia or hypoplasia of the odontoid): observation. Posterior C1-C2 fusion if symptoms of myelopathy.
- Type I: stable fractures that are managed nonoperatively (eg, cervical orthosis).
- **Type II in young — halo immobilization.** Surgery if risk factors for nonunion. II in elderly — surgery preferred. Cervical orthosis if not surgical candidates (no halo immobilization in the elderly).
- Type III — cervical orthosis (eg, halo brace).

BURST (JEFFERSON) FRACTURE OF THE ATLAS C1 ARCH

- **Bilateral fractures of both the anterior & posterior arches of the atlas (C1).**

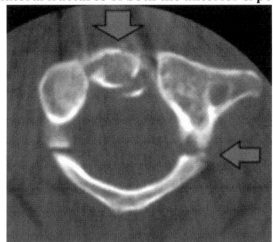 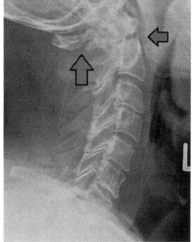

Jefferson burst fracture of C2 and fracture of the odontoid

James Heilman, MD, CC BY-SA 4.0 <https://creativecommons.org/licenses/by-sa/4.0>, via Wikimedia Commons

ODONTOID PROCESS (DENS) FRACTURE

- **Fracture at the base of the odontoid process (dens) where it attaches to C2**

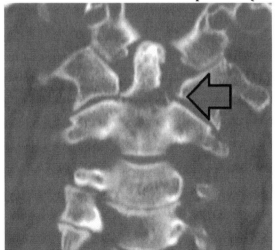

CERVICAL BURST FRACTURE

- Burst fracture of the fifth cervical vertebra with dislocation of the left C4/5 facet joint. Significant retropulsion with severe narrowing of the central canal.

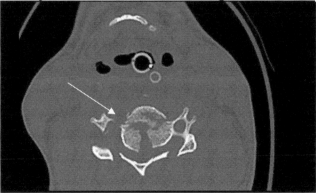

Case courtesy of Domenico Nicoletti, Radiopaedia.org, rID: 37420

FLEXION TEARDROP FRACTURE

- **Anterior displacement of a wedge-shaped fracture fragment** (teardrop shape of the **antero-inferior portion** of the superior vertebral body). **Often associated with loss of vertebral height.**
- Most commonly occurs in the **lower cervical spine**.

MECHANISM OF INJURY

- **Extreme hyperflexion & compression** causes the vertebral body to collide with an inferior vertebral body resulting in disruption of the posterior longitudinal spinal ligament at the level of the injury.
- **Highly unstable**: **may cause** **Anterior spinal cord syndrome** & quadriplegia.

CLINICAL MANIFESTATIONS

- Neck pain. **Anterior cord syndrome symptoms,** quadriplegia.

MANAGEMENT

- **Surgical decompression** due to it highly unstable nature.

EXTENSION TEARDROP FRACTURE

- Triangular-shaped avulsion fracture of the antero-inferior corner of the vertebral body as a result of rupture of the anterior longitudinal ligament. May be seen in Osteoporosis (anterior osteophytes).
- **Most common at C2.** May be seen at C5–C7 with diving accidents (may cause Central cord syndrome).
- Extension teardrop fractures are unstable in extension & stable in flexion.

MECHANISM OF INJURY

- **Abrupt neck hyperextension: the anterior longitudinal ligament avulses the antero-inferior corner from the remainder of the vertebral body, producing a triangular-shaped fragment.**
- The 'teardrop' appears similar to the Flexion teardrop fracture — both cause an anteroinferior vertebral fragment. However, the **extension teardrop is not usually associated with loss of vertebral height, is not as severe (the vertebral body is not displaced), & can cause Central cord syndrome** (not a common occurrence) vs. Anterior cord seen in Flexion teardrop fractures.
- **May cause neck pain. Usually neurologically intact. May have symptoms of Central cord syndrome.**

MANAGEMENT

- **Immobilization in a hard collar** in most cases as the injury is mechanically stable.

FLEXION TEARDROP FRACTURE	EXTENSION TEARDROP FRACTURE
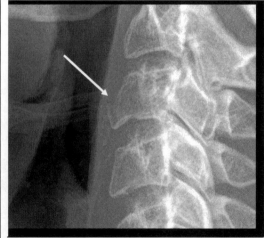	
On plain lateral radiographs, the fractured vertebra appears to be divided into a smaller anterior fragment and a larger posterior piece.	Anteroinferior vertebral fragment. The vertical height of the fragment usually equal or greater than its width.
A vertebra with a flexion teardrop fracture **may lose height from compression.**	The **extension teardrop is not usually associated with loss of vertebral height.**

BURST FRACTURES

- Burst fracture due to nucleus pulposus of the intervertebral disc being forced into the vertebral body, causing it to shatter or 'burst' outwards. Usually as a result of a vertical compression injury.

MECHANISM OF INJURY
- **Axial loading injury causing vertebral compression injuries of the cervical & lumbar spine (eg, diving and motor vehicle accidents).** Displacement of bony fragments may go into the canal.
- Stable: all the ligaments are intact and usually no posterior displacement of the fracture segment.
- Unstable: >50% compression of the spinal cord, >50% loss of vertebral height, >20 degrees of spinal angulation, or associated neurologic deficits. **May cause incomplete or complete spinal cord injury (eg, Anterior cord syndrome).**

DIAGNOSIS
- **Radiographs: comminuted vertebral body and loss of vertebral height** (depicted as a vertical fracture on the AP view). [see photo on page 703].

MANAGEMENT
- **Surgical correction due to instability** — eg, anterior decompression (corpectomy) and reconstruction using a bone graft strut stabilized with a plate and screws.

SUBCLAVIAN-VERTEBRAL ARTERY STEAL SYNDROME

- **Signs and/or symptoms** that occur due to **reversal of blood flow (retrograde) from the vertebral artery diverted to the ipsilateral arm during arm use as a result of decreased flow in the subclavian artery (stenosis or occlusion)** proximal to the origin of the vertebral artery.
- The vertebral artery serves as a collateral to supply blood to the arm. In SSS, the blood flow to the arm is at the expense of the vertebrobasilar circulation.

ETIOLOGIES
- **Atherosclerosis of the subclavian/innominate artery most common**. AV malformations.
- Takayasu arteritis, dissecting aortic aneurysm, Giant cell arteritis, anterior Thoracic outlet syndrome.

CLINICAL MANIFESTATIONS
Most patients are asymptomatic ("subclavian steal" not syndrome), is an incidental finding.
- **Symptoms of arm arterial insufficiency: arm claudication with exercise; arm pain, paresthesias, fatigue, or numbness.** Symptoms of effort fatigue are more common than neurologic symptoms.
- **Symptoms of vertebrobasilar insufficiency with arm use** (including exercise, head movements) — eg, **dizziness, lightheadedness, vertigo, presyncope, syncope, neurologic deficits,** binocular diplopia, nystagmus, tinnitus, disequilibrium, weakness, drop attacks, gait abnormalities.

PHYSICAL EXAM
- **Blood pressure difference between the arms**: reduction of brachial systolic blood pressure in the affected arm ≥15 mmHg compared to the unaffected arm.
- Radial pulse may diminish with arm elevation or arm exercise; or delayed compared to other side.

DIAGNOSIS
- **Duplex ultrasound** can reveal proximal subclavian artery stenoses and demonstrate reversal of flow in the ipsilateral vertebral artery, if present. Continuous wave Doppler US.
- **Angiography for confirmation** — Magnetic resonance (MR) angiography, CT angiography, or Digital subtraction angiography (DSA) may be used if US nondiagnostic or for confirmation.

MANAGEMENT
- **Atherosclerotic SSS: usually managed conservatively** — risk reduction (eg, control of blood pressure, dyslipidemia, Diabetes; smoking cessation). Treat underlying cause if nonatherosclerotic.
- **Severe cases: Revascularization: endovascular (angioplasty and stenting) &/or surgical bypass** (eg, carotid-subclavian bypass or subclavian-carotid transposition).

ANTERIOR CORD SYNDROME

- Incomplete spinal cord syndrome predominantly affecting the anterior two-thirds of the spinal cord.

MECHANISM OF INJURY
- **[1] Hyperflexion injury: most commonly seen after burst fractures of the vertebral bodies, especially with hyperflexion injuries.**
- **[2] Vascular injury**: ischemia secondary to compression of the anterior spinal artery, aortic surgery.
- **Disc herniation**, crush injury, compression from a hematoma.

CLINICAL MANIFESTATIONS
- Both the spinothalamic and corticospinal tracts are involved since they are located in the anterior aspect of the spinal cord. The symptoms are almost always bilateral.

Motor deficits:
- **Motor deficits (eg, motor paralysis) below the lesion, especially the lower extremities.** May vary from paraplegia to quadriplegia.
- Autonomic dysfunction: ± Bladder or bladder dysfunction, hypotension, sexual dysfunction.

Sensory deficits:
- **Loss of temperature, pain, & light touch sensation at & below the level of the lesion.**

Spared:
- **Posterior column preservation: proprioception (position), deep pressure, light touch, tactie sensation, and vibration sensation are intact.**

MANAGEMENT
- In addition to the usual care for spinal cord injury, treatment of the Anterior cord syndrome involves stabilization or removal of any structure that exerts increased pressure on the anterior aspect of spinal cord. **Poor recovery prognosis**: return of useful motor function seen in only 10%-16%.
- Laminectomy may be necessary to decompress the spinal cord.

CENTRAL CORD SYNDROME

- Most common incomplete cord syndrome.

MECHANISM OF INJURY
- **Hyperextension injury most common** (eg, whiplash, forward fall while striking the chin and having the neck extend backward at the time of the fall). Vascular.
- **Older patients with degenerative spine disease and cervical spondylolysis** (stress defect).

CLINICAL MANIFESTATIONS
Motor deficits:
- **Bilateral motor paresis in the upper extremities, especially distal extremities (hands) > lower extremities.** Decreased strength and, to a lesser degree, decreased pain and temperature sensation more in the upper than lower extremities. This is because the upper limb tracts are central (medial) compared to the thoracic & lower extremity (which are more lateral), while sacral segments lie on the most lateral aspect. Spastic paraparesis or spastic quadriparesis may also occur.

Sensory deficits:
- **Loss of temperature, pain, or burning sensation classically in a shawl distribution (cape-like) distribution across the upper back & down their posterior upper extremities.** Degree of motor weakness with lower limbs stronger than upper limbs and sacral sensory sparing (because the lower extremities and sacral tracts of the spinothalamic and corticospinal tracts are more lateral).
- **Bladder dysfunction with sacral sparing. Vibration & position sensation are usually preserved.**
- Variable sensory deficits below the level of injury (eg, weakness; pain, temperature, and sensory loss; reflex loss (eg, triceps). Central cord is the most common of the partial cord syndromes.
- Variable prognosis 50%-75% of patients with CCS show some neurologic improvement.

BROWN-SÉQUARD SYNDROME

- **Functional hemisection of the spinal cord.**

MECHANISM OF INJURY
- **Most common with <u>penetration trauma</u> (eg, gunshot, stab wound, impalement).** Blunt trauma.
- Disc or bone herniation or hematomas causing lateral cord compression. Spinal cord tumor, ischemia, infection, hematoma, decompression sickness, fracture, dislocation, Multiple sclerosis.

CLINICAL MANIFESTATIONS
- **<u>Contralateral deficits</u>: <u>temperature & pain sensory deficits</u> usually ~2 levels below injury** (since the fibers of the spinothalamic tract cross over in the spinal cord at the level of their nerve roots).
- **<u>Ipsilateral deficits</u>: "MVP" <u>M</u>otor, <u>V</u>ibration, <u>P</u>roprioception deficits** below the lesion; Ipsilateral hemiparesis & motor weakness (ipsilateral corticospinal tract carries motor function to the same side of the body distal to the lesion & the posterior column fibers have not crossed the midline yet).
- May be associated with Horner syndrome (ptosis, miosis, and anhidrosis) if lesion at or above T1.
- <u>Good prognosis</u>: 90% of patients regaining function of the bowel and bladder as well as the ability to walk in closed injuries.

POSTERIOR CORD SYNDROME

ETIOLOGIES
- **Most common: B12 deficiency, late Neurosyphilis, Multiple sclerosis.** Extension-type injuries.

CLINICAL MANIFESTATIONS
- **<u>Proprioception deficits</u> <u>loss of position and vibratory sense</u> below the level of the injury — decreased coordination of voluntary movements, poor balance, unsteady gait, and falls.**
- **<u>Sensory ataxia:</u> vibration and fine touch deficits.**
- Bowel and or bladder dysfunction.

ANTERIOR CORD SYNDROME
Because ANT couldn't walk to the bathroom in the TeePee, he peed his pants when his bladder busted into flecks.

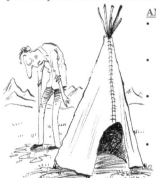

ANT = Anterior Cord Syndrome
- **Couldn't walk:** lower extremity motor deficit
- **TeePee** = loss of <u>T</u>emperature & <u>P</u>ain sensation
- **Peed his pants** = bladder dysfunction, lower extremity involvement
- **Flex** = flexion compression injuries common mechanism

BROWN SEQUARD SYNDROME
The MVP on the winning side was oblivious 2(to) the stabbing heat of the pain of defeat from the losing side.

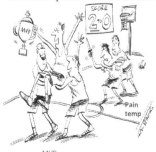

Ipsilateral deficits
- **MVP** = Motor, Vibratory and Proprioception deficits

Contralateral deficits
- pain & temperature **deficits** occurring usually 2 levels below the level of injury.

Mechanism
Stabbing: penetration injuries

CENTRAL CORD SYNDROME
Because Maleficent developed frostbite when she extended her hand to touch the cold window pane, she couldn't put on her shawl with her weak hands.

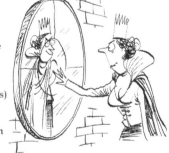

Extension **injuries**

loss of pain & temperature sensation

upper extremity > lower extremity (especially hands)

Shawl = shawl distribution

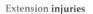

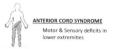

ANTERIOR CORD SYNDROME
Motor & Sensory deficits in lower extremities

CENTRAL CORD SYNDROME
Motor & Sensory deficits in upper extremities in a "shawl" distribution

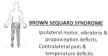

BROWN SEQUARD SYNDROME
Ipsilateral motor, vibratory & propioception deficits.
Contralateral pain & temperature deficits

DEFICITS
MOTOR
SENSORY
VIBRATORY PROPRIOCEPTION

	ANTERIOR CORD	CENTRAL CORD	POSTERIOR CORD	BROWN SÉQUARD
MECHANISM OF INJURY	• MC after blowout vertebral body burst fractures (flexion). • Anterior spinal artery injury or occlusion. • Direct anterior cord compression. • Aortic dissection, SLE, AIDS.	• Hyperextension injuries (ex 50% occur c MVA), falls in elderly, gun shot wounds, tumors, cervical spinal stenosis, syringomyelia. • MC incomplete cord syndrome. • It affects primarily the central gray matter (including the spinothalamic tracts).	• Rare • Damage to posterior cord or posterior spinal stenosis.	• Unilateral hemisection of the spinal cord • MC after *penetrating trauma* (tumors may cause it) • Rare injury.
DEFICITS	**Motor deficit:** • *lower extremity > upper* (corticospinal) **Sensory deficit:** • pain, temperature (spinothalamic tract) • light touch • May develop *bladder dysfunction* (retention, incontinence)	**Motor deficit:** • *upper extremity > lower**. The distal portion of the upper extremity more severe involvement (ex. hands) from corticospinal involvement. **Sensory deficit:** • pain, temperature (spinothalamic tract) deficit greater in the upper extremity > lower extremity. Sometimes described as a *"shawl" distribution.*	• *Loss of proprioception & vibratory sense only**	**Ipsilateral deficits:** - *Motor* (lateral corticospinal tract) - *Vibration & proprioception* (dorsal column) **Contralateral deficits:** - *pain & temperature* (lateral spinothalamic tract) usually 2 levels below the injury (where the spinothalamic tract crosses at the spinal cord level)
PRESERVATION	**Preserved:** • Proprioception, vibration, pressure (dorsal column spared) • Light touch preservation.	**Preserved:** Proprioception, vibration, pressure (dorsal column spared)	**Preserved:** • Pain & light touch. • No motor deficits	
	Anterior Cord Syndrome	Central Cord Syndrome	Posterior Cord Syndrome	BROWN SÉQUARD

CARPAL TUNNEL SYNDROME

- **Median nerve entrapment & compression** as is passes through the carpal tunnel at the wrist.
- Multifactorial — increased pressure in the intracarpal canal may directly injure the nerve, impair axonal transport, or compress vessels in the perineurium, leading to median nerve ischemia.

INCREASED INCIDENCE
- **Female gender** (3 times more common than in males), **Diabetes Mellitus, Pregnancy** (especially the 3rd trimester), Hypothyroidism. Rheumatological: Rheumatoid arthritis, Osteoarthritis, connective tissue diseases, use of Aromatase inhibitors. Obesity. Peak incidence 45-60 years of age.
- Occupations with repetitive wrist extension & flexion (eg, typing), forceful exertion, & vibration.

CLINICAL MANIFESTATIONS
- **Sensory symptoms: pain or paresthesias (numbness, tingling) in a median nerve distribution — palmar aspect of the first 3 digits & radial half of the fourth digit, typically worse at night** (may wake the patient up from sleep), flexing or extending the wrists (eg, driving, typing, holding a phone). The pain may be relieved shaking the hand/wrist.
- Patients may complain their hands fall asleep or that things slip from their fingers without their noticing (loss of grip, dropping things).
- Autonomic symptoms: tight or swollen feeling in the hands and/or temperature changes (eg, hands being cold/hot all the time). Sensitivity to changes in temperature (cold) and difference in skin color.
- Motor: in more severe cases, hand clumsiness & weakness — eg, loss of power, especially with precision grips involving the thumb — eg, difficulty holding objects, turning keys or doorknobs, buttoning clothing, opening jar lids.

Physical examination:
- ⊕ **Durkan test (carpal tunnel compression test)** symptom reproduction with pressing thumbs over the carpal tunnel and holding pressure for 30 seconds. **Most sensitive test to diagnose CTS.**
- ⊕ **Phalen test if flexion of both wrists for 30-60 seconds reproduces the symptoms** (pain and/or paresthesias along the median nerve distribution). The patient fully flexes the palms at the wrist with the elbow in full extension to provide extra pressure on the median nerve.
- ⊕ **Tinel test if percussion of the median nerve produces symptoms** (pain and/or paresthesias along the median nerve distribution). Less sensitive than the Phalen test.
- Sensory deficits: median nerve distribution palmar aspect of the 1st 3 digits & radial one half of the 4th.
- **Motor signs: thenar muscle atrophy or weakness of thumb abduction & opposition if advanced.**

DIAGNOSIS
Clinical diagnosis but can be confirmed by electromyography & nerve conduction velocity studies.
- **Nerve conduction studies: can be used to confirm the diagnosis, determine the severity of nerve compression, exclude other etiologies, or determine the need for surgical intervention.** The classic finding is impaired median nerve conduction across the carpal tunnel.
- Electromyography: **needle electromyography often used as a supplement with nerve conduction studies to exclude other conditions** (eg, radiculopathy, polyneuropathy, plexopathy).

MANAGEMENT
- **Conservative: volar splint in neutral position or slight flexion (eg, volar/cock up splint) worn at nighttime initial management** for a minimum of 3-4 weeks, NSAIDs, avoiding repetitive wrist movements. Corticosteroid injection if patient refuses splinting at night.
- Glucocorticoids: oral or injection — **glucocorticoid injection is an alternative to splinting** for short-term relief of symptoms (lasts 1-3 months) or if no response to initial management.

Surgical decompression:
- Indications: most patients with CTS with **refractory disease or severe median nerve injury (eg, significant axonal degeneration on nerve conduction studies, denervation on needle EMG, thenar atrophy).**

SELECTED REFERENCES

Jankovic J. Parkinson's disease: clinical features and diagnosis. J Neurol Neurosurg Psychiatr. 2008;79(4):368-76.

Zochodne DW. Autonomic involvement in Guillain-Barré syndrome: a review. Muscle Nerve. 1994;17(10):1145-55.

Conti-fine BM, Milani M, Kaminski HJ. Myasthenia gravis: past, present, and future. J Clin Invest. 2006;116(11):2843-54.

Saidha S, Eckstein C, Calabresi PA. New and emerging disease modifying therapies for multiple sclerosis. Ann N Y Acad Sci. 2012;1247:117-37.

Mackenzie C. Dysarthria in stroke: a narrative review of its description and the outcome of intervention. Int J Speech Lang Pathol. 2011;13(2):125-36.

Abboud H, Ahmed A, Fernandez HH. Essential tremor: choosing the right management plan for your patient. Cleve Clin J Med. 2011;78(12):821-8.

Jankovic J. Parkinson's disease: clinical features and diagnosis. J Neurol Neurosurg Psychiatr. 2008;79(4):368-76.

Walker FO. Huntington's disease. Lancet. 2007;369(9557):218-28.

Hughes RA, Wijdicks EF, Barohn R, et al. Practice parameter: immunotherapy for Guillain-Barré syndrome: report of the Quality Standards Subcommittee of the American Academy of Neurology. Neurology. 2003;61(6):736-40.

Maddison P, Newsom-davis J. Treatment for Lambert-Eaton myasthenic syndrome. Cochrane Database Syst Rev. 2005;(2):CD003279.

Nakahara J, Maeda M, Aiso S, Suzuki N. Current concepts in multiple sclerosis: autoimmunity versus oligodendrogliopathy. Clin Rev Allergy Immunol. 2012;42(1):26-34.

Maher AR, Maglione M, Bagley S, et al. Efficacy and comparative effectiveness of atypical antipsychotic medications for off-label uses in adults: a systematic review and meta-analysis. JAMA. 2011;306(12):1359-69.

Cruccu G, Biasiotta A, Di rezze S, et al. Trigeminal neuralgia and pain related to multiple sclerosis. Pain. 2009;143(3):186-91.

Easton JD, Saver JL, Albers GW, et al. Definition and evaluation of transient ischemic attack: a scientific statement for healthcare professionals from the American Heart Association/American Stroke Association Stroke Council; Council on Cardiovascular Surgery and Anesthesia; Council on Cardiovascular Radiology and Intervention; Council on Cardiovascular Nursing; and the Interdisciplinary Council on Peripheral Vascular Disease. The American Academy of Neurology affirms the value of this statement as an educational tool for neurologists. Stroke. 2009;40(6):2276-93.

Zink BJ. Traumatic brain injury outcome: concepts for emergency care. Ann Emerg Med. 2001;37(3):318-32.

Pelonero AL, Levenson JL, Pandurangi AK. Neuroleptic malignant syndrome: a review. Psychiatr Serv. 1998;49(9):1163-72.

Tyler KL. Herpes simplex virus infections of the central nervous system: encephalitis and meningitis, including Mollaret's. Herpes. 2004;11 Suppl 2:57A-64A.

Rozenberg F, Deback C, Agut H. Herpes simplex encephalitis : from virus to therapy. Infect Disord Drug Targets. 2011;11(3):235-50.

The International Classification of Headache Disorders: 2nd edition. Cephalalgia. 2004;24 Suppl 1:9-160.

Bonte FJ, Harris TS, Hynan LS, Bigio EH, White CL. Tc-99m HMPAO SPECT in the differential diagnosis of the dementias with histopathologic confirmation. Clin Nucl Med. 2006;31(7):376-8.

Singer HS. Tourette syndrome and other tic disorders. Handb Clin Neurol. 2011;100:641-57.

Clay shoveler's fracture: Case courtesy of David Cuete, Radiopaedia.org, rID: 22568

Extension teardrop fracture: Moquito 17 at the English language Wikipedia [GFDL (www.gnu.org/copyleft/fdl.html) or CC-BY-SA-3.0 (http://creativecommons.org/licenses/by-sa/3.0/)], via Wikimedia Commons.

Flexion teardrop fracture:

CHAPTER 11 – PSYCHIATRY/ BEHAVIORAL SCIENCE

PREMENSTRUAL DYSPHORIC DISORDER (PMDD)

- **Premenstrual syndrome (PMS):** cluster of physical, behavioral and mood changes with cyclical occurrence during the luteal phase of the menstrual cycle.
- **Premenstrual dysphoric disorder (PMDD): severe PMS with functional impairment where anger, irritability, & internal tension are prominent** (DSM V diagnostic criteria).

CLINICAL MANIFESTATIONS
- **Physical: abdominal bloating & fatigue most common;** breast swelling pain, or tenderness; weight gain, headache, changes in bowel habits; muscle or joint pain.
- **Emotional: irritability most common, anger, internal tension, anxiety, feeling on edge,** hostility, aggressiveness, **mood swings, sudden depressed mood,** sense of hopelessness, self-critical thoughts, **increased sensitivity to rejection,** libido changes, feeling overwhelmed or out of control.
- **Behavioral:** food cravings, change in appetite, poor concentration, noise sensitivity, loss of motor senses, diminished interest in usual activities, easy fatigability, decreased energy, sleep changes.

DIAGNOSIS
- **Symptoms occurring 1-2 weeks before menses (luteal phase), relieved within 2-3 days of the onset of menses plus at least 7 symptom-free days during the follicular phase.**
- For majority of women with PMDD, symptoms are the most severe 2 days prior to onset of menses.
- Patient should record a diary of symptoms for >2 cycles.

MANAGEMENT
- Lifestyle modifications: stress reduction & exercise most beneficial. Caffeine, alcohol, cigarette, & salt reduction. NSAIDs, vitamins B6 & E.
- **SSRIs first-line medical therapy (eg, Fluoxetine, Sertraline, controlled-released Paroxetine).** Continuous use or only during the luteal phase only (started on cycle day 14 to onset of menses).
- **Oral contraceptives (especially Drospirenone-containing combined OCPs) can be used in patients who do not want to take SSRIs &/or who desire contraception.**
- Gonadotropin-releasing hormone (GnRH) agonist therapy for ovulation suppression with estrogen-progestin addback if no response to SSRIs or OCPs.

SUICIDE

RISK FACTORS
- Plan: **previous attempt strongest single predictive factor** (70% of people who committed suicide succeeded on their first try). Organized plan > no organized plans.
- Access to firearms is an increased risk.
- Gender: **females attempt suicide more than men, but men are more successful at committing suicide.**
- Age: increases with age. **Elderly white men have the highest risk for Suicide in the US.**
- Race: whites > blacks.
- Psychiatric disorders: majority who attempt or commit suicide have underlying psychiatric disorders.
- Substance abuse: increased risk.
- Marital status: **alone** > never married > widowed > separated or divorced > married without children > married with children (marriage is protective).
- Others: positive family history of suicide, history of impulsivity, chronic illness. Among highly skilled workers, physicians are at an increased risk of suicide.

MANAGEMENT
- Assuring the patient's safety to prevent the patient from committing suicide.
- Admission and psychiatric evaluation.
- Once safety is established, treatment is aimed at diagnosing and treating any underlying mental disorder, including psychotherapy.

ANXIETY DISORDERS

PANIC ATTACKS

- **Fear response**: sudden, abrupt, discrete episode of intense fear, anxiety, or discomfort that usually peaks within 10 minutes & usually resolves within 1 hour (most end within 30 minutes).
- Patients may feel anxious for hours after the attack.

CLINICAL MANIFESTATIONS
- **≥4 of the following symptoms of <u>sympathetic system overdrive</u>** — sense of impending doom or dread (hallmark):

  PANIC ATTACK SYMPTOMS: sympathetic overdrive

1. Dizziness	6. Shortness of breath	11. Palpitations, increased heart rate
2. Trembling	7. Chest pain/discomfort	12. Nausea or abdominal distress
3. Choking feeling	8. Chills or hot flashes	13. Depersonalization (being detached from
4. Paresthesias	9. Fear of losing control	oneself) or derealization (feelings of unreality)
5. Sweating	10. Fear of dying	

MANAGEMENT OF ACUTE ATTACK
- **Benzodiazepines first-line medical management for an acute Panic attack** (eg, **Alprazolam**, Lorazepam, Diazepam, Clonazepam). Watch for dependence or abuse.
- **With a Panic attack (even in patients with Panic disorder), one must rule out potentially life-threating conditions (eg, Myocardial infarction, thyrotoxicosis, Aortic dissection etc.). Workup may include ECG, thyroid function tests, and urine toxicology screen,** as needed.
- Panic attacks are a feature of many different anxiety disorders but is not a disorder in & of itself.

PANIC DISORDER

- Average age of onset in early to mid 20s. Greater risk if a first degree relative is affected.
- Up to 65% of patients with Panic disorder also have major depression or other disorders.
- More common in females compared to males (2:1). 1-3% of the population.

DIAGNOSTIC CRITERIA
- **<u>Recurrent, unexpected panic attacks</u>** (at least 2 attacks) may or may not be related to a trigger.
- At least one of the following must occur for at least 1 month: ❶ **Panic attacks often followed by persistent concern about future attacks, ❷ persistent worry about the implication of the attacks** (eg, losing control) or ❸ **significant maladaptive behavior related to the attacks.**
- Symptoms are not due to substance use, medical condition (eg, thyroid, hypoglycemia, cardiac), or other mental disorder.

Specifiers:
- **Agoraphobia: anxiety about being in places or situations from which escape may be difficult** (eg, open spaces, enclosed spaces, crowds, public transportation, or outside of the home alone). Agoraphobia now seen as a separate entity from Panic disorder (can occur with other disorders).

MANAGEMENT
- **The main approaches to the treatment of Panic disorder include both [1] psychological (eg, Cognitive behavioral therapy) &/or [2] pharmacological interventions as the most effective management.**
- **<u>Cognitive Behavioral Therapy (CBT):</u>** adjunctive treatment that focuses on thinking & behavior (eg, relaxation, desensitization, examining behavior consequences etc.). Psychotherapy alone may be used in mild cases as initial therapy. **Pharmacotherapy + CBT most effective.**
- **<u>Pharmacotherapy:</u> SSRIs first-line (eg, Paroxetine, Sertraline, Fluoxetine).** May initiate therapy with SSRIs + Benzodiazepines (or Gabapentin), then taper and discontinue the Benzodiazepine. **The SNRI Venlafaxine is also used.** TCAs are options if SSRI/SNRIs are ineffective.
- **<u>Acute panic attacks:</u> Benzodiazepines (eg, Alprazolam) or Gabapentin for rapid relief** of acute symptoms as needed; tapered off when antidepressants take effect. Watch for abuse or dependence.

AGORAPHOBIA

- **Intense fear or anxiety about being in places or situations from which escape or obtaining help may be difficult if panic-like symptoms occur or that cause helplessness, incapacitation, or embarrassment** (eg, open spaces such as bridges, enclosed spaces, crowds, public transportation, shopping malls, or being outside of the home).
- Although **Agoraphobia is commonly seen with Panic disorder**, Agoraphobia is now seen as a separate entity from Panic disorder & can occur with other psychiatric disorders.
- The triggering situation causes anxiety or fear out of proportion to the potential danger of the situation. **Often associated with a range of agoraphobic avoidance.**
- **Symptoms last at least 6 months, cause significant social or occupational dysfunction,** & not better explained by another disorder, medical condition, medication, or substance use.
- <u>Risk factors:</u> strong genetic factor & may follow a traumatic event.

MANAGEMENT
- <u>**Similar to Panic disorder:**</u> Cognitive behavioral therapy &/or SSRIs (eg, Paroxetine, Fluvoxamine, Sertraline) or SNRIs (eg, Venlafaxine).

GENERALIZED ANXIETY DISORDER (GAD)

- More common in females than males 2:1. Onset of symptoms usually occurs in early 20s.
- Comorbidity with major depression or other anxiety disorders in the majority of cases of GAD.
- **<u>Multifocal worry:</u>** eg, finance, family, health, interpersonal relationships, work, minor matters, the future.
- <u>Somatic symptoms</u> may occur (eg, nausea, epigastric pain, headaches, fever, muscle tension, racing heartbeat).

DIAGNOSTIC CRITERIA
- **[A] <u>Excessive anxiety and worry</u> (apprehensive expectation), occurring a majority of days (more days than not) for <u>at least 6 months</u>, about a number of and various events or activities** (such as work or school performance). **It is not episodic (as in panic disorders), situational (as in phobias), nor focal.**
- [B] **<u>Uncontrollable or difficult to control</u>**: the individual finds it difficult to control the worry.
- [C] **The anxiety and worry are associated with ≥3 of the following 6 symptoms (with at least some symptoms having been present for more days than not for the past 6 months):** (1) restlessness or feeling keyed up or on edge; (2) being easily fatigued; (3) difficulty concentrating or mind going blank; (4) irritability; (5) muscle tension, (6) Sleep disturbance [difficulty falling or staying asleep, or restless, unsatisfying sleep].
- [D] **The anxiety, worry, or physical symptoms cause clinically significant distress or impairment in social, occupational, or other important areas of functioning.**
- [E] The disturbance is not attributable to the physiological effects of a substance (eg, a drug of abuse, a medication) or another medical condition (eg, hyperthyroidism).
- [F] The disturbance is not better explained by another mental disorder.

MANAGEMENT
The combination of psychotherapy + pharmacotherapy is more effective than either alone.
- **<u>Antidepressants (eg, SRIs)</u>** — SSRIs (eg, Fluoxetine, Paroxetine, Escitalopram, Sertraline) or SNRIs (eg, Duloxetine, Venlafaxine) are first-line agents for General anxiety disorder (GAD).
- **<u>Partial response to SRI:</u> <u>Buspirone</u> augmentation can be used if partial response to SRIs &/or CBT treatment (does not cause sedation).** Gabapentin is another alternative.
- Benzodiazepines can be used as adjunctive therapy for short-term use only until long-term therapy takes effect. Watch for dependence or abuse.
- <u>Beta-blockers</u> (eg, Propranolol) may be used to help control autonomic symptoms (eg, palpitations, diaphoresis, tachycardia) of panic attacks or performance anxiety.
- <u>Tricyclic antidepressants</u> (TCAs) & MAO inhibitors may be used if above medications are not helpful.

<u>Psychotherapy:</u>
- **<u>Cognitive-behavioral therapy</u> (CBT) preferred therapy for anxiety disorders.** Psychodynamics.

BUSPIRONE

- <u>Mechanism of action:</u> partial serotonin (5HT-1A) receptor agonist & dopamine receptor antagonist.
<u>Indications:</u>
  - **Generalized anxiety disorder: selective anxiolytic with minimal CNS depressants effects (does not cause sedation** or affect driving skills), **does not potentiate the CNS depression of alcohol** (useful in alcoholics & almost negligible abuse or addiction potential), **& does not have anticonvulsant or muscle relaxant properties**. Takes 1-2 weeks to take full effect.
  - <u>Adverse effects:</u> headache, dizziness, GI symptoms, restless legs syndrome, extrapyramidal symptoms.

SOCIAL ANXIETY DISORDER (formerly Social phobia)

- Most common type of phobia (eg, public speaking).
<u>DIAGNOSTIC CRITERIA</u>
  - [A] **Disabling, persistent (≥6 months) intense excessive fear of social or performance situation in which the person is exposed to the scrutiny of others** for fear of embarrassment (eg, **public speaking, meeting new people, eating or drinking in front of people, using public restrooms**).
  - [B] **The individual fears he or she will act in a way or show anxiety symptoms that will be negatively evaluated** (will be **humiliating or embarrassing** or lead to rejection or offend others).
  - [C] **The social situations almost always provoke fear or anxiety (expected attacks).**
  - [D] **The social situations are avoided or endured with intense fear or anxiety.**

<u>MANAGEMENT</u>
  - **Psychotherapy (individual Cognitive behavioral therapy) is the mainstay of treatment for Social anxiety disorder and other phobias** (desensitization, relaxation, insight-oriented therapy).
  - **Pharmacotherapy: SRIs: SSRIs (eg, Fluoxetine, Sertraline) or SNRIs (eg, Venlafaxine).** Adjunctive use of Benzodiazepines can be used until full effect of SRIs for patients with need of faster relief.
  - Moderate-severe cases benefit from combination pharmacotherapy & psychotherapy. Gabapentin.
  - <u>Performance only SAD:</u> **Medication treatment is often prescribed on an "as needed" basis for performance-only SAD, such as [1] Beta-blockers (eg, Propranolol, Atenolol) preferred or [2] Benzodiazepines (eg, Clonazepam or Lorazepam)** [potential for misuse, tolerance, dependence].

SPECIFIC PHOBIAS

- <u>Specific phobia:</u> an anxiety disorder characterized by significant fear of a specific object or situation that leads to endurance of the anxiety and/or avoidance of the feared object or situation.

<u>DIAGNOSTIC CRITERIA</u>
  - **[A] Persistent (≥6 months) intense fear or anxiety of a specific situation** (eg, heights, flying), **object** (eg, pigeons, snakes, blood) or **place** (eg, hospital).
  - [B] **Exposure to the situation triggers an immediate fear response.**
  - [C] **The fear is out of proportion to any real danger or threat.**
  - [D] **The phobic object or situation is actively avoided when possible or endured (tolerated) with intense fear or anxiety.**
  - **[E] Everyday activities must be impaired by distress or avoidance** of the situation or object.
  - [F] Not due to substance use, medical condition, or other mental disorder.

<u>SPECIFIERS</u>
  - <u>Animal</u> (eg, spiders, dogs, mice), <u>situational</u> (eg, airplanes, elevators), <u>natural environment</u> (eg, heights, thunder, water), <u>blood-injection injury</u> (injuries, needle injections, or blood), & other.

<u>MANAGEMENT</u>
  - **Exposure & desensitization therapy treatment of choice for Specific phobia** (most effective).
  - Short-term benzodiazepines or Beta-blockers can be used in some patients.

MOOD (AFFECTIVE) DISORDERS

MAJOR DEPRESSIVE DISORDER (MDD)/UNIPOLAR DEPRESSION

- Risk factors: family history, **female**: male (2:1). Peak onset of age in the 20s.

PATHOPHYSIOLOGY
- **Alteration in neurotransmitters** — serotonin, epinephrine, norepinephrine, dopamine, acetylcholine, & histamine. Genetic factors.
- Neuroendocrine dysregulation: adrenal, thyroid, or growth hormone dysregulation.
- 15% of patients commit suicide (especially men 25-30y & women 40-50y). Higher suicide rates in patients with a detailed suicide plan, white males >45y, & concurrent substance abuse.
- Patient Health Questionnaire (PHQ)-2 form for initial screen. If positive, may use PHQ-9 form.

DIAGNOSTIC CRITERIA
- **At least 2 distinct episodes of ≥5 associated symptoms (must include either depressive mood or anhedonia)** almost every day for most of the days for **at least 2 weeks:** depressive mood, anhedonia, fatigue almost all day, insomnia or hypersomnia, feelings of guilt or worthlessness, recurring thoughts of death or suicide, psychomotor agitation or retardation (restlessness or slowness), significant weight change (gain or loss), decreased or increased appetite, & decreased concentration or indecisiveness. Not associated with mania or hypomania.
- **The symptoms must cause significant distress or impairment (social or occupational).**
- The symptoms are not due to substance use, bereavement, or medical conditions.
- **[A] At least 5** associated symptoms [must include either **(1) depressive mood OR (2) anhedonia]** almost every day for most of the days for at least 2 weeks: **(1) depressed mood most of the day, nearly every day**, as indicated by either subjective report (eg, feels sad, empty, hopeless) or observation made by others (eg, appears tearful); **(2) Anhedonia - markedly diminished interest or pleasure in all, or almost all, activities most of the day, nearly every day; (3) Significant weight loss when not dieting or weight gain** (eg, a change of >5% of body weight in a month), or decrease or increase in appetite nearly every day; **(4) insomnia or hypersomnia** nearly every day; **(5) psychomotor agitation or retardation** nearly every day; **(6) Fatigue or loss of energy** nearly every day; (7) feelings of worthlessness or excessive or inappropriate guilt (which may be delusional) nearly every day (not merely self-reproach or guilt about being sick); (8) diminished ability to think or concentrate, or indecisiveness, nearly every day (either by subjective account or as observed by others); (9) recurrent thoughts of death (not just fear of dying), recurrent suicidal ideation without a plan, or a suicide attempt or specific plan.
- **[B] The symptoms must cause significant distress or impairment in social, occupational, or other important areas of functioning.**
- [C] Not attributable to physiologic effects of a substance, bereavement, or another medical condition.
- [D] The occurrence of the major depressive episode is not better explained by seasonal affective disorder, schizophrenia, schizophreniform disorder, delusional disorder, or other specified and unspecified schizophrenia spectrum and other psychotic disorders.
- **[E] There has never been a manic episode or a hypomanic episode.**

MANAGEMENT
- **Psychotherapy** (eg, **Cognitive behavioral therapy, interpersonal therapy,** & supportive therapy).
- **Pharmacological therapy: SSRIs first-line medical management (eg, Sertraline).** If no effect after 4 weeks, switch to another SSRI or SNRI.
- **Second line: SNRIs (eg, Duloxetine, Venlafaxine); Bupropion.**
- Other alternatives: Tricyclic antidepressants, Tetracyclics, MAO inhibitors.
- **Electroconvulsive therapy (ECT): rapid response in patients unresponsive to medical therapy, unable to tolerate pharmacotherapy, or for rapid reduction of symptoms in patients with severe symptoms (eg, refuse to eat/drink or acutely suicidal).** Safe in pregnancy & in the elderly.

SUBTYPES "COURSE SPECIFIERS" OF MDD

1. **SEASONAL AFFECTIVE DISORDER/SEASONAL PATTERN:** the presence of depressive symptoms at the same time each year (eg, most common in the fall or winter "winter blues" – due to reduction of sunlight & cold weather). **Management: SSRIs, light therapy, Bupropion.**
2. **ATYPICAL DEPRESSION:** shares many of the typical symptoms of major depression but patients experience **mood reactivity (improved mood in response to positive events).** Symptoms include significant weight gain/appetite increase, hypersomnia, heavy/leaden feelings in arms or legs & oversensitivity to interpersonal rejection. Management: **MAO inhibitors.**
3. **MELANCHOLIA:** characterized by anhedonia (inability to find pleasure in things), lack of mood reactivity, depression, severe weight loss/loss of appetite, excessive guilt, psychomotor agitation, or retardation & sleep disturbance (increased REM time & reduced sleep). Sleep disturbances may lead to early morning awakening or mood that is worse in the morning.
4. **CATATONIC DEPRESSION:** motor immobility, stupor, extreme withdrawal, purposeless motor activity.

SELECTIVE SEROTONIN REUPTAKE INHIBITORS (SSRIs)

Fluoxetine, Paroxetine, Citalopram, Escitalopram, Sertraline, Fluvoxamine, Vilazodone.
Mechanism of action:
- **Increase CNS serotonin activity by inhibiting presynaptic serotonin reuptake:** block the serotonin (5HT1A) transporter, prolonging extracellular serotonin within the synaptic cleft.
- Little or no effect on dopamine, norepinephrine (adrenergic), histamine, or acetylcholine.
- SSRIs cause a lower frequency of anticholinergic, sedating, & cardiovascular adverse effects but possibly greater incidence of GI symptoms, sleep impairment, & sexual dysfunction than do TCAs.
Indications:
- **SSRIs first-line medical therapy for depression, PTSD, Obsessive compulsive disorder, Panic disorder, Premenstrual dysphoric disorder, & Anxiety disorder in most cases** — effective, relatively mild adverse effects, and less toxic in overdose compared to other antidepressants (because they don't affect norepinephrine, acetylcholine, histamine, or dopamine as much).
- **Antidepressants take 4-6 weeks for maximum efficacy.** If no response, switch to another SSRI.
- **Fluoxetine: only FDA-approved antidepressant to treat Bulimia.** Has a long-half life (2-4 days) compared to other SSRIs (~1 day). Because of the longer half-life, there is a longer washout period for switching to MAOI (5 weeks) compared to other SSRIs (≥2 weeks). **Lowest risk of weight gain.**
Adverse effects:
- **GI distress: nausea most common adverse effect, diarrhea. Headache,** changes in energy level (fatigue, restlessness, irritability). Xerostomia. Escitalopram has less weight gain vs. Paroxetine.
- **Sexual dysfunction** (eg, decreased libido, anorgasmia). Treatment options for sexual dysfunction include (1) lowering the antidepressant dose if feasible; (2) switching to another antidepressant (eg, Bupropion, Mirtazapine); (3) augmenting with either Bupropion or Phosphodiesterase-5 inhibitor.
- **CNS stimulation** anxiety, **insomnia. Weight changes (eg, weight gain),** SIADH, Serotonin syndrome.
- **Increased suicidality in children & young adults <25y (black box warning).** Follow-up usually at 2 weeks is recommended because suicide risk is greatest following initial use of antidepressants.
- Of the SSRIs, **Paroxetine has more sexual dysfunction, antihistaminic activity, & more significant anticholinergic activity (can cause more dry mouth, dizziness, and weight gain).**
- **QT prolongation: especially Citalopram (avoid Citalopram in patients with long QT syndrome).**

- **Exam tip:**
- **In general, SSRIs are first-line medical therapy in most cases** because they are effective, have relatively mild adverse effects, and are less toxic in overdose compared to other antidepressants.
- **On average, antidepressants take 4-6 weeks to reach maximum efficacy.**
- In patients not responsive to initial SSRI therapy after 4-6 weeks, switch to another SSRI.
- **Duloxetine first-line if depression + neuropathic pain.*** TCAs also great for neuropathic pain.
- **Bupropion may be preferred if patient is fearful of sexual dysfunction or weight gain;** also good for **smoking cessation.** Mirtazapine also has less sexual effects but is associated with weight gain.

CNS stimulants: MAOIs, SSRIs, & Bupropion; Sedation: TCAs, Mirtazapine, Trazodone.

SEROTONIN & NOREPINEPHRINE REUPTAKE INHIBITORS (SNRIs)

Duloxetine, Venlafaxine, Desvenlafaxine, Levomilnacipran, Milnacipran.

Mechanism of action:

- **Block presynaptic reuptake of both norepinephrine & serotonin, enhancing the actions of both neurotransmitters** responsible for affecting mood. They also increase dopamine levels.
- Venlafaxine has less affinity for the Norepinephrine transporter than Desvenlafaxine or Duloxetine.

Indications:

- **Duloxetine may be used as first line agent, particularly in patients with significant <u>fatigue or neuropathy pain syndromes</u>* in association with depression** (eg, neuropathic pain, diabetic neuropathic pain, Fibromyalgia). General anxiety disorders, Depression. SNRIs alternative to SSRIs.

Adverse effects:

- **Safety, tolerability, & adverse effect profile similar to those of SSRIs: hyponatremia (SIADH), GI symptoms, headache, fatigue, sleep impairment, xerostomia, sexual dysfunction, suicidality.**
- **<u>Norepinephrine effects</u>: sweating, dizziness,** dry mouth, constipation. **Avoid using Venlafaxine in patients with uncontrolled or labile Hypertension since <u>Venlafaxine can cause Hypertension</u>.* Monitor blood pressure every 2-6 months after initiating treatment.**
- Venlafaxine can cause abnormal bleeding, altered platelets. Pharyngitis.
- <u>Anticholinergic:</u> (dizziness, dry mouth, constipation), CNS stimulant effects, Serotonin syndrome.

Contraindications & cautions:

- MAOI use, renal or hepatic impairment, seizures. Avoid abrupt discontinuation. Use with caution in patients with Hypertension or Glaucoma. ↑risk of Serotonin syndrome with SNRIs + St John's Wort.

BUPROPION

Mechanism of action: **(Atypical antidepressant)**

- **<u>Norepinephrine Dopamine reuptake inhibitor:</u> (NDRI)** — Bupropion's activity is not fully understood but Bupropion is a relatively weak inhibitor of the neuronal presynaptic uptake of norepinephrine & dopamine; **primary mechanism of action is thought to be noradrenergic and/or dopaminergic (also responsible for most of Bupropion's adverse effects).**
- Has minimal serotonin effects such as nausea and weight gain and no activity at histamine (H1) receptors, **so doesn't cause sedation (<u>Bupropion is a CNS stimulant</u>).**
  It is also a <u>nicotine antagonist</u>. This effect, in addition to increasing dopamine concentration in the nucleus accumbens, makes it useful for the **<u>management of nicotine dependence</u>.**
- Has an exceptionally short half-life, requiring frequent dosing.

Indications:

- Major depressive disorder & Seasonal affective disorder (Wellbutrin). **Can be used with SSRIs.**
- **<u>Bupropion is associated with less GI symptoms, weight gain, & sexual adverse effects</u> compared to SSRIs & SRNIs (useful in depressed patients who are fearful of sexual adverse effects or weight gain).*** It causes weight loss initially, but this effect is not usually sustained.
- Mirtazapine & Bupropion are often prescribed as monotherapy or as augmenting agents when patients develop sexual adverse effects due to other antidepressants (SSRIs, SNRIs, TCAs, MAOIs).
- **<u>Smoking cessation</u>: Useful in depressed smokers also interested in smoking cessation and in patients attempting to withdraw from Nicotine dependence** (marketed as Zyban).

Adverse effects:

- **The most serious adverse effects of Bupropion are a <u>lowered seizure threshold</u> and potential worsening of suicidal ideation (especially in adolescents & young adults <25 years).**
- <u>Noradrenergic activity:</u> **<u>CNS stimulant like adverse effects</u> (eg, insomnia, agitation, anxiety),** tachycardia, dizziness, diaphoresis, headache, **dry mouth,** constipation, hypertension, tremor.
- <u>Dopaminergic activity:</u> **nausea, increased psychosis at high doses.** Avoid abrupt withdrawal.
- <u>Respiratory:</u> pharyngitis, rhinitis.

Contraindications:

- **<u>Epilepsy or conditions with increased seizure risk</u>** (eg, **eating disorders, such as Bulimia & Anorexia** or patients undergoing abrupt discontinuation of alcohol, benzodiazepine, barbiturate, or antiepileptic medications). Avoid in patients with MAO inhibitor use in the past 14 days.

<u>CNS stimulants</u>: MAOIs, SSRIs, & Bupropion; <u>Sedation</u>: TCAs, Mirtazapine, Trazodone.

TRICYCLIC ANTIDEPRESSANTS (TCAs)

Tertiary amines: **Amitriptyline, Clomipramine, Imipramine, Doxepin, Amoxapine**
Secondary amines: **Desipramine, Nortriptyline,** Maprotiline

- Amitriptyline & Imipramine form active metabolites, Nortriptyline and Desipramine, respectively.

Mechanism of action:

- **Inhibit reuptake of both serotonin (5-HT) & norepinephrine,** increasing the concentration of these neurotransmitters in the synaptic cleft, resulting in their antidepressive effects.
- Additionally, they act as **competitive antagonists on post-synaptic alpha-adrenergic (alpha-1 & alpha-2), muscarinic (cholinergic), and histaminergic (H1) receptors.**

Indications:

- **Depression (not first line),** insomnia, **neuropathies, & pain disorders** (eg, Diabetic neuropathic pain, Post-herpetic neuralgia) due to their sodium channel blocker effects.
- **Used less often because of their adverse effect profile & severe toxicity with overdose.**
- **Clomipramine is FDA-approved for Obsessive-compulsive disorder (OCD)** in ages ≥10 years.
- **Insomnia and anxiety due to their sedative effects.**
- Migraine prophylaxis (Amitriptyline; Doxepin), Urge incontinence, Bipolar affective disorders, acute panic attacks, phobic disorders, Attention deficit hyperactivity disorder.
- **Nocturnal enuresis (eg, Imipramine) after the failure of Desmopressin in children.**

Adverse effects:

- **Anticholinergic (antimuscarinic) effects** most common: **dry mouth,** constipation, urinary retention, tachycardia, mydriasis, orthostatic hypotension; confusion or hallucinations in elderly. **Amitriptyline & Doxepin are the most anticholinergic.**
- **Antihistamine (H1) effects — sedation and drowsiness (lassitude, fatigue, confusion), increased appetite, weight gain, and confusion.**
- Alpha-1 adrenergic receptor blockade: **orthostatic hypotension, dizziness,** reflex tachycardia.
- Serotonergic effects: **sexual dysfunction** — erectile/ejaculatory dysfunction in males; anorgasmia.
- **Prolonged QT interval (best indicator of toxicity). Lowered seizure threshold, & SIADH.**
- **Increased suicidality in adolescents and young adults <25 years of age.** Serotonin syndrome.
- Contraindications/cautions: Use of MAO Inhibitors, recent MI/cardiac conditions, seizure history.

Overdose:

- **Anticholinergic symptoms**: tachycardia, dry mouth, mydriasis, hyperreflexia, **warm flushed dry skin, hyperthermia,** gastrointestinal complaints, urinary retention, confusion, and agitation.
- **3 C's: Cardiotoxicity: wide complex tachycardia** (Quinidine-like Na^+ channel blocker effects), **Convulsions (seizures)** or other neurologic symptoms (eg, respiratory depression), & **Coma.**
- **Management: Cardiotoxicity: IV Sodium bicarbonate*** (to reverse Na+ blocking effects of TCAs). **Seizures: Benzodiazepines first line.** Phenytoin is contraindicated (due to Na+ blockade).

TRICYCLIC ANTIDEPRESSANTS	SPECIFIC FACTS
TERITIARY AMINES	• **Most antihistaminic (sedating) [Doxepin & Amitriptyline]; most anticholinergic, & antiadrenergic: higher toxicity with TCA overdose.**
Amitriptyline	• **Useful in neuropathies & chronic pain** due to its sodium channel blocking properties. Insomnia [has sedating effects (antihistaminic effects)].
Doxepin	• Good for chronic pain. Sleep aid in low doses (antihistaminic effects).
Imipramine	• **Useful for Enuresis in children** and Panic disorder.
Clomipramine	• **Useful in Obsessive compulsive disorder (most serotonin specific).**
SECONDARY AMINES	• **Least anticholinergic, antiadrenergic & antihistaminic (less sedating) of the TCAs.**
Desipramine	• **Least sedating (least antihistaminic) and least anticholinergic.**
Nortriptyline	• Good for chronic pain. **Best tolerated, especially in the elderly.** • **Least likely to cause orthostatic hypotension.**

Sedation: **TCAs, Mirtazapine, Trazodone;** CNS stimulants: **MAOIs, SSRIs, & Bupropion.**

TETRACYCLIC (MIRTAZAPINE)
Mechanism of action: Atypical antidepressant
- **Alpha-2 adrenergic receptor antagonist:** tetracyclic antidepressant that has antagonist effects on the central presynaptic alpha-2-adrenergic receptors involved in feedback inhibition, which causes an **increased release of the amines serotonin & norepinephrine from nerve endings**.
- **High affinity for histamine H1 receptors (leading to its sedative, calming properties);** antagonist postsynaptic serotonin receptors (5-HT2A, 5-HT2C, and 5-HT3), leading to the remaining serotonin concentration left to interact with the free 5-HT1A receptor. Muscarinic receptor antagonist.

Indications:
- **Depression, especially patients with insomnia or significant weight loss** (has appetite stimulating & sedating properties). **Fewer sexual adverse effects*** vs. SSRIs, SNRIs, and MAOIs.
- **Anxiety disorders** (has anxiolytic properties). May be used with Trazodone.

Adverse effects:
- **Antihistaminic: drowsiness, sedation most common*** (54%), **weight gain (appetite stimulant).***
- Dry mouth, constipation, tremor, dizziness, & agranulocytosis. Transaminitis (increased LFTs).
- Increased risk of suicidality in children, adolescents, and young adults.
- Contraindications: Use with MAO inhibitors (may result in Serotonin syndrome).

Sedation: TCAs, Mirtazapine, Trazodone; **CNS stimulants:** MAOIs, SSRIs, & Bupropion.

NONSELECTIVE MAO INHIBITORS
Nonselective: Tranylcypromine, Phenelzine, Isocarboxazid; **MAO B only:** Selegiline (at low doses).
Mechanism of action:
- Blocks breakdown of neurotransmitters (**increased levels of norepinephrine, serotonin,** dopamine [MAO-B], epinephrine, & tyramine) **by inhibiting monoamine oxidase (MAO).**
- **Indications: Refractory or atypical** depression or **refractory** anxiety disorders.

Adverse effects:
- **Orthostatic hypotension most common;** insomnia, anxiety, weight gain, & sexual dysfunction.
- **CNS stimulants:** MAOIs, SSRIs, & Bupropion; **Sedation:** TCAs, Mirtazapine, Trazodone.
- **Hypertensive crisis after ingesting foods high in tyramine (eg, aged or fermented cheese, all aged, smoked, pickled, or cured meats/poultry/fish, red wine,** draft beer, & chocolates). Nonselective MAO inhibition prevents the breakdown of tyramine, leading to hypertension.

Drug interactions:
- **Increased risk of Serotonin syndrome** if MAO inhibitors are combined with SSRIs, SNRIs, St. John's wort, MDMA, cocaine, Meperidine, Tramadol, & Dextromethorphan.
- **Wait at least 2 weeks before switching from MAO inhibitors to SSRIs or vice versa (5 weeks for Fluoxetine due to its longer half-life).** MAOI + TCAs may cause delirium & hypertension.

SEROTONIN MODULATORS (SEROTONIN RECEPTOR ANTAGONISTS & AGONISTS)
Trazodone, Nefazodone, Vilazodone, and Vortioxetine.
Mechanism of action:
- **Serotonin antagonist & agonists:** postsynaptic serotonin 5-HT2A & 5-HT2C receptor inhibitors (inhibit both serotonin transporter & serotonin type 2 receptors). **Weakly inhibit presynaptic serotonin uptake.** Some of the active metabolites are serotonin receptor agonists.
- **Sedative effects: Alpha-1 adrenergic receptor antagonism leads to sedation.** Trazodone also reduces levels of other neurotransmitters associated with arousal effects, such as serotonin (5-HT-2A receptor), noradrenaline, dopamine, acetylcholine, & histamine.

Indications:
- **Antidepressant with anxiolytic & hypnotic effects (useful for insomnia).** Low dose (sleep aid).
- Unlike SSRIs, Trazodone does not affect REM sleep or cause anxiety, insomnia, sexual adverse effects.

Adverse effects:
- **Sedation (most common),*** dizziness, dry mouth, nausea, orthostatic hypotension, headache.
- **Priapism*** rare but classic with Trazodone. Increased suicidality <25y of age. Cardiac arrhythmias.
- **Nefazodone has a black box warning for rare but serious fulminant Hepatitis.**

Sedation: TCAs, Mirtazapine, Trazodone; **CNS stimulants:** MAOIs, SSRIs, & Bupropion.

SEROTONIN SYNDROME (SEROTONIN TOXICITY)

- Potentially life-threating syndrome due to **increased serotonergic activity in the CNS.**

ETIOLOGIES

- **Serotonergic antidepressants**: SSRIs, SNRIs, TCAs, & MAO inhibitors, Bupropion, St. John's wort.
- Increased release of serotonin: Cocaine, MDMA (ecstasy), Amphetamines (eg, Dextroamphetamine, Methamphetamine, Fenfluramine, Dexfenfluramine, Phentermine), and Mirtazapine.
- Impaired serotonin reuptake from the synaptic cleft into the presynaptic neuron: **Meperidine, Tramadol, Triptans, Dextromethorphan, cocaine, MDMA (ecstasy), 5-HT3 receptor antagonists (eg, Dolasetron, Granisetron, Ondansetron, Palonosetron), Cyclobenzaprine, Methylphenidate, Metoclopramide.** Lithium. **Linezolid** (is a MAO inhibitor).
- Increased serotonin formation: **Triptans**, Tryptophan, Oxitriptan.

CLINICAL MANIFESTATIONS

- Symptoms most commonly develop rapidly after initiation or change in precipitating drug: 30% within 1 hour, 60% within 6 hours, and nearly all patients with toxicity within 24 hours of exposure.
- **Cognitive effects: mental status changes — anxiety, agitation, confusion,** disorientation, agitated delirium, hallucinations, hypomania. CNS stimulatory effects including seizures.
- **GI serotonin effects: nausea, vomiting, increased bowel sounds, & diarrhea.**

PHYSICAL EXAMINATION:

- **Autonomic instability — hyperthermia (temperature >38°C), tachycardia, hypertension, diaphoresis,** vomiting, and diarrhea. Severe cases may be associated with rapid swings in blood pressure and pulse and cardiovascular instability.
- **Neuromuscular hyperactivity: tremor, spontaneous or inducible clonus,** ocular clonus (slow, continuous, horizontal eye movements), **hypertonia (increased DTR & hyperreflexia), muscle rigidity,** bilateral Babinski, akathisia (restlessness). Lower extremity involvement most severe.
- **Mydriasis (dilated pupils),** dry mucous membranes, ↑'ed bowel sounds, flushed skin, diaphoresis.

DIAGNOSIS

- Clinical diagnosis based on the Hunter criteria.

MANAGEMENT OF MILD

- **Immediate discontinuation of offending drug(s) most important initial step.**
- **In mild cases, discontinuation of inciting medications, supportive care, and sedation with Benzodiazepines is usually sufficient.**
- Supportive care mainstay of therapy to help normalize vital signs — supplemental oxygen to maintain SaO2 ≥94%, IV fluids for volume depletion, continuous cardiac monitoring.
- **Benzodiazepines for agitation, to reduce hyperthermia, and to correct mild increases in heart rate & blood pressure;** Refractory/severe Hypertension: Esmolol, Nicardipine, or Nitroprusside.
- IV fluids & cooling measures for Hyperthermia. Antipyretics such as Acetaminophen are ineffective because increased muscular activity causes hyperthermia in Serotonin syndrome.

MANAGEMENT OF MODERATE

- **As above + Cyproheptadine (a serotonin antagonist) to improve autonomic instability.** Cyproheptadine is indicated if Benzodiazepines and supportive care fail to improve agitation and correct vital signs. Adverse effects of Cyproheptadine: may cause sedation and transient hypotension that is responsive to intravenous fluids.
- Immediate sedation, paralysis, and tracheal intubation may be indicated in hyperthermic patients who are critically ill, whose temperature is above 41.1°C (antipyretics are ineffective).
- Hypotension is often treated with IV fluids alone. Hypotension from MAOIs may need treatment with low dose direct-acting sympathomimetics (eg, Epinephrine, Phenylephrine, Norepinephrine).

BIPOLAR I DISORDER

- <u>Risk factors:</u> **family history (1st-degree relatives) strongest risk factor** (10 times more likely).
- 1% of population. Average age of onset is 20s - 30s. New onset rare after 50y. More common in men.
- The earlier the onset, the greater likelihood of psychotic features & the poorer the prognosis.

DIAGNOSTIC CRITERIA
- **<u>At least 1 Manic or mixed episode</u> (only requirement).** The manic episodes often cycle with occasional depressive episodes, but *major depressive episodes are not required for the diagnosis.*
- **Mania:** abnormal & persistently <u>elevated, expansive, or irritable mood</u> at least <u>1 week</u> (or less **if hospitalization is required) with <u>marked impairment of social/occupational function.</u>** ≥3: **<u>Mood:</u>** euphoria, irritable, labile, or dysphoric; **<u>Thinking:</u>** racing, flight of ideas, disorganized, easily distracted, expansive or grandiose thoughts (highly inflated self-esteem). Judgment is impaired (eg, spending sprees); **<u>Behavior:</u>** physical hyperactivity, pressured speech, decreased need for sleep (may go days without sleep), increased goal directed activity. Excessive involvement in activities that have a high potential for painful consequences (eg, engaging in unrestrained buying sprees, sexual indiscretions, risk-taking or foolish business investments). Excessive speech.
- Psychotic symptoms (paranoia, delusions, hallucinations) may be seen in these patients.
- Symptoms not due to medical condition or substance use.

MANAGEMENT
Mood stabilizers (eg, Lithium, Valproic acid) &/or second-generation (atypical) antipsychotics are often used for Bipolar disorder. Carbamazepine may be used without an antipsychotic.
- **[1] Mood Stabilizers:** First line agents include Lithium (acute mania & long-term management Lithium also decreases suicide risk), Lamotrigine; Valproic acid. Valproic acid & Carbamazepine are also useful for rapid cycling or mixed features. **Lithium generally avoided in renal disease; Valproate generally avoided in liver disease.**
- **[2] 2nd-generation (atypical) antipsychotics:** (eg, **Quetiapine. Aripiprazole, Olanzapine, Risperidone**) are effective as monotherapy or as adjunctive therapy to mood stabilizers — combination of mood stabilizers and antipsychotics is faster & more effective than monotherapy.
- **Psychotherapy:** cognitive, behavioral & interpersonal. Good sleep hygiene recommended.
- **Bipolar depression:** The FDA has approved 4 psychotropics in the setting of acute bipolar depression: **Lurasidone, Quetiapine, Cariprazine, & the Olanzapine-Fluoxetine combination.** Bipolar depression often persists longer, and it is very challenging to treat, needing a different approach from that used in unipolar depression. Valproate may be used if refractory.
- Antidepressant therapy may be used as adjunct to mood stabilizers for severe depression, but **<u>antidepressant monotherapy may precipitate mania or hypomania in Bipolar disorder</u>**.

ACUTE MANIA
- **Mood stabilizers (eg, Lithium, Valproic acid) &/or Antipsychotics (eg, Risperidone or Olanzapine > Haloperidol).**
- Antipsychotics or benzodiazepines can be used for acute psychosis or agitation.
- **<u>Electroconvulsive therapy (ECT)</u>** especially helpful for refractory or life-threatening acute mania or depression (also best treatment for pregnant women with manic episodes). Decreased suicidality.

	MANIA/MIXED	MAJOR DEPRESSION
BIPOLAR I	Yes	Typical but not required.
BIPOLAR II	HYPOmania only (no mania)	Yes
CYCLOTHYMIA	No (but may have periods of mood elevation)	No. Associated with relatively mild depressive episodes.
MAJOR DEPRESSIVE DISORDER	No	Yes
PERSISTENT DEPRESSIVE DISORDER (DYSTHYMIA)	No	Usually mild but can meet criteria for major in some cases.

"Mixed" symptoms = simultaneous occurrence of ≥3 manic (or hypomanic) symptoms + depression.

LITHIUM

Mechanism of action:
- Exact mechanism unknown; thought to alter neuronal sodium transport and influence the reuptake of serotonin &/or norepinephrine. Inhibits phosphoinositol recycling in neurons (affecting mood).

Indications:
- **Bipolar disorder** (both manic & depressive episodes). **Acute mania (mood stabilizer).**
- **Lithium decreases suicide risk.**
- Schizoaffective disorder

Adverse effects:
- **Endocrine:** hyperparathyroidism, hypercalcemia, hypermagnesemia, sodium depletion, **AVP/ADH resistance (nephrogenic Diabetes insipidus),** increased thirst (should drink 8-10 glasses of water daily). **Hypothyroidism — monitor TFTs while on Lithium therapy.**
- **Neurologic: tremor is common**, headache, sedation, seizures.
- GI: nausea, vomiting, diarrhea, weight gain.
- Cardiac: edema, arrhythmias, and ECG changes. Hematological: Leukocytosis
- **Narrow therapeutic index: prior to initiating therapy, a basic ECG, chemistries, thyroid function, beta-hCG, and CBC should be performed**. Initially levels should be checked after 5 days then every 2-3 days until therapeutic. Once therapeutic, monitor plasma levels every 4-8 weeks. Therapeutic range is 0.8-1.2. **Levels may be toxic if > 1.5**. ECG performed on initiation if >50 years.

Contraindications:
- **Pregnancy** — may be associated with **Ebstein anomaly** if taken during the first trimester.
- **Severe renal disease (may increase Lithium levels),** cardiac disease.

Drug interactions:
- **Blood level is increased** by dehydration, thiazides, tetracyclines, nonsteroidal anti-inflammatory drugs (NSAIDs), Angiotensin converting enzyme inhibitors (ACEIs), and loop diuretics — they impair renal function & may increase Lithium in the blood to toxic levels.
- Blood level decreased by bronchodilators, Verapamil, Theophylline, carbonic anhydrase inhibitors.

CYCLOTHYMIC DISORDER

- **Similar to Bipolar II but is less severe** — [1] hypomanic symptoms that fall short of meeting criteria for a full hypomanic episode and [2] mild to moderate depressive symptom episodes that fall short of meeting criteria for Major depressive or Bipolar disorders. Fluctuating mood.
- ~1/3 will eventually develop Bipolar disorder. May coexist with Borderline personality disorder.

DIAGNOTIC CRITERIA
- **Characterized by ≥2 consecutive years** of prolonged, milder elevations and milder depressions in mood that do **not** meet the criteria for either (1) full hypomanic episodes or (2) major depressive episodes. ≥1 year in children and adolescents. Criteria for mania never met.
- The symptoms recur over a time interval of at least 2 consecutive years, during which **patients are symptomatic at least half the time (present for more days than not) and are not symptom-free for more than 2 consecutive months** (stability of mood cannot have exceeded any length of time longer than 2 consecutive months).
- **Major depressive, manic, hypomania, or mixed episodes do not occur**
- In addition, the symptoms cause significant distress or psychosocial impairment at some point.
- Symptoms are not the direct result of a substance (eg, drug of abuse or medication) or another medical condition. Specifier: mood symptoms are marked by anxious distress.

MANAGEMENT
- **Mood stabilizers (eg, Lamotrigine, Valproic acid, Lithium) &/or second–generation antipsychotics (eg, Quetiapine, Aripiprazole, Olanzapine, Risperidone).** Psychotherapy.
- Valproate helpful if anxiety is dominant, Lamotrigine if the anxious-depressive polarity is more prominent, and Lithium for significant affective intensity.

BIPOLAR II DISORDER

DIAGNOSTIC CRITERIA FOR BIPOLAR II

- **History of <u>at least 1 major depressive episode</u> + at least 1 <u>hypomanic</u> episode.** Mood fluctuation. Any current or prior Manic episode or mixed episode makes the diagnosis Bipolar I.
- **<u>Hypomania</u>: abnormal & persistently elevated, expansive, or irritable mood at least 4 days that (1) does not require hospitalization, (2) is <u>not</u> associated with marked impairment of social/occupational function,** & (3) not associated with psychotic features. At least 3 symptoms affecting mood, thinking, or behavior (symptoms otherwise similar to Manic episodes).
- At least 2 years in adults (at least 1 year in children/adolescents). 0.5% prevalence.

DIAGNOSTIC CRITERIA (HYPOMANIA)

- **[A] <u>Mood disturbance</u>: A distinct period of abnormally and persistently elevated, expansive, or irritable mood and abnormally and persistently increased activity or energy, lasting at least 4 consecutive days** and present most of the day, nearly every day.
- [B] During the period of mood disturbance & increased energy & activity, 3 (or more) of the following (4 if the mood is only irritable) have persisted, represent a noticeable change from usual behavior, & have been present to a significant degree: (1) Inflated self-esteem or grandiosity; (2) Decreased need for sleep (eg, feels rested after only 3 hours of sleep); (3) More talkative than usual or pressure to keep talking; (4) Flight of ideas or subjective experience that thoughts are racing; (5) Distractibility (eg, attention too easily drawn to unimportant or irrelevant external stimuli); (6) Increase in goal-directed activity (either socially, at work or school, or sexually) or psychomotor agitation; (7) Excessive involvement in activities that have a high potential for painful consequences (eg, engaging in unrestrained buying sprees, sexual indiscretions, or foolish business investments).
- [C] The episode is an unequivocal change uncharacteristic of the individual when not symptomatic.
- [D] The disturbance in mood and the change in functioning are observable by others.
- **[E] The episode is (1) not severe enough to cause marked impairment in social or occupational functioning or (2) to necessitate hospitalization.**
- [F] Not attributable to the physiological effects of a substance (eg, a drug of abuse or medication)

MANAGEMENT

- **[1] <u>Mood stabilizers</u> (eg, Lamotrigine, Lithium, Valproic acid, or Carbamazepine) &/or [2] <u>second-generation antipsychotics</u> (eg, Quetiapine, Aripiprazole, Olanzapine, Risperidone).**
- <u>Psychotherapy</u>: cognitive, behavioral & interpersonal. Good sleep hygiene recommended.

PERSISTENT DEPRESSIVE DISORDER (DYSTHYMIA)

- DSM V combined Dysthymia & Chronic major depressive disorder into PDD.
- More common in women. Onset often in childhood, adolescence, or early adulthood.

DIAGNOSTIC CRITERIA

- **[A] <u>Chronic depressed mood</u> (required) for <u>at least 2 years</u> in adults** (at least 1 year in children/adolescents) that lasts most of the day, more days than not.
- **[B] At least 2 of the following conditions present** — insomnia, hypersomnia, fatigue or low energy, low self-esteem, decreased or increased appetite, hopelessness, poor concentration, indecisiveness.
- **[C] In that 2-year period, the patient is <u>not symptom free for >2 consecutive months at a time</u> during the 2-year period.** May have major depressive episodes or meet the criteria for Major depressive disorder continuously.
- [D] Never have had a manic episode (rules out Bipolar I) or hypomanic episode (rules out cyclothymic disorder).

MANAGEMENT

A combination of psychotherapy & pharmacotherapy is more efficacious than either alone.

- **Pharmacotherapy: SSRIs**, SNRIs, Bupropion, Mirtazapine, TCAs, & MAO inhibitors.
- <u>Psychotherapy</u>: interpersonal, cognitive, and insight-oriented therapy. Less effective than meds alone.

PSYCHOGENIC NONEPILEPTIC SEIZURES [PNES]

- Seizures are events that may resemble epileptic seizures but are not associated with any change in brain electrical/neuronal activity or reduced perfusion to the brain.
- Psychogenic nonepileptic seizures are events thought to have mainly psychologic origins. They may result as a conversion reaction triggered by underlying psychological distress or malingering.

EPIDEMIOLOGY
- More common in women, especially with a history of physical or sexual abuse.
- Patients with PNES often have other psychiatric disorders, epilepsy, developmental disabilities, recurrent medical evaluations for unexplained somatic complaints, and other conditions.

CLINICAL MANIFESTATIONS
Convulsive PNES most common type (may present similar to a tonic clonic seizure):
- The event consists of a fall if the patient is upright. Certain behaviors such as side-to-side turning or tremors of the head with low frequency and high amplitude, **asynchronous "thrashing movements"** of the limbs, **forcible ictal eye closure** (unlike Epileptic seizures, in which they eyes are usually open), asymmetric large amplitude shaking or twitching movements of the limbs, back arching, odd movements (eg, flailing), pelvic thrusting, & longer duration occur more in PNES
- Unlike an Epileptic seizure, there is usually no tonic phase (eg, initiating cry), hurtful fall, incontinence. Postictally, there are no changes in behavior, confusion, or neurologic findings.

Swoon PNES:
- This form may be similar to a syncopal episode. Events are associated with a fall to the ground or "slump" to one side if sitting, with little or no movement. The eyes are usually closed, and the patient is unresponsive. Prolonged events are almost always PNES. should be ascertained that an eyewitness account extends from before the beginning until after the end of the event, as many epileptic seizures are followed by a period where the patient lies still.

DIAGNOSIS
- **Simultaneous Video & EEG monitoring** useful when historic features are nondiagnostic. Generalized tonic-clonic seizures always produce marked EEG abnormalities during and after the seizure.
- **Measurement of serum prolactin** levels may also help to distinguish between epileptic and psychogenic seizures. Most generalized seizures and some focal seizures are accompanied by a rise in serum prolactin 10-20 minutes after a seizure, whereas psychogenic seizures are not. However, prolactin has limited usefulness because levels are normal after an epileptic seizure in ~50% and prolactin levels can be elevated for other reasons (eg, medications).

MANAGEMENT
- Once established, the diagnosis of PNES should be discussed with the patient in a supportive, nonjudgmental way. Antiepileptic medications should be gradually discontinued, with appropriate supervision in patients with no Epilepsy.
- Neurologic follow-up should be continued after a diagnosis of PNES to monitor the safe withdrawal of antiseizure medications, answer patient concerns, & reassess if new events appear.
- **Psychological intervention** main therapy, including Cognitive behavioral therapy (CBT) but may not be beneficial.

ABUSE & NEGLECT

INTIMATE PARTNER ABUSE

- According to the CDC, 1 in 4 women and 1 in 7 men will experience physical violence by their intimate partner at some point during their lifetimes. About 1 in 3 women and nearly 1 in 6 men experience some form of sexual violence during their lifetimes.
- **A woman who leaves an abusive partner has a 70% greater risk of being killed by the abuser in that immediate period after leaving compared to staying.**
- Abuse during pregnancy can make up about 10% of pregnant pregnancy-related hospital admissions.
- Barriers to screening include lack of privacy, low self-esteem, fear, and sensitive nature of intimate partner violence.
- Clues to violence: contusions to breast, chest, abdomen, face, neck, musculoskeletal injuries, and "accidental" injuries, delay to seek care for injuries. They may have multiple injuries in various stages of healing. Patients may have nonspecific general symptoms (eg, fatigue & headache).
- On confrontation of a potential victim [1] validate the abuse without blaming the victim, [2] assess the patient's current safety (including emergency escape plan), [3] thoroughly document history and physical examination findings in case they are required for a police report, [4] provide resources.

MANAGEMENT
- All healthcare facilities should have a plan that includes screening, assessing, and referring patients for intimate partner violence.
- Once suspected, patients should be addressed directly with a nonthreatening question to confirm if intimate partner abuse has occurred. If it has occurred, then alternatives should be discussed with referral if the patient accepts as it is the patient's right to accept or refuse help.

SEXUAL ABUSE

- According to the National sexual Violence Resource Center, more than one-quarter to one-third of female children have experienced sexual abuse before 18 years of age.
- Common ages of sexual abuse is between ages 9-12 years.
- **Perpetrators are most commonly males, and most are relatives to the child or known by the child** (have access).
- ~33% of sexual offenders were once themselves victims of sexual abuse.
- Any of the following should increase the index of suspicion for child abuse — children that exhibit sexual knowledge, initiate sex acts with peers, show knowledge of sexual acts, bruises, pain, or pruritus in the genital or anal area, or evidence of a sexually transmitted infection.

PHYSICAL ABUSE

- Abuser often female and usually the primary caregiver.
- Signs may include cigarette burns, burns in a stocking glove pattern, lacerations, healed fractures on radiographs, subdural hematoma, multiple bruises, or retinal hemorrhages.
- Hyphema or retinal hemorrhages seen in shaken baby syndrome.

CHILD ABUSE & NEGLECT

- Child neglect is the most common form of Child abuse.
- Failure to provide the basic needs of a child (eg, supervision, food, shelter, affection, education) etc.
- Signs include malnutrition, withdrawal, poor hygiene, and failure to thrive; injuries, burns, or lacerations that do no align with the history or repetitive may be suggestive of abuse (eg, round burns suggestive of cigarette burns, donut shaped burns, subdural or retinal hemorrhages).
- Management: child protective services; youth and children services to protect from further abuse.

ELDER ABUSE

- Actions or failures to act, perpetrated by those with an ongoing relationship involving an expectation of responsibility toward the victim.

Warning signs:
- Skin findings: skin tears, abrasions, lacerations, burns, and bruises that are insufficiently explained or occur in unusual locations may suggest elder physical abuse. Injuries from the use of restraints.
- Fractures: spiral fractures of long bones and fractures in sites other than the wrist; Fractures of the face, ulna, ribs, or multiple fractures at various stages of healing.
- Malnutrition (eg, weight loss, poor nutrition), dehydration (eg, fecal impaction, dry mucous membranes, sunken eyes), orthostatic changes, tachycardia., pressure ulcers.
- Neglect may include poor hygiene, poor personal care, lack of eyeglasses or hearing aids, withholding food, medicine, or misusing their finances.
- Sexual abuse is suspected in the presence of soiled clothing, genital or rectal injuries or bleeding, evidence of drugging, or a lack of or delay in seeking medical attention.
- Psychological abuse can be perpetrated by verbal abuse, threats, or insults.

MANAGEMENT
Most states have similar reporting protocols for elder abuse similar to child abuse.
- Interventions: If a health care worker has reason to believe that an older adult is the victim of elder abuse or self-neglect, appropriate reporting should be promptly initiated. Careful and immediate documentation should be made of observations that support a finding of elder abuse. The APS agencies and the courts are obliged to use the least-restrictive alternative when an individual's autonomy is impacted in order to protect that person.
- Resources – Community-dwelling older adults may be offered resources and protection in the United States by state Adult Protective Services (APS) agencies.

RAPE

- Act of sexual aggression that may be perpetrated on a spouse, a known partner, or a stranger.
- Forced participation in any sexual acts can result in psychological sequelae, including PTSD, depression, anxiety, appetite or sleep disturbances, and a myriad of emotions.

Approach to the patient:
- Evaluation of the sexual assault victim should be performed by a trained forensic provider, if feasible. A detailed forensic history should be documented. Evaluation should include psychological assessment, evaluation of areas of trauma, and examination of the breasts and pelvic and anorectal areas. Colposcopy should be performed, when possible, to detect genital trauma.
- **Forensic evaluation**: A rape evidence collection kit, with detailed instruction and containers for specimen collection. The victim should be evaluated as soon as possible after an assault, but evidence may be collected at later times depending upon factors. All procedures should be documented, clothing saved, and samples taken.
- Laboratory testing: should include pregnancy testing in females of childbearing age. Baseline serology for syphilis and hepatitis B, HIV counseling should be provided. Drug screening may be warranted if the victim was found unconscious or has amnesia for any time surrounding the event.
- **Empiric STI treatment** – In a sexual assault victim, treating empirically for gonorrhea, chlamydia, and trichomoniasis (eg, Ceftriaxone 500 mg by intramuscular injection, Doxycycline 100 mg by mouth twice daily for 7 days, and Metronidazole 500 mg by mouth twice daily for 7 days). Post-exposure prophylaxis against HIV infection should be given to a victim of sexual assault.
- **Emergency contraception** can be offered to the patient (eg, Ulipristal acetate, Levonorgestrel, Mifepristone, Copper or Levonorgestrel IUD).
- **Acute crisis counseling** with a mental health professional and follow-up counseling scheduled.

DELUSIONAL DISORDER

- **[1] The presence of ≥1 <u>nonbizarre delusions</u> for at least a month in an individual who, except for the delusions and their behavioral ramifications, [2] does not appear odd or bizarre and is not markedly functionally impaired** (eg, no accompanying prominent hallucinations, thought disorder, mood disorder, significant flattening of the affect, or dementia).
- Nonprominent hallucinations and odd behaviors related to the delusional theme may be present.

DEFINITIONS
- **<u>Delusion</u>: fixed belief of an external reality despite evidence to the contrary.**
- **<u>Nonbizarre delusion</u>: false belief that is plausible (could occur) but highly unlikely** — eg, being poisoned, followed, infected, loved at a distance, deceived by a spouse, or having a disease.

EPIDEMIOLOGY
- ~0.03% of the general population experience persistent, relatively fixed delusions in the absence of the characteristic features of other psychotic disorders, such as Schizophrenia.
- Mean age of onset is ~40 years, but the range is from 18 years to 90 years.
- Depression has been the most commonly observed co-occurring condition; anxiety can also occur.
- Risk factors include a family history of Paranoid personality disorder and sensory impairment.

DIAGNOSTIC CRITERIA
- **[A] At least 1 delusion, lasting at least 1 month** (see next page for Delusion types).
- **[B] Criterion A for Schizophrenia are not met — there should <u>not</u> be significant hallucinatory experiences, marked thought disorder, prominent negative symptoms, thought disorder, or psychosocial deterioration.** Hallucinations, if present, are not prominent & are related to the delusional theme.
- **[C] Apart from the delusion and its ramifications, behavior is not obviously odd or bizarre & there is no significant impairment of function.** An individual's cultural beliefs merit consideration before coming to the diagnosis.
- **[D]** If manic or major depressive episodes have occurred, these have been brief relative to the duration of the delusional periods.
- **[E]** Not explained by another psychiatric disorder, medical condition, medications, or substance use.

MANAGEMENT
- **<u>Atypical (2nd-generation) antipsychotics</u> first-line medical management (eg, Ziprasidone, Aripiprazole).**
- **<u>Individual psychotherapy</u>** (eg, Cognitive behavioral, Supportive) **may be additive in some patients rather than group therapy**, as patients are often suspicious and sensitive around their delusions.
- Because of the lack of insight, patients often refuse to see a mental health clinician and usually reject antipsychotic medication &/or psychotherapy, making treatment challenging.

EXAM TIP **PSYCHOTIC DISORDERS**
- Disorder of abnormal thinking, behavior, & emotion. **The duration of symptoms is important.**

<u>Schizophrenia diagnostic criteria:</u>
- **≥2 of the following symptoms** — positive symptoms, negative symptoms, grossly disorganized or catatonic behavior **<u>for at least 6 months</u>.**

<u>Schizophreniform:</u>
- Symptoms of Schizophrenia but **duration between <u>1- 6 months</u>.**

<u>Brief psychotic disorder:</u>
- At least 1 psychotic symptom with onset & remission **<<u>1 month.</u>**

<u>Schizoaffective disorder:</u>
- **Schizophrenia + mood disorder** (major depressive or manic episode).

SCHIZOPHRENIA

- **Disorder of abnormal thinking, behavior, & emotion.**
- ~1% of population. Men & women are affected equally but men present earlier (early to mid 20s) compared to late 20s as seen in women. Rarely initially presents before 15 or after 55 years.
- **Strong genetic predisposition** — 50% concordance among monozygotic twins. 40% risk if both parents have schizophrenia. 12% risk if a first-degree relative is affected.
- Substance use is common — nicotine most common (>50%), alcohol, cannabis, and cocaine.
- **Better prognosis: later age at onset, acute onset, positive symptoms,** good social support, female gender, few relapses, good premorbid function, mood symptoms, & no family history.
- **Worse prognosis: early age of onset, gradual onset, negative symptoms,** poor social support, male gender, many relapses, poor premorbid function.

PATHOPHYSIOLOGY
- **Several studies postulate that the development of Schizophrenia results from abnormalities in multiple neurotransmitters, such as dopaminergic, serotonergic**, and alpha-adrenergic hyperactivity or glutaminergic and GABA hypoactivity.
- The **positive symptoms are thought to be due to excess dopamine in the mesolimbic pathway;** negative symptoms due to dopamine imbalance in the mesocortical pathway.

LABORATORY EVALUATION
- Urine toxicology to rule out reversible causes for symptoms, such use of recreational drugs.
- ECG: check baseline QTc interval before starting antipsychotic.
- Serum labs: CBC, electrolytes including calcium & magnesium (rule out delirium & hyperglycemia), LFTs, thyroid stimulating hormone (rule out hypothyroidism), 24-h cortisol (rule out Hypercortisolism), fasting glucose to rule out metabolic causes & have a baseline. HIV & Syphilis.

DIAGNOSTIC CRITERIA
- **[1] ≥2 of the following 5 symptoms at least 6 months — positive symptoms, such as (1) hallucinations, (2) delusions, (3) disorganized speech, (4) grossly disorganized or catatonic behavior; (5) negative symptoms** (eg, diminished emotional expression or avolition).
- **[2] At least 1 of these symptoms must be hallucination, delusion, or disorganized speech & must manifest for at least a 1-month period.**
- **[3] Must impair function in one or more major areas of life** (eg, work, social or interpersonal relationships, self-care) substantially below the level achieved prior to the onset of symptoms.
- Symptoms not due to the effects of a substance, medication, or medical condition

HALLUCINATIONS **Auditory**	Sound or a voice. Voice often in "3rd person" or can be command hallucinations. **Auditory hallucinations (most common type).**
Visual	Simple (flashing light) or complex (eg, seeing faces).
Olfactory	Stench or foul smells common.
Tactile	Insects on skin or being touched.
Somatic	Sensation arising from within the body.
Gustatory	Can be a part of persecutory delusions (tasting poison in food).

DELUSIONS	A fixed belief held with strong conviction despite evidence to the contrary
Persecutory	Person or force is interfering with them, observing them or wishes harm to the patient
Reference	Random events take on a personal significance (directed at them).
Control	Some agency takes control of the patient's thoughts, feelings & behaviors.
Grandiose	Unrealistic beliefs in one's powers & abilities.
Nihilism	Exaggerated belief in the futility of everything & catastrophic events.
Erotomania	Believes another person is in love with them.
Jealousy	Somebody is suspected of being unfaithful.
Doubles	Believes a family member or close person has been replaced by an identical double.

Positive symptoms: these symptoms are "added to" normal behavior
- **Hallucinations** (sensory perception without physical stimuli) — **auditory most common,** visual, gustatory, tactile, olfactory, or somatic.
- **Delusions** (firmed, fixed beliefs despite evidence to the contrary) — **persecutory, grandiose,** reference, control, nihilism, erotomania, doubles, & jealousy.
- **Disorganized speech** — thoughts are disconnected & tangential rambling.
- Behavioral disturbances.

Negative symptoms: these symptoms "take away" from normal behavior. **6 As** –
- **Absence of normal cognition** — impairment in attention, working memory, & executive function.
- **Affect flattening** — poor eye contact, unchanging facial expression, little change in affect, little spontaneous movement, lack of vocal inflections.
- **Alogia** — poverty of speech, increased latency of response.
- **Avolition** (lack of will) — poor hygiene & grooming, anergy, failure of proper role responsibilities.
- **Anhedonia** — lack of interest in stimulating activities, intimacy, or sex.
- **Asociality** — failure to engage with others socially, socially withdrawn.

Not part of diagnostic criteria but findings asked on exams:
Neuroimaging:
- **CT scan** — **ventricular enlargement** (lateral & third); **decreased cortical volume** & grey matter.
- PET scan — hypoactive frontal lobes, hyperactivity in the basal ganglion.

MANAGEMENT OF SCHIZOPHRENIA
- **Second-generation (atypical) antipsychotics** first-line management for Schizophrenia — eg, **Risperidone, Aripiprazole, Olanzapine, Quetiapine, Ziprasidone, Cariprazine, & Lurasidone.** Mechanism of action **Serotonin & Dopamine antagonists (SDAs): serotonin (5-HT2A and 5-HT1A) antagonists & dopamine antagonists (D4 & D3 > D2 receptors) in the ventral striatum** (Clozapine and Quetiapine are weak D2 antagonists), as well as histamine, muscarinic (cholinergic), and alpha-adrenergic antagonism. They calm the patient, blunt emotional responses, reduce hallucinosis and aggressive and impulsive behavior, while leaving cognitive functions relatively intact. Lower risk of extrapyramidal adverse effects but increased risk of metabolic adverse effects. **Clozapine is not used first-line but is the most effective medication for treatment-resistant psychosis** (eg, after 2 medications have been tried). Medications should be tried for at least 4 weeks before efficacy is determined. **Aripiprazole is unique in that it is a partial agonist at the dopamine (D2) and serotonin 5-HT1A receptors and an antagonist at the serotonin 5-HT2A receptor.**
- First-generation (typical) antipsychotics: (eg, **Haloperidol,** Droperidol, Fluphenazine, Chlorpromazine, Perphenazine, & Thioridazine). **Most effective drugs for positive symptoms (due to dopamine antagonism).** Minimal effect on negative symptoms but **increased risk of extrapyramidal symptoms (EPS), Tardive dyskinesia, & Neuroleptic malignant syndrome.**
- Behavioral therapy & family therapy.
- Long-acting IM versions of Risperidone, Fluphenazine, Paliperidone, Aripiprazole, or Haloperidol can be used in patients who don't take their oral medications regularly. Lithium.

ACUTE PSYCHOSIS
- Emergency: — **Risperidone or Aripiprazole are appropriate choices due to their relatively favorable side effect profiles**; Paliperidone can be used.
- **Severely agitated psychotic:** IM **Olanzapine, Ziprasidone, or Aripiprazole may be used (Diphenhydramine or Benztropine often given to reduce the risk of dystonia and severe EPS). IM Haloperidol may be used but has more adverse effects.** Sometimes, if clinically needed, they are given with a benzodiazepine such as Diazepam, Clonazepam, or Lorazepam to control behavioral disturbances and non-acute anxiety [eg, Haloperidol 5mg, Lorazepam 2 mg, & Benztropine 2 mg IM].
- **Hospitalize patient.** Urine toxicology to rule out substance abuse & routine labs.

ANTIPSYCHOTIC	SPECIFIC FACTS
Risperidone	• One of the most commonly agents prescribed for Schizophrenia. • Long-acting injectable form. **Greater incidence of movement disorders**.
Quetiapine	• **Lower incidence of movement disorders (extrapyramidal symptoms).**
Olanzapine	• **Higher incidence of <u>weight gain, dyslipidemia, & Diabetes mellitus</u>.** • Olanzapine & Clozapine have the highest risk of metabolic abnormalities. • Orthostatic hypotension, transaminase elevations.
Clozapine	• **Not first-line due to <u>increased risk of agranulocytosis & myocarditis</u>.** • **Best drug for medication-refractory Schizophrenia.** • Decreased incidence of suicide and depression.
Ziprasidone	• **Higher risk of <u>prolonged QT interval.</u>** • **Less likely to cause significant weight gain**. Must be taken with food.
Aripiprazole	• Unique mechanism – partial dopamine (D2) & 5-HT1A agonism. • **Little or no hyperglycemia, dyslipidemia, hyperprolactinemia, or weight gain vs others.** Less sedation but **<u>increased risk of Akathisia</u>.**
Lurasidone	• Safer for use in pregnancy. Less sedation. Must be taken with food. • Can be used in Bipolar depression. Higher risk of Akathisia.

ADVERSE EFFECTS OF ALL ANTIPSYCHOTICS

Extrapyramidal symptoms (EPS):

- **<u>EPS</u> due to dopamine blockade in nigrostriatal pathway, especially with the first-generation (typical agents) Haloperidol and Fluphenazine due to higher affinity for the D2 receptor.**
- Second-generation (atypical) antipsychotics are associated with less EPS and anticholinergic side effects as compared to traditional antipsychotics.
- **<u>Acute dystonia</u> muscle spasms of the face, neck, tongue, and other muscles** leading to abnormal movements or postures as well as trouble swallowing. Most common within 3-4 hours to days of use. **Management: Anticholinergics (Benztropine, Diphenhydramine,** Trihexyphenidyl).
- **<u>Parkinsonism</u>** resting tremor, rigidity, bradykinesia. Occurs within 3 days – weeks. **Management: Anticholinergics (Benztropine, Diphenhydramine,** Trihexyphenidyl).
- **<u>Akathisia</u> sustained feeling of motion or restlessness** may occur after a month – 3 months of use. <u>Management:</u> **Benzodiazepines &/or Beta blockers**. Anticholinergic (Benztropine).
- **<u>Tardive dyskinesia</u> repetitive, involuntary, stereotypical movements like grimacing, chewing, lip-smacking, writhing movement of hands**. TD is most common in older women after at least 6 months of therapy, usually after years. <u>Management:</u> **stop high potency D2 blockers and switch to atypicals (Clozapine preferred — Clozapine is unusual in that it suppresses Tardive dyskinesia) or Quetiapine.** Vitamin E has been shown to prevent further deterioration of Tardive dyskinesia. **Valbenazine and Deutetrabenazine may also help TD.**

Hyperprolactinemia:

- **Dopamine 2 receptor (D2) blockade in the tuberoinfundibular pathway results in hyperprolactinemia** (normally dopamine inhibits prolactin). Prominent with Risperidone.

Metabolic adverse effects: 2nd generation > 1st generation.

- **Hyperlipidemia, weight gain, hyperglycemia, and hypertension**.
- **Dyslipidemia, significant weight gain, and hyperglycemia due to a diabetogenic action occur with several of the second-generation agents, especially Olanzapine and Clozapine**.
- Aripiprazole has little or no tendency to cause hyperglycemia, hyperprolactinemia, or weight gain.
- **<u>Aripiprazole & Ziprasidone</u> associated with <u>LOWEST amount of weight gain & dyslipidemia</u>**.

QT prolongation

- **Prolonged QT can be seen with most of the atypicals, especially Quetiapine and Ziprasidone.**
- **Thioridazine,** a low-potency typical antipsychotic, is associated with prolonged QT and increased incidence of Ventricular arrhythmias.

Anti-HAM effects: AntiHistamine, AntiAdrenergic, and AntiMuscarinic (anticholinergic) effects.
- **AntiHistaminic effects: weight gain and sedation** especially with Chlorpromazine and less with Aripiprazole, Lurasidone, and Haloperidol. Weight gain (5H1 and 5HT-2 blockade).
- **AntiAdrenergic effects: Orthostatic hypotension** (due to alpha adrenoreceptor blockade). Sexual side effects, and tachycardia.
- **AntiMuscarinic (anticholinergic) effects include dry mouth, constipation, urinary retention, and visual problems are often pronounced with the use of Thioridazine and Chlorpromazine, as well as Clozapine and most of the atypical drugs but not with Ziprasidone or Aripiprazole.** Confusion due to blockage of the muscarinic receptors.

Neuroleptic malignant syndrome (NMS):
- **Suspect NMS if ≥2 of the 4 cardinal clinical features [1] mental status change, [2] rigidity, [3] fever, or [4] dysautonomia appear in the setting of antipsychotic use or dopamine withdrawal.**
- Malignant hyperthermic syndrome characterized by **lead pipe muscle rigidity**, impairment of sweating, hyperpyrexia (high fever), autonomic instability (unstable vital signs), increased WBCs, Rhabdomyolysis (increased creatine kinase, hyperkalemia), **hyporeflexia.**
- Management: **immediate discontinuation of the antipsychotic (first line),** supportive (IV fluids & cooling blankets), **start Benzodiazepines** (Lorazepam, Diazepam) **& add Dantrolene if moderate to severe** (Dantrolene is a muscle relaxant blocks calcium & most effective for the rigidity & fever). **May have to add Dopamine agonists (Bromocriptine, Amantadine).**

NEUROLEPTIC MALIGNANT SYNDROME

Fever (most common presenting symptom) + **"ALTERED"** mental status
Autonomic instability - tachycardia, tachypnea, hyperthermia, fever, blood pressure changes, hypersalivation, diaphoresis & **incontinence**.
Lead-pipe muscle rigidity – almost universal.
Tremor
Elevated WBC (leukocytosis) & CPK, LDH & LFTs (rhabdomyolysis)
Regular-sized pupils (distinguishes it from mydriasis in Serotonin syndrome)
Excessive sweating (diaphoresis)
Delirium (altered mental status changes), **Decreased DTR** (hypOreflexia)

Management:
- **Prompt immediate discontinuation of the antipsychotic** (first-line),
- supportive: IV fluids and cooling blankets
- **Benzodiazepines (eg, Lorazepam or Diazepam) (especially if agitated), along with Dantrolene** in moderate to severe cases (Dantrolene is a muscle relaxant most effective for the rigidity and fever).
- **Dopamine agonists:** (eg, Bromocriptine, Amantadine) may be added.

FIRST-GENERATION ANTIPSYCHOTICS

High-potency antipsychotics (descending order)	Advantages	Disadvantages
Haloperidol Fluphenazine Perphenazine	Fewer side effects of sedation and hypotension Able to use long-acting depot injections Can be given IM in acute situations	High association with extrapyramidal symptoms
Chlorpromazine	Lower frequency of extrapyramidal side effects	Greater incidence of anticholinergic effects, sedation. Corneal deposits
Thioridazine		Retinal deposits Prolonged QT

CLOZAPINE

- Benefits:
    - **(1) most effective medication for treatment-resistant psychosis** (eg, after at least 2 medications have been tried for at least 6 weeks), probably due to its significant D4 and 5HT2 receptor-blocking actions.
    - **(2) decreased suicide risk** and decreased incidence of depression.
    - **(3) useful for patients who develop Tardive dyskinesia** — Clozapine is unusual in that it suppresses Tardive dyskinesia.
- **Clozapine is not used first-line due to its adverse effects of Myocarditis, agranulocytosis (1-2%), & seizures**, especially at higher doses. **Increased weight gain, sedation, & hyperglycemia.**
- Indications: treatment resistant Schizophrenia — Clozapine may be indicated if symptoms still persist after 6 weeks of therapy with 2 different antipsychotics, one of which is a second generation.
- Monitoring: Before initiating treatment with Clozapine, the patient's baseline absolute neutrophil count must be $1500/mm^3$ or greater for the general population. **Clozapine should be regularly monitored with CBC measurements for the duration of therapy.**

TRAUMA & STRESSOR-RELATED DISORDERS

ACUTE STRESS DISORDER

- **Acute stress disorder (ASD) is characterized by acute stress reactions that may <u>occur in the initial month</u> after a person is exposed to a traumatic event (threatened death, serious injury, sexual violation, etc.), lasting for <u>3 days–30 days</u>.**

DIAGNOSTIC CRITERIA
- **[1] Symptoms similar to PTSD except the traumatic event occurred < 1 month ago and the symptoms last 3 days <u>up to 1 month</u> after the trauma exposure.**
- [2] The symptoms include intrusive symptoms, avoidance, increased arousal, and negative alterations in thought and mood (see PTSD for list of symptoms).
- [3] The disturbance causes clinically significant distress or impairment in social, occupational, or other important areas of functioning.
- [4] The disturbance is not attributable to the physiological effects of a substance (eg, medication or alcohol) or another medical condition.

MANAGEMENT
- **<u>Cognitive behavioral therapy:</u> <u>Counseling & Trauma-focused cognitive-behavioral therapy (CBT)</u> as first-line treatment of patients with acute stress disorder (ASD) rather than other psychotherapies or medication** because by definition the symptoms will resolve in 1 month.
- Exposure, a component of trauma-focused CBT, has been found to be more effective when provided as monotherapy than cognitive restructuring in patients with ASD.
- **If symptoms > 1 month, treat as PTSD.**
- Pharmacotherapy: For patients with ASD and acute, intense anxiety, agitation, or sleep disturbance in the immediate period following the traumatic event, adjunctive treatment with a Benzodiazepine rather than other medications may be considered but should be limited to 2-4 weeks.

- **EXAM TIP**
- Posttraumatic stress disorder (PTSD) and Acute stress disorder (ASD) have the same symptoms. The difference is time of event & duration of symptoms.
- **ASD: trauma occurs < 1 month AND symptoms < 1 month in duration.**
- **PTSD: trauma occurred at any time in the past >1 month OR symptoms > 1 month.**

POSTTRAUMATIC STRESS DISORDER (PTSD)

- **Long-lasting anxiety response**: PSTD is a syndrome resulting from exposure to real, threatened, or perceived serious or life-threatening injury (**traumatic or catastrophic event**) with **symptoms lasting > 1 month &/or the event occurred >1 month ago.**

DIAGNOSTIC CRITERIA
- **[A] Stressor: Exposure to actual or threatened death, serious injury, or sexual violence** via (1) direct experience of the traumatic event, (2) witnessing the event in person, (3) learning the event happened to someone close (family member or friend) or (4) experiencing extreme or repeated exposure to aversive details of the traumatic event (eg, military combat, sexual or physical assault, childhood sexual abuse, natural disasters, sudden death of a loved one, severe medical illness).
- **[B] Recurrent intrusions: Presence of at least 1 of the following intrusion symptoms** after the event that may lead to significant distress or impairment in function (eg, occupational, social, or other areas). **Re-experiencing: >1 month** of recurrent intrusions, such as **repetitive recollections (eg, distressing dreams, nightmares, memories) & dissociative reactions** (eg, **flashbacks** in which the person feels/acts as if the event is recurring), leading to physiologic distress &/or physiologic reactions. **Intense distress at exposure to cues relating to the trauma**; or physiological reactions to cues relating to the trauma.
- **[C] Active avoidance of triggering stimuli** associated with the traumatic event (reminders of the events, such as memories, feelings, people, places, objects).
- **[D] Negative alterations in mood: ≥2 negative alterations in cognition & mood**: inability to remember an important aspect of the event, dissociative amnesia, negative feelings of self, world or others, **anhedonia, intense negative emotions** (eg, horror guilt, anger or shame, self-blame, sadness, guilt), **dissociation** (eg, feelings of detachment from oneself or reality), or inability to experience or express positive emotions.
- **[E] Alterations in arousal & reactivity: at least 2 arousal & reactivity symptoms: angry outbursts, irritable behavior, reckless or self-destructive behaviors, hypervigilance, sleep disturbances, concentration issues, & exaggerated startle response.**
- **[F] Duration: Symptoms last >1 month. Traumatic event occurred anytime in the past** (may occur immediately after the trauma or with delayed expression).
- [G] The disturbance causes significant functional impairment or distress in various areas of life, such as social or occupational.
- [H] Symptoms not the direct cause of a substance or another medical condition.

MANAGEMENT
Behavioral therapy:
- **For most adults newly treated for PTSD, first-line treatment with a Trauma-focused psychotherapy that includes exposure rather than a serotonergic reuptake inhibitor (SRI) is often recommended.**
- **Trauma-focused psychotherapy is considered as the first-line treatment** in adults as well as children, and it includes **Trauma-focused CBT (cognitive-behavioral therapy),** Eye movement desensitization and reprocessing (EMDR), Cognitive processing therapy, and Imaginal exposure.

Pharmacotherapy:
- **Serotonergic reuptake inhibitor (SRI): SSRIs first-line medical treatment** (eg, **Sertraline & Paroxetine are FDA-approved;** Citalopram, Sertraline, Fluoxetine) **or SNRIs (eg, Venlafaxine).** Tricyclic antidepressants (eg, Imipramine). MAO inhibitors. May be augmented with atypical antipsychotics.
- **Trazodone may be helpful for insomnia.**
- **Prazosin is an alpha-1 agonist that can be an augmenting agent to SRIs; may be used to reduce nightmares, sleep disturbance, and some symptoms, such as hypervigilance (off-label use).**
- Prazosin and Clonidine are useful in decreasing trauma-related nightmares.
- Clonidine and Guanfacine may be used for agitation.

ADJUSTMENT DISORDER

- **Adjustment disorder occurs when <u>maladaptive behavioral or emotional symptoms</u> develop after a stressful or <u>non-life-threatening</u> event** — eg, relationship issues (eg, divorce, breakups, marital problems, getting married), death of a loved one, work issues (eg, loss of a job, failing to meet goals), having a baby, serious health issues, school issues, financial difficulties.

CLINICAL MANIFESTATIONS:
- **One or both of the following — [1] <u>marked distress out of proportion to the severity</u> of stressor and/or [2] <u>significant impairment</u> in areas of functioning (eg, occupational, social, etc.).**
- <u>Common stressors</u> in adults include job loss, physical illness, leaving home, divorce, new parenthood; in children, parenteral rejection or divorce, moving homes or school, school issues are common.
- May manifest as depressed mood, lack of enjoyment, anxiety, hopelessness, disturbance of conduct, nervousness, anxiety, desperation, feeling overwhelmed and thoughts of suicide, performing poorly in school/work etc.

DIAGNOSTIC CRITERIA
- **Maladaptive emotional or behavioral reaction to an identifiable stressor or a non-life-threatening event that causes a disproportionate response** than would normally be expected **<u>beginning within 3 months of the stressor</u>** (does not include bereavement) & **<u>resolves usually within 6 months of the stressor</u>.**
- These symptoms produce either excessive distress in relation to the event or significant impairment in daily functioning.
- The stress-related disturbance does not meet criteria for another mental disorder.

MANAGEMENT:
- **<u>Supportive psychotherapy</u> initial management of choice,** including individual or group therapy.
- Medications may be used in selected cases, but they are not the preferred treatment.
- Patients may self-medicate with alcohol or other drugs.

PROGNOSIS
- Unlike major depression, Adjustment disorder is caused by an outside stressor and generally resolves once the individual is able to adapt to the situation.

MALINGERING

- **[1] Intentional falsification or exaggeration** of signs & symptoms of a medical or psychiatric illness for **[2] <u>external (secondary) gain</u>** — eg, **financial gain (insurance money, lawsuits), food, shelter,** avoidance of prison, school, work, military services, to obtain drugs (eg, narcotics).
- **Malingering is NOT a mental illness.**
- Malingering should be suspected in the presence of any combination of the following: medicolegal presentation, marked discrepancy between the claimed distress and the objective findings, lack of cooperation during evaluation and in complying with prescribed treatment, or presence of an antisocial personality disorder.

Both factitious disorder and Malingering are associated with intentionally faking signs and symptoms.
- The difference is that in **Malingering, they <u>feign illness for secondary gain</u> whereas in Factitious disorder the primary motive is to 'assume the sick role' & get sympathy.**

SOMATIC SYMPTOM & RELATED DISORDERS

- Somatic symptom and related disorders are diagnoses characterized by prominent somatic concerns, distress, and impaired functioning.

SOMATIC SYMPTOM DISORDER (Formerly Somatization Disorder)

- **Chronic condition in which the patient has [1] <u>prominent physical symptoms</u> involving at least 1 body system, but [2] no physical cause found on workup and [3] is associated with significant distress or functional impairment (excessive thoughts, feelings, &/or behaviors).**
- May or may not be associated with other medical condition. An event may precede the symptoms.

EPIDEMIOLOGY
- **Most common in young women** (10:1) with onset usually before 30 years age.
- **Risk factors:** Older age, unemployment, history of sexual abuse, fewer years of education, & lower socioeconomic status.

CLINICAL MANIFESTATIONS
- **<u>Excessive thoughts, feelings, or behaviors related to the somatic physical symptoms</u>** — disproportionate & persistent thoughts about the seriousness of the symptoms, persistently high level of anxiety about symptoms or health, or excessive time & energy devoted to the symptoms & health concerns. **Patients often express lots of concerns regarding their symptoms and chronically perseverate over them.**
- They frequently seek treatment from many medical providers, resulting in extensive lab work, diagnostic procedures, hospitalizations, and/or surgeries.
- **The symptoms may change but the disorder persists.**

DIAGNOSTIC CRITERIA
- **[A] ≥1 vague physical symptoms that result in significant distress or significant disruption of daily life.** These symptoms cannot be explained by a physical or medical cause. At least 2 symptoms increase the likelihood of somatization disorder.
- [B] At least 1 of the followings: (1) <u>thoughts</u> disproportionate and persistent thoughts about the seriousness of one's symptoms; (2) <u>emotions</u>: persistently high level of anxiety about health or symptoms; (3) <u>behaviors</u> such as excessive time and energy devoted to these symptoms.
- [C] **The state of being symptomatic is persistent (<u>usually >6 months</u>),** although any one of the somatic symptoms may not be continuously present (the specific symptoms may shift over time).
Specifiers:
- **With predominant pain** (previously Pain disorder in DSM IV) & Persistent.

MANAGEMENT
- **<u>Supportive care:</u> <u>Regularly-scheduled appointments</u> with a single provider for close follow-up and develop a therapeutic alliance with the patient** in which the primary care clinician offers continued reassurance, acknowledge health fears, communicate and coordinate care with other clinicians, improve coping skills while not dismissing their fears, evaluate for and treat diagnosable general medical disease, limit diagnostic tests and referrals to specialists, educate patients about coping with health anxiety, and other supportive care.
- **<u>Psychotherapy</u> (eg, Cognitive behavioral therapy) and when possible, the psychiatrist should work closely with the patient's primary care provider**. Patients may be reticent to seek mental health counseling because they truly believe there is an organic cause.
- Pharmacologic therapy should be limited, but antidepressants can be initiated to treat psychiatric comorbidities (anxiety, depressive symptoms, obsessive-compulsive disorder). Selective serotonin reuptake inhibitors (SSRIs) and Serotonin-norepinephrine reuptake inhibitors (SNRIs) have shown efficacy with an improvement of SSD compared to placebo.

ILLNESS ANXIETY DISORDER (formerly HYPOCHONDRIASIS)

- **Illness anxiety disorder is characterized by <u>excessive concern or preoccupation about having or developing a serious, undiagnosed general medical disease.</u>**
- Illness anxiety disorder is in the category called Somatic symptom and related disorders, which are diagnoses characterized by prominent somatic concerns, distress, and impaired functioning.

EPIDEMIOLOGY
- Most common in early adulthood (onset usually 20-30 years of age); rarely begins after the age of 50y.
- **Comorbid disorders — Generalized anxiety disorder (71%) and Depressive disorders** [Dysthymia (persistent depressive disorder in 45%), Unipolar major depression (43%)], phobias (43%), Panic disorder (17%), and Substance use disorder (17%).

CLINICAL MANIFESTATIONS
[1] Excessive concern about an illness:
- **The patient's distress comes primarily from an unfounded fear of having a disease rather than physical symptoms**, and persists despite appropriate physical examination, medical workup, and laboratory testing that are negative.
- Patients may be preoccupied with a particular diagnosis (eg, cancer or HIV infection), a bodily function (eg, bowel movements), normal variation in function (eg, in heart rate or blood pressure), or vague somatic sensation (eg, "tired heart").

[2] Minimal to nonexistent somatic symptoms
- **Physical symptoms are not present, or they are minimal and often represent a misperception of normal bodily sensations** (distinguishes it from Somatic symptom disorder).

DSM V DIAGNOSTIC CRITERIA
Requires each of the following criteria:
- [A] **Preoccupation with having or developing a serious illness**.
- [B] **Somatic symptoms are not present, or if present, mild in intensity**. If a general medical illness is present or the risk for acquiring a medical illness is high (eg, strong family history), the preoccupation is clearly excessive.
- [C] High level of anxiety about health and a low threshold for becoming alarmed about one's health.
- [D] Either of the following: **1. Excessive health-related behaviors**, such as repeatedly checking oneself for signs of illness **or 2. Maladaptive avoidance of situations** (eg, visiting sick family members, doctor appointments, or hospitals, doctor shopping) or activities (eg, exercise) that are thought to represent health threats.
- [E] **Preoccupation with illness or behaviors is present for at least 6 months** (the specific illness that is feared may change over time).
- [F] The illness preoccupation is not better explained by other mental disorders such as somatic symptom disorder, generalized anxiety disorder, or somatic type of delusional disorder.

MANAGEMENT
Supportive health care:
- **The primary care clinician generally plays the central role in managing patients. Management includes regularly scheduled appointments with close follow-up and develop a therapeutic alliance.**
Psychotherapy:
- **Cognitive behavioral therapy CBT) first-line management for Somatic symptom disorder.**
- <u>Second line</u>: a different psychotherapy .
- <u>Third line</u>: Antidepressant medications.
- Comorbid anxiety & depressive disorders should be treated with SSRIs or other antidepressants.

FUNCTIONAL NEUROLOGICAL SYMPTOM DISORDER (CONVERSION DISORDER)

- **Functional neurological symptom disorder is characterized by <u>neurologic symptoms</u> (eg, weakness, abnormal movements, or nonepileptic seizures) that are inconsistent with a neurologic disease, but cause distress and/or impairment.**
- **Formerly known as Conversion disorder** (patients "convert" their psychological distress into neurological symptoms).

EPIDEMIOLOGY
- 2-3 times more common in women.
- Onset at any age but more common in adolescence or early adulthood.
- High incidence of comorbid depressive, anxiety, or neurological disorder.
- Often preceded by a traumatic event.

CLINICAL MANIFESTATIONS
- **At least 1 symptom of neurologic dysfunction (voluntary motor or sensory) that cannot be explained fully by a neurological condition.**
- Patients are often calm or seem unconcerned about the deficits (*la belle indifference*).
- **Symptoms are <u>NOT</u> intentionally produced or feigned (no evidence of deceptive behavior).**
Motor dysfunction:
- **Paralysis, aphonia, mutism, psychogenic nonepileptic seizures, gait abnormalities,** involuntary abnormal movements, tics, weakness, swallowing, globus sensation (lump in throat).
Sensory dysfunction:
- **Blindness,** anesthesia, paresthesias, visual changes, & deafness. Speech deficits, sensory symptoms.
Physical examination:
- The diagnosis rests upon positive clinical findings that indicate the symptom is incongruent with anatomy, physiology, or known diseases, or is inconsistent at different times.

DIAGNOSTIC CRITERIA
- **[A] At least 1 symptom of neurologic dysfunction (altered voluntary motor or sensory function) that cannot be explained clinically & not explained by another medical or psychiatric condition.**
- [B] **Clinical findings that demonstrate incompatibility between the symptom and recognized neurologic or general medical conditions** (eg, Hoover's sign of functional limb weakness or a positive entrainment test for functional tremor).
- [C] The symptom or deficit is not better explained by another medical or mental disorder.
- [D] **The symptom or deficit causes significant distress, psychosocial impairment, or other important areas of functioning, or warrants medical evaluation.**
Specifiers:
- With weakness or paralysis
- With abnormal movement (eg, tremor, dystonic movement, myoclonus, gait disorder)
- With swallowing symptoms; with speech problems (eg, dysphonia, slurred speech)
- With attacks or seizures
- With anesthesia or sensory loss
- With special sensory symptoms (eg, visual, olfactory, or hearing disturbances)
- With mixed symptoms

MANAGEMENT
- **<u>Patient education</u> about the illness first-line treatment,** including helping the patient understand without judgment that the symptoms are being taken seriously, self-help techniques, follow-up.
- Physical therapy second line for those with motor symptoms.
- **<u>Cognitive behavioral therapy</u>** with or without physical therapy if education not successful. Insight-oriented therapy.

FACTITIOUS DISORDER

- **[1]** <u>Intentional</u> **falsification or exaggeration of signs & symptoms of medical or psychiatric illness for [2] "<u>primary gain</u>" (inner need to be seen as ill or injured and assume the role of a sick patient) but NOT for external rewards** (aka secondary gain, as seen in Malingering).

EPIDEMIOLOGY
- May be at least 1% of hospitalized patients. More common in women.
- Higher incidence in hospital and health care workers (who have learned how to feign symptoms).
- Many patients have a history of illness and hospitalization, as well as childhood physical or sexual abuse. May be associated with personality disorders.

CLINICAL MANIFESTATIONS
- **Intentional creation or exaggeration of symptoms of illness** self-induced, feigned, or **exaggerated symptoms** — eg, may hurt themselves to bring on symptoms, alter diagnostic tests, lie, or mimic symptoms [fever (by heating the thermometer), may inject themselves with substances to make themselves sick, pseudoseizures, volitional tremors, etc.]. Medical history may be dramatic but inconsistent.
- **May be willing or eager to undergo surgery repeatedly or painful tests in order to obtain sympathy.** They may "hospital hop", use other aliases, or go to different cities to access care. They often have extensive knowledge about medical terminology, hospitals, or great detail about their "illness" (may even work in healthcare). They may provide inconsistent information.

DIAGNOSTIC CRITERIA
- **[A] <u>Identified deception</u>: Intentional falsification or exaggeration of signs & symptoms of a medical or psychiatric illness for "<u>primary gain</u>" (motivation of their actions is to assume the sick role to get sympathy).**
- [B] Induction of an injury or disease with intent to deceive. The deceptive behavior is evident even in the **absence of obvious external rewards (as seen in Malingering).**
- [C] Presentation of the individual or another individual (imposed on another).
- [D] Behavior is not explained by another psychiatric disorder (eg, Delusional disorder).

MANAGEMENT
- Inform and discuss with patients about the diagnosis of Factitious (confrontation) with compassionate feedback, provide reassurance that support is available (eg, psychiatry referral) without being judgmental.
- <u>Factitious disorder imposed on self</u>: Psychotherapy is standard treatment.
- **<u>Factitious disorder imposed on another</u>: considered abuse** — child or adult protective services.

- **<u>Exam tip:</u>**
- These 5 disorders seem similar so look for these clues to differentiate them:
- <u>Somatic symptom disorder:</u> physical symptoms (at least 1 body system) with no cause on workup + no intentional falsification (they believe they are ill).
- <u>Functional neurologic disorder:</u> neurologic symptoms or deficits (sensory or motor) with no cause on workup + no intentional falsification (they believe they are ill).
- <u>Illness anxiety:</u> preoccupation one has an undiagnosed serious illness (but little to no symptoms of the illness) + no intentional falsification (they believe they are ill).
- <u>Factitious disorder:</u> intentional falsification of symptoms for primary gain (assuming the sick role or sympathy).
- <u>Malingering:</u> intentional falsification of symptoms for secondary (external) gain (eg, money, shelter, etc.).

OBSESSIVE-COMPULSIVE & RELATED DISORDERS

OBSESSIVE-COMPULSIVE DISORDER (OCD)

- **OCD is characterized by [1] <u>obsessions</u> (bothersome intrusive thoughts that elicit a feeling of discomfort) and/or [2] <u>compulsions</u> (rituals, repetitive actions, or mental acts to relieve the discomfort of the obsessions) that are time-consuming, distressing, and impairing.**
- The obsessions are usually **<u>ego-dystonic</u>** (inconsistent with one's own personal beliefs).
- **Mean age of onset 20y with 50% often present in childhood & adolescence** (onset rare after 50y).

PATHOPHYSIOLOGY
- **Theorized due to abnormal communication between the basal ganglia (eg caudate nucleus), orbitofrontal cortex, and the anterior cingulate gyrus; serotonin involved.**
- May be associated with the triad of "uncontrollable urges" — OCD, ADHD, & Tic disorders (Tourette).

CLINICAL MANIFESTATIONS
4 major patterns:
- **[1] <u>Contamination</u>** — compulsion may include cleaning, washing, or avoidance of contaminant.
- **[2] <u>Pathologic doubt or harm</u>** — eg, forgetting to unplug iron or turn off the stove, with the compulsion being checking multiple times to avoid potential danger.
- **[3] <u>Symmetry/precision</u>** — with the compulsion being ordering, counting, rearranging, repeating.
- **[4] <u>Intrusive obsessive thoughts</u>** — (eg, fear of aggression/harm), doubts, sexual or religious fears with or without compulsion (eg, reassurance-seeking).

(DSM-5) diagnostic criteria:
- [A] **Presence of obsessions, compulsions, or both: Obsessions as defined by: (1) Recurrent and persistent thoughts, urges, or images that are experienced, at some time during the disturbance, as intrusive and unwanted, and that in most individuals cause marked anxiety or distress; (2) The individual attempts to ignore or suppress such thoughts, urges, or images**, or to neutralize or replace them with some other thought or action (eg, by performing a compulsion). **Compulsions as defined by: (1) Repetitive behaviors (eg, hand washing, ordering, checking) or mental acts (eg, praying, counting, repeating words silently) that the individual feels driven to perform in response to an obsession,** or according to rules that must be applied rigidly; **(2) The behaviors or mental acts are aimed at preventing or reducing anxiety or distress or preventing some dreaded event or situation;** however, the behaviors or mental acts are not connected in a realistic way to neutralize or prevent the obsession, or are clearly excessive.
- [B] **<u>The obsessions &/or compulsions are time-consuming</u> (eg, >1 hour per day)** or cause clinically significant distress or impairment in social, occupational, or other areas of functioning.
- [C] The obsessive-compulsive symptoms are not attributable to the physiological effects of a substance (eg, a drug of abuse, a medication) or another medical condition.
- [D] The disturbance is not better explained by the symptoms of another mental disorder.
Specifiers include patient's insight and presence/history of a tic disorder.

MANAGEMENT
- **<u>Cognitive behavioral therapy:</u> first-line therapy of OCD — exposure & response prevention (CBT/ERP),** psychoeducation.
- <u>Pharmacotherapy:</u> **SSRIs first-line medical therapy** (eg, **Fluoxetine, Fluvoxamine, Sertraline, Paroxetine**) — higher doses needed compared to depressive disorders; Tricyclic antidepressants **(Clomipramine because it is the most serotonin specific)**, SNRIs (eg, Venlafaxine). Augmentation therapy with antipsychotics. **Pediatric patients: approved SSRIs are Fluoxetine, Fluvoxamine, & Sertraline.** Paroxetine, Citalopram, & Escitalopram are not used in the pediatric population.
- Combination of cognitive behavioral therapy and pharmacotherapy more effective than either alone.
- <u>Severely debilitating or resistant:</u> psychosurgery (cingulotomy) or Electroconvulsive therapy (ECT).

BODY DYSMORPHIC DISORDER

- **Body dysmorphic disorder (BDD)** is characterized by **excessive preoccupation with at least 1 perceived flaw or defect in one's physical appearance in which the individual believes they look abnormal, ugly, unattractive, or deformed that is not observable by others or appears slight to others in comparison.**
- This preoccupation often causes them to be ashamed or feel self-conscious, leading to functional impairment or significant distress.
- **May commit repetitive acts and behaviors in response to this preoccupation** of physical flaw/defect (mirror checking, skin picking, seeking reassurance) or mental acts (comparison to others), which are usually difficult to control and are not pleasurable.

EPIDEMIOLOGY
- Average age of onset 15 years of age.
- May be associated with anxiety disorder or depression.

CLINICAL MANIFESTATIONS
- Patients with BDD may present to mental health clinicians as well as clinicians, often for nonspychiatric cosmetic management of their perceived flaws (eg, dermatologists, plastic surgeons, etc.).
- The most common concerns revolve around the patient's skin, hair, nose, breasts, eyes, and stomach. Men are more commonly preoccupied with balding and genital size; Women are more preoccupied with areas with body fat (eg, hips, breasts, legs, buttocks, and waist).

DIAGNOSTIC CRITERIA
- **[A] Preoccupation with at least one nonexistent or slight defect in physical appearance (eg, thinks about the perceived defects for at least 1 hour per day).**
- **[B] Concerns about appearance lead to repetitive behaviors (eg, mirror checking, excessive grooming, or skin picking) or mental acts (eg, comparing one's appearance with that of others)** at some point during the course of the illness.
- **[C] Clinically significant distress or psychosocial impairment** resulting from the appearance concerns.
- [D] Appearance preoccupations are not better explained by an eating disorder.

SPECIFIERS
Insight:
- Fair to good — Patient recognizes that the beliefs about physical appearance are probably not true (good insight) or that they may or may not be true (fair insight).
- Poor — Patient thinks that the beliefs are probably true.
- Absent (delusional beliefs) — Beliefs are firmly held despite what others think.
Muscle dysmorphia
- If patients with BDD are preoccupied with the belief that their body build is too small or insufficiently muscular.
BDD with Panic attacks:
- If BDD triggers panic attacks (eg, after seeing oneself in the mirror).

MANAGEMENT
- **Antidepressants (eg, SSRIs) &/or Cognitive behavioral therapy tailored specifically to BDD.**
- **SSRIs: Fluoxetine, Sertraline or Escitalopram.** Fluvoxamine or Paroxetine are alternatives.
- **Augmentation therapy** if no full relief with SSRIs, add-on therapy may include a second-generation antipsychotic (eg, Aripiprazole, Buspirone, a glutamate modulator, or Clomipramine).
- **TCAs (eg, Clomipramine) are an alternative to SSRIs.**

TRICHOTILLOMANIA (HAIR PULLING DISORDER)

EPIDEMIOLOGY
- 1-2% of the adult population. **More common in women** (10:1).
- Onset usually at puberty and often associated with a stressful event.
- **Increased incidence of comorbid OCD, excoriation (skin picking disorder) & Major depressive disorder.**

CLINICAL MANIFESTATIONS
- **Difficulty resisting an urge to control pulling their hair out.** Hair loss usually involves the scalp, eyebrows, or eyelashes. May include facial, axillary, or pubic hair.

Physical examination:
- **Trichoscopy: decreased hair density, coarse hairs in the affected area and broken hair of different lengths, short vellus hairs.**
- May have a **round patch of alopecia on the vertex with a tonsure pattern ("Friar tuck sign").**

DIAGNOSTIC CRITERIA
- **[A] Recurrent pulling of hair, resulting in hair loss. Usually involves the scalp, eyebrows, or eyelashes. May include facial, axillary, or pubic hair.**
- **[B] Repeated attempts to stop or minimize hair pulling.**
- [C] Causes significant distress or impairment in daily functioning.
- [D] Not due to another medication, medical condition, or psychiatric disorder.

MANAGEMENT
- **Cognitive behavior therapy (CBT) first line therapy — eg, habit reversal training.**
- Pharmacologic management: SSRIs, second generation antipsychotics, N-acetylcysteine, or Lithium

HOARDING DISORDER

EPIDEMIOLOGY
- **Most prevalent in the elderly population but behavior often begins in the early teens** (mean age at onset of hoarding symptoms around 16.5 years old).

DIAGNOSTIC CRITERIA
All 6 criteria must be met:
- **[A] Persistent difficulty discarding possession, regardless of their actual value resulting in accumulation of a large number of possessions that may clutter living spaces.**
- [B] Difficulty is due to the need to save the possessions with distress associated with discarding them.
- [C] The difficulty discarding possessions results in the accumulation of possessions that congest and clutter active living areas and substantially compromises their intended use. If living areas are uncluttered, it is only because of the interventions of third parties (eg, family members, authorities).
- [D] The hoarding causes clinically significant distress or impairment in social, occupational, or other important areas of functioning (including maintaining a safe environment for self and others).
- [E] The hoarding is not attributable to another medical condition.
- (F) The hoarding is not better explained by the symptoms of another mental disorder.

MANAGEMENT
Psychotherapy
- **Cognitive behavioral therapy specific for hoarding first-line treatment (very difficult to treat).**

Resistant to initial CBT:
- **Cognitive remediation rather than pharmacologic management, is recommended for individuals who do not respond to initial treatment with CBT.**
- Pharmacologic management: SSRIs can be used (not as effective unless concurrent OCD).

NARCOLEPSY

- Long-term neurological disorder characterized by decreased ability to regulate sleep-wake cycles.
- Elements of sleep interfere with wakefulness and elements of wakefulness interferes with sleep.

CLINICAL MANIFESTATIONS

- **Chronic daytime sleepiness: patients are prone to fall asleep throughout the day and develop sudden sleep attacks (rapid dozing off without warning), often at inappropriate times.**
- **Cataplexy: emotionally triggered transient loss of muscle tone** (eg, excitement, laughter, anger). **The muscle weakness often begins in the face** (eg, slack, ptosis, hypotonic face with an open mouth) and often affects the neck and knees. Patients may develop bilateral weakness or paralysis.
- **Hypnagogic hallucinations: Hallucinations when falling asleep or awakening** (eg, vivid visual, tactile, or auditory hallucinations).
- **Sleep paralysis:** complete inability to move for 1-2 minutes immediately after waking or before falling asleep. May develop other sleeping disorders (eg, fragmented sleep, Obstructive sleep apnea).

WORKUP

- Thorough medical history, history and physical examination, sleep history, and neurologic examination. Workup usually includes both polysomnography and multiple sleep latency testing.
- **Polysomnography:** excludes alternative and/or coexisting causes of daytime sleepiness.
  Narcolepsy: spontaneous awakenings, mild reduced sleep efficiency, increased light non-REM sleep, REM sleep within 15 minutes after the onset of sleep (healthy individuals usually experience REM sleep 80-100 minutes after the onset of sleep).

- **Multiple sleep latency test:** identifies the sleep onset rapid eye movements and measure the mean sleep latency. The patient is placed in a sleep-inducing environment & instructed to try to fall asleep.
  - On average, healthy patients fall asleep within 10-15 minutes.
  - Narcolepsy: often fall asleep < 8 minutes. The naps include **sleep onset rapid eye movements.**
  - Prior to testing, patients should discontinue antidepressants 3 weeks prior (4 weeks for Fluoxetine) and stimulants or psychoactive medications should be stopped 1 week prior.

MANAGEMENT

- **Sleep hygiene: Daytime naps & regular, adequate sleep schedule, caffeine & alcohol avoidance are the mainstays of nonpharmacologic therapy.** These improves alertness & function.
- **Mild to moderate sleepiness — initial trial of Modafinil (wake-promoting medication).** Reasonable first-line wake-promoting medications include Armodafinil, Pitolisant, & Solriamfetol. **Modafinil:** improves control of sleepiness, promotes wakefulness early into the evening.
  - Mechanism: exact mechanism unknown but thought to inhibit dopamine reuptake, increasing dopaminergic signaling. Adverse effects: headache, dry mouth, diarrhea, decreased appetite, nausea, increased blood pressure (used cautiously with arrhythmia or heart disease).
  Solriamfetol: oral selective dopamine and norepinephrine reuptake inhibitor, improving wakefulness. Similar adverse effects to Modafinil.
- **Severe/disabling sleepiness — For patients with severe and disabling sleepiness with or without cataplexy, treatment with Oxybates** rather than other wake-promoting medications may be indicated. Alternatives in patients who are not candidates for oxybates include Solriamfetol or moderate to high doses of stimulants (Methylphenidate, Amphetamines) or combination therapy.

Cataplexy
- **REM-suppressing medications:** eg, Fluoxetine, Venlafaxine, Atomoxetine. Sodium oxybate alternative.
- **Residual cataplexy —** For patients with mild to moderate sleepiness who respond well to a first-line wake-promoting agent but have disruptive cataplexy, add a REM-suppressing medications — serotonergic antidepressant with anti-cataplexy effects (eg, Venlafaxine). An alternative is to add or switch to Pitolisant. For more severe cataplexy, Oxybates can be added.
- **Sleepiness and cataplexy: Oxybates (eg, Sodium oxybate or mixed oxybate sales) and Pitolisant.**

PARASOMNIAS THAT OCCUR UPON AROUSAL FROM NREM SLEEP

- Confusional arousals, Sleep terrors, and Sleepwalking are usually seen in toddlers and school-aged children. ≥1 of these parasomnias may occur in the same child.
- Most patients show gradual, spontaneous resolution of the events over months to years. However, sleepwalking has a greater tendency to continue into adolescence compared with sleep terrors or confusional arousals.
- **Management:** patients & their parents should be **reassured that parasmonias are benign**, usually resolve within a few years, and discuss environmental safety issues to prevent harm or self-injury. Avoiding sleep deprivation may reduce the frequency of sleep terrors.
- Sleepwalking may require cautious short-term use of long-acting benzodiazepine for safety considerations if severe (eg, Clonazepam).

CLINICAL FEATURE	SLEEP (NIGHT) TERROR	CONFUSIONAL AROUSAL	SLEEPWALKING
Age of onset	2-10 years of age	2-10 years of age	5-12 years of age
Peak time of occurrence	First one-third of night sleep	First one-third of night sleep (2-3 hours of sleep onset).	First one-third of night sleep
Behavior during event	• **Arousal (abrupt wakening from sleep) with panicky screams or crying accompanied by <u>fear and signs of autonomic arousal</u>,** such as **tachycardia, sweating, flushed face, rapid breathing, agitation,** and inconsolable (may become more agitated when consoled). • The child may jump out of bed as if running away from an unseen threat. • Patients with sleep terror disorder have **<u>no recollection of a dream or the episode</u>,** which causes distress or impairment in social or occupational functioning.	• **Whimpering, crying, moaning, may utter words** (eg, "no" "go away"). • **Sitting up in bed,** • **Appear distressed or inconsolable.** • Usually none of the signs of autonomic arousal (eg, sweating, flushed face, etc.) • Has no recollection of the event.	• **Walking around in the house.** • May be quiet or agitated. • **Unresponsive to verbal commands.** • Inappropriate behaviors may be seen. • May injure themselves by unconsciously carrying out behaviors (eg, leaving the house). • Autonomic dysfunction may also occur (eg, sweating and flushing of the face).
EEG during event	Slow-wave sleep with rhythmic theta or delta activity	Slow-wave sleep with rhythmic theta or delta activity	Slow-wave sleep with rhythmic theta or delta activity
Duration	10-20 minutes	10-30 minutes	10-20 minutes
Frequency	3-4/week to 1-2/month	3-4/week to 1-2/month	3-4/week to 1-2/month

FEEDING AND EATING DISORDERS

OBESITY

- **Body mass index (BMI) ≥30 kg/m² or body weight ≥20% over the ideal weight.**

COMPLICATIONS
- Obesity increases risk for coronary disease, Diabetes mellitus II, breast & colon cancers.
- ~50% of patients experience Binge eating episodes

MANAGEMENT
- <u>Lifestyle behavioral modification:</u> exercise & dietary changes, group therapy for weight management.
- <u>Medical therapy:</u> antidepressants if there is underlying depression. Treat any complications.
- **<u>Weight loss medications</u>: Subcutaneous Tirzepatide or Semaglutide first line; Liraglutide.** <u>Alternatives</u>: **Phentermine-Topiramate**; Naltrexone-Bupropion; Orlistat (decreases fat digestion). Lorcaserin ± Liraglutide. Avoid Phentermine if cardiovascular disease or uncontrolled Hypertension.
- **<u>Surgical options</u>: gastric bypass, gastric sleeve, gastric banding, & bariatric surgery.** Candidates include adults with a BMI ≥35 kg/m², or a BMI of 30-34.9 kg/m² with type 2 diabetes mellitus.
- <u>SCREENING:</u> USPSTF recommends for screening all adults and children age ≥6 years.

BINGE-EATING DISORDER

- **Eating disorder characterized by [1] <u>frequent & recurrent binge eating episodes</u>** associated negative psychological & social problems **[2] <u>without compensatory behaviors</u> of Bulimia nervosa.**
- May have low impulse control activity in the prefrontal cortex, inferior frontal gyrus, and insula.

EPIDEMIOLOGY
- Binge eating disorder is more common in women than men. More common in obese individuals.

CLINICAL MANIFESTATIONS
- **<u>Weight fluctuations</u> (eg, weight gain);** may be triggered by stress, mood changes, or emotions.
- **<u>Ego-dystonic</u> (troublesome to the patient and patients are embarrassed by their binge eating).** Dysphoria can occur after a binge, along with remorse and self-loathing.

DIAGNOSTIC CRITERIA
- **[A] <u>Recurrent episodes of binge eating</u> — recurrent episodes characterized by eating within a discrete time (eg a 2-hour period) an unusually large amount of food** (more than most people would in a similar period) with **<u>lack of control during an overeating episode.</u>** Binge eating episodes are marked by at least 3 of the following: eating more rapidly than normal, eating until feeling uncomfortably full, eating large amounts of food when not feeling physically hungry, eating alone because of embarrassment by the amount of food consumed, and feeling disgusted with oneself, depressed, or guilty after overeating.
- **[B] Episodes occur, on average, at least once a week for 3 months.**
- **[C] <u>No regular use of inappropriate compensatory behaviors</u>** (eg, purging, fasting, or excessive exercise) as are seen in Bulimia nervosa and they are not as fixated on their body shape or weight.
- [D] Binge eating does not occur solely during the course of Bulimia nervosa or Anorexia nervosa.

MANAGEMENT
- **<u>Psychotherapy</u> (eg, Cognitive behavioral therapy) with a strict diet & coordinated exercise program first line.** Interpersonal and Dialectic behavioral therapy. SSRIs may also be added.
- **<u>For overweight or obese patients with BED</u>** who do not have access to psychotherapy, decline it, or do not respond to it, **alternatives include (1) behavioral weight loss therapy or (2) SSRIs or (3) use of Topiramate, Zonisamide, or Lisdexamfetamine for those with marked obesity.**

BULIMIA NERVOSA

- Eating disorder characterized by [1] <u>frequent and recurrent binge eating</u> combined with [2] <u>inappropriate compensatory behaviors</u> **to counteract weight gain** (eg, purging with vomiting, laxatives, diuretics, enemas, fasting, caloric restriction, excessive exercise).

Anorexia vs. Bulimia:
- Both cause overevaluation of body shape & weight. Both can engage in purging &/or binge-eating.
- **Unlike Anorexia, patients with Bulimia nervosa [1] <u>usually maintain a normal weight (or may be overweight)</u> & [2] their compensatory behaviors are <u>ego-dystonic</u> (troublesome to the patient** and patients are embarrassed by their binge eating). Dysphoria can occur after a binge, along with remorse and self-loathing. [3] the severe weight loss that occurs in Anorexia nervosa is accompanied by anatomic and physiologic sequelae that are not found in Bulimia nervosa.

EPIDEMIOLOGY
- More common in females 10:1.
- **Average onset of age in the late teens (mean age 12.4 years) or early adulthood.**
- <u>Risk factors</u>: jobs or hobbies that require rapid gain or loss of weight (eg, wrestling and bodybuilding) or emphasize a thin body type (eg, ballet, running, cheerleading, diving).
- **High incidence of comorbid mood disorders**, anxiety or impulse control disorders, substance use, prior physical/sexual abuse, and increased prevalence of borderline personality disorder.

CLINICAL MANIFESTATIONS
- Patients with Bulimia nervosa develop sore throat (from vomiting), headache, fatigue, abdominal pain, bloating, constipation, or irregular menstruation (including Amenorrhea).
- Symptoms are usually exacerbated by stressful conditions. **Sense of <u>lack of control during eating episodes</u>.**
- Patients with Bulimia nervosa may engage in (1) caloric restriction, (2) binge eating, and (3) self-induced vomiting. The binge-eating episode triggers further caloric restriction, which results in intense hunger and increases the probability of an additional binge eating episode.

Episodes of binge eating:
- (1) **Patients eat portions more significant than what most people would consume in a similar period (usually < 2 hours) and under comparable conditions.**
- (2) **<u>Sense of lack of control</u>:** During the eating episodes, patients feel they have no control over their eating and are unable to curb the servings they consume. The episode of bingeing usually continues until the patient is uncomfortable or painfully full.

Compensatory behaviors:
- Binging episodes are followed by inappropriate compensatory behavior to prevent weight gain: self-induced vomiting, misuse of medications, such as laxatives, diuretics, insulin, or thyroid hormone; extreme physical activity, excessive exercise, or fasting.

Restrictive behaviors:
- Patients often restrict their diet between binge eating episodes to influence body weight or shape.

Medical complications:
- Medical complications, including metabolic alkalosis, dehydration, constipation, and cardiac arrhythmias. Esophageal erosions and tears may occur due to vomiting.
- **Cardiac arrhythmias due to electrolyte disturbances (eg, hypokalemia) can be lethal.**

PHYSICAL EXAMINATION
- **Common physical examination signs associated with Bulimia nervosa include hypotension, dry skin, and signs of self-induced vomiting. Patients are normal weight or overweight.**
- Bulimia nervosa can also be associated with hypotension, dry skin, hair loss, edema, & epistaxis.

Self-induced vomiting:
- **Teeth pitting or enamel erosion (from vomiting), dental caries.**
- **<u>Russell's sign</u>: calluses on the dorsum of the hand from self-induced vomiting.**
- **Parotid gland hypertrophy and swelling.**

LABORATORY FINDINGS
- <u>Comprehensive metabolic panel</u>: **Hypokalemia, hypomagnesemia** (electrolyte imbalance may lead to cardiac arrhythmias). Hyponatremia. Hypoalbuminemia.
- **Increased amylase** (due to salivary gland hypertrophy + vomiting). Transaminitis.
- **Metabolic alkalosis (hypochloremic hypokalemic Metabolic alkalosis) from vomiting-induced volume depletion.** Metabolic acidosis may be seen with laxative abuse.
- Female patients should undergo a pregnancy test (hCG). Female patients with secondary amenorrhea should have testing for luteinizing hormone (LH), prolactin, and follicle-stimulating hormone (FSH) to assess for possible additional contributors to amenorrhea.
- <u>Stool or urine laxative tests</u>: Lab tests are available to test for stool or urine Bisacodyl, emodin, aloe-emodin, and rhein. However, a positive test for a stool or urine laxative is not necessary to establish the diagnosis.

ECG:
- QT-interval prolongation, especially in the setting of hypokalemia, indicates serious risk for cardiac arrhythmias

DIAGNOSTIC CRITERIA
- **[A] <u>Recurrent episodes of binge eating</u> — recurrent episodes characterized by eating within a discrete time (eg a 2-hour period) an unusually large amount of food** (more than most people would in a similar period) with **lack of control during an overeating episode.**
- **[B] <u>Compensatory behaviors:</u> Recurrent inappropriate attempts to compensate for overeating and prevent weight gain: <u>Purging type</u> — primarily engages in self-induced vomiting, diuretic, laxative or enema abuse. <u>Restrictive type</u> — reduced calorie intake, dieting, fasting, excessive exercise, & diet pills.**
- **[C] The binge-eating and compensatory behaviors occur at least one a week for 3 months**. May be triggered by stress or mood changes.
- **[D] Self-evaluation is excessively influenced by body shape and weight**. Excessive concern & preoccupation with body weight and shape, which strongly influence the patient's self-esteem.
- [E] The disturbance does not occur exclusively during an episode of Anorexia nervosa.

MANAGEMENT
Psychotherapy:
- **<u>Cognitive Behavioral Therapy</u> (CBT) has been shown to be the most effective psychotherapy in managing Bulimia nervosa. The primary objective of treatment is cessation of the binging and purging behaviors and control of concern about body weight.** CBT mainly focused on core behaviors and cognitive problems, including binge eating episodes, inappropriate compensatory behaviors, and constant concern with body shape.
- Nutritional counseling and education. Group therapy, Interpersonal therapy, and family therapy.
- **Combination psychotherapy & pharmacotherapy more effective than either alone.**
Pharmacotherapy:
- **<u>Fluoxetine</u> is the only FDA-approved medication for Bulimia nervosa — has been shown to reduce the binge-purge cycle (60-80 mg/day).** Fluoxetine associated with cardiovascular adverse effects especially if electrolyte abnormalities are present. **Adverse effects of SSRIs common adverse effects include nausea, diarrhea, headache, insomnia (CNS stimulation).**
- <u>Second line pharmacotherapy</u>: In patients who do not respond to Fluoxetine, other SSRIs (Sertraline, Escitalopram, or Fluvoxamine) may be used.
- <u>Third-line pharmacotherapy</u>: other antidepressants (eg, Trazodone) or Topiramate.
- **<u>Bupropion is contraindicated in Bulimia nervosa & other eating disorders</u> due to the increased risk of seizures.**
<u>Stabilization</u>
- Always stabilize the patient's volume status and replete electrolytes prior to psychiatric therapy.
- Normal saline or Lactated ringer's administration for Hypochloremic hypokalemic metabolic alkalosis from vomiting induced volume depletion, may be indicated.

ANOREXIA NERVOSA

- Anorexia nervosa is characterized by an abnormally low body weight, intense fear of gaining weight, distorted perception of body weight and shape, & preoccupation with body weight, body image, & being thin.
- **Body mass index (BMI) ≤18.5 kg/m² OR body weight <85% of ideal weight.**
- **Anorexia nervosa is ego-syntonic (their behaviors are acceptable to them and are in harmony with their self-image goals).**

EPIDEMIOLOGY
- **Most common in teenage girls (14-18y). 90% are women.** Prevalence: 1% in females; 0.1% males.
- **Frequently seen in conditions or sports requiring thinness, revealing attire, or weight classes** (eg, athletes, figure skating, cheerleading, ballet, dancers, running, wrestling, diving, etc.).
- 60% incidence of comorbid depression. Rate of suicide is ~12% per 100,000 per year.
- **Anorexia nervosa has the highest mortality rate of all psychiatric conditions due to medical complications (eg, arrhythmias,** cardiac failure), suicide, starvation, or substance use.

CLINICAL MANIFESTATIONS
- **3 core features: [1] restriction of energy intake, [2] preoccupation with weight: intense fear of gaining weight, preoccupation with their weight, their body image, and being thin, and [3] distorted perception of body weight.** They may describe calorie counting or portion control.
- **Common symptoms include amenorrhea, cold intolerance, constipation, fatigue, irritability, or extremity edema.**
- Severe cases: **bradycardia & hypotension can cause dizziness;** hypothermia.
- **Hypogonadotropic hypogonadism: Amenorrhea and loss of libido is common due to Hypogonadotropic hypogonadism** (eg, decreased estrogen in women, decreased testosterone in men).

2 subtypes:
- **Restrictive type: strict, reduced calorie intake, dieting, fasting, excessive exercise, & diet pills.** No regular engagement in binge-eating or purging behavior. Many exercise compulsively for extended periods of time and may increase exercise activity after food intake if they feel they have "overeaten".
- **Binge eating/purging type: primarily engages in self-induced vomiting as well as diuretic, laxative use, or enema abuse.** They may intermittently binge eat, often followed by purging.

PHYSICAL EXAMINATION
- Emaciation, hypotension (may be orthostatic), **Sinus bradycardia (classic finding),** loss of body fat; skin or hair changes, such as dry and scaly skin, alopecia, **increased lanugo (fine soft body hair type commonly found on newborns),** muscle wasting, arrhythmias, Osteopenia.
- **Body mass index (BMI) ≤18.5 kg/m² OR body weight <85% of ideal weight.**

Self-induced vomiting:
- Salivary gland (eg, parotid gland) hypertrophy and edema may be seen in those who engage in self-induced vomiting. Dental enamel erosion may also be seen.
- **Russel's sign: calluses on the dorsum of the hand from self-induced vomiting.**

COMPLICATIONS
- Cardiovascular: **Sinus bradycardia, hypotension,** dilated cardiomyopathy, electrolyte abnormalities, electrolyte-induced arrhythmias, QTc prolongation, mitral valve prolapse, pericardial effusion.
- Endocrine: hypothalamic hypogonadism (decreased estrogen, decreased testosterone, and amenorrhea); Osteopenia, Osteoporosis. Hematologic: cytopenias, including a normocytic normochromic anemia or leukopenia, bone marrow hypoplasia/aplasia.
- Neurologic: cognitive impairment, brain atrophy, peripheral neuropathy (mineral and vitamin deficiencies). Gastrointestinal: constipation (laxative abuse), gastroparesis.

DIAGNOSTIC CRITERIA
- **[A] <u>Restriction of calorie intake</u> relative to requirements, leading to significantly low body weight** (<minimally normal, or in children, minimally expected) for age, sex, & physical health.
- **[B] <u>Intense morbid fear of gaining weight</u> or becoming fat or persistent behaviors to prevent weight gain,** even though at a significantly low weight.
- **[C] <u>Distorted body image</u>** — self-perception of being overweight (even though they are underweight), undue influence of weight or shape on self-evaluation, or persistent lack of recognition of the seriousness of the current low body weight.

Specify type: Restrictive type or Binge eating/purging type.

Specify current severity:
- Mild – BMI 17-18.49 kg/m²; Moderate – BMI 16-16.99 kg/m²; Severe – BMI 15-15.99 kg/m²; Extreme – BMI <15 kg/m².

LABORATORY EVALUATION
- **Basic labs:** eg, CBC, complete metabolic profile, 25-hydroxyvitamin D, testosterone (males), thyroid-stimulating hormone (TSH), urine testing (hCG [females] and drugs, either illicit or prescription), & coagulation panel.
- **ECG** recommended to assess for life-threatening arrhythmias and for prolonged QT interval.
- **Hypokalemia** due to GI loss from laxatives, diuretics, and/or vomiting.
- **Elevations of blood urea nitrogen (BUN) and serum creatinine** (from dehydration), hypoglycemia.
- **Hypochloremic metabolic alkalosis** (from vomiting).
- Hypogonadotropic hypogonadism (low estrogen and/or testosterone), hypothyroidism, transaminitis, normochromic normocytic anemia.

MANAGEMENT
- **The cornerstone of treatment for patients acutely ill with Anorexia nervosa is <u>nutritional rehabilitation plus psychotherapy</u>.** Treatment involves Cognitive-behavioral therapy (CBT), Cognitive analytic therapy, family therapy (eg, Maudsley approach — the gold standard for treatment of Anorexia nervosa in teenagers), and **supervised weight programs.**
- Behavioral modifications establish healthy eating habits & positive behavior reinforcement. **Clinical improvement measured by weekly weight gain [eg, 1 pound (0.45 kg/week)],** increasing BMI, patient motivation to change, increased body image satisfaction, & improvement of depression.

Medical stabilization:
- Patients may be treated as an outpatient with intensive therapy (eg, 2-3 hours/weekday) and partial hospitalization (6 hours per day) unless they require hospitalization.
- Hospitalization indications: <70% ideal body weight, BMI <14-15 kg/m², medical complications (eg, dehydration), unstable vital signs (eg, pulse <40/min, BP <80/60 mmHg, light-headedness, orthostatic changes), Hypothermia, Dysrhythmia, severe edema, acute food refusal, suicidality.

Nutritional rehabilitation:
- **Most common complication is <u>Refeeding syndrome</u>** — decreased phosphate from starvation + phosphate demand from refeeding (increased insulin triggers intracellular uptake of phosphate & phosphate use to make ATP) **leads to hypophosphatemia (<2 mg/dL), hypokalemia, hypomagnesemia, marked edema, cardiac complications (CHF, edema),** Rhabdomyolysis, seizures, hemolysis, or respiratory insufficiency due to fluid & electrolyte shifts during refeeding.
- Refeeding syndrome may be prevented by judiciously avoiding very rapid increases in the number of daily calories ingested and close monitoring during refeeding to assess for complications.

Pharmacotherapy:
- Pharmacotherapy is not used initially. **For acutely ill patients not gaining weight with nutritional rehabilitation plus psychotherapy, add-on treatment with <u>Olanzapine</u>** 2.5 mg to 10 mg/day, rather than other medications (Olanzapine helps with weight gain and is the preferred medication).
- Not acutely ill + co-morbid psychiatric condition: combination psychotherapy + SSRI preferred.
- **<u>Bupropion is contraindicated in Anorexia and other eating disorders</u> due to increased seizure risk.**

PERSONALITY DISORDERS

- **Cluster A:** SOCIAL DETACHMENT with unusual behaviors: WEIRD, ODD, ECCENTRIC BEHAVIOR.

SCHIZOID PERSONALITY DISORDER

- Lifelong pattern of <u>voluntary social withdrawal, isolation, & anhedonic introversion</u>.

EPIDEMIOLOGY
- **The disorder occurs more often in men than in women and may be more severe in men.**
- Estimates of the prevalence of Schizoid personality disorder in the general population vary with the criteria used, ranging from 0.5%-7%.
- SPD doesn't appear to have a strong genetic relationship to Schizophrenia.

DSM-5 DIAGNOSTIC CRITERIA
- [A] **A pervasive pattern of detachment** from social relationships and a restricted range of expression of emotions in interpersonal settings, beginning by early adulthood and present in a variety of contexts, as indicated by ≥4 of the following: 1. **Neither desires nor enjoys close relationships,** including being part of a family. 2. Almost always **chooses solitary activities.** 3. Has **little, if any, interest in having sexual experiences with another person.** 4. **Takes pleasure in few, if any, activities.** 5. **Lacks close friends or confidants** other than first-degree relatives (if any). 6. **Appears indifferent to the praise or criticism of other**s. 7. **Shows emotional coldness, detachment, or flattened affectivity.**
- [B] Does not occur exclusively during the course of Schizophrenia, a bipolar disorder or depressive disorder with psychotic features, another psychotic disorder, or autism spectrum disorder and is not attributable to the physiological effects of another medical condition.

MANAGEMENT
- **Psychotherapy:** first line management for Personality disorders: Cognitive behavioral therapy, behavioral, psychoanalysis.** Management is difficult based on the little value the patients see with establishing a relationship with others, little perceived distress, and the tendency of these patients and lack of insight for individual psychotherapy. May only seek help due to family insistence.
- May find group therapy threatening. May benefit from daily programs or drop-in centers.
- <u>Pharmacological management</u> only if patient suffers from concomitant depression or psychosis.

PANCE PREP PEARL OF THE WEEK
SCHIZOID PERSONALITY DISORDER
Lifelong pattern of voluntary social withdrawal & anhedonic
introversion (constricted affect). **Most common in males.**

Think **Schizoids AVOID** people
Anhedonic – little pleasure in activities or relationships.

Voluntary social withdrawal – **prefers to be alone** (unlike avoidant PD). No
desire for close or sexual relationships, prefers solitary activities.

Odd-appearing or eccentric but lacks the bizarre or idiosyncratic thinking seen
with Schizotypal or Schizophrenia.

Introvert – **loner "hermit-like behavior",** quiet. Indifference to the praises and
criticisms of others.

Detached, flat, cold, constricted affect

SCHIZOTYPAL PERSONALITY DISORDER

- **Characterized by odd, eccentric, bizarre behavior, and peculiar thought patterns suggestive of Schizophrenia without psychosis (no delusions or hallucinations).**
- Usually, early adulthood onset with manifestations beginning in childhood and adolescence.
- **Small percentage may develop Schizophrenia & certain family traits of this disorder predominate in first-degree relatives with Schizophrenia.**

CLINICAL MANIFESTATIONS
[1] Cognitive-perceptual
- **Odd beliefs/magical thinking** — Magical thinking is the belief that unrelated events are causally connected despite the absence of any plausible causal link between them accepted by the individual's subculture, particularly as a result of supernatural or paranormal phenomena (belief in clairvoyance, telepathy, superstition, bizarre fantasies, control of external events with one's mind).
- **Unusual perceptual experiences and bodily illusions** — seeing a halo or aura surrounding someone; experiencing the presence of an unseen force or being; bodily illusions (eg, one's body appears to be changing in shape or proportion); déjà vu; and bizarre dissociative experiences (feeling one is falling into a "different dimension").
- **Ideas of reference** — **misinterpretation of incidents and events as having direct personal reference to oneself** (excluding delusions of reference), such as a global event indicating a personal sign for them to change their life. **Paranoia/suspiciousness** — Suspiciousness and paranoia can vary widely. They can range from persistent and overt hostility, guardedness, and evasiveness to pleasant and agreeable compliance and deference intended to avert potential reprisal.

[2] Oddness/disorganized
- **Distorted cognition & reasoning** — **May have hygiene, attire, and social behaviors that are eccentric, unconventional, idiosyncratic, or somewhat neglected or impoverished.** Speech and thought process can be vague, unelaborate, circumstantial, metaphorical, or stereotyped but not grossly incoherent or blocked. Psychomotor expressions of affect are commonly constricted.

[3] Interpersonal
- **Chronic social anxiety** — **Pervasive discomfort with close relationships** (increased social anxiety, may have few close friends).
- **Social anhedonia** — The lack of close friends is thought to be due a deficit in finding social interactions gratifying and distress related to "making sense" of the range of affects elicited by social interaction and interpersonal closeness.

DIAGNOSTIC CRITERIA
≥ 5 of the following 9:
- **Cognitive-perceptual**: (1) **Ideas of reference** (excluding delusions of reference); (2) Odd beliefs or magical thinking that influences behavior and is inconsistent with subcultural norms (eg, superstitiousness, belief in clairvoyance, telepathy, or "sixth sense"; in children and adolescents, bizarre fantasies or preoccupations); (3) Unusual perceptual experiences, including bodily illusions; (4) Suspiciousness or paranoid ideation.
- **Oddness:** (5) Odd thinking and speech (eg, vague, circumstantial, metaphorical, overelaborate, or stereotyped); (6) Inappropriate or constricted affect; (7) Behavior or appearance that is odd, eccentric, or peculiar.
- **Interpersonal:** (8) Lack of close friends or confidants other than first-degree relatives; (9) Excessive social anxiety that does not diminish with familiarity and tends to be associated with paranoid fears rather than negative judgments about self.

MANAGEMENT
- **Psychotherapy first-line treatment for Personality disorders** — **Cognitive behavioral therapy (CBT) to help develop social skills training**, individual, or group therapy. Pyschoanalysis.
- Pharmacologic: short term low-dose antipsychotics for psychotic episodes or if suspiciousness occurs.

PARANOID PERSONALITY DISORDER

- **Pervasive pattern of excessive distrust & suspiciousness of others, and often interpret their motives as malevolent.**

EPIDEMIOLOGY
- <u>Prevalence</u>: 1–4% of the general population.
- Individuals with a PPD rarely seek treatment on their own. They are usually referred by family members, coworkers, or employers.
- Begins in early adulthood. More commonly diagnosed in males.
- Higher incidence if family members of Schizophrenics.

CLINICAL MANIFESTATIONS
- **The hallmark feature of Paranoid personality disorder is the presence of <u>generalized distrust or suspiciousness.</u> They tend to bear grudges, are easily slighted, and are overly sensitive.**
- These patients are often unsuccessful in intimate relationships because of their suspiciousness (pathologically jealous) without justification.
- **They consistently project blame their own difficulties and problems onto others, externalizing their own emotions while paying keen attention to the emotions and attitudes of others.**
- Patients with a Paranoid personality disorder are formal, skeptical, and mistrustful and may exhibit either poor or fixated eye contact. There is often underlying hostility and resentment.

DIAGNOSTIC CRITERIA
- **[A] Pervasive distrust and suspicion of others with interpretation of their motives as malevolent**, beginning by early adulthood and indicated by **≥4 of the following 7**: (1) Suspects, without sufficient basis, that others are exploiting, harming, or deceiving them; (2) Is preoccupied with unjustified doubts about the loyalty or trustworthiness of friends or associates; (3) Is reluctant to confide in others because of unwarranted fear that the information will be used maliciously against them; (4) Reads hidden demeaning or threatening meanings into benign remarks or events; (5) Persistently bears grudges (eg, is unforgiving of insults, injuries, or slights); (6) Perceives attacks on their character or reputation that are not apparent to others and is quick to react angrily or to counterattack; (7) Has recurrent suspicions, without justification, regarding fidelity of spouse or partner.
- [B] Does not occur exclusively during the course of Schizophrenia, Bipolar disorder, or Depressive disorder with psychotic features, or another psychotic disorder and is not attributable to the physiological effects of another medical condition.

MANAGEMENT
Psychotherapy
- **<u>Cognitive behavioral therapy (CBT)</u>: first-line treatment for Personality disorders — however, often difficult to treat and patients rarely initiate treatment as they lack trust,** and therefore rarely enter treatment unless there is another coexisting emotional disorder, such as a mood or anxiety disorder, or coercion from a family member or employer. Psychoanalysis.
- **Patients may be suspicious of group therapy so it should be avoided** due to their lack of basic trust and suspiciousness, and misinterpretation of others' statements.
- Paranoid personality disorder patients sometimes present for treatment with family members as couples. These patients often feel that the therapist and family members are working against them, making it difficult to work with them.

Pharmacological therapy:
- Short-term antipsychotics if severe or if psychosis occurs.

COURSE & PROGNOSIS
- This condition usually has a chronic course, causing lifelong marital and job-related problems.

CLUSTER B DISORDERS
ANTISOCIAL PERSONALITY DISORDER

- **Pervasive socially irresponsible, exploitative, & guiltless behaviors that deviate sharply from the norms, values, & laws of society, often violating the rights of others.**

EPIDEMIOLOGY

- 1-4% of the population. 3-5 times more common in males.
- Persons with ASPD have high rates of other psychiatric diagnoses (eg, substance misuse, mood and anxiety disorders, attention deficit hyperactivity disorder, learning disabilities.
- **History of Conduct disorder: APD is the adult continuation of childhood Conduct disorder.**

CLINICAL MANIFESTATIONS

- Patients diagnosed with Antisocial personality disorder often exploit and violate the rights of others, and break rules to meet their own needs. Seen in many areas of their lives (eg, family relations, marriage, school, work, military service).
- **They are impulsive, deceitful, and often violate the law without regard (may commit criminal acts).** Their deceitful nature may be masked and they may seem charming at first.
- They are frequently skilled at reading social cues and can appear charming and normal to others who meet them for the first time and do not know their history.

DIAGNOSTIC CRITERIA

- **[A] Must be at least 18 years old and must have history by 15 years of age of violating the rights of others consistent with Conduct disorder.**

≥3 of the following 7:

- **(1) Failure to conform to social norms with disregard & violation of the rights of others or committing unlawful acts.**
- (2) Irritability or aggressive towards others (eg, repeated assaults or fights).
- (3) Exploiting others for personal gain (eg, lying, manipulating, or deceitful acts).
- (4) Recklessness & disregard for the safety of self or others (eg, drunk driving common).
- (5) Impulsivity or failure to plan ahead.
- (6) Lack of remorse for actions.
- (7) Irresponsibility or failure to maintain work or honor financial obligations.

MANAGEMENT

- **Cognitive behavioral therapy (CBT): first-line treatment for Personality disorders — establishing limits. However, psychotherapy & pharmacotherapy often ineffective.**
- Avoid medications with abusive potential due to high comorbidity with substance use disorders.
- Severe ASPD (psychopathy): address comorbid disorders and aggressive behaviors.

PANCE PREP PEARL OF THE WEEK
ANTISOCIAL PERSONALITY DISORDER

"CORRUPTS"

*Conduct disorder history by 15 years of age & patients must be at least
    18 years of age to be diagnosed.

At least 3 of the following 7 DSM V criteria:

*Obligations (work, financial) are not honored

*Reckless and disregard the safety of others (eg, drunk driving)

*Remorselessness (lacks remorse for actions)

*Use others and Untruthful (deceitful) – exploits others for personal gain
    (eg, lying, manipulating, or deceitful acts).

*Planning not meditated - impetuous and impulsive, with lack of planning

*Temper – irritable or aggressive towards others (repeated assaults, fights).

*Society laws violated, Social norms disregarded & violation of the rights
    of others or committing unlawful acts.

BORDERLINE PERSONALITY DISORDER (BPD)

- Borderline personality disorder (BPD) is characterized by <u>instability of interpersonal relationships, self-image, & emotions</u>; hypersensitivity to rejection, as well as by impulsivity, causing significant impairment or subjective distress.

<u>EPIDEMIOLOGY</u>
- <u>Prevalence of BPD</u>: 1–2% general population & 20% of the psychiatric inpatients. Most common in women.
- **Comorbid mood disorders:** Patients with Borderline personality disorder have been shown to have higher rates of moos disorders, anxiety disorders, & other psychiatric disorders.

<u>CLINICAL MANIFESTATIONS</u>
Core features:
- **The hallmark features of Borderline personality disorder (BPD) are [1] <u>instability</u> of interpersonal relationships, self-image, moods, & behavior as well as [2] <u>marked impulsivity</u>.**
Interpersonal difficulties:
- **Unstable relationships with others, identity disturbance, and chronic <u>emptiness (fear or abandonment)</u>.** Relationships begin with intense attachments and end with the slightest conflict.
- **Patients with BPD often have stormy relationships, especially with people to whom patients are close.**
- <u>Splitting:</u> **"<u>Black and white thinking</u>" — patients use rigid classifications and tend to view others as all good or all bad, a phenomenon known as "splitting".** Rigidly classifying other people as good or bad can lead the patient to shift between extreme points of view and to selectively attend to information in a way that confirms his or her current opinion.
Affective dysregulation:
- **Affective lability (<u>mood swings</u>), excessive anger, & <u>efforts to avoid abandonment.</u>**
Behavior dysregulation: impulsivity, suicidality, and self-injurious behavior:
- <u>Impulsivity</u> **— impetuous and self-damaging behavior is common. Patients abuse substances, binge eat, engage in unsafe sex, spend money irresponsibly, and drive recklessly.**
- <u>Nonsuicidal self-injury</u> **— patients may engage in self-injurious behavior that is not intended as suicide, such as self-mutilation (eg, cutting or burning themselves).**

<u>DSM V DIAGNOSTIC CRITERIA</u>
- **[A] A pervasive pattern of instability of interpersonal relationships, of self-image, and affects as well as marked impulsivity beginning by early adulthood and present in a variety of contexts** as indicated by **≥5 of the following 8:**
- **[B]** (1) Frantic efforts to avoid real or imagined abandonment (not including suicidal or self-mutilating behavior); (2) a pattern of unstable and intense interpersonal relationships characterized by alternating between extremes of idealization and devaluation; (3) Identity disturbance: Markedly and persistently unstable self-image or sense of self; (4) Impulsivity in at least two areas that are potentially self-damaging, for example, spending, substance abuse, reckless driving, sex, binge eating, etc.; (5) Affective instability caused by a marked reactivity of mood, for example, intense episodic dysphoria, anxiety, or irritability, usually lasting a few hours and rarely more than a few days; (6) Chronic feelings of emptiness; (7) Inappropriate, intense anger, or difficulty controlling anger, for example, frequent displays of temper, constant anger, recurrent physical fights; (8) Transient paranoid ideation or severe dissociative symptoms.

<u>MANAGEMENT</u>
- **Psychotherapy: first-line treatment for BPD — <u>Dialectical behavior therapy</u> (DBT)** for the most regressed patients or for those with high levels of self-destructiveness. **Cognitive behavioral therapy (CBT).** Mentalization-based, Transference-focused, or schema-focused therapies.
- Medications such as SSRIs, mood stabilizers, and antipsychotics have shown limited effectiveness in trials aiming at control of symptoms such as anxiety, sleep disturbance, depression, or psychotic symptoms.

PANCE PREP PEARL OF THE WEEK

BORDERLINE PERSONALITY DISORDER

Think of the "B"s

* Cluster B disorder ("dramatic, wild, erratic, impulsive & emotional")

* "Bat" - mood swings'.*

* 'Black & white thinking': thinks in extremes "all good" or "bad" - no middle ground (splitting).

* Blown up (intense) reaction that is disproportionate to the event.

* Broken: unstable relationships & fear of abandonment (Breaking up)

* Bad behavior: Impulsivity in self-damaging behaviors: suicide, self-mutilation, substance abuse, reckless driving, binge eating, spending. Bad sense of self

MANAGEMENT: Behavioral therapy: cognitive, dialectical

PANCE PREP PEARL OF THE WEEK

HISTRIONIC PERSONALITY DISORDER

Think of the 'H"s for Histrionic

•Hey look at me - attention-seeking, "Overly emotional, dramatic, seductive."

•Hissy fits - self-absorbed, 'temper tantrums" efforts to draw attention to themselves with need to be the center of attention.

•Hysterical: theatrical and dramatic

•Come Hither: often inappropriate, sexually provocative, seductive

•Hype me up - seeks reassurance & praise often. May believe their relationships are more intimate than they are.

MANAGEMENT: Behavioral therapy: eg, cognitive, dialectical

HISTRIONIC PERSONALITY DISORDER

- **Histrionic personality disorder is characterized by being overly emotional, dramatic, seductive (sexual provocativeness), and attention-seeking.**

EPIDEMIOLOGY
- The overall prevalence of Histrionic personality disorder has been estimated as 1–3% in the general population.
- Histrionic personality disorder tends to be diagnosed more frequently in women and is often overlooked and underdiagnosed in men.

CLINICAL MANIFESTATIONS
- **The hallmark feature of Histrionic personality disorder is the deliberate use of excessive, superficial emotionality and sexuality to draw attention, evade unpleasant responsibilities, and control or manipulate others.**
- **Appearance**: attention seeking; large concern of appearance & attractiveness and may include revealing or seductive clothing, suggestive or extensive tattoos, brightly colored hair, and eccentric hairstyles.
- **Behaviors** may include hypersexual gestures, flirtatious behaviors, and acting out to gain the spotlight. They display exaggerated displays of emotions and are self-indulgent. HPD patients feel best when they are the center of attention, and they become disappointed when the attention and focus shift off of them (they may feel devalued when not in the spotlight).
- **Reward dependence**: desire to cater to behaviors in response to social reward cues. Individuals with HPD have very high reward.
- **Speech:** Individuals with HPD often speak loudly and dramatically and may include dramatic anecdotes. Although descriptions of events may be passionate and colorful, they tend to be imprecise and lack detail, with the information obtained being more impressionistic than specific.
- **Emotions are characteristically labile, and they may exhibit <u>childlike regressive behaviors</u> (eg, temper tantrums, tearful outbursts, or dramatic accusations when upset) to provoke a reaction such as guilt, sympathy, or acquiescence from those around them. Theatric level of emotional reactions.**
- **Thought process:** In individuals with HPD, the thought process is usually linear but limited in range and logic. **They are often easily suggestible and can be easily persuaded from their thought processes to others around them.**
- Repression of anger and other disturbing affects. Anger tends to be expressed indirectly or fleetingly.

DSM V CRITERIA
A pervasive pattern of excessive emotionality and attention seeking, beginning by early adulthood and present in a variety of contexts, as indicated by ≥5 of the following:
- (1) Is uncomfortable in situations in which they are not the center of attention;
- (2) Interaction with others is often characterized by inappropriate sexually seductive or provocative behavior;
- (3) Displays rapidly shifting and shallow expression of emotions;
- (4) Consistently uses physical appearance to draw attention to self;
- (5) Has a style of speech that is excessively impressionistic and lacking in detail;
- (6) Shows self-dramatization, theatricality, and exaggerated expression of emotion;
- (7) Is suggestible (eg, easily influenced by others or circumstances); or
- (8) Considers relationships to be more intimate than they actually are.

MANAGEMENT
- **Psychotherapy (eg, supportive, problem-solving, interpersonal, group) is the treatment of choice for patients with Histrionic personality disorder.**
- Pharmacotherapy to treat associated depressive or anxious symptoms as necessary.

NARCISSISTIC PERSONALITY DISORDER

- **Grandiose often excessive sense of self-importance, superiority, need for attention & admiration, & lack of empathy (may fluctuate between grandiose and vulnerable states).**
- Additional features of the disorder include problems with self-definition, self-esteem regulation, and affective reactivity.

EPIDEMIOLOGY
- **More common in men** than women. Occurs in <1% of the general population.

CLINICAL MANIFESTATIONS
- **The hallmarks of the NPD are grandiosity, a notable lack of empathy, and a lack of consideration for others. There also is hypersensitivity to evaluation by others.**
- <u>Grandiosity</u> — **exaggerated sense of self-importance & inflated self-image, viewing themselves as entitled & superior to others** & deserving of extra special treatment or admiration. They show devaluation, disdain, contempt, & deprecation of others. Arrogant, haughty attitudes & behaviors.
- <u>Excessive need for admiration</u> — **constant need to experience themselves as the center of attention**, regardless of the setting, perpetually grabbing the limelight and monopolizing social conversations. When attention is not forthcoming, or others receive the attention they feel they themselves deserve, they may feel slighted, mistreated depleted, and enraged. **Because they are highly vulnerable to criticism, they may react to rejection or criticism with rage.**
- <u>Superficial & exploitative relationships</u> — **will exploit and manipulate others for self-gain** (eg, recognition, status), associated with markedly superficial relationships, Often envious of others or belief that others are envious of them. Difficulty with attachment and dependency.
- <u>Lack of empathy</u> — lacks capacity to empathize with the needs of others.
- <u>Identity disturbance</u> — **a sense of self that is relatively stable, but highly superficial, extremely rigid, and often fragile;** stability is tied on maintaining the view that one is exceptional & by receiving constant external feedback of superiority, with vulnerability when such feedback isn't given (they become depressed when they do not receive the recognition they think they deserve). **Vulnerability to life transitions (eg, mid-life crisis).** Chronic feelings of emptiness & boredom.
- **Because they place a high value on youth and power, the aging process can be extremely difficult challenging for individuals with NPD** (may become depressed or have mid-life crises).

DSM 5 DIAGNOSTIC CRITERIA
Pervasive pattern of grandiosity (either overt or covert), excessive need for admiration, superficial and exploitative relationships, and lack of empathy, with ≥5 of the following:
- (1) Exaggerated sense of self-importance.
- (2) Preoccupation with fantasies of unlimited money, success, brilliance, etc.
- (3) Belief that they are "special" or unique and can associate only with other high-status individuals.
- (4) Requires excessive admiration.
- (5) Has sense of entitlement.
- (6) Takes advantage of others for self-gain.
- (7) Lacks empathy.
- (8) Envious of others or believes others are envious of them.
- (9) Arrogant or haughty.

<u>Not in DSM-5:</u>
- Identity disturbance, difficulty with attachment and dependency, Chronic feelings of emptiness and boredom, and vulnerability to life transitions.

MANAGEMENT:
- <u>**Psychotherapy** initial treatment of choice</u> — Manualized psychotherapy, Transference-focused psychotherapy, Supportive psychotherapy, Schema-focused therapy.
- <u>Cognitive-perceptual disturbances:</u> atypical antipsychotics — Aripiprazole, Risperidone, Quetiapine.
- <u>Impulsivity, recklessness, or behavioral dyscontrol:</u> mood stabilizer — Lithium or Lamotrigine.

CLUSTER C DISORDERS

- **Cluster C:** ANXIOUS, WORRIED & FEARFUL.

AVOIDANT PERSONALITY DISORDER

- **Characterized by a pervasive pattern of social inhibition due to an intense fear of rejection, with a longing to relate to others, affecting their daily lives.**

EPIDEMIOLOGY:
- ~2% of the general population. Closely related to Social anxiety disorder.

CLINICAL MANIFESTATIONS
- Avoidant personality disorder is characterized by [1] an <u>inferiority complex</u> coupled with a [2] <u>coexisting fear of rejection</u>, which manifests behaviorally as <u>widespread avoidance of social interaction.</u>
- Unlike Schizoid personality disorder in which patients *prefer* to be alone, patients with Avoidant personality *desire* relationships but fear rejection because they are timid, shy, and lack confidence.

DSM 5 DIAGNOSTIC CRITERIA
A pervasive pattern of <u>social inhibition, feelings of inadequacy, and hypersensitivity to negative evaluation</u>, beginning by early adulthood and present in a variety of contexts, as indicated by ≥4 of the following 7:
- (1) Avoids occupational activities that involve significant interpersonal contact because of **fears of criticism, disapproval, or rejection.**
- (2) Is **unwilling to get involved with people unless certain of being liked.**
- (3) Shows caution and/or restraint within intimate relationships because of the fear of being shamed or ridiculed.
- (4) Is **preoccupied with being criticized or rejected in social situations.**
- (5) Is inhibited in new interpersonal situations because of **feelings of inadequacy.**
- (6) Views self as socially inept, personally unappealing, inadequate, or inferior to others.
- (7) Is **reluctant to take personal risks** or engage in any new activities that may prove embarrassing.

MANAGEMENT
Psychotherapy: first line management of Personality disorders.
- Social training, Cognitive behavioral therapy, or group therapy. Interpersonal therapy (ITP) may be beneficial for overcoming social anxiety and developing trust.

PANCE PREP PEARL OF THE WEEK
AVOIDANT PERSONALITY DISORDER

A pervasive pattern of social inhibition, feelings of inadequacy, and hypersensitivity to negative evaluation, beginning by early adulthood and

DSM 5 CRITERIA At least 4 of the following: **AFRAIDS**

- **A**voids occupational activities that involve significant interpersonal contact because of fears of criticism, disapproval, or rejection.
- **F**ears being criticized or rejected in social situations.
- **R**eluctant to take personal risks or to engage in any new activities because they may prove embarrassing.
- **A**fraid to get involved with people unless certain of being liked.
- **I**nhibited in new interpersonal situations due to feelings of inadequacy.
- **D**eficient sense of self makes them view themselves as inferior to others, inadequate, personally unappealing, and socially inept.
- **S**hows caution and/or restraint within intimate relationships because of the fear of being shamed or ridiculed.

DEPENDENT PERSONALITY DISORDER

- **Characterized by the [1] <u>inability to assume responsibility, dependent or submissive, needy, & clinging</u> behavior, [2] fear of being alone and abandoned, & [3] <u>difficulty making day to day decisions</u>.** ~2% of the general population. More common in women.
- Juvenile medical conditions or Separation anxiety disorder may increase the likelihood of DPD.

CLINICAL MANIFESTATIONS

- **<u>Dependent behavior</u>: Psychological dependence on others to meet their emotional** they have poor self-confidence and have an **excessive need to be taken care of** — manifests as **passive and clingy behavior with lack of self-confidence, specifically feeling unable to care for oneself.**
- **<u>Fear of separation</u>** due to their overwhelming dependence on other people, they are submissive with **increasing appeasement & submissiveness when relationships are threatened** (may accepting imposition from others and tolerating poor treatment, to avoid disapproval or being rejected).
- **<u>Difficulty making day to day decisions</u>:** overdependence and allowance of others to make decisions for them because they need constant approval from other people. They tend to place needs and opinions of others above their own as they do not have the confidence to trust their decisions.
- **<u>Pessimistic outlook on life</u>** — Generally people with DPD expect the worst out of situations or believe that the worst will happen. They are more introverted & sensitive to criticism.

DSM-5 DIAGNOSTIC CRITERIA

A pervasive and excessive need to be taken care of that leads to submissive, needy, and clinging behavior and fears of separation, beginning by early adulthood and present in a variety of contexts, as indicated by ≥5 of the following:

- (1) Has difficulty making everyday decisions without external help (eg, excessive amount of advice and reassurance from others).
- (2) Needs others to assume responsibility for most major areas of their life.
- (3) Has difficulty expressing disagreement with others because of fear of loss of support or approval. (Note: Do not include realistic fears of retribution).
- (4) Has difficulty initiating projects or doing things on their own (because of a lack of self-confidence in judgment or abilities rather than a lack of motivation or energy).
- (5) Goes to extreme lengths to obtain approval, nurturance, and support from others to the point of volunteering to do things that are unpleasant.
- (6) Uncomfortable/helpless when alone with exaggerated fears of being unable to care for themselves.
- (7) Urgently seeks another relationship as a source of care and support when a close relationship ends.
- (8) Is unrealistically preoccupied with fears of being left to take care of themselves.

DIFFERENTIAL DIAGNOSIS

- <u>Dependent vs. Borderline PD:</u> both are afraid of abandonment, but **DPD responds to the fear with increasing appeasement and submissiveness when relationships are threatened and seeks another relationship to maintain their dependency;** whereas the patient with BPD reacts with rage and feelings of emptiness. **Interpersonal relationships of people with Dependent personality disorder are more stable and last longer than those of people with BPD.**
- <u>Dependent vs. Histrionic:</u> both are dependent on others but patients with DPD have more stable, long-lasting relationships, whereas patients with HPD are often unable to maintain long relationships.
- <u>Dependent vs. Avoidant PD:</u> Patients with DPD grow extreme in their need to be around someone all the time, while someone with Avoidant personality disorder will withdraw from society entirely when their fear of being seen as inadequate predominates.

MANAGEMENT

- **<u>Psychotherapy:</u> first-line management of Dependent personality disorder** — **cognitive behavioral therapy, social skills training, and assertiveness skills treatment of choice.**
- <u>Pharmacological therapy</u> may be used to treat comorbid anxiety or depression.

OBSESSIVE-COMPULSIVE PERSONALITY DISORDER

- Characterized by pervasive pattern of <u>perfectionism, inflexibility, and orderliness</u> with <u>intense focus on & preoccupation with order and details, without obsessions or compulsions</u>.
- 2 times more common in men. 2-7% prevalence.

CLINICAL MANIFESTATIONS

- **Pervasive pattern of perfectionism & inflexibility that they become preoccupied with orderliness, neatness, control, & unimportant details that they often fail to complete tasks in a timely fashion** (relentless pursuit of perfection often becomes counterproductive — inefficiencies due to excessive focus, missing deadlines, requests time extensions to refine work).
- <u>Ego syntonic behavior</u>: **they don't see anything wrong with their thoughts or behaviors or are aware their behavior causes issues).** They believe their way of thinking & doing things is the only correct way & everyone else is wrong (vs. Obsessive compulsive disorder, which is ego dystonic).
- <u>Affect</u>: **They often appear as serious, stiff, rigid, and formal, with a constricted affect.**
- They often feel righteous, indignant, and angry; they find it hard to express their feelings. They can experience anxiety and depression. They may micromanage or take over the entire workload.
- <u>Poor interpersonal skills</u>: **They are often successful professionally but have poor interpersonal skills (impaired ability to function with others).** They often feel the need to be in control and have difficulty forming and maintaining close relationships with others. They often face social isolation.

DSM-5 DIAGNOSTIC CRITERIA

A pervasive pattern of preoccupation with orderliness. Perfectionism, and mental and interpersonal control, at the expense of flexibility, openness, and efficiency, beginning by early adulthood and present in a variety of contexts, as indicated by at least 4 of the following:

- (1) preoccupation with details, rules, lists, minute details, order, organization, or schedules to the extent that the primary goal of the activity is lost.
- (2) perfectionism that interferes with task completion in a timely fashion (eg, is unable to complete a project because their own overly strict standards are not met).
- (3) excessive devotion to work, morals, ethics, and productivity to the exclusion of leisure activities and friendships (not accounted for by obvious economic necessity).
- (4) Is overconscientious, scrupulous, and inflexible about matters of morality, ethics, or values (not accounted for by cultural or religious identification).
- (5) inability to discard worn-out, worthless, or useless objects even if there is no sentimental value.
- (6) hesitant and reluctant to delegate tasks or to work with others unless they submit to exactly their way of doing things for fear it won't be done right.
- (7) Adopts a miserly spending style toward both self and others; money is viewed as something to be hoarded for future catastrophes.
- (8) rigid, stubborn, or restricted affect.

DIFFERENTIAL DIAGNOSIS

- <u>Obsessive-compulsive disorder:</u> Patients with OCPD do not have recurrent obsessions or compulsions classically seen with OCD. Also, the symptoms of OCPD are ego-syntonic, whereas they are ego-dystonic in OCD and they are aware they have a problem in OCD.
- <u>Narcissistic personality disorder:</u> both conditions focus on assertiveness and achievement, but OCPD patients are motivated but perfectionism and the work itself whereas NPD patients are motivated by status.

MANAGEMENT

- **Psychotherapy initial treatment of choice for Personality disorders, including OCPD — eg, social training, cognitive behavioral therapy**, group therapy. Psychodynamic therapy.
- <u>Pharmacotherapy:</u> May be indicated if comorbid conditions are present. SSRIs most commonly used.

GRIEF REACTION

- Altered emotional state as a response to a major loss (eg, death of a loved one).

5 stages of grief: Denial, anger, bargaining, depression, & acceptance (the stages are not linear).

- **Denial** often occurs in the early days after bereavement as a temporary defense, experienced consciously or subconsciously, in which a person feels numb, downplays their symptoms, or carry on as if nothing has happened ("I feel fine") or minimizes the situation. They may feel the presence of the person who died, hear their voice, or even "see" them (simple hallucinations).

- **Anger** response to the feeling that death is cruel and unfair, especially when the feeling is the person died before time or there were future plans together. They may feel angry towards the person who has died, or angry at themselves for things they did or didn't do before the death.

- **Bargaining:** in trying to deal with the difficulty that it is hard to accept that there's nothing they can do to change things, they make deals or going over what happened, asking a lot of "what if" questions, wishing they could go back and change things with the hope for a different outcome.

- **Depression**: sadness and longing with intense pain that come in waves over many months or years.

- **Acceptance** coming to terms with the situation. They may never "get over" it but the pain may ease, and they can find more meaning to life and the loss of life.

Normal grief: usually resolves within 6 months to 1 year.

- It peaks usually within the first couple of months after the loss. **Usually characterized by intense emotions, appetite or sleep disturbances, guilt, weight loss.**

- Symptoms may include illusions or simple hallucinations of the deceased that the patient understands is not real. Patients are usually able to function.

- **Abnormal grief: Severe symptoms, symptoms >1 year or positive suicidal ideation,** psychosis, illusions, or hallucinations that the patient perceives are real.

- Persistent complex bereavement disorder: only one considered a mental disorder. Severe grief reactions that persist >1 year (or 6 months in children) after the death of the bereaved.

MANAGEMENT

- Psychotherapy. Short course of Benzodiazepines may be needed for insomnia in some.

PHARMACOTHERAPY FOR SMOKING CESSATION		
TREATMENT	**INDICATIONS**	**ADVERSE EFFECTS**
VARENECLINE	• **More effective than either Bupropion or combination NRT.** • **Mechanism of action: partial nicotine receptor agonist** (blocks nicotine from binding, reducing reward effects).	• **Nausea (most common),** headache • **Disorder sleep: Insomnia & abnormal dreams.** • **Increased suicidality** • **Neuropsychiatric conditions.**
NICOTINE REPLACEMENT THERAPY **Long-acting NRT** Nicotine patch **Short acting NRT** nasal spray, gum, inhaler, lozenge	• Less cravings & daytime withdrawal symptoms • Long-acting may be combined with short-acting to improve efficacy.	• **No significant adverse effects;** safe in almost all patients. • GI: nausea, vomiting, abdominal pain, diarrhea. • **Headache** • Local irritation (eg, patch)
BUPROPION	• **Less post cessation weight gain** • Norepinephrine & Dopamine reuptake inhibitor (NDRI) that **reduces nicotine cravings and withdrawal symptoms.** • **Good for Major depressive disorder.**	• **Contraindicated in patients with reduced seizure threshold, including eating disorders.** • **Psychosis at high doses.**

DRUG ABUSE/DEPENDENCE

TOBACCO USE/DEPENDENCE

EPIDEMIOLOGY
- **Smoking is the most important modifiable risk factor in the US for preventable pulmonary, cardiac, and cancer deaths and the leading cause of preventable death in the US and worldwide.** Smoking cessation should be discussed with all smokers at every clinical contact.

CLINICAL MANIFESTATIONS
- <u>Effects:</u> restlessness, anxiety, insomnia, and increase in gastrointestinal motility.

Nicotine toxicity
- **Acute toxicity from overdosage of caffeine or nicotine includes <u>excessive CNS stimulation</u>** with tremor, insomnia, nervousness; cardiac stimulation with arrhythmias and respiratory paralysis.
- Cigarette smoking during pregnancy is associated with low birth weight, SIDS, & postnatal effects.

Nicotine withdrawal:
- **The anxiety and mental discomfort experienced from discontinuing <u>nicotine</u> are major hindrances to quitting the habit** — symptoms include intense nicotine craving, dysphoria, restlessness, anxiety, irritability, poor concentration, sleep abnormalities (eg, insomnia), headache, mood depression, increased appetite, weight gain, chest tightness, and inability to socialize.

MANAGEMENT OF DEPENDENCE
- **Includes counseling, motivational interviewing, support therapy, and Cognitive behavioral therapy as part of the management, often with medical management.** Combination therapy most effective than any single treatment. Relapse after abstinence is common.
- **First-line pharmacotherapies for smoking cessation include [1] Nicotine replacement therapy (NRT), [2] Varenicline, and [3] Bupropion.** For the general population, the choice among the therapies is based largely on patient preference, with a few notable exceptions for patients with comorbidities or contraindications to certain drugs.
- Pharmacotherapy is usually recommended for at least 3 months. If there is no response to initial therapy, switching to another first-line therapy is indicated.

Regimen options:
- **For most patients, treatment with either [1] Varenicline or [2] a combination of two Nicotine replacement products (a patch which a long-acting form, plus a short-acting form such as the gum or lozenge) is first-line pharmacologic therapy;** the choice depends upon patient preference after shared clinical decision-making. In studies, **Varenicline produced higher quit rates than Bupropion or the Nicotine patch, which were comparable in efficacy.**
- Combination treatment with Varenicline and Nicotine patch is also an option when selecting initial therapy.
- Bupropion appears to be somewhat less effective than combination NRT or Varenicline. However, Bupropion is a reasonable alternative first-line choice if the patient had short-term success with Bupropion in a previous quit attempt, if cost is an issue, if the patient has Depression that would also benefit from treatment, or if the patient wishes to temporarily avoid post-cessation weight gain.

Considerations for special populations:
- **Varenicline is associated with depression and suicidal ideation;** thus, patients with a history of depression should be closely monitored.
- **<u>Bupropion:</u> reasonable alternative in patients with Depression or worried about weight gain.**
- <u>Cardiovascular disease</u> — Varenicline, NRT, and Bupropion are all options. NRT is often used in hospitalized patients with CVD due to its widespread ability and rapid relief of symptoms.
- **<u>Seizures</u> — Bupropion is contraindicated in patients with a seizure disorder or a predisposition to seizures, as it reduces the seizure threshold (eg, eating disorders such as Bulimia nervosa, Anorexia nervosa, alcohol withdrawal).** Varenicline and NRT are options for patients with seizure disorders.

- <u>Pregnancy</u> — For all pregnant individuals who smoke, a behavioral counseling program. In addition, for pregnant individuals who smoke heavily or are unable to quit with behavioral counseling alone, adjunctive pharmacotherapy with Nicotine replacement therapy (NRT) may be needed. Bupropion is a reasonable alternative to NRT as adjunctive pharmacotherapy. Because of lack of safety data, Varenicline is not usually used for smoking cessation in pregnant individuals.

VARENICLINE
<u>Mechanism of action:</u>
- **Blocks the nicotine receptors (nAChR), reducing nicotine activity.**
- **Partial agonist of the alpha4 beta-2 subtype nicotinic receptors that mimics the effects of nicotine, reducing the reward effect and preventing withdrawal symptoms.**

<u>Efficacy:</u>
- In studies, Varenicline produced higher quit rates than bupropion or the Nicotine patch, which were comparable in efficacy.

<u>Initiation:</u>
- **Therapy should begin 1 week prior to quit date and continued 4 months after quit date.**

<u>Adverse effects:</u>
- **Nausea most common,** headache, insomnia, **increased suicidality, neuropsychiatric conditions.**

NICOTINE REPLACEMENT THERAPY (NRT)
- Nicotine replacement therapy with gum, nasal sprays, transdermal patches, inhaler, & lozenges allows for tapering.

<u>Indications:</u>
- Nicotine replacement therapy (NRT) is for those who want to quit smoking, as abruptly stopping can cause withdrawal symptoms and cravings.
- Using NRT helps one to reduce the motivation of smoking cigarettes because the body still gets nicotine from another safer method.

<u>Dosing:</u>
- The initial dosing for Nicotine replacement therapy is usually based on the number of cigarettes smoked per day.
- Heavier smokers should use an increased strength/dose of nicotine therapy.

Regimens:
- **2 Nicotine replacement products (a patch which a long-acting form and gives a basal rate of nicotine, plus a short-acting form such as the gum or lozenge) is first-line pharmacologic therapy**; The patch is used to provide sustained withdrawal symptom relief for 24 hours; the short-acting nicotine product is added to be used "as needed" to control any breakthrough cravings or other withdrawal symptoms.
- When using NRT, combination NRT is considered standard of care; however, using single-type NRT may be a reasonable alternative based on cost, side effect profiles, and patient preference.

BUPROPION
- **Antidepressant drug often used in combination with nicotine tapering therapy.**

<u>Mechanism of action:</u>
- **<u>Norepinephrine-Dopamine reuptake inhibitor</u>** increases brain levels of dopamine in the nucleus accumbens and norepinephrine, simulating the effect of nicotine on these neurotransmitters; **reduces nicotine cravings and withdrawal symptoms. It also acts as a nicotine antagonist.**

<u>Adverse effects:</u>
- **<u>CNS stimulation</u>** (noradrenergic effects): increased anxiety, insomnia, **dry mouth,** hypertension, headache, tremor. **Increased risk of seizures (lowers seizure threshold).**
- <u>Dopaminergic effects</u>: **nausea, increased psychosis at high doses.**

Contraindications:
- **<u>Increased seizure risk</u>: Epilepsy or conditions with increased seizure risk (eg, eating disorders such as Bulimia & Anorexia,** or patients undergoing abrupt discontinuation of alcohol).

OPIOID INTOXICATION

- Opiates: a drug derived from alkaloids of the opium poppy (eg, Heroin).
- Opioid: The class of drugs that includes opiates, opioid peptides, and all synthetic and semisynthetic drugs that mimic the actions of the opiates.

Opioid agonists:
- Strong: Fentanyl, Heroin, Morphine, Meperidine, Hydromorphone, Hydrocodone, Methadone.
- Moderate: Oxycodone, Hydrocodone, Codeine.
- Other: Dextromethorphan (antitussive); Loperamide and Diphenoxylate (antidiarrheal agent).

OPIOID INTOXICATION
Euphoria & sedation:
- **Most of the adverse effects of the opioid analgesics (eg, nausea, vomiting, constipation, respiratory depression) are predictable extensions of their pharmacologic effects.**
- **A triad of [1] respiratory depression (most specific sign), [2] pupillary constriction** (not always), **& [3] comatose state is characteristic of Opioid intoxication.**
- Drowsiness, impaired social functioning, impaired memory, slow or slurred speech, & coma.
- Drug interactions involving opioid analgesics are additive CNS depression with ethanol, sedative hypnotics, anesthetics, antipsychotic drugs, tricyclic antidepressants, and antihistamines.
- Meperidine, Tramadol, and Tapentadol have also been implicated in Serotonin syndrome when used with Selective serotonin reuptake inhibitors (SSRIs).

Physical examination findings:
- **Respiratory depression (decreased respiratory rate <12/minute) most specific sign. Decreased tidal volume, shallow breathing, hypopnea, & bradypnea.** May develop Biot's breathing (groups of quick, shallow inspirations followed by regular or irregular periods of apnea).
- **Altered and/or depressed mental status** — may range from euphoria to coma. Lethargy.
- **Pupillary constriction (narcotics are miotics).** Meperidine may be associated with normal pupils.
- **Bradycardia.** Decreased bowel sounds.
- **Histamine release may cause mild hypotension, nausea, vomiting, flushing.**
- Patients on long-term narcotics may develop constipation (opioid receptors in the GI tract reduce GI motility), hypothermia.

DIAGNOSIS
- Diagnosis of overdosage is confirmed if intravenous injection or nasal insufflation of Naloxone, an antagonist of the opioid receptors, results in prompt signs of recovery. Rule out hypoglycemia.

MANAGEMENT OF OPIOID INTOXICATION
- **Support airway & breathing first step** (monitor depth and rate of ventilation). Airway protection must be maintained. **Adequate ventilation (oxygenation) with a bag valve mask should be provided BEFORE Naloxone is given. Assisted ventilation with a bag valve mask is utilized until Naloxone reverses the respiratory depression** in patients with low respiratory rates of apnea. Endotracheal intubation if unable to maintain airway.
- **Opioid antagonists, such as Naloxone (short-acting) and other therapeutic measures, especially ventilatory support.** Nalmefene or Naltrexone are alternatives.
- **Naloxone is an opioid receptor antagonist used in acute intoxication or overdose to acutely reverse the effects of opioids. Onset of action ~2 minutes IV preferred (~5 minutes IM),** SQ & nasal insufflation preparation of Naloxone to treat opioid overdose promptly. ~30-60 minutes duration of action. Most commonly used in patients with respiratory depression. A second IV dose can be administered every 2 to 3 minutes.

Prevention of recurrent opioid overdose:
- Initiation of opioid agonist therapy (eg, Buprenorphine) associated with decreased all-cause and opioid-related mortality. Other harm reduction strategies: take-home Naloxone, substance use disorder programs, recovery specialist referral, & distributing sterile injection equipment.

OPIOID WITHDRAWAL

- Signs and symptoms of withdrawal begin as early as 4-12 hours after the last dose of a short-acting opioid; often delayed 24-48 hours after cessation of a longer-acting opioid (eg, Methadone). Withdrawal symptoms typically peak within 24-48 hours of onset and persist for several days with short-acting agents and up to two weeks with Methadone.
- **Symptoms**: **lacrimation, rhinorrhea, pruritus, nausea, vomiting, abdominal cramping, diarrhea, sweating, yawning, joint pains (arthralgias), myalgias, dysphoria, restlessness, craving for opioid.** Withdrawal is often unpleasant but is not life threatening.
- **Physical examination**: **piloerection (goose bumps), pupillary dilation (mydriasis), yawning, diaphoresis, increased bowel sounds, flu-like symptoms (eg, rhinorrhea, sneezing). CNS activation: hypertension, tachycardia, tachypnea.**

MANAGEMENT
Opioid withdrawal:
- **Symptomatic control: Clonidine (decreases sympathetic symptoms), Loperamide for diarrhea, Dicyclomine for abdominal cramps, & NSAIDs for joint pains & muscle cramps.**
- Benzodiazepines may be helpful in some cases of mild withdrawal.
- **Severe symptoms can be treated with detox with Methadone or Buprenorphine + Naloxone.**
Long-term management of dependence:
- Methadone maintenance program. **Suboxone (Buprenorphine + Naloxone), or Naltrexone.**
- **Naloxone, Nalmefene, and Naltrexone are pure opioid receptor antagonists that have few other effects at doses that produce marked inhibition of agonist effects.**

Methadone
- Mechanism of action: long-acting opioid receptor agonist used in the control withdrawal from opioid in patients with opioid addiction. Can be used in pregnant opioid-dependent women. Given orally.
- Indications: In withdrawal states, Methadone permits a slow tapering of opioid effect that diminishes the intensity of abstinence symptoms, and the prolonged action of Methadone blocks the euphoria inducing effects of doses of shorter acting opioids (eg, Heroin, Morphine).
- Adverse effects: can cause prolonged QT interval.
Buprenorphine; Buprenorphine + Naloxone
- Mechanism of action: **mixed agonist-antagonist. Partial mu opioid receptor agonist. Suboxone is a combination of Buprenorphine + Naloxone** (Naloxone prevents intoxication from IV injection).
- Indications: **[1] acute withdrawal states**: Buprenorphine has an even longer duration of action and can reduce withdrawal symptoms for 24 to 36 hours; 4-8 mg SQ. **[2] long-term management of opioid dependence: partial agonist (ceiling exists for its potential to cause respiratory depression), minimizes effects of opioids, long duration of action, & high affinity with partial activity at the mu opioid receptor.** Clinically supervised while initiating treatment.
- **Start Buprenorphine when the patient is abstinent from opioids (eg, in the withdrawal period)** — as a partial opioid agonist, Buprenorphine induces withdrawal symptoms in patients who have full agonists in their system because it will displace the full agonist but with reduced opioid effect.
Naltrexone
- Mechanism of action: competitive opioid antagonist. Naltrexone decreases the craving for ethanol and is approved for adjunctive use in alcohol dependency programs. Oral or monthly depot injection.
- Adverse effects: Precipitates withdrawal if used within 7 days of heroin use.
Other:
- Unlike the older drugs, two new antagonists, Methylnaltrexone and Alvimopan, do not cross the blood-brain barrier. These agents block adverse effects of strong opioids on peripheral mu receptors, including those in the gastrointestinal tract responsible for constipation, with minimal effects on analgesic actions and without precipitating an abstinence syndrome.
- Naloxegol, a pegylated form of Naloxone, is also used to reverse opioid constipation.

ALCOHOL WITHDRAWAL

UNCOMPLICATED ALCOHOL WITHDRAWAL:

- **Uncomplicated = no seizures, hallucinosis, or delirium tremens.**
- **Onset: 6–36 hours after last drink (time may vary).** Symptoms of mild withdrawal resolve within 1-2 days (24-48 hours) if the symptoms do not progress, usually with recovery.
- Clinical manifestations: **increased CNS activity — hand tremors, shaking, restlessness, anxiety, irritability, minor agitation, insomnia, diaphoresis, palpitations, tachycardia, hypertension, headache, GI (nausea, vomiting, diarrhea, loss of appetite), alcohol craving.**
- Physical signs include sinus tachycardia (heart rate >120 beats/min), systolic hypertension, hyperactive reflexes, and tremor.
- Some patients with mild withdrawal will go on to develop additional manifestations of withdrawal, such as alcohol hallucinosis, withdrawal seizures, or withdrawal delirium (delirium tremens).
- **Patients can have withdrawal seizures or hallucinosis without symptoms of mild withdrawal.**

WITHDRAWAL SEIZURES:

- **Onset: 6–36 hours after drinking either stops or is significantly reduced.** Usually generalized tonic-clonic type, occurring singly or in clusters of 2-3; seen in 10-30% of patients in withdrawal.
- Most commonly occurs as a single brief episode.
- Risk factors may include concurrent withdrawal from Benzodiazepines or other sedative-hypnotic drugs; other risk factors include relatively low potassium and platelet levels.

ALCOHOLIC HALLUCINOSIS:

- **Onset: 12–24 hours after the last drink and resolves in another 24-48 hours.**
- Clinical manifestations: **visual (most common; often seeing insects or animals in the room), auditory, and/or tactile hallucinations. Unlike withdrawal delirium, Alcoholic hallucinosis is associated with [1] a clear sensorium (no altered cognition) & [2] normal vital signs usually.**
- The risk for Alcohol hallucinosis may be related to genetic factors and/or decreased thiamine absorption.

WITHDRAWAL [DELIRUM (DELIRIUM TREMENS (DTs)]:

- Onset: **2–5 days after last drink** and reported to occur in 1 - 4% of patients hospitalized for alcohol withdrawal and has a 5% mortality rate. **Most common between 48-96 hours after the last drink.**
- Risk factors: age >30 years, prior DTs increase risk.
- Clinical manifestations: **rapid-onset, fluctuating disturbance of attention and cognition — delirium (altered sensorium), hallucinations, agitation. Abnormal vital signs (eg, tachycardia, hypertension, fever, drenching sweats). Patients are often diaphoretic.**

6-12 hours after last drink	12-48 hours after last drink	2-5 days after last drink
Tremulousness	Hallucinations Seizure	Delirium tremens
Mild withdrawal **Autonomic hyperactivity** • **Anxiety, tremors** • Agitation, restlessness • Diaphoresis, palpitations • Insomnia • GI upset (N/V) • Intact orientation • Headache • Alcohol craving • Loss of appetite • Sinus tachycardia Systolic hypertension, • Hyperactive reflexes	**Seizures (6-48 hours):** • Single or generalized tonic clonic **Alcoholic Hallucinosis (12-24h):** • (1) Visual, auditory, or tactile • **(2) Clear sensorium:** **Intact orientation** **(3) Stable vital signs**	**Delirium tremens 48-96 hours:** • **(1) Altered sensorium:** **confusion, agitation,** hallucinations, **disorientation.** • **(2) Abnormal vital signs** - fever (hyperthermia) - tachycardia - hypertension - diaphoresis

LABORATORY & OTHER TESTING

- Laboratory testing usually includes complete blood count, serum electrolytes, including potassium, magnesium, and phosphate, glucose, creatinine, liver function tests, amylase and lipase, blood alcohol level, urine drug testing, which should include testing for benzodiazepines, cocaine, and opioids. Urine human chorionic gonadotropin test for premenopausal women.
- ECG: An electrocardiogram is suggested for patients over 50 years or if there is a history of cardiac problems.

MANAGEMENT

- **Supportive management: medical treatment, IV hydration, nutritional supplementation, continuous monitoring of vital signs & symptoms, & hospitalization** to prevent or complications of withdrawal and cardiac arrhythmias. **Alcohol withdrawal can be fatal.**
- Vitals monitoring: Abnormal vital signs indicate the progression of the withdrawal due to the autonomic nervous system becoming unstable (eg, tachycardia, hypertension, and tachypnea).

IV Benzodiazepines:

- **Benzodiazepines are used to treat the psychomotor agitation most patients experience during withdrawal & to prevent progression** from minor withdrawal symptoms to more severe ones. eg, **IV Diazepam, IV Lorazepam, oral Chlordiazepoxide, & oral Oxazepam.**
- Mechanism of action: **potentiates GABA-mediated CNS inhibition.** Alcohol mimics GABA at the receptor sites (GABA is the most abundant inhibitory neurotransmitter in the CNS) so Alcohol withdrawal causes increased CNS activity.
- Benzodiazepines are titrated until they patient is slightly somnolent & then gradually tapered.
- **Lorazepam (shorter half-life) or Oxazepam (no active metabolites) preferred in patients with advanced cirrhosis or alcoholic hepatitis** (Chlordiazepoxide may cause over titration).

Other:

- **IV fluids, IV thiamine (B1), magnesium, multivitamins (including B12 & folate), & electrolyte repletion.** Repleting thiamine (B1) can reduce the risk of Wernicke encephalopathy.
- Electrolyte and fluid abnormalities should be corrected.
- Beta blockers can be used to treat the elevated blood pressure and tachycardia associated with alcohol withdrawal. Delirium tremens refractory to Benzodiazepines: Phenobarbital or Propofol.

ALCOHOL DEPENDENCE

- Alcohol abuse becomes dependence when withdrawal symptoms develop or tolerance.

CAGE ALCOHOL SCREENING

≥2 considered a positive screen.

Cutdown	Have you felt the need to cut down on drinking?
Annoyed	Have people told you that they were annoyed at you when you drink?
Guilt	Have you ever felt guilty about your drinking?
Eye opener	Have you ever needed an eye opener to start your day or reduce jitteriness?

MANAGEMENT

- Supportive: psychotherapy: eg, individual, group (eg, Alcoholics Anonymous); Inpatient & residential rehabilitation programs.
- **Disulfiram (Antabuse)** can be a deterrent to alcohol use.
  - Mechanism of action: **inhibits aldehyde dehydrogenase (enzyme needed to metabolize alcohol),** leading to increased acetaldehyde when coupled with alcohol intake ⇨ **uncomfortable symptoms including hypotension, palpitations, flushing, hyperventilation, dizziness, nausea, vomiting, & headache.**
  - Contraindications: cardiovascular disease, diabetes mellitus, hypothyroidism, epilepsy, kidney, or liver disease.
- **Naltrexone:** opioid antagonist that reduces alcohol craving & reduces alcohol-induced euphoria.
- Gabapentin, Topiramate.

COCAINE INTOXICATION AND WITHDRAWAL

COCAINE INTOXICATION

- Cocaine can be snorted, swallowed, injected, or smoked.

CLINICAL MANIFESTATIONS
CNS effects:

- **Cocaine produces a stimulant effect via inhibition of the reuptake of the CNS neurotransmitters dopamine, norepinephrine, and epinephrine in the synaptic cleft (has marked Amphetamine-like effects).**
- Dopamine plays a role in the "reward" system of the brain.
- The euphoria, self-confidence, and mental alertness produced by Cocaine are short-lasting and positively reinforce its continued use.

Cardiovascular effects:

- The primary actions of Cocaine on the cardiovascular system are from alpha- and beta-1-adrenoceptor stimulation, resulting in **increased heart rate, systemic arterial pressure, myocardial contractility, and arterial vasoconstriction (eg, coronary arteries)**, major determinants of myocardial oxygen demand.
- **Cocaine toxicity may cause tachycardia, dysrhythmia, hypertension, and coronary vasospasm, which can result in acute coronary syndrome, stroke, and death.**
- **Tachycardia:** Excess catecholamine release can lead to tachycardia. Cocaine causes sodium channel blockade (unlike Methamphetamine), which **may trigger refractory tachydysrhythmias & re-entry ventricular arrhythmias.**
- **Hypertension:** Cocaine-induced hypertension results from excess monoamines, such as dopamine, norepinephrine, and epinephrine, in the central nervous system and peripheral circulation, causing alpha- and beta-adrenergic stimulation. Like Methamphetamine, **Cocaine prevents the reuptake of catecholamines, increasing sympathetic tone, causing hypertension and coronary vasospasm.**
- **Thrombosis:** Cocaine-induced platelet activation and thrombus formation caused by alpha-adrenergic- and adenosine diphosphate-mediated increase in platelet aggregation may result in macro- and microvascular occlusion, ischemia, and increased risk of cardiac dysrhythmia.
- Long-term use of Cocaine can also alter cardiac histology leading to fibrosis, myocarditis, and contraction band necrosis.

CLINICAL MANIFESTATIONS

- **CNS stimulation & autonomic hyperactivity: elevated or euphoric mood, psychomotor agitation, paranoia, pressured speech, emotional lability, altered mental status.**
- Nausea, vomiting & seizures. Chest pain &/or dyspnea. Abdominal pain (mesenteric ischemia).

Physical examination:

- **Sympathetic hyperactivity — increased motor activity, tremor, flushing, hyperthermia (may be as high as 45oC), diaphoresis, cold sweats, & pupillary dilation (mydriasis).**
- **The excess catecholamines may cause hypertension, tachycardia, agitation, and aggression** (however, bradycardia &/or hypotension may also be seen).
- **Increased bowel sounds and diaphoresis helps to distinguish Cocaine toxicity from Anticholinergic toxicity,** which presents with dry skin and decreased bowel sounds.

Severe intoxication:

- **Respiratory depression, arrhythmias, hypertension, seizures, repetitive behaviors (eg, picking at skin), agitation, aggression, hallucinations, and paranoia.**
- **Deaths from Cocaine are usually the result of cardiac arrest, arrhythmias, stroke, myocardial infarction, seizures, or respiratory arrest.** Cardiac toxicity is partly due to blockade of norepinephrine reuptake by Cocaine; its local anesthetic action contributes to the production of seizures. The powerful vasoconstrictive action of Cocaine may lead to severe hypertensive episodes, resulting in myocardial infarcts and strokes.

DIAGNOSIS

- Depending on the patient's presentation, laboratory testing for suspected Cocaine toxicity may include complete blood count, comprehensive chemistry panel, troponin, B-type natriuretic peptide, creatinine kinase, urinalysis, urine toxicology screen, and electrocardiogram.
- Creatine kinase and Urinalysis may detect myoglobinuria if Rhabdomyolysis is suspected.
- A urine drug screen is a must to detect other illicit substances. Most cocaine disappears from the body within 24 hours, but the metabolite, benzoylecgonine, may persist for weeks. This metabolite can also cause neurotoxicity. Troponin if myocardial infarction is suspected.
- An ECG should be done if the patient has chest pain, dyspnea, irregular pulse, or hypoxia.

MANAGEMENT

- Patients with Cocaine toxicity need to be stabilized, and the ABCDEs should be assessed. The treatment should be based on clinical symptoms, and physical restraints should be avoided.
- **<u>Benzodiazepines</u> are first-line management of cocaine-induced agitation, hyperthermia, and cardiovascular toxicity as they decrease CNS sympathetic outflow.**

<u>Mild:</u> **Reassurance and Benzodiazepines.**

<u>Severe agitation or psychosis:</u>

- **<u>Benzodiazepines</u> first-line treatment with agitation** (eg, Diazepam 5-10 mg IV every 3-5 minutes until agitation is controlled). **Antipsychotics such as Haloperidol and Olanzapine may also be useful**.
- Diphenhydramine is often added to enhance sedation and as prophylaxis against dystonia and akathisia. A common example of this is the "B-52" with its combination of Haloperidol (5 mg), Diphenhydramine (50 mg), and Lorazepam (2 mg). Do <u>not</u> place the patient in restraints (may lead to Rhabdomyolysis).

<u>Cardiovascular effects:</u>

- **<u>Benzodiazepines</u> (eg, Lorazepam or Diazepam) first line because most of the cardiovascular effects (eg tachycardia, tachydysrhythmia, hypertension, chest pain) in cocaine toxicity are centrally mediated via the sympathetic system** & they decrease CNS & sympathetic activity.
- <u>Phentolamine</u>, an alpha blocker, may be used in patients with refractory or symptomatic cocaine-induced hypertension to counteract the alpha-adrenergic vasoconstrictive effects of cocaine.
- Nitroglycerin or Nitroprusside are suitable alternative medications for the management of refractory hypertension because they are vasodilators without beta blocking effects. Nitroglycerin also helpful for Myocardial infarction.
- Non-dihydropyridine calcium channel blockers (eg, Diltiazem and Verapamil) have been shown to reduce hypertension, but not tachycardia. Dihydropyridines (eg, Nifedipine) should be avoided due to the potential for reflex tachycardia.
- **If a beta-blocker is used, a mixed alpha-1/beta blocker (eg, Labetalol) is often preferred over the other beta blockers** to prevent "unopposed alpha-stimulation".

<u>Hyperthermia:</u>

- <u>External cooling methods</u>: eg, Cooling blankets and possibly ice baths. Tepid water misting with convection cooling from a fan may be used.

COCAINE WITHDRAWAL

- The abstinence syndrome associated with withdrawal from Cocaine is similar to that after <u>Amphetamine</u> discontinuance. The symptoms are mild and non-life threatening.
- **Cocaine craving with resultant dysphoria, apathy, irritability, marked depression, anhedonia, sleep disturbance [insomnia initially followed by <u>hypersomnia</u> (excessive sleep)], disorientation, increased appetite,** difficulty concentrating, psychomotor slowing.
- <u>Physical signs</u> musculoskeletal pain, tremors, chills, involuntary motor movement, and possibly bradycardia (vitals are often normal).
- **Patients may develop nightmares, <u>suicide ideation</u>,** headache, and increased irritability.

MANAGEMENT

- **Mainly symptomatic; individual or group counseling.** Intensive outpatient program for more severe symptoms. Hospitalization may be required for severe psychiatric symptoms.

PHENCYCLIDINE (PCP) INTOXICATION

- **Phencyclidine (PCP) is a dissociative anesthetic and hallucinogenic drug that is a NMDA glutamate receptor antagonist (also known as "angel dust").**
- Can be ingested orally, injected intravenously, inhaled, or smoked.

CLINICAL MANIFESTATIONS
Short onset of action with a brief duration (1-4 hours).
- **Symptoms of PCP intoxication:** PCP blocks the uptake of dopamine and norepinephrine, leading to sympathomimetic effects — **eg, severe agitation, hyperthermia, hypoxia, nystagmus, hypertension, tachycardia, confusion, hallucinations, delusions, violent behavior, seizures, bronchodilation, muscle rigidity, ataxia, and coma.**
- **Psychotomimetic: Psychomotor agitation, rage,** impulsiveness, fear, homicidality, delirium. **PCP intoxication often leads to bizarre and often violent behavior, hallucinations, delusions of physical prowess, and a diminished perception of pain.** Impaired judgment often leads to reckless behavior, and often leads to **traumatic injuries**. Detachment of surroundings.

Neuropsychiatric findings:
- CNS signs and symptoms are common and vary widely. Patients may be alert with bizarre behavior, agitated or violent, or sedated, even present in a comatose state.
- Adrenergic stimulation is classic, but patients may exhibit CNS stimulation or depression.
- Complications: Hypertension, hyperthermia, seizures, Rhabdomyolysis, hypoglycemia, coma.

PHYSICAL EXAMINATION
- **Multidirectional nystagmus (vertical, horizontal, or rotary).**
- **Marked hypertension, tachycardia,** ataxia, erythematous and dry skin.

MANAGEMENT
- **Supportive care:** eg, airway, breathing and circulation monitoring, placement in a low stimulus (quiet environment with low lights).
- Physical restraints may be necessary initially and several staff members are often needed to control patients agitated from PCP. Chemical sedation should be administered as rapidly as possible.
- **Parenteral Benzodiazepines (eg, Diazepam, Lorazepam, Midazolam) are the first line agents for chemical sedation if agitated, hyperthermic, for PCP-induced hypertension & seizures, and to protect against seizures.**
- Antipsychotics (eg, Haloperidol 5 mg or Droperidol 2.5 mg) may be used as adjunctive therapy if Benzodiazepine does not adequately control symptoms of agitation and psychosis. Brief physical restraints may be required in some cases of severe agitation.
- Treatment of complications — after adequate sedation, the patient with PCP intoxication should be carefully examined for secondary injuries and associated trauma.

MARIJUANA INTOXICATION & WITHDRAWAL

CLINICAL MANIFESTATIONS OF MARIJUANA INTOXICATION
- **Euphoria, giddiness, anxiety, disinhibition, intensification of sensory experiences, dry (cotton) mouth, increased appetite, motor impairment, conjunctival injection (red eye), tachycardia, blood pressure changes,** tachypnea, fear, depression, psychosis & hallucination, nystagmus, ataxia.
- Chronic use can lead to cognitive performance issues.

MANAGEMENT
- Treatment is usually not needed. Symptomatic management if needed.
- Hyperemesis syndrome: Chronic severe emesis in chronic users. Managed with cessation of marijuana use and antiemetics (Ondansetron & Metoclopramide).

MARIJUANA WITHDRAWAL
- Irritability, insomnia, depression, restlessness, diaphoresis, diarrhea, & twitching 24-48 hours after cessation.

	INTOXICATION		WITHDRAWAL	
	BEHAVIORAL/MOOD EFFECTS	PSYCHOLOGICAL EFFECTS	ONSET	SYMPTOMS
ETHANOL **BENZODIAZEPINES**	Disinhibition *Depression:* slurred speech, impaired judgment & somnolence. Ataxia. Labile Mood: erratic behavior, aggression *Flumazenil used to treat benzodiazepine intoxication**	Prolonged reaction time, muscular incoordination, facial flushing **Chronic:** - **Wernicke's encephalopathy:** triad of ataxia, confusion & oculomotor palsy (due to thiamine/B1 deficiency). - **Korsakoff syndrome** amnesia (both retrograde & antegrade) - Hepatomegaly, palmar erythema, cirrhosis, Dupuytrens contractures, gynecomastia, testicular atrophy. - Increased mean corpuscular volume	6-24 hours 6 – 48 hours 2 – 5 days	*Increased CNS activity* tremor*, insomnia, nausea, vomiting, anxiety, tachycardia, hypertension, increased respirations Seizures, hyperreflexia *DELIRIUM TREMENS: altered sensorium:* tactile, visual or auditory hallucinations (ex. formication – "something crawling" on them) especially at night, altered mental status, seizures, coma, death. *Often occurs when hospitalized for a nonrelated illness.*
STIMULANTS **COCAINE** **AMPHETAMINES**	• *Initial:* elevated/euphoric mood, restlessness, pressured speech • **Psychosis:** mild ⇔ anxiety. Paranoia, *aggression, agitation,* hallucinations (Ex tactile, auditory) • *Treat cocaine intoxication with benzodiazepines,* neuroleptics & blood pressure reduction.	• Neurologic: ↑motor activity, headache, tremor, flushing, hyperthermia, cold sweats, nausea, vomiting, seizures • *SYMPATHETIC STIMULATION:* sweating, tachycardia, *hypertension, pupillary dilation*,* peripheral vasoconstriction, myocardial infarction. • Compulsive & stereotyped behavior (ex. picking at skin), rhabdomyolysis.	Varied onset	Craving with resultant dysphoria, agitation, anxiety, diaphoresis, *hypersomnia, increased appetite.* Neurologic: nightmares, *suicide ideation*,* headache, irritability, extreme fatigue, muscle cramps.
OPIOIDS & **NARCOTICS**	• **Euphoria & sedation:** impaired social functioning, impaired memory, drowsiness, slow or slurred speech. *Naloxone (Narcan) used to treat opioid intoxication**	• *Pupillary constriction** (narcotics are miotics). • *Respiratory depression,* bradycardia, hypotension,* coma, nausea, vomiting, hypothermia. • Chronic: pruritus & constipation (opioid receptors in GI tract decreases motility).	6-24 hours (Methadone may take longer)	Neurologic: psychomotor agitation, anxiety, irritability, twitching, yawning dysphoria, insomnia, diaphoresis Vitals: hyperthermia, hypertension, tachycardia Flulike sx: *rhinorrhea*,* myalgias, chills, *piloerections** (Goosebumps). GI: nausea, vomiting, diarrhea Ocular: *pupillary dilation*, tearing*
NICOTINE	• Nausea, vomiting, diarrhea, abdominal pain, headache	Tremor, tachycardia, salivation	Usually begin within 24h after last use	Psychomotor: anxiety, restlessness, bradycardia, increased appetite & craving
CANNABIS	• Euphoria, giddiness. • Psychosis in some cases.	Dry mouth (cotton-mouth), conjunctival erythema, tachycardia, hypotension	Usually on seen with heavy usage	Irritability insomnia, restlessness, diaphoresis, diarrhea, twitches.
PCP	• Impulsiveness, homicidality, psychosis, delirium, seizures, *nystagmus*			Depression, irritability, anxiety, sleep problems
LSD	• Visual hallucinations & synesthesias (seeing sound as color), delusions, pupillary dilation			

MDMA (ECSTASY)

- **MDMA (3,4-methylenedioxymethamphetamine), commonly called "Ecstasy" or "Molly", is a common illicit drug used, especially in adolescents and young adults.**

CLINICAL MANIFESTATIONS
- **Desired effects of MDMA** include increased alertness, reduced fatigue, euphoria, increased sexual arousal, disinhibition, enhanced sensory perception, retrieval of repressed memories, feelings of increased physical and mental powers, emotional closeness to others. These effects begin about 1 hour after oral ingestion, peak within 2 hours and usually lasts 4-6 hours.

Adverse effects:
- **Stimulant effects** include agitation, anxiety, disorientation, nausea, diaphoresis, blurry vision, tachycardia, and hypertension, all of which usually resolve spontaneously within a few hours.
- **Serotonergic effects** bruxism (grinding teeth or jaw clenching), restless legs, feelings of restlessness, hyperactivity, insomnia, difficulty concentrating, and possibly Serotonin syndrome.
- Serious adverse effects are less common but may include severe hypertension, severe tachycardia, hyperthermia, delirium, and psychomotor agitation.
- Life-threatening complications can occur, including **hyperthermia, dehydration,** intracranial hemorrhage, myocardial infarction, aortic dissection, dysrhythmias, **Rhabdomyolysis**, seizure, DIC, and Serotonin syndrome. **Hyponatremia** (increased physical activity & sympathomimetic effects result in hyperthermia and can result in Rhabdomyolysis; patients have increased thirst and hyperthermia, so they often consume large amounts of water, in addition to SIADH caused by MDMA, all resulting in severe Hyponatremia, resulting in cerebral edema, seizures, and death).
- Initial workup in severe cases may include CBC, coagulation studies, basic metabolic panel (if hyponatremia, order serum osmolality). creatine kinase, ECG, point of care glucose, Acetaminophen and salicylate blood concentrations, pregnancy testing in women of childbearing age.

MANAGEMENT
- **Severe Hypertension and psychomotor agitation** — Benzodiazepines (eg, Lorazepam 1-2 gm IV push) until the patent is sedated or the Hypertension is controlled. Nitroprusside or Phentolamine may be used in refractory Hypertension. Beta-blockers are avoided because they may result in unopposed alpha-adrenergic stimulation (causing a paradoxical increase in blood pressure).
- Gastrointestinal decontamination with activated charcoal is recommended for patients with recent MDMA intoxication (eg, <1 hour of ingestion) who are not sedated & can protect their airway.
- **Treatment of Hyponatremia** Hypertonic saline (3%) used for severe symptomatic hyponatremia (serum sodium usually <120 mEq/L) to rapidly reduce cerebral edema. Obtundation may require endotracheal intubation & the use of routine induction or paralytic agents. Mild hyponatremia can be managed with fluid restriction alone, often with sodium levels normalizing in 12-24 hours.
- **Butyrophenones (eg, Haloperidol, Droperidol) should <u>not</u> be used to sedate patients with MDMA toxicity.** Butyrophenones interfere with heat dissipation, prolong the QTc interval, and may decrease the seizure threshold.

CONDUCT DISORDER

- **Persistent pattern of disruptive behaviors that deviate sharply from the age–appropriate norms and <u>violates the rights of other humans & animals</u>, including aggressive behaviors.**

EPIDEMIOLOGY
- Lifetime prevalence 9%. More common in males.
- **High incidence of comorbid ADHD and/or Oppositional defiance disorder (ODD).**
- **May progress to Antisocial personality disorder in adulthood.**

CLINICAL MANIFESTATIONS
- **These individuals engage in physical and/or sexual violence, lack empathy for their victims, and may lack remorse for committing crimes.**

4 main group of behaviors: **"BADD"**
- **<u>B</u>reaking (violation) of rules** or age-appropriate norms: running away, skipping school (truancy), mischief, pranks, very early sexual activity.
- **<u>A</u>ggressive conduct:** physical fights, bullying or intimidating behavior, cruelty to others or animals, using a weapon, forcing someone into sexual activity, rape, or molestation.
- **<u>D</u>estructive conduct:** intentionally destroying property (vandalism), fire setting (arson).
- **<u>D</u>eceitfulness:** lying, theft, shoplifting, delinquency.

Gender differences:
- <u>Males:</u> Higher risk of fighting, stealing, fire setting, and vandalism.
- <u>Females:</u> Higher risk of lying, running away, sex-work, and substance use.

DIAGNOSTIC CRITERIA
- **Persistent pattern of recurrent violation of the rights of others or age-appropriate societal norms** with ≥3 behaviors over the last year and at least one incidence within the last 6 months:
- **[1] Aggression to humans or animals** — threatens, intimidates, or bullies others, use of a weapon, robbery, **physically cruelty or aggression to animals or humans,** sexual violence.
- **[2] Destruction of property** — **engages in fire setting, vandalism,** etc.
- **[3] Deceitfulness or theft** — lies to obtain goods and favors, burglary (eg, breaks into buildings, cars, or homes etc.), steals the properties of others, property loss. Lacks remorse for actions.
- **[4] Serious violation of rules** — runs away from home, stays out past curfew late at night, engages in truancy (often before 13 years old).
- **<18 years of age.**

MANAGEMENT
- **Multimodal:** **behavioral modification** (eg, more adaptive behaviors to deal with stressors, anger management training, problem-solving skills), community (eg, school) and family involvement, parent management training (eg, enforcing rules and setting limits).
- Pharmacotherapy to treat psychiatric comorbidities (eg, stimulants and non-stimulants for the treatment of ADHD), antidepressants for depression, mood stabilizers for the treatment of aggression, mood dysregulation, and bipolar disorder.

PROGNOSIS
Good prognosis:
- Positive relationship with at least 1 parent
- adolescent onset of symptoms
- female gender
- good interpersonal skills
- high IQ, good academic performance.

Poor prognosis:
- Onset of symptoms prior to 10 years
- Low IQ, poor academic performance.

ATTENTION-DEFICIT HYPERACTIVITY DISORDER (ADHD)

- **Neurodevelopmental disorder characterized by persistent [1] <u>inattention</u> (problems paying attention), [2] <u>impulsivity</u> (difficulty controlling behaviors), &/or [3] <u>hyperactivity</u> that is not age appropriate.**

EPIDEMIOLOGY
- <u>Prevalence</u>: 10% of children and 4.5% of adults. Many continue to have symptoms as adults (inattentiveness > hyperactivity).
- Male > females with a 2:1 ratio. Females present more often with inattentive symptoms.
- **Other psychiatric disorders often co-occur with ADHD in adults, including 67% comorbid with Conduct and Oppositional defiant disorders;** mood and anxiety disorders, substance use disorder, and intermittent explosive disorder. Learning disabilities and tic disorders are often seen.

ETIOLOGY
- The etiology of ADHD is related to a variety of factors, including genetic and an environmental component.
- <u>Genetics</u>: Siblings have twice the risk of having ADHD than the general population.
- <u>Environmental</u>: viral infections, smoking during pregnancy, nutritional deficiency, and alcohol exposure in the fetus have also been explored as possible causes of the disorder.

PATHOGENESIS
- **Dopamine and Norepinephrine play a key role in the areas of the brain responsible for regulating attention and executive function.**
- Neuroimaging reveals evidence of structural brain abnormalities among ADHD patients. The most common findings are smaller volumes in the frontal cortex (eg, anterior cingulate gyrus and prefrontal cortex reduction), cerebellum, and subcortical structures and abnormalities in the prefrontal (especially right fronto-subcortical) and parietal circuits.

CLINICAL MANIFESTATIONS
- <u>Children</u>: persistent (1) <u>inattention</u> (problems paying attention), (2) <u>impulsivity</u> (difficulty controlling behaviors), &/or (3) <u>hyperactivity</u> that is not age appropriate.
- In adults, however, these core symptoms may be missing, and they may manifest as other problems such as procrastination, mood instability, and low self-esteem. They will likely be more impulsive in nature or inattentive, as the hyperactivity symptoms can be better controlled.

DIAGNOSTIC CRITERIA
- **[A] A persistent pattern of inattention and/or hyperactivity-impulsivity that interferes with functioning or development, as characterized by 1 and/or 2:**
  - **1. At least 6 inattentive symptoms**: difficulty maintaining attention, does not appear to listen, fails to pay close attention to details, makes careless mistakes, easily distracted, loses things, forgetful in daily activities, struggles to follow instructions has difficulty with organization, avoids or dislikes tasks that require a lot of thinking. **and/or**
  - **2. At least 6 hyperactivity/impulsivity symptoms**: difficulty in engaging in activities quietly, fidgets with hands or feet, runs around or climbs excessively in childhood, extreme restlessness in adults, difficulty remaining seated, squirms in chair, acts as if driven by a motor, blurts out answers before questions have been fully asked, interrupts others, difficulty waiting/taking turns.
- **[B] Several inattentive or hyperactive-impulsive symptoms were present prior to age 12 years.**
- **[C] Several inattentive or hyperactive-impulsive symptoms are present in two or more settings** (eg, at home, school, or work; with friends or relatives; in other activities).
- **[D]** There is clear evidence that the symptoms interfere with, or reduce the quality of, social, academic, or occupational functioning.
- **[E]** The symptoms are not due to physiological effects of a substance, another medical or neurological condition (eg, traumatic brain injury), or another mental disorder.

3 subcategories:

- **Combined**: If both Criterion A1 (inattention) and Criterion A2 (hyperactivity-impulsivity) are met for the past six months.
- **Predominantly inattentive**: If Criterion A1 (inattention) is met but Criterion A2 (hyperactivity-impulsivity) is not met for the past six months.
- **Predominantly hyperactive/impulsive**: If Criterion A2 (hyperactivity-impulsivity) is met and Criterion A 1 (inattention) is not met for the past six months.

MANAGEMENT
Multimodal approach:

- Behavior modification techniques, social skills training, educational accommodations (eg, classroom modifications, executive function coaching, parental psychoeducation, parent management training, and medications. **CBT adjunct therapy for school-aged children, adolescents, and adults.**
- **Preschool-aged children** aged 4-5 years) — parent (or caregiver) training in behavior management (PTBM).

PHARMACOLOGICAL MANAGEMENT

- **School-aged children (≥6 years) & adolescents who meet diagnostic criteria — medications, with or without behavioral/psychologic interventions first-line therapy.**
- Medications are the most effective treatment for decreasing core symptoms but should be used in combinations with educational and behavioral interventions.

Stimulants:

- Indications: **stimulants are first-line and mainstay medical treatment of choice for ADHD — eg, Methylphenidate, Dexmethylphenidate, Amphetamine &/or Dextroamphetamine.** Stimulants are preferred to other medications because of rapid onset of action record of safety and efficacy.
- Mechanism of action: **Norepinephrine and dopamine reuptake inhibitors (presynaptic membranes), increasing norepinephrine and dopamine levels,** resulting in increased frontal lobe activity & impulse control. Amphetamines also directly release dopamine. Dopamine is a neurotransmitter associated with motivation, pleasure, attention, and movement. For many people with ADHD, stimulant medications increase executive function, boost concentration and focus, while reducing hyperactive and impulsive behaviors.
- Although Amphetamines may be slightly more efficacious, **Methylphenidate is better tolerated.**
- Adverse effects: **decreased appetite and insomnia (most common); weight loss, poor growth**, changes in blood pressure, dizziness, nightmares, psychosis, **bone loss**, risk of dependency **(diversion and misuse), tics (rare).**
- **Stimulant withdrawal symptoms: fatigue, hypersomnia, hyperphagia (increased appetite) and vivid dreams.**

Nonstimulants:

- **Atomoxetine & Viloxazine (selective norepinephrine reuptake inhibitors) are alternatives to stimulants and may be more appropriate for patients with a history of illicit substance use or household members with a history of illicit substance use, concern about abuse or diversion,** or a strong caregiver preference against stimulant medication. **Atomoxetine is less effective than stimulants but well tolerated.**
- Mechanism of action: **Selective norepinephrine reuptake inhibitors.** Dopamine & Norepinephrine play a key role in the areas of the brain responsible for regulating attention & executive function.
- Adverse effects: dry mouth decreased appetite, insomnia.

Alpha-2 adrenergic agonists:

- **(eg, Guanfacine, Clonidine),** are usually used when children respond poorly to a trial of stimulants or selective norepinephrine reuptake inhibitors, have unacceptable side effects, or have significant coexisting conditions. Less effective than stimulants.
- Adverse effects: hypotension, dizziness, sedation (Clonidine > Guanfacine), weight gain, dizziness.

Antidepressants:

- Bupropion: Norepinephrine and dopamine reuptake inhibitor.
- Venlafaxine: Serotonin and norepinephrine reuptake inhibitor.

AUTISM SPECTRUM DISORDER

- **Spectrum of developmental disorders characterized by [1] impairment in social interaction or communication, [2] restricted, repetitive stereotyped behaviors, as well as other signs leading to impaired social functioning.**

EPIDEMIOLOGY:
- Male: female 4:1.
- **Symptoms usually recognized between 12-24 months old.**

ETIOLOGY:
Multifactorial:
- Prenatal neurological insults (eg, infections, drugs), advanced paternal age, and low birth weight.
- 15% of ASD cases are associated with a known genetic mutation. **Fragile X syndrome is the most commonly known single gene cause of ASD.** Other genetic causes of ASD: Down syndrome, Rett syndrome, and tuberous sclerosis.
- Untreated Phenylketonuria results in Autism in 50% of patients. Association with Epilepsy.

CLINICAL MANIFESTATIONS:
- **ASD should be considered if there is a rapid deterioration of social and/or language skills during the first 2 years of life.**
- **ASD is characterized by (1) Atypical social communication and (2) Restricted, repetitive patterns of behavior, interests, or activities.**
- **Social interaction difficulties:** significant emotional discomfort or detachment (eg, avoiding eye contact, no response to cuddling or affection).
- **Impaired communication:** either inability to communicate or has the ability to communicate but chooses not to in social settings. Difficulties in understanding what is not explicitly stated (eg, metaphors, humor in jokes etc.).
- **Restricted, repetitive, stereotyped behaviors** & patterns of activities (eg, peculiar interest in objects, rigid, inflexible thought patterns), repetitive motor patterns.
- Other signs: persistent failure to develop social relationships, failure to show preference to parents over other adults; unusual sensitivity to visual, auditory or olfactory stimuli; unusual attachments to ordinary objects. Savantism (unusual talents).
- The gold standards of assessment are the Autism Diagnostic Interview-Revised and the Autism Diagnostic Observation Schedule.

DSM 5 DIAGNOSTIC criteria:

A diagnosis of ASD requires **all** of the following 5:

[1] Atypical social communication:

- Persistent deficits in social communication and social interaction in multiple settings; demonstrated by deficits in all 3 of the following (either currently or by history):
- **Social-emotional reciprocity** (eg, failure to produce mutually enjoyable and agreeable conversations or interactions because of a lack of mutual sharing of interests, lack of awareness or understanding of the thoughts or feelings of others).
- **Nonverbal communicative behaviors used for social interaction** (eg, difficulty coordinating verbal communication with its nonverbal aspects [eye contact, facial expressions, gestures, body language, and/or prosody/tone of voice]).
- **Developing, maintaining, and understanding relationships** (eg, difficulty adjusting behavior to social setting, lack of ability to show expected social behaviors, lack of interest in socializing, difficulty making friends even when interested in having friendships).

[2] Restricted, repetitive patterns of behavior, interests, or activities:

- Restricted, repetitive patterns of behavior, interests, or activities; demonstrated by at least 2 of the following (either currently or by history):
- **Stereotyped or repetitive movements, use of objects, or speech** (eg, stereotypies such as rocking, flapping, or spinning); echolalia (repeating parts of speech; repeating scripts from movies or prior conversations).
- **Insistence on sameness, unwavering adherence to routines, or ritualized patterns of verbal or nonverbal behavior** (eg, ordering toys into a line).
- **Highly restricted, fixated interests that are abnormal in strength or focus** (eg, preoccupation with certain objects [trains, vacuum cleaners, or parts of trains or vacuum cleaners]); perseverative interests (eg, excessive focus on a topic such as dinosaurs or natural disasters).
- **Increased or decreased response to sensory input or unusual interest in sensory aspects of the environment** (eg, adverse response to particular sounds; apparent indifference to temperature; excessive touching/smelling of objects.

Other criteria:

- **[3] The symptoms must impair function** (eg, social, academic, completing daily routines).
- **[4] The symptoms must be present in the early developmental period**. However, they may become apparent only after social demands exceed limited capacity; in later life, symptoms may be masked by learned strategies.
- **[5] The symptoms are not better explained by intellectual disability** (formerly referred to as mental retardation) or global developmental delay.

MANAGEMENT

- **Autism spectrum disorder (ASD) is a chronic condition that requires a comprehensive treatment approach — Referral for neuropsychologic testing, applied behavior analysis, behavioral modification strategies.** Treatment programs should be monitored to ensure appropriate response to therapy.
- Applied behavioral analysis: For Autism spectrum disorders (ASD), applied behavior analysis can be adapted for each individual, can be done at home or school, and can include one-to-one play therapy.
- Management must be individualized according to the child's age and specific needs. Treatment of ASD focuses on behavioral and educational interventions that target the core symptoms.
- **The primary treatment goals include (1) decrease patient deficits and family distress, (2) maximize functioning, move the child toward independence, and (3) improve the quality of life.**
- Pharmacologic interventions may be used as an adjunct to address medical or psychiatric comorbidities. Alpha-2 agonists (eg, Clonidine, Guanfacine) and low-dose atypical antipsychotic medications (eg, Risperidone, Aripiprazole) may help reduce disruptive behavior, aggression, and irritability.

OPPOSITIONAL DEFIANT DISORDER

- **Type of childhood disruptive behavior characterized by a persistent pattern of negative, angry or resentful, or irritable mood, argumentative or defiant behavior, & intentional vindictiveness or spitefulness (eg deliberately trying to annoy others)** associated with distress in the patient or close contacts or impairs ability to function in social, school, work, or other settings.

Characteristics:
- These interpersonal difficulties involve **at least 1 non-sibling (usually an authority figure).**
- **Disorder in which children are generally defiant towards authority but is <u>not</u> associated with physical aggression, violating others' basic rights, or breaking laws** (unlike Conduct disorder).

EPIDEMIOLOGY
- ~3% prevalence.
- Onset often in the preschool years; seen more often in boys before adolescence.
- 50% associated with ADHD; increased incidence of comorbid substance use.
- May occasionally lead to Conduct disorder (CD). Although ODD may precede CD, most do not develop CD.

DSM 5 DIAGNOSTIC CRITERIA
- **Characterized by at least 4 symptoms present <u>at least 6 months</u> (with at least one individual that is not a sibling).**
- **<u>Angry or irritable mood</u>** — eg, loses temper often, anger or resentment, often blames others for their misbehaviors & negative attitude.
- **<u>Argumentative or defiant behavior</u>** — breaks rules, often blames others for their behavior, **argues with authority figures,** & deliberately annoys or aggravates others.
- **<u>Vindictiveness:</u>** or spiteful at least 2 times in the past 6 months.
- **Behaviors are associated with distress in the individual or others, or negatively impact functioning.**
- Behaviors nor accounted for or explained by the diagnosis of another psychiatric disorder.

Specifier:
- Mild is for one setting, moderate is for two settings, and severe is for three or more settings.

MANAGEMENT
Psychotherapy:
- **Behavioral modification therapy, problem-solving skills, conflict management training.**
- **<u>Parent management training</u>:** educating parents child management (parenting skills, parent-child interaction therapy, setting limits, and enforcing consistent rules).
- Medications may be used to treat comorbid conditions (eg, ADHD).

EXAM TIP
Both ODD and Disruptive mood dysregulation disorder are associated with a disruptive and angry child, blaming others, or refusing to follow rules.
ODD is associated with intent behind their behavior.
Children with DMDD do not do it on purpose and may feel remorseful after outbursts.

DISRUPTIVE MOOD DYSREGULATION DISORDER

- **DMDD is a childhood disorder characterized by frequent temper outbursts along with a persistently irritable mood in between outbursts.**
- Criteria require that symptoms be present for at least twelve months, be present in multiple settings, and have an onset before the age of ten.
- While ODD and DMDD share symptoms of chronic irritable mood and temper outbursts, irritable mood in between outbursts persists in DMDD, and the severity of temper outbursts are more severe.

DISSOCIATIVE IDENTITY DISORDERS (DID)

- **Marked discontinuity in identity & loss of personal agency with <u>fragmentation into ≥2 distinct identities or personality states.</u>** The symptoms of the disruption of the identity may be self-reported and/or observed by others.
- Gaps in the recall of events may occur for everyday and not just for traumatic events.

EPIDEMIOLOGY
- Most common in women.
- Psychiatric conditions commonly comorbid with DID include posttraumatic stress disorder, sexual abuse, borderline personality disorder, substance abuse, depression, and somatoform disorder.
- **DID has been most commonly conceptualized as occurring among individuals predisposed to dissociation who experience severe trauma during childhood.**

CLINICAL MANIFESTATIONS
- The presence of ≥2 distinct personality states and recurrent gaps in recall of personal information or events (alterations in affect, behavior, consciousness, perception, cognition, and/or sensory-motor functioning).
- **Distinct personality states in DID are reported to be experienced by the patient or others as having different characteristics (eg, ages, genders, sexual orientation, and abilities).**

Other dissociative symptoms observed in patients with DID include:
- **<u>Dissociative amnesia:</u> <u>Inability to recall important personal information</u> (eg, autobiographical, an event, personal identity, or history), usually of a traumatic or stressful nature.**
- **<u>Dissociative fugue:</u> amnesia is associated with wandering or traveling (abrupt change in geographic location)** with loss of identity or inability to recall the past. Before determining this diagnosis, neurologic testing must be done to rule out seizures or brain tumor as the cause. Patients often report that they have periods of time (most often hours) that they cannot remember. From secondary reports, these periods may be associated with certain mood states or behaviors (eg, angry outbursts).
- **<u>Depersonalization</u>** – feeling of detachment or estrangement from oneself (eg, feeling outside of one's body or that one is observing oneself from the outside).
- **<u>Derealization</u>** –feeling that the external world is strange or unreal.
- <u>Self-alteration</u> – sense that one part of oneself is markedly different from another part of oneself.
- <u>Trance state</u> –narrowing of awareness of one's immediate surroundings or stereotyped behaviors or movements that are experienced as being beyond one's control.

DSM-5 diagnostic criteria for dissociative identity disorder (DID):
- [A] **Disruption of identity characterized by two or more distinct personality states**, which may be described in some cultures as an experience of possession. The disruption in identity involves marked discontinuity in sense of self and sense of agency, **accompanied by related alterations in affect, behavior, consciousness, memory, perception, cognition, and/or sensory-motor functioning**. These signs and symptoms may be observed by others or reported by the individual.
- [B] Recurrent gaps in the recall of everyday events, important personal information, and/or traumatic events that are inconsistent with ordinary forgetting.
- [C] The symptoms cause clinically significant distress or impairment in social, occupational, or other important areas of functioning.
- [D] The disturbance is not a normal part of a broadly accepted cultural or religious practice. Note: In children, the symptoms are not better explained by imaginary playmates or other fantasy play.
- [E] The symptoms are not attributable to the physiological effects of a substance (eg, blackouts or chaotic behavior during alcohol intoxication) or another medical condition.

MANAGEMENT OF DISSOCIATIVE DISORDERS
- Psychotherapy.

CHAPTER 12 – DERMATOLOGIC SYSTEM

ROSACEA

- **Chronic acneiform skin condition with [1] vascular (eg, telangiectasias, flushing, erythema) and [2] inflammatory manifestations (papules, pustules, phymatous skin changes).**
- Face most commonly involved. Most commonly presents in adulthood (women aged 30-50 years).
- <u>Etiology:</u> unclear etiology — persistent vasomotor instability, capillary vasodilation, and abnormal pilosebaceous activity.

TRIGGERS
- **Alcohol, hot or cold weather, hot drinks, hot baths, spicy foods, sun exposure,** & medications.

CLINICAL MANIFESTATIONS
- **<u>Transient centrofacial erythema</u> (nose, medial cheeks, chin), or flushing, often accompanied by a feeling of warmth in the skin, burning or stinging sensation,** subtle transient facial swelling (swelling may persist for days). Episodes usually last for <5 minutes (may spread to the neck and chest). In patients with moderate to highly pigmented skin, centrofacial erythema may be subtle.
- **<u>Acne-like rash</u> non-comedogenic inflammatory papules & pustules with a dry appearance (including roughness and scaling)** primarily localized to the central face. Inflammation may extend outward beyond the follicular unit to form plaques. Skin coarsening may occur.
- **<u>Telangiectasias</u>**: visible, enlarged, cutaneous blood vessels predominantly located on the central face, especially on the cheeks. Eyelid telangiectasias.
- **<u>Ocular symptoms</u>: may include ocular erythema, tearing,** foreign body sensation, burning, itching, photophobia, and blurred vision. May occur with or independent of skin findings.

PHYSICAL EXAMINATION
- Transient or persistent skin erythema, inflammatory papules or pustules, <u>telangiectasias</u>, or hyperplasia of the connective tissue (eg, skin coarsening).
- **<u>Absence of comedones</u> (blackheads) and presence of neurovascular symptoms distinguishes Rosacea from Acne vulgaris.**
- **<u>Phymatous change</u>** characterized by sebaceous gland hypertrophy & fibrosis — skin thickening with irregular contours. **A red enlarged nose (rhinophyma)** is the most common site of involvement.

DIAGNOSIS
- Usually clinical. Biopsy definitive but rarely needed.

MANAGEMENT
- **<u>Lifestyle modifications:</u> initial step.** Management begins with the use of mild cleansing agents and moisturizing regimens, education on avoidance of triggers, as well as photoprotection with wide-brimmed hats and broad-spectrum mineral-based sunscreens (zinc oxide or titanium dioxide) with minimum sun protection factor of ≥30. Avoid astringents, toners, abrasives, fragrances, and sensory stimulants (eg, camphor, menthol, alcohol, acetone).
- **<u>Mild-moderate papulopustules:</u> topical Metronidazole** (0.75% and 1% gel or cream), **Azelaic acid or topical Ivermectin first line for papulopustules.** <u>Alternatives:</u> Topical Sulfur-sodium Sulfacetamide or topical anti-acne antibiotics (eg, topical Minocycline; topical Macrolides).
- **<u>Moderate-severe papulopustules:</u> systemic oral antibiotics (eg, Tetracycline, Doxycycline, Minocycline)**; can also be used for disease not responsive to topical therapy. Improvement can be maintained by topical therapy or Subantimicrobial dose oral Doxycycline. Laser therapy.
- <u>Refractory cases:</u> Oral Isotretinoin may be used in cases refractory to topical and oral treatment.
- **<u>Facial erythema:</u> topical Brimonidine 0.33% gel** — alpha-2 adrenergic receptor agonist causes vasoconstriction. Topical Oxymetazoline (alpha-1 agonist). Laser or intense pulsed light therapy.
- **<u>Telangiectasia</u> vascular laser therapy** (pulsed dye laser, intense pulsed light, near infrared laser, Nd:YAG laser) effective in treating facial erythema and telangiectasia but does not treat papulopustular lesions.

ACNE VULGARIS

- Inflammatory skin condition associated with papules and pustules involving the pilosebaceous units.
- Pathophysiology: 4 main factors — follicular hyperkeratinization, increased sebum production, *Cutibacterium acnes* (formerly *Propionibacterium*) overgrowth, & and inflammatory response.

CLINICAL MANIFESTATIONS
- Commonly seen in areas with increased sebaceous glands — eg, face, neck, trunk, and proximal upper extremities.
- **Noninflammatory: Acne lesions consisting of open and closed comedones.** Comedones are small, noninflammatory bumps from clogged pores.
- **Open comedones (blackheads) due to <u>incomplete</u> blockage** — noninflammatory papules <5 mm with a central, dilated, follicular orifice containing gray, brown, or black keratotic material.
- **Closed comedones (whiteheads) due to <u>complete</u> blockage** — noninflammatory; <5 mm, dome-shaped, smooth, skin-colored, whitish or grayish papules.
- **Inflammatory: papulopustular acne** — inflamed, relatively superficial papules and pustules, often surrounded by inflammation and typically <5 mm in diameter.
- Skin pigmentation may mask the hallmark erythema of inflamed lesions in patients with highly pigmented skin.
- **Nodular (cystic) acne: Deep-seated, inflamed, often tender, large papules (≥5 mm) or nodules ≥5 mm.** Often heals with scarring (often evident on examination).

DIAGNOSIS
- **Mild:** comedones + small, scattered amounts of papules &/or pustules without scarring.
- **Moderate:** comedones + larger amounts of papules &/or pustules.
- **Severe:** nodular (>5 mm) or cystic acne.

MANAGEMENT
- General Skin care — utilize gentle skin cleansers rather than soaps or scrubs with lower pH (eg, 5.5 to 7) to minimize skin irritation and dryness; avoid aggressive scrubbing of the skin; use of noncomedogenic skin care and cosmetic products, and avoidance of picking of Acne lesions.

Mild comedonal acne:
- **Topical retinoid monotherapy first-line for mild and exclusively comedonal Acne vulgaris — Tretinoin, Adapalene (best tolerated),** Tazarotene, Trifarotene. Adverse effects include local erythema, irritation, dryness and flaking of the skin, pruritus, and stinging, especially during the first month of therapy.
- Topical acid alternatives Azelaic acid, Salicylic acid, or Glycolic acid.

Mild papulopustular & mixed (comedonal and papulopustular):
- **A combination of topical retinoid & topical antimicrobial therapy first-line therapy for almost all patients with mild Acne. [1]** topical retinoid and topical antimicrobial(s) [eg, Benzoyl peroxide alone or Benzoyl peroxide ± topical Clindamycin] OR **[2]** Benzoyl peroxide & topical antibiotic (if patient is unable to tolerate a retinoid or prefer a simpler treatment regimen). Topical Erythromycin or topical Dapsone are alternative antimicrobials.
- **Topical retinoids are the best comedolytic agents, indicated for acne of any severity (noninflammatory and inflammatory Acne) and preferred option for maintenance therapy.**
- Topical & systemic antibiotics should be used only in combination with Benzoyl peroxide (to reduce resistance) and retinoids and for a maximum of 12 weeks. Topical antibiotics are more effective when used in conjunction with topical retinoids.
- Severe: add oral antibiotics.

Mild comedonal (noninflammatory) acne: topical therapy mainstay:	Mild papulopustular & mixed:	Moderate papulopustular & mixed:	Severe:
• (1) Topical retinoid (eg, Tretinoin, Adapalene, Tazarotene, Trifarotene)	• (1) topical retinoid AND (2) topical antimicrobial (Benzoyl peroxide ± topical Clindamycin) OR	• (1) topical retinoid AND	• Oral Isotretinoin monotherapy
	OR	• (2) topical antimicrobial (Benzoyl peroxide ± topical Clindamycin) AND	OR
• (2) Alternatives: Topical acids: Salicylic, azelaic, or glycolic acids	• Benzoyl peroxide + topical antibiotic	• (3) Oral antibiotic	• (1) topical retinoid AND • (2) topical antimicrobial (Benzoyl peroxide ± topical Clindamycin) AND • (3) Oral antibiotic

Moderate:

Consider systemic therapy (eg, oral antibiotics, hormonal agents, oral Isotretinoin).

- **Systemic (oral) antibiotics are added to topical treatment (eg, Benzoyl peroxide and/or a topical retinoid) for moderate and severe Acne and forms of inflammatory Acne that are resistant to topical treatments. First-line oral agents include Minocycline and Doxycycline.** The use of oral macrolides (eg, Erythromycin, Azithromycin) should be limited to patients who cannot use Tetracyclines (eg, pregnant women or children <8 years). Trimethoprim-sulfamethoxazole and Trimethoprim use should be restricted to patients who are unable to tolerate Tetracyclines or in treatment-resistant patients.
- Maintenance therapy: After treatment goals are attained, oral antibiotics should be replaced with topical retinoids for maintenance therapy.
- **Combined oral contraceptives** can be used to treat inflammatory and noninflammatory acne in women with adult-onset acne or perimenstrual flare-ups.

Severe (refractory nodular acne):

- **Oral Isotretinoin is used for severe, recalcitrant acne.** Because of the risk of teratogenicity, patients, pharmacists, and prescribers must register with the U.S. Food and Drug Administration–mandated risk management program, iPledge, before implementing Isotretinoin therapy. **Adverse effects: include dry skin and lips (most common),** dry eyes, **high teratogenicity, increased triglycerides & cholesterol,** arthralgias, myalgias, hepatitis, leukopenia, premature long bone closure, photosensitivity, worsening of Diabetes mellitus, headache, Idiopathic intracranial hypertension, fatigue, & **possible psychiatric effects (eg, depression, suicidal thoughts).**

Acne scars:
- Trichloroacetic acid, derma roller, micro-needling, or fractional CO_2 laser. As an adjunct, subcutaneous injections of collagen can be used.
- **Hyperpigmentation: Topical Hydroquinone** is available in 3-4% strength in prescription doses. It functions by inhibiting melanin production and twice-daily use is recommended to reduce skin discoloration.

ISOTRETINOIN

Mechanism of action:
- Affects all 4 of the pathophysiologic mechanisms of Acne — **most effective medication for Acne vulgaris**.

Indications:
- Usually reserved for severe or refractory acne.

Adverse effects:
- **Dry skin and lips (most common),** dry eyes.
- **Highly teratogenic** — must obtain at least 2 pregnancy tests prior to initiation of treatment & monthly while on treatment, must commit to 2 forms of contraception (used at least 1 month prior to initiation & 1 month after it is discontinued).
- **Increased triglycerides & cholesterol,** arthralgias, myalgias, hepatitis, leukopenia, & premature long bone closure.
- Photosensitivity, worsening of Diabetes mellitus, headache, Idiopathic intracranial hypertension, fatigue, & possible psychiatric effects.
- Due to the severe risk of teratogenesis, prescribers and patients in the US must sign up for iPledge.

FOLLICULITIS

- **Superficial hair follicle infection or inflammation.**
- <u>Risk factors:</u> more common in men, prolonged use of antibiotics, topical corticosteroids

ETIOLOGIES
- ***Staphylococcus aureus* most common cause of Folliculitis.**
- Other gram-positive & gram negatives and fungi (eg, *Malassezia* species), and *Demodex* mites.
- ***Pseudomonas aeruginosa* is the most common cause of Hot tub-related Folliculitis.** Commonly seen 8-48 hours after exposure to water in a **contaminated spa, whirlpool, swimming pool, or hot tub (especially if it is made of wood).**

CLINICAL MANIFESTATIONS
- **Singular or clusters of perifollicular papules and/or pustules with surrounding erythema on hair bearing skin. Often pruritic.**
- **Hot tub Folliculitis: small** (2–10 mm), **tender, pruritic, pink to red papules, papulopustules or nodules** around the hair follicles within 1-4 days after exposure. May have flu-like symptoms (eg, malaise, low grade fever).

MANAGEMENT
- **Mild:** Mild *S. aureus* **Folliculitis may resolve without antibiotic treatment.** For patients with known or suspected *S. aureus* folliculitis that **persists and involves a limited area of skin, Topical antibiotics (eg, topical Mupirocin or Clindamycin,** Erythromycin, or Benzoyl peroxide).
- **Severe or refractory: Systemic (oral) antibiotics** — eg, **Cephalexin or Dicloxacillin.** If MRSA is suspected: Trimethoprim-sulfamethoxazole, Clindamycin, or Doxycycline.
- <u>Gram negative:</u> Daily acetic acid or topical Benzoyl peroxide (usually resolves without treatment).
- **Hot tub Folliculitis: No treatment needed in most cases** — usually spontaneously resolves within 7–14 days without treatment. **Oral Ciprofloxacin if persistent.**
- <u>Fungal folliculitis:</u> Oral antifungal therapy is the mainstay of therapy.
- *Demodex* folliculitis: antiparasitic agents (eg, Permethrin, oral Ivermectin).

PERIORAL DERMATITIS [PERIORIFICIAL DERMATITIS]

RISK FACTORS
- **History of topical corticosteroid use;** may worsen initially when steroids are discontinued.
- Fluorinated toothpaste, cinnamon-flavored chewing gum, oral contraceptive therapy.
- **Most commonly seen in young adult women 20–45 years of age.**

CLINICAL MANIFESTATIONS
- **Multiple erythematous grouped small inflammatory papules, papulopustules, or papulovesicles or erythematous scaling around the mouth, nose, or eyes,** which may become confluent into plaques with scales. May have satellite lesions.
- **Characteristically spares the skin adjacent to the vermillion border of the lip.**
- Uncommonly, it may affect the periorbital or paranasal skin.

DIAGNOSIS
- Perioral dermatitis is usually diagnosed clinically; skin biopsy may be performed in atypical cases.

MANAGEMENT
- **Discontinuation of topical corticosteroids and avoidance of other skin irritants** (eg, cosmetics and irritating skin care products). Self-limited.
- **Mild disease topical therapy: Topical Calcineurin inhibitors** (eg, **Pimecrolimus), Metronidazole** (cream or gel), **or Erythromycin first line medical therapy.** Clindamycin, Tacrolimus, Azelaic acid.
- **Extensive or refractory: Oral: Tetracyclines** (eg, Doxycycline , Minocycline). Oral Erythromycin in children <8 years, during pregnancy, or nursing mothers. <u>Alternative:</u> Oral Azithromycin.

ERYTHEMA MULTIFORME

- **Type IV hypersensitivity reaction** of the skin often following infections or medication exposure.
- Most common in young adults 20-40 years but may occur at any age.

RISK FACTORS

- **Infections** most common cause — **Herpes simplex virus** most common, *Mycoplasma pneumoniae* **(especially in children),** *S. pneumoniae.*
- Medications: (<10%) — eg, **sulfa drugs, beta-lactams, Phenytoin, Phenobarbital,** Allopurinol, etc.
- Malignancy, autoimmune, & idiopathic.

CLINICAL MANIFESTATIONS

- **Target lesions:** — 3 components: **raised (papular) lesions [1] dusky central area or blister, [2]** a dark red inflammatory zone **surrounded by a pale ring of edema, & [3] an erythematous halo on the extreme periphery** of the lesion. Most common on acral surfaces (hands, feet, elbows, and knees) & spreads centripetally.
- **Negative Nikolsky sign (no epidermal detachment).** Often febrile.
- **Minor:** target lesions distributed acrally with **no mucosal membrane involvement.**
- **Major:** target lesions acrally progressing centrally + **mucosal membrane involvement** (oral, genital, or ocular). **No epidermal detachment.**

DIAGNOSIS: Usually clinical. Biopsy or Direct immunofluorescence studies if the diagnosis is not clear.

MANAGEMENT

- Cutaneous remove offending drugs, topical steroids, oral antihistamines, analgesics, skin care.
- Oral nondisabling: Topical Corticosteroid + Lidocaine + Diphenhydramine + antacid mouthwash for oral lesions. EM typically resolves in ~2 weeks.
- Oral disabling: Systemic corticosteroids if severe. Antibiotics if Mycoplasma-related. Oral Acyclovir.

STEVENS-JOHNSON SYNDROME (SJS) & TOXIC EPIDERMAL NECROLYSIS (TEN)

- Stevens-Johnson syndrome (SJS) & Toxic epidermal necrolysis (TEN) are **severe mucocutaneous reactions characterized by detachment of the epidermis & extensive necrosis.**
- **SJS:** sloughing involving **<10%** of the body surface involvement. **TEN: >30%** body surface area.

RISK FACTORS

- **Medications most common cause especially** sulfonamides **& anticonvulsants (eg, Lamotrigine), Allopurinol,** NSAIDs & COX-2 inhibitors, antipsychotics, & antibiotics.
- Infections less common (eg, *Mycoplasma pneumoniae*, HIV, HSV). Malignancy, idiopathic.

CLINICAL MANIFESTATIONS

- Prodrome of fever & URI symptoms followed by **widespread flaccid bullae** beginning on the trunk & face.
- **Pruritic atypical targetoid lesions (erythematous flat/macules with purpuric centers)** or diffuse erythema (macules becoming vesicles & bullae) with involvement of **≥1 mucous membrane + involvement with epidermal detachment (positive Nikolsky sign).**
- **The skin is often tender to touch (large painful erosions).** The lesions start on the face & thorax before spreading to other areas (palms and soles rarely involved).
- Ocular involvement common (corneal ulceration or uveitis). Pulmonary (bronchitis, pneumonitis).

DIAGNOSIS: Clinical. Biopsy: full thickness skin necrosis supports the diagnosis but not necessary.

MANAGEMENT

- **Supportive therapy: Prompt discontinuation of causative agent. Treat like severe burns** — burn unit admission, pain control, prompt withdrawal of offending medications, fluid & electrolyte replacement, wound care (eg, gauze, petroleum).
- Cyclosporine adjunctive treatment if started 24-48 hours within symptom onset.

DISORDERS OF THE HAIR AND NAILS

ALOPECIA AREATA

- **Nonscarring <u>immune-mediated</u> hair loss** targeting the anagen hair follicles, (scalp most common).
- **Commonly associated with other autoimmune disorders** (eg, thyroid, Addison's disease, SLE).

CLINICAL MANIFESTATIONS
- **Smooth, discrete, circular patches of complete hair loss** that develop over a period of weeks (painless and not pruritic). No erythema, inflammation, or scarring.

Physical examination:
- **<u>Exclamation point hairs</u> — short hairs broken off a few mm from the scalp with <u>tapering near the proximal hair shaft</u> (exclamation point appearance!)** at the margins of the patches. In some cases, hair loss may be diffuse. Hair regrowth may occur (fine white hair regrowth). No erythema, inflammation, or scarring seen.
- **<u>Nail abnormalities</u>:** pitting ~30%, nail fissuring, trachyonychia (roughening of the nail plate), etc.

DIAGNOSIS
- Mainly a clinical diagnosis. Biopsy may be performed in cases when the diagnosis is uncertain.
- <u>Punch biopsy</u>: definitive — peribulbar lymphocytic inflammatory infiltrates surrounding the follicles.

MANAGEMENT
- **<u>Local:</u> intralesional corticosteroids first-line.** Topical corticosteroids or Anthralin. Observe if mild.
- <u>Extensive:</u> JAK inhibitors (eg, oral Baricitinib or Ritlecitinib). Systemic corticosteroids.

Prognosis:
- May spontaneously resolve or progress to Alopecia totalis (complete scalp hair loss) or Alopecia universalis (complete hair loss on the scalp & body, including the eyelashes). Relapse is common.

ANDROGENETIC ALOPECIA

- Genetically predetermined progressive loss of the terminal hairs on the scalp in a characteristic distribution (pattern).
- Most common type of hair loss in men & women. Gradual in onset & usually occurs after puberty.

PATHOPHYSIOLOGY
- **Dihydrotestosterone (DHT) is the key androgen leading to Androgenetic alopecia.** Activation of the androgen receptor shortens the anagen (growth phase) in the normal hair growth cycle.
- Pathologic specimens show decreased anagen to telogen ratio.

CLINICAL MANIFESTATIONS
- Varying degrees of hair thinning & nonscarring hair loss. In males, it begins as **bitemporal thinning of the frontal scalp then involves the vertex, anterior, and mid scalp.** In women, it is seen as thinning of the hair between the frontal and vertex of the scalp without affecting the frontal hairline.

DIAGNOSIS: **usually clinical.** Dermoscopy — miniaturized hair and brown perihilar casts.

MANAGEMENT
- **<u>Topical Minoxidil:</u> best used if recent onset Alopecia involving a smaller area or if the patient does not want systemic therapy.** Requires a 4–6-month trial before noticing improvement and must be used indefinitely. <u>Mechanism:</u> widens blood vessels, allowing more blood oxygen and nutrients to promote the anagen (growth) phase. <u>Adverse effects:</u> pruritus & local irritation with flaking.
- **<u>Oral Finasteride:</u> 5-alpha reductase type 2 inhibitor** — androgen inhibitor (inhibits the conversion of testosterone to dihydrotestosterone). <u>Adverse effects:</u> decreased libido, sexual or ejaculatory dysfunction. Increased risk of high-grade prostate cancer. Category X.
- <u>Hair transplant</u> is effective if the patient has a sufficient number of donor plugs. Laser therapy.

ONYCHOMYCOSIS

- **Nail infections caused by fungi (dermatophytes, yeast, or nondermatophyte molds).**
- Most commonly affects the great toe.

ETIOLOGIES
- Dermatophytes — Trichophyton & Epidermophyton genera (***Trichophyton rubrum* most common**). *Candida albicans* (more likely to affect fingernails) & nondermatophyte molds.

RISK FACTORS
- Increasing age, tinea pedis (including close contacts), Psoriasis, occlusive shoes, & immunodeficiency.

CLINICAL MANIFESTATIONS
3 variants: distal lateral, superficial white, and proximal.
- Distal subungual onychomycosis most common clinical subtype.
- **Begins with white, yellow, or brown discoloration of the distal corner of the nail that may gradually spread to involve the entire width of the nail.**
- Nail that is opaque, thickened, discolored, and/or cracked. Subungual hyperkeratinization.

DIAGNOSIS
- Because only 50% of dystrophic nails are due to fungal infection, **confirmation of fungal infection is essential prior to treatment** [a rapid test (eg, KOH wet mount preparation, histopathologic examination with a PAS stain, or PCR) + **Fungal culture**].
- **Periodic acid-Schiff test most sensitive test and rapid** (performed on nail plate clippings).
- Fungal cultures: If the KOH preparation or PAS stain is positive, confirming Onychomycosis, a nail sample for fungal culture on Sabouraud's medium identifies the causative organism.

MANAGEMENT
- Management can be initiated if KOH or PAS is positive while waiting for cultures.
- **Systemic antifungals Oral Terbinafine first line for dermatophytes (most effective treatment).** Itraconazole for both dermatophytes & Candida.
  - **Systemic antifungals associated with hepatotoxicity & drug-drug interactions.** Transaminase levels should be checked at baseline prior to initiating therapy and then repeated at six weeks to monitor for liver enzyme abnormalities or hepatic toxicity.
  - Contraindications include alcohol use & Hepatitis.
- Topical antifungal: Efinaconazole, Tavaborole, and Ciclopirox are topical options if oral agents are contraindicated or not desired.
- Yeast and nondermatophyte mold onychomycosis: Itraconazole primary treatment of this variant. Oral Terbinafine may be used in some.

PARONYCHIA

- **Acute:** Infection of the lateral & proximal nail folds (periungual), including the tissue that borders the root and sides of the nail for **<6 weeks duration.** Chronic: >6 weeks.

ETIOLOGIES
- **Skin flora:** _**Staphylococcus aureus**_ **most common** (especially if rapid), _Streptococcus pyogenes._
- Oral flora if associated with nail biting.
- _Candida_ species associated with Chronic paronychia.

PATHOPHYSIOLOGY
- Most commonly occurs after penetrating skin trauma (eg, dishwashing, biting nails, cuticle damage during manicures, ingrown nails, hangnails).

CLINICAL MANIFESTATIONS
- **Rapid onset of painful erythema & swelling to the proximal and/or lateral nail folds,** usually within 2-5 days following minor local trauma (eg, manicuring, infection, structural abnormalities, inflammatory disease, or occupational). May have purulent discharge or superficial abscess.
- Physical examination: painful, erythematous, swollen, and tender area around the proximal or lateral nail folds at the cuticle. An area of fluctuance or visible pus under the nail fold if abscess is present.

MANAGEMENT
Paronychia without abscess:
- **Mild:** **warm water or antiseptic soaks (eg, Chlorhexidine, Povidone-iodine for 10-15 minutes)** followed by topical anti-staphylococcal antibiotics (eg, triple antibiotics, Bacitracin, or Mupirocin).
- **Moderate:** **oral antibiotics — Cephalexin or Dicloxacillin** first-line or if no response to topicals. Amoxicillin-clavulanic acid or Clindamycin used if associated with nail biting (anaerobic coverage).
- **MRSA risk factors: Trimethoprim-sulfamethoxazole DS, Clindamycin, or Doxycycline.**
Paronychia with abscess:
- **Incision & drainage alone mainstay of treatment, followed by warm soaks.** If there is a significant extension of Cellulitis, oral antibiotics for 5 days may be prescribed.
- **Drainage via elevation** is performed by insertion of an 11-blade scalpel or 18-gauge needle into the eponychium and paronychium parallel to the nail until pus begins to drain.

FELON (PULP SPACE INFECTION)

- **Closed-space infection of the fingertip pulp space.** A Paronychia can progress to a Felon.

ETIOLOGIES
- **Skin flora:** _**Staphylococcus aureus**_ **most common** (especially if rapid), _Streptococcus pyogenes._

PATHOPHYSIOLOGY
- Most commonly occurs after penetrating skin trauma (eg, biting nails, cuticle damage, splinters etc.).
- An abscess develops in the small fingertip pulp compartments.

CLINICAL MANIFESTATIONS
- **Severe throbbing pain, erythema, swelling, and fluctuance to the pad of the fingertip.**

MANAGEMENT
- **Fluctuant: incision and drainage (single volar longitudinal or high lateral incision) performed by a hand specialist.**
- Early without fluctuance: elevation, warm water or saline soaks, & oral antibiotics (eg, Cephalexin or anti-staphylococcal Penicillin).

BROWN RECLUSE SPIDER BITE

- Most common in the Southwestern & Midwestern US.
- Brown recluse spiders (*Loxosceles reclusa*) may have a **violin pattern** on its anterior cephalothorax.

PATHOPHYSIOLOGY
- **Brown recluse venom is cytotoxic & hemolytic (causes local tissue destruction)** — local symptoms, can be **necrotic**, and associated with lack of severe systemic symptoms (Loxoscelism).

CLINICAL MANIFESTATIONS
- **Local effects: local burning & erythema at the bite site for 3-4 hours followed by blanching of the affected area (due to vasoconstriction)** followed by an erythematous margin around the ischemic center **"red halo" for 24-72 hours followed by a hemorrhagic bulla that undergoes eschar formation. 10% may develop** skin necrosis. Usually heals by secondary intention.
- Systemic effects: some may develop fever, chills, nausea, vomiting, or a morbilliform rash.

MANAGEMENT
Supportive: local wound care & pain control is the mainstay of management.
- **Local wound care:** clean the affected area with soap & water, apply cold packs to the bite site (avoid freezing the tissue). If possible, keep the affected body part in elevated or neutral position. **Most wounds heal spontaneously** within days to weeks. **Antivenom is not needed.**
- **Pain control:** NSAIDs (or opioids if more severe). Tetanus prophylaxis if needed.
- Dermal necrosis: debridement (if needed) should be delayed until the lesion is demarcated and clinically stable. In some cases, it may lead to better wound healing. Dapsone has been used in the past.
- Antibiotics only if a secondary infection develops (treat like Cellulitis).

BLACK WIDOW SPIDER BITE

PATHOPHYSIOLOGY
- **Neurotoxin production: Black widow spider (*Latrodectus Hesperus*) produces a neurotoxin** that causes release of Acetylcholine and Norepinephrine.
- **Characteristic red hourglass shape on the underside of its belly.**

RISK FACTORS
- Outdoor activities, gardening, sleeping outside, etc.

CLINICAL MANIFESTATIONS
- **Latrodectism: local symptoms — pain at the bite site with the onset of** systemic & neurologic symptoms **within 30 minutes to 2 hours — muscle pain (most prominent feature), spasms, & rigidity, & CNS excitation.** Muscle pain most common in the extremities, back, chest, & abdomen.
- **Usually self-limited** with resolution within 1-3 days.

PHYSICAL EXAM
- **Classic appearance of bite: blanched circular patch with a surrounding red perimeter and central punctum (target lesion).** No necrosis. Local diaphoresis or lymphadenopathy may occur.

MANAGEMENT
- **Mild: wound care & pain control** — gently clean the area with mild soap & water. NSAIDs for analgesia, and tetanus prophylaxis, if needed.
- Moderate to severe: **above + muscle relaxants for spasms** (eg, **Benzodiazepines,** Methocarbamol).
- Antivenom reserved for patients not responsive to the above medications. Antivenom is not always readily available and if given, usually given after a consult with a toxicologist.

PARVOVIRUS B19 INFECTION (ERYTHEMA INFECTIOSUM/FIFTH'S DISEASE)

- **Parvovirus B19** — Parvovirus B19 infects & destroys reticulocytes, leading to a decrease or transient halt in erythropoiesis (this can lead to Aplastic crisis); Ag-Ab complex may deposit in the joint.
- Transmission: respiratory droplets, vertical transmission; 5–10-day incubation period.

CLINICAL MANIFESTATIONS: 2 classic syndromes – EI in children; arthralgias in older children/adults.
- **[1] Erythema infectiosum (Fifth's disease)**: Nonspecific viral symptoms (eg, coryza, fever, malaise, headache, diarrhea) for 2-5 days, followed by **erythematous malar rash with a "slapped cheek" appearance & circumoral pallor** for 2-4 days. **The malar rash may be followed by a lacy (reticular) maculopapular rash on the trunk or extremities** (especially upper) that usually spares the palms and soles, resolving in 2-3 weeks. Most common in children 4-10 years of age.
- **[2] Arthralgias or arthritis: most common manifestation in adults (especially women),** although it can be seen in older children. Usually symmetric and most commonly involves the small joints of the hands, wrists, knees, and feet. **May develop a rash (but not usually on the face).**
- **[3] Aplastic crisis: Parvovirus B19 can cause transient Aplastic crisis** (temporary suspension of erythropoiesis leading to severe anemia), especially with underlying heme abnormalities, (eg, Sickle cell disease, Hereditary spherocytosis, G6PDD). Pure red cell aplasia if immunocompromised.
- **[4] Hydrops fetalis &/or feral demise** if pregnant women become infected with Parvovirus B19.

DIAGNOSIS: usually a clinical diagnosis in children. Serologies — eg, Parvovirus-specific IgM antibody.
- DNA probe, NAAT, or quantitative PCR in serum or bone marrow helpful in patients with Transient aplastic crisis, chronic Pure red cell aplasia, and for those who are immunocompromised.

MANAGEMENT OF ERYTHEMA INFECTIOSUM
- **No treatment or supportive**: anti-inflammatories (Acetaminophen or NSAIDs). Self-limited disease.

RUBEOLA (MEASLES)

- ETIOLOGY: **Measles (Rubeola) virus, part of the Paramyxovirus family.**
- Transmission: respiratory droplets, person to person, or airborne. Incubation period: 6-21 days.

CLINICAL MANIFESTATIONS
- **[1] URI prodrome malaise, anorexia, high fever + 3 Cs — cough, coryza (nasal obstruction, sneezing, sore throat), & conjunctivitis.** ± followed by Koplik spots.
- **[2] Koplik spots: small 1-3 mm pale white/blue papules with an erythematous base on the buccal mucosa opposite the second molars** (pathognomonic). May precede the rash by 48 hours.
- **[3] Exanthem: morbilliform (maculopapular), brick-red rash begins at hairline & neck,** spreads cephalocaudally & centrifugally (down & out) then **darkens & coalesces. Rash usually lasts 7 days.**
- Headache, abdominal pain, vomiting, diarrhea, myalgia, lymphadenopathy, and pharyngitis.
Complications:
- **Diarrhea (most common), Otitis media (5-10%),** Conjunctivitis, Secondary skin infection.
- Serious: **Pneumonia most common cause of Measles-related deaths in children.** Encephalitis.

DIAGNOSIS
- Primarily a clinical diagnosis. Measles-virus specific IgM antibodies.
- PCR of viral ribonucleic acid from throat, nasopharyngeal, or urine samples.

MANAGEMENT
- **Supportive mainstay of treatment of Measles** — antipyretics (eg, Acetaminophen, Ibuprofen), oral hydration, & treatment of bacterial superinfections and other complications.
- **Vitamin A reduces morbidity & mortality in children with severe Rubeola or if malnourished.**
- Measles immune globulin (for individuals at high risk for complications).
- **Prevention: MMR vaccine 2 doses — 1 dose given at 12-15 months; second dose at 4-6 years.**

HAND, FOOT, AND MOUTH DISEASE

- **Coxsackie virus (especially type A16) most common cause.** Coxsackie virus is an Enterovirus that is part of the Picornavirus family.
- Most common in children <7 years of age but can affect any age group.
- <u>Transmission:</u> primarily fecal-oral and oral-oral. Oral and respiratory secretions or vesicle fluid.
- Most cases occur in the summer & early fall.

CLINICAL MANIFESTATIONS
- Mild fever, URI symptoms, anorexia, malaise, & decreased appetite starting 3-5 days after exposure.
- **[1] Oral enanthem (anterior cavity): erythematous macules that become painful oral vesicles surrounded by a thin halo of erythema that undergo shallow ulceration (especially buccal mucosa & the tongue). Sore throat & oral pain may affect oral intake.** Followed by exanthem.
- **[2] Exanthem:** greyish-yellow vesicular, macular, or maculopapular nonpruritic, nontender skin lesions on the distal extremities (often including the palms and soles). Less commonly, vesicles may be seen on the torso and face. Fever, when present, is usually <38.3°C (101°F).

DIAGNOSIS
- Mainly a clinical diagnosis.
- Coxsackievirus-specific immunoglobulin A. Viral culture.

MANAGEMENT
- <u>Supportive:</u> **antipyretics (eg, Acetaminophen, Ibuprofen), hydration.** Topical Lidocaine. HFMD usually resolves within 7 days. Once the fever resolves, children can return to daycare.

COMPLICATIONS
- **Coxsackievirus type A: Hand, foot, and mouth disease; Herpangina, Aseptic (viral) meningitis.**
- **Coxsackievirus type B: Myocarditis, Pericarditis, Aseptic (viral) meningitis.**
- <u>Both:</u> Guillain–Barré syndrome (GBS). Aseptic meningitis most common with Enterovirus 71.

HERPANGINA

- Primarily caused by **Coxsackie virus, especially type A** (A1-A6, A8, A10). Coxsackie virus is an Enterovirus that is part of the Picornavirus family.
- Most common in children 3-10 years of age.
- Most common in summer & early fall.

CLINICAL MANIFESTATIONS
- **<u>Fever, mouth pain, & oral vesicles or ulcers without skin lesions</u>:** sudden onset of **high fever, <u>stomatitis</u> — discrete small yellow white papulovesicular lesions on the <u>posterior pharynx</u> (soft palate, uvula, anterior tonsillar pillars, tonsils, posterior pharyngeal wall) that ulcerate** before healing (**<u>small, yellow or white ulcers with red rims</u>**). **May interfere with oral intake.** Anorexia due to pain common.
- Pharyngitis, odynophagia, cervical lymphadenopathy.
- In older children, may be accompanied with malaise, headache, vomiting, neck stiffness, or back stiffness.

DIAGNOSIS
- Mainly a clinical diagnosis.
- Coxsackievirus-specific immunoglobulin A. Viral culture.

MANAGEMENT
- **<u>Supportive:</u> self-limited — antipyretics (eg, Acetaminophen, Ibuprofen), oral hydration.**
- Complications are rare but can include Aseptic meningitis & Guillain-Barré syndrome.

CELLULITIS

- **Acute spreading infection of the <u>deeper dermis & subcutaneous tissues (eg, fat)</u>.**
- Bacterial entry usually occurs after a break in the skin, such as underlying skin conditions (eg, Impetigo, Tinea), trauma (eg, bites, wounds, pressure ulcers, cuts), surgical wounds, etc.

<u>ETIOLOGIES</u>
- **<u>Group A *Streptococci*</u> most common cause of Cellulitis.**
- ***Staphylococcus aureus* second most common cause. <u>Dog or cat bites</u>: *Pasteurella multocida*.**

<u>CLINICAL MANIFESTATIONS</u>
- **<u>Localized</u> macular skin erythema (flat margins) poorly demarcated (indistinct borders), edema, warmth, and/or tenderness.** Lower extremity most frequently involved.
- <u>Systemic symptoms</u> not as common — eg, fever, chills, regional lymphadenopathy, myalgias, vesicles, bullae hemorrhage. May develop lymphangitis (streaking).

<u>DIAGNOSIS:</u> primarily a clinical diagnosis.

<u>MANAGEMENT</u>
- **<u>Oral antibiotics:</u> Cephalexin, Cefadroxil, & Dicloxacillin are first line agents.** Amoxicillin.
- **<u>Penicillin allergy:</u> Trimethoprim-sulfamethoxazole. <u>Alternatives:</u> Clindamycin**, Linezolid.
- **<u>IV antibiotics:</u> Cefazolin, Nafcillin, Oxacillin.** Ampicillin-sulbactam, Ceftriaxone, & Clindamycin.
- **<u>Cat bite (*Pasteurella multocida*)</u>: Amoxicillin-clavulanate;** <u>Penicillin allergy</u>: Doxycycline.
- **<u>Dog or human bite:</u> Amoxicillin-clavulanate.** Trimethoprim-sulfamethoxazole + Metronidazole; Clindamycin + either Ciprofloxacin or Trimethoprim-sulfamethoxazole. **<u>IV:</u> Ampicillin-sulbactam**; Ceftriaxone plus Metronidazole.

<u>MRSA:</u>
- **<u>Cellulitis with MRSA risk factors</u>: Trimethoprim-sulfamethoxazole in addition to Cephalexin (TMP-SMX good for Staph but does not cover Streptococcus).** <u>Risk factors</u>: purulent Cellulitis, MRSA colonization, Cellulitis associated with an abscess or extensive puncture wounds, recent hospitalization, history of intravenous drug use. **<u>Alternatives:</u> Clindamycin or Linezolid.**
- <u>IV:</u> **Vancomycin** or Daptomycin. Linezolid & Ceftaroline often reserved when other agents not used.

ERYSIPELAS

- **Variant of Cellulitis involving the <u>upper dermis & superficial cutaneous lymphatics</u>.**

<u>ETIOLOGIES</u>
- **<u>Group A *Streptococcus*</u> (*S. pyogenes*) most common.** *Staphylococci.*

<u>CLINICAL MANIFESTATIONS</u>
- **Intensely erythematous, <u>raised indurated area with sharply demarcated borders</u>** between the involved & uninvolved tissue, **tenderness, & warmth. Often shiny or glistening. Intense pain.**
- **Most commonly involves the lower extremities (90%), arm** (5%), **face** (2.5%) or skin with impaired lymphatic drainage. Ear involvement (Milian's ear sign) may be seen.
- **<u>Systemic manifestations</u> are common (eg, fever, chills, malaise, leukocytosis), unlike Cellulitis.**

<u>DIAGNOSIS</u>
- Clinical. Ultrasound with Gram stain and culture of expressed fluid if underlying abscess.

<u>MANAGEMENT</u>
- **<u>Oral</u>: Penicillin V potassium, Amoxicillin, Cephalexin, Cefadroxil, Dicloxacillin.**
  <u>Penicillin allergy</u>: Clindamycin, Trimethoprim-sulfamethoxazole, or Linezolid.
- **<u>IV:</u> Cefazolin, Ceftriaxone**, or Flucloxacillin may be required if systemic symptoms are present.
- **<u>MRSA:</u> IV Vancomycin used if Penicillin allergy or if MRSA is suspected.**

LYMPHANGITIS

- **Inflammation of the lymphatic channels due to infectious or noninfectious causes.**
- It can be a complication of a distal infection that gains access to the lymphatic vessels, spreading towards regional lymph nodes.

CLINICAL MANIFESTATIONS
- **<u>Red, tender streaks</u> rapidly progressing, extending proximally from the site of Cellulitis.**
- **May involve regional lymph nodes** (lymphadenitis) or systemic symptoms (eg, fever & chills).

MANAGEMENT
- Based on the underlying cause. It should be treated like the underlying etiology.

MANAGEMENT IF ASSOCIATED WITH CELLULITIS
- **Oral antibiotics: Cephalexin, Cefadroxil, Dicloxacillin are first line agents.** Amoxicillin.
- **PCN allergy: Trimethoprim-sulfamethoxazole. Alternatives: Clindamycin,** Linezolid.
- **IV antibiotics: Cefazolin, Nafcillin, Oxacillin.** Ampicillin-sulbactam, Ceftriaxone, & Clindamycin.

MRSA:
- **Cellulitis with MRSA risk factors: Trimethoprim-sulfamethoxazole in addition to Cephalexin (TMP-SMX good for Staph but does not cover Streptococcus).** <u>Risk factors:</u> purulent Cellulitis, MRSA colonization, Cellulitis associated with an abscess or extensive puncture wounds, recent hospitalization, history of intravenous drug use. **Alternatives: Clindamycin or Linezolid.**
- <u>IV</u>: **Vancomycin** or Daptomycin. Linezolid & Ceftaroline often reserved when other agents not used.

FURUNCLE & CARBUNCLE

- **<u>Furuncle (abscess)</u>: deep infection of the hair follicle** (in contrast to Folliculitis, which is superficial).
- <u>Carbuncle</u> is a coalescence or interconnection of several furuncles into a single mass with purulent drainage from multiple follicles.

ETIOLOGIES:
- ***Staphylococcus aureus* most common cause of an Abscess.** Streptococcus second most common.

CLINICAL MANIFESTATIONS
- **Erythematous, tender, <u>indurated nodule with fluctuance</u>** (abscess) may have a central plug.
- ± surrounding Cellulitis. Systemic symptoms (eg, fever or chills) not common.

WORKUP
- Usually a clinical diagnosis. Routine culture of debrided material is not necessary in healthy patients who do not receive antibiotics. Cultures may be obtained in high-risk patients.

MANAGEMENT
- **<u>Incision and drainage alone</u> mainstay of treatment for <u>most uncomplicated Abscesses</u>. It is reasonable not to administer antibiotic therapy in otherwise healthy patients who have small (eg, <2 cm) abscesses and no other comorbidities.** Warm moist compresses with a dry covering if not fluctuant or as adjunctive treatment for open and draining abscesses.
- **Antibiotics typically reserved for associated extensive surrounding Cellulitis, Cellulitis associated with purulent drainage in the absence of drainable Abscess, signs of systemic infection (eg, associated with fever or chills, rapid progression), skin abscess ≥2 cm,** recurrent or persistent Furunculosis, multiple lesions, major comorbidities or immunosuppression, inadequate clinical response to incision and drainage alone.

Patients with purulent infection should be managed with empiric therapy for infection due to MRSA, pending culture results:
- **<u>Oral regimens</u>: Trimethoprim-sulfamethoxazole, Doxycycline, Minocycline, or Clindamycin.**
- **<u>Parenteral therapy of MRSA</u>: Vancomycin (preferred). Daptomycin is an alternative.** Linezolid & Ceftaroline are usually reserved for when first line agents cannot be used to reduce resistance.

IMPETIGO

- **Highly contagious superficial vesiculopustular skin infection;** common on the face & extremities.
- Most common bacterial skin infection in children; highest incidence 2-6 years of age.

RISK FACTORS
- Poor personal hygiene, poverty, crowding, warm & humid weather, and skin trauma.

3 TYPES
- **[1] Nonbullous (Impetigo contagiosa): most common type — nonpainful, pruritic, superficial papules, vesicles (blisters), & pustules with weeping, later resulting in "thick honey-colored, golden crusts."** Leaves behind denuded areas. Occurs typically at sites of superficial skin trauma (eg, insect bite), primarily on **exposed surfaces of the face & arms.** Associated with regional lymphadenopathy. Extensive disease may be associated with systemic symptoms (eg, fever).
  Staphylococcus aureus **most common cause. Group A *Streptococcus* second most common.**

- **[2] Bullous: rapidly forming vesicles that form large bullae filled with clear or yellow fluid that later become dark and turbid, with subsequent rupture, leaving behind thin brown "varnish-like crusts."** Fever, diarrhea. The trunk is the most common site of involvement. Rare (usually seen in newborns or young children). If seen in adults, consider underlying HIV infection.
  Staphylococcal aureus **most common cause** (some strains produce exfoliative toxin A that destroys a protein in the epidermal desmosomes, cleaving the superficial skin layer).

- **[3] Ecthyma: ulcerative pyoderma caused by Group A *Streptococcus* — "punched-out" ulcers covered with yellow crusts, surrounded by raised violaceous margins;** often heals with scarring. Rare.

DIAGNOSIS
- **Clinical. Gram stain and culture** of pus or exudate can identify *S. aureus* or GAS as the cause.

MANAGEMENT
- **Mild (limited to small area): Topical antibiotics — eg, topical Mupirocin initial drug of choice or topical Retapamulin** (improvement of the lesions should begin within 3-5 days of starting antibiotics). Wash the area gently with soap & water. Good skin hygiene.
- **Extensive disease (eg, >5 lesions) &/or systemic symptoms (eg, fever): systemic antibiotics — Cephalexin or Dicloxacillin.** Penicillin allergy: Macrolides (eg, Erythromycin, Clarithromycin).
- Community-acquired MRSA: Trimethoprim-Sulfamethoxazole, Doxycycline, or Clindamycin.

COMPLICATIONS
- **Cellulitis most common (10%). 5% may develop poststreptococcal Glomerulonephritis.**
- Impetigo does not lead to Rheumatic fever.

CYST	FISSURE	MACULE	**MACULE:** flat nonpalpable lesion <10mm.

MACULE: flat nonpalpable lesion <10mm.
PATCH: flat nonpalpable lesion >10 mm.

PAPULE: solid, raised lesions <5mm in diameter.
NODULE: solid, raised lesions >5mm in diameter.

NODULE   PAPULE   POLYP

PLAQUE: raised, flat-topped lesion >10mm.

VESICLE: circumscribed, elevated fluid-filled lesion <5mm.
BULLA: circumscribed, elevated fluid-filled lesion >5mm.

PUSTULE   VESICLE   WHEAL

PUSTULE: pus-filled vesicle or bulla.
WHEAL: transient, elevated lesion (local edema).
PETECHIAE: small punctate hemorrhages that don't blanch.

DERMATOPHYTOSIS

- **Fungal skin & hair infections** caused by Trichophyton, Microsporum, and Epidermophyton.
- Infects keratinized tissues in the stratum corneum of the skin, hair & nails by ingesting keratin.

TINEA CAPITIS
- **Superficial fungal infection of the scalp hairs primarily caused by the dermatophyte species Trichophyton and Microsporum.** "Ringworm" is a common term.

ETIOLOGIES
- ***Trichophyton tonsurans*, the cause of black dot, is most common in the United States (90%).**
- ***Microsporum canis*** a primary cause of Tinea capitis in central and southern Europe, China, Russia, & Australia. *Microsporum* infections result from exposure to infected dogs or cats and may produce a greater inflammatory response than *Trichophyton* infections.

RISK FACTORS
- Poor hygiene, direct contact. **More common in African-Americans.**
- **Most common in pre-pubertal boys 3-14 years of age** but can occur at any age.

CLINICAL MANIFESTATIONS
There are 3 types of Tinea capitis: black dot, gray patch, and favus.
- **Patches of alopecia with black dots: multiple black dots representing the distal broken hair shafts resulting from endothrix infection.**
- **Scaly patches with alopecia: single or multiple scaly patches with hair loss** is the more common presentation of ectothrix infections (eg, *M. canis*). Erythema and pruritus may occur.
- **Kerion**: severe form of resulting from an intense immune response to the infection. — **inflammatory boggy edematous plaque or nodule with pustules, thick crusting, and/or drainage**, with a suppurative Folliculitis. **Often painful and tender and may lead to scarring alopecia**. Most commonly in children 5-10 years of age; rare in infancy.
- **Favus**: distinct clinical presentation of Tinea capitis resulting from infection with *T. schoenleinii* (and rarely other dermatophytes). **In favus, perifollicular erythema progresses to the characteristic development of cup-shaped, yellow crusts called scutula** (contains fungi, neutrophils, dried serum, and epidermal cells). Deep-seated oozing nodules, abscesses, crusting, or scutula.
- **Lymphadenopathy: palpable cervical &/or suboccipital lymphadenopathy** — frequent finding.

DIAGNOSIS
- **Clinical diagnosis** — children with risk factors presents with scaling, alopecia (hair loss), especially if cervical adenopathy and scaling with black dots are present.
- **Potassium hydroxide (KOH) 20% preparation: rapid method for confirming the presence of a dermatophyte infection (eg, Tinea capitis) via visualization of fungal elements (eg, fungal hyphae & spores).** It can be performed by scraping the black dots (broken hairs).
- Wood's lamp: no fluorescence with *Trichophyton spp.*; Fluorescence with Microsporum.
- Culture: definitive diagnosis.

MANAGEMENT
- **Oral Griseofulvin: first-line treatment (preferred over Terbinafine if known or suspected secondary to *Microsporum* species; also used for *Trichophyton*)** for 6-12 weeks. **Can cause hepatitis**, GI, headache, & Disulfiram reaction. Griseofulvin better absorbed with fatty food (eg, peanut butter). **LFTs & CBC should be obtained if treatment duration is >8 weeks.**
- **Alternative: Oral Terbinafine — also has good coverage for *Trichophyton* species.**
      Less commonly used — oral Itraconazole or Fluconazole.
- Lifestyle: use of antifungal shampoos by all house members; avoid sharing hats, clippers, and combs.
- Adjunctive treatment includes topical antifungals (eg, Selenium sulfide 1 or 2.5%, Ketoconazole 2% shampoo, or Ciclopirox 1%) at least twice weekly to decrease the number of spores.

TINEA PEDIS (ATHLETE'S FOOT)

- *Trichophyton rubrum, T. mentagrophytes/interdigitale* complex, and *Epidermophyton floccosum.*
- Most common in adolescents and young men. Most common dermatophyte infection
- <u>Transmission:</u> direct contact (eg, walking barefoot in gyms/swimming pool areas), occlusive wear.

CLINICAL MANIFESTATIONS

- **<u>Interdigital:</u> most common — pruritic, erythematous erosions or scales between the toes (may be associated with interdigital fissures with white maceration or peeling).** Most common in the third and fourth digital interspaces. **Itching, stinging, or burning of interdigital web.**
- <u>Hyperkeratotic</u>: diffuse hyperkeratotic rash involving the soles, lateral and medial surfaces of the feet with a "moccasin" distributive pattern.
- <u>Vesiculobullous (inflammatory):</u> pruritic vesicular or bullous eruption with underlying erythema, especially involving the medial surfaces of the foot (may be painful).

DIAGNOSIS

- Clinical diagnosis. **<u>KOH prep:</u> of skin scraping most common initial test — segmented hyphae.**
- <u>Culture:</u> definitive diagnosis.

MANAGEMENT

- **<u>Topical antifungals</u> first-line (eg, Butenafine, Tolnaftate, Ciclopirox, azoles)** — 4-week duration. **Terbinafine 1% cream x 1 week. Naftifine.** Burrow's solution added for Hyperkeratotic lesions.
- Oral Terbinafine, Fluconazole, or Itraconazole if topical medications are ineffective. Griseofulvin.
- Clean shoes with antifungal spray; keep cool/dry. Topical Nystatin is not effective.

TINEA CRURIS (JOCK ITCH)

- **Superficial fungal infection of the groin or inner thighs (crural folds) of the stratum corneum.**

ETIOLOGIES

- **Fungi of the Trichophyton genera (<u>*T. rubrum* most common</u>)** or *Epidermophyton floccosum.*

RISK FACTORS

- Males, copious sweating (eg, close contact sports, wearing tight clothing), immunocompromised.
- Tinea pedis may be the source of infection.

CLINICAL MANIFESTATIONS

- **Pruritus hallmark. Annular hyperpigmented patches or plaques, diffuse erythema to the inner thighs or groin with a sharply demarcated raised border** that may have tiny vesicles. Spreads centrifugally, with partial central clearing and a slightly elevated, erythematous or hyperpigmented, sharply advancing border. May spread to the perineum or perianal areas. Spares the scrotum.

DIAGNOSIS

- Clinical diagnosis based on history and physical.
- **<u>KOH prep:</u> best initial diagnostic test** — scrapings from lesion reveals segmented hyphae.
- <u>Fungal cultures</u> definitive diagnosis.

MANAGEMENT

- **<u>Topical antifungals</u> first-line — Clotrimazole, Butenafine, Terbinafine,** azoles (eg, Ketoconazole), Ciclopirox, Tolnaftate. In addition, use of desiccant powders in the inguinal area with the avoidance of tight-fitting clothing and noncotton underwear. Putting on socks before underwear.
- <u>Oral antifungals:</u> if topical ineffective or extensive — Terbinafine or Griseofulvin.

ID REACTION [AUTOECZEMATIZATION (DEMATOPHYTID REACTION)]

- **<u>Idiosyncratic reaction:</u> inflammatory dermatitis at [1] <u>sites DISTANT from the primary dermatophytosis</u>** (Type IV hypersensitivity in response to the fungi); **[2] <u>absence of fungal elements in the lesions</u>** (negative KOH testing), & **[3] <u>resolution when primary infection clears</u>.**
- **The Id reaction presents as intensely pruritic, papulovesicular eruptions, usually on the feet or hands, erythema nodosum, or annular erythema.**

TINEA CORPORIS

- **Superficial fungal infection of the body (trunk, legs, arms, or neck)** other than the feet, hands, groin, nails, hands, or the scalp.

ETIOLOGIES

- Fungi of the **Trichophyton and Microsporum** genera (***T. rubrum* most common**).
- *T. tonsurans* is a common cause of Tinea corporis gladiatorum (Tinea corporis in athletes who have skin-to-skin contact, such as wrestlers).

TRANSMISSION

- **Direct contact — common in preadolescents** (eg, wrestlers), contact with fomites.
- Infection from other animals (eg, kittens and puppies). Infection from another part of the body.

CLINICAL MANIFESTATIONS

- **Single or multiple pruritic, erythematous, scaly, circular, or oval plaques or patches with central clearing with well-defined raised advancing scaly borders** that spread outwardly.
- Multiple plaques may coalesce. Pustules may develop.

DIAGNOSIS

- **Potassium hydroxide (KOH prep): best initial test — scrapings from lesion reveals segmented hyphae.**
- Culture: definitive diagnosis (slower method).

MANAGEMENT

- **Limited disease: Topical antifungals first-line: "azoles" (eg, Clotrimazole, Ketoconazole), Butenafine, Terbinafine, Naftifine, Ciclopirox, or Tolnaftate.** Usually treated for 1-3 weeks.
- **Topical treatment ineffective or extensive disease: Oral (systemic) antifungals — Itraconazole or Terbinafine.** Griseofulvin or Fluconazole second-line systemic therapies. Nystatin not effective.

INTERTRIGO

- Inflammatory condition of the **intertriginous areas (two skin surfaces in close proximity) such as inguinal folds, axilla, intergluteal folds, & inframammary folds. *Candida spp.* most common.**

RISK FACTORS

- **Moisture & friction: warm moist environment** (eg, **skin folds,** hyperhidrosis, incontinence, **obesity**), **immunocompromised** (eg, **Diabetes mellitus, HIV**), maceration, constrictive clothing.
- Can be a complication of Irritant diaper dermatitis.

CLINICAL MANIFESTATIONS

- **Pruritus,** burning, & tingling in the skin folds and flexural surfaces. Pain if maceration occurs.

Physical examination

- **Erythematous "beefy red" macerated, moist plaques** & erosions with peripheral scaling and **erythematous satellite lesions (papules and pustules).** The groin is the most common site.
- Burning, tenderness, pruritus, and a malodor may be associated with the lesions.

DIAGNOSIS

- **Usually clinical.** When the diagnosis is uncertain, Wood's lamp examination, potassium hydroxide preparation (KOH), or skin biopsy is used. Fungal cultures definitive. Fasting glucose (rule out DM).
- **KOH preparation of skin scrapings — budding yeast ± pseudohyphae.** Direct microscopy.

MANAGEMENT

- **Topical antifungals azole creams first-line (eg, Clotrimazole, Ketoconazole, Miconazole)** due to their antifungal, antibacterial, and anti-inflammatory properties.
- Topical corticosteroids may be adjunctive to topical antifungals. Oral antifungals in severe cases.
- **Prevention: proper hygiene, keeping intertriginous areas cool and dry. Weight loss (if needed).**

ERYTHRASMA

- **Superficial infection caused by _Corynebacterium minutissimum_, part of the normal skin flora.**
- Erythrasma occurs in healthy adults, but individuals with immunodeficiency (eg, Diabetes mellitus, HIV), humid conditions, hyperhidrosis, and obesity are risk factors.
- Coinfection with dermatophytes or _Candida_ may occur.

CLINICAL MANIFESTATIONS
- **Interdigital most common presentation — scaly, macerated, moist skin in the toe web spaces.** Erythrasma is usually asymptomatic. Mildly pruritus, scaling, or erythema. Skin discoloration.
- **Intertriginous: erythematous to brown macules or plaques that may coalesce into larger patches with sharp borders in the groin, axillae, inframammary areas, or umbilicus. May be macerated with overlying fine scaling and wrinkling ("cigarette paper-like").**

DIAGNOSIS
- **Wood's lamp — coral-red fluorescence confirms the diagnosis.** Gram stain of skin scraping.
- **Potassium hydroxide (KOH) preparation of a skin scraping** with microscopic examination to assess for concomitant dermatophyte infection in patients with interdigital involvement.

MANAGEMENT
- **Localized Erythrasma topical therapy: topical Clindamycin or topical Erythromycin** for 14 days.
- **Extensive erythrasma systemic antibiotics** — oral Clarithromycin or Erythromycin.

BEDBUG BITES

- Bedbugs are obligate, blood-feeding parasitic insects _(Cimex lectularius_ and _Cimex hemipterus)_ that inhabit human dwellings.
- Spread of infestation can occur through transportation of items containing the bedbugs (eg, travel or acquisition of used furniture), or through direct movement of bedbugs through dwellings.
- Bedbugs do not live on humans. They inhabit cracks and crevices of mattresses, cushions, bed frames, or other structures. Bedbugs are attracted to carbon dioxide and the heat of the body host and generally feed at night, inflicting painless bites on exposed area while the victim sleeps.

CLINICAL MANIFESTATIONS
- Skin reactions to bedbugs vary, ranging from no reaction to pruritic papules or wheals, purpuric macules, or bullae. **Bites typically occur on the face, neck, hands, & arms** or other exposed areas.
- **The classic appearance of a bedbug bite reaction is a 2-5 mm erythematous papule or wheal with a central hemorrhagic punctum.**
- Reactions are typically noticed upon awakening or within a few days after the bites. Usually follows a **linear or zigzag configuration of bites in a group of 3-5 blood meals, often described as "breakfast, lunch, and dinner/supper"** (classic but not consistent finding).
- When to suspect?: potential exposure (recent travel, residence within building with known bedbug infestation). Cohabitants may have similar symptoms.

DIAGNOSIS
- Confirmation of the diagnosis of Bedbug bites requires detection of bedbugs in the victim's environment. **Inspection of the victim's residence by a professional pest control service.**

INFESTATION MANAGEMENT
- **Management of Bedbug infestation** eradication of the infestation via a professional pest control service management. The primary methods include application of insecticides and heat treatment.
- **Patient management not mandatory because Bedbug bites resolve spontaneously.** Pruritus: **Low- or medium-potency topical corticosteroid** (eg, Triamcinolone acetonide 0.1%) or oral antihistamine.

SCABIES

- A highly contagious skin infection due to the mite **_Sarcoptes scabiei_ via direct skin to skin contact.**
- **Female mites burrow into the skin to lay eggs, feed, & defecate** (scybala are the fecal particles that precipitate a hypersensitivity reaction in the skin). They cannot survive off the human body >4 days.

CLINICAL MANIFESTATIONS
- **Intense generalized pruritus especially at night or after a hot shower or bath.**
- Infected patients may remain asymptomatic for up to 4-6 weeks after initial infestation.

Physical examination:
- **Multiple small erythematous papules with excoriations.**
- **Linear burrows (pathognomonic) — serpiginous white lines often found in the intertriginous zones, including the scalp & web spaces** between the fingers & toes. Usually spares neck & face.
- **Erythematous pruritic papules, vesicles, or nodules on the scrotum, glans or penile shaft, or body folds pathognomonic.**
- **Young children and infants often show heavy involvement of the palms and soles and all aspects of the fingers.** Head usually spared in adults but may be involved in very young children.
- Crusted Scabies: high mite burden in immunocompromised patients — plaques or papules with overlying, prominent, adherent scales and crusts.

DIAGNOSIS
- Clinical. **Microscopy of skin scraping: definitive diagnosis — visualization of mites, ova, or feces from skin scraping under microscopy.**

MANAGEMENT
- **Topical: Permethrin topical drug of choice.** Applied topically from the neck down for 8-14 hours before showering. A repeat application after 1 week is recommended. Safe in pregnancy and lactation. Alternatives: Benzyl benzoate, Precipitated sulfur, Spinosad, and Ivermectin.
- **Oral Ivermectin alternative initial treatment** for nonpregnant adults who prefer oral treatment or is unable to apply topical therapy, or in severe cases. Not used in children <15 kg.
- **Pruritus:** Diphenhydramine or Hydroxyzine.
- **Lindane: DO NOT use after bath/shower (causes seizures** due to increased absorption through open pores). Contraindications: **Teratogenic, not used if & in children <2 years.**
- **All clothing, bedding etc. should be placed in a plastic bag at least 72 hours then washed & dried using heat.** All close contacts should be treated simultaneously as well.

PEDICULOSIS (LICE)

PUBIC LICE (CRABS)
- Pediculosis pubis (also known as *Phthiriasis pubis*).

TRANSMISSION:
- Usually sexually transmitted (especially in teenagers and young adults).

CLINICAL MANIFESTATIONS:
- **Pruritus of the involved area is the chief complaint. Nits may be seen.**

DIAGNOSIS
- Clinical diagnosis (visual of lice or nits). Microscopic examination of hair shafts.

MANAGEMENT
- **Topical Permethrin 1% or Pyrethrins first-line.** Treatment repeated after 9-10 days if lice remain.
- Sexual partners should be treated simultaneously.
- Clothing and bedding should be laundered in hot water.
- Alternative agents: Malathion lotion or oral Ivermectin.

HEAD LICE (*Pediculus humanus capitis*)

- Transmission: direct contact (person to person). Fomites (hats, headsets, clothing, bedding etc.).
- **Head lice: girls** > boys. Less common in Black individuals.
- Outbreaks commonly affect children 3-12 years old; warmer and & humid weather.

CLINICAL MANIFESTATIONS:
- **Intense itching** (especially occipital area), **papular urticaria near lice bites.**

Physical examination:
- Visualization of crawling nymphs or adult lice. The presence of nits alone does not confirm infestation.
- **Nits: white, oval-shaped egg capsules at the base of the hair shafts.**

MANAGEMENT
- **Permethrin topical drug of choice.** Capitis: Permethrin shampoo left on x 10 minutes. **A fine-tooth wet comb should be used to remove the nits.** Pubis/Corporis: Permethrin lotion for at least 8-10 hours. Safe in children at least 2 months of age. **Reapplication in 9-10 days recommended to destroy any newly hatched lice.** Permethrin is a neurotoxic synthetic pyrethroid that affects sodium transport across neuronal membranes causing respiratory paralysis of arthropods.
- Petroleum jelly can be used in addition to Permethrin to suffocate the lice.
- **Malathion is a first-line alternative to Permethrin.** Malathion is an organophosphate cholinesterase inhibitor that causes paralysis in arthropods. Requires 8-12 hour treatment period.
- Benzyl alcohol, Spinosad and topical Ivermectin. Spinosad has ovicidal activity, so combing to remove the nits is not necessary. **Lindane rarely used to its adverse effect — neurotoxic** (headaches, seizures, so do not use after shower or a bath). Usually avoided in children.
- **Oral Ivermectin can be used in cases that are refractory to topical therapies.**

AFTERCARE:
- **Contact items (eg, bedding & clothing) should be laundered in hot water with detergent & dried in a hot drier for 20 minutes.** Toys that cannot be washed are placed in air-tight plastic bags x 14 days.
- Avoid sharing contact items. Prophylactic treatment for individuals who share bedding.

BODY LICE (*Pediculus humanus corporis*)

TRANSMISSION
- Usually sexually transmitted.
- **Strongly related to poor body hygiene** — eg, homeless population, prisons, crowded unsanitary conditions, natural disasters, refugees from war.

PATHOPHYSIOLOGY
- Unlike head & pubic lice, body lice do not live on the skin.
- Body lice live and lay their eggs in seams of clothing or bedding and move to the skin only to feed.

DISEASE TRANSMISSION
- **Body lice can be a vector for diseases to humans, such as relapsing fever, epidemic typhus, and Trench fever.**

CLINICAL MANIFESTATIONS
- **Pruritus is usually the chief complaint** (reaction to the louse saliva) & excoriations.

DIAGNOSIS: clinical — identification of the louse or its nits in clothing, especially in the seams.

MANAGEMENT
- **Hygiene improvement first-line treatment** — bathe thoroughly.
- Infested clothing and bedding should be heat washed, dry cleaned, or discarded. Ironing especially in the seams will also destroy lice.
- Permethrin 5% cream (8–10-hour application) may be added if there are a few nits on body hair.

PIGMENT DISORDERS

VITILIGO

- Acquired skin disorder characterized by **skin depigmentation without evidence of inflammation.**

PATHOPHYSIOLOGY:
- **Autoimmune destruction of melanocytes, leading to skin depigmentation** thought to be play a major role. **Vitiligo is associated with other autoimmune diseases (eg, thyroid disease).**

CLINICAL MANIFESTATIONS
- **Irregular discrete (well-defined) milky white macules & patches of** total depigmentation.
- Commonly involves the dorsum of the hands, fingers, axilla, face, body folds, & genitalia.
- **Nonsegmental: includes the generalized, acrofacial or acral, mucosal, & universal subtypes.**
- Segmental Vitiligo — dermatomal or quasi-dermatomal pattern, most frequently along the distribution of the trigeminal nerve.

DIAGNOSIS
- Clinical diagnosis. Wood's lamp: fluorescence. Biopsy rarely needed — loss of epidermal melanocytes.

MANAGEMENT
- **Localized (<10%):** mid- to high-potency topical corticosteroids (except face). **Alternative:** Topical calcineurin inhibitors, eg, Tacrolimus [great for facial involvement and does not cause skin atrophy]. Cosmetic camouflage. Sunscreen. JAK inhibitor: Topical Ruxolitinib.
- **Disseminated & >20-25%:** systemic phototherapy (narrow band UVB) + topical or oral corticosteroids. Laser therapy, grafts, & cultured epidermal suspensions effective on limited areas.
- Rapidly progressive, nonsegmental: (eg, depigmented macules spreading over a few weeks or months) — oral Glucocorticoids and/or Narrowband ultraviolet B (NBUVB).
- **Stable, segmental:** topical therapies — eg, topical corticosteroids, topical calcineurin inhibitors, targeted phototherapy, and surgical therapy.

MELASMA & CHLOASMA

- **Hypermelanosis (hyperpigmentation) of sun exposed areas of the skin.**

RISK FACTORS
- **Increased estrogen exposure (OCPs, pregnancy, women).** Women with darker complexions.
- **Sunlight exposure: sun exposure** & exposure to phototoxic drugs. Family history.

CLINICAL MANIFESTATIONS
- **Mask-like hypermelanotic (light brown to gray brown) symmetrical macules and patches,** especially on the face & neck. Chloasma = Melasma during pregnancy.
- Dermal melasma has a bluish-grey appearance.

DIAGNOSIS
- Clinical diagnosis. Woods lamp may help to determine the pattern of pigment deposition. Appearance is unchanged under black light in dermal Melasma. May be enhanced in epidermal Melasma.
- Histology: increased melanin deposition in all layers of the epidermis and in the dermis.

MANAGEMENT
- **Sun protection:** sunscreen, iron oxide sunscreen, avoidance of the sun, wearing a wide-brimmed hat.
- **[1] Mild Melasma: Hydroquinone 4% cream** first-line bleaching agent. Other bleaching agents: Azelaic acid, Topical retinoids. Chemical peels are an option if no response to topical agents.
- **[2] Moderate to severe Melasma: Triple therapy** often used = (1) Fluocinolone acetonide 0.01% + (2) Hydroquinone 4% + (3) Tretinoin 0.05%. Laser therapy may help for dermal Melasma.
- **[3] During pregnancy (Chloasma) & if breastfeeding: Broad spectrum sunscreen & sun avoidance treatment of choice if pregnant (Hydroquinone & Tretinoin are contraindicated).**

MOLLUSCUM CONTAGIOSUM

- **Benign infection with Molluscum contagiosum virus [MCV] DNA poxvirus in *poxviridae* family.**

<u>TRANSMISSION</u>
- <u>Highly contagious</u> — direct contact (skin to skin) most common & autoinoculation. Fomites.
- Most common in school-aged children, sexually active adults, & patients with HIV.
- MCV-1 most common in children; MCV-2 most common in patients with HIV.

<u>CLINICAL MANIFESTATIONS</u>
- **Single or multiple firm dome-shaped, flesh-colored to pearly-white, waxy, painless papules 2-5 mm in diameter with <u>central umbilication.</u>** Common on the face, lower abdomen, & genitals.
- **Curd-like material may be expressed from the center if lesion is squeezed** (central keratin plug).

<u>DIAGNOSIS</u>
- Usually a clinical diagnosis. In adults, it may be an indicator of HIV.
- **<u>Histology: Henderson-Paterson bodies</u> — keratinocytes containing eosinophilic cytoplasmic inclusion bodies.**

<u>MANAGEMENT</u>
- **<u>No treatment</u> needed in most cases (spontaneous resolution in 3-9 months usually).**
- **Adolescents and adults with sexually transmitted molluscum contagiosum in the genital region may be treated to avoid spread of the disease to others.**
- **<u>Curettage</u> — first line when therapy when <u>rapid resolution</u> is indicated.**
- **Cryotherapy, Cantharidin or Podophyllotoxin.** Electrodesiccation. Imiquimod. Topical retinoids.
- Care should be taken to reduce risk of transmission to others: lesions in areas that are likely to come in contact with others should be **<u>covered with clothing or a watertight bandage.</u>**
- **Affected individuals do not need to be excluded from contact sports activities <u>provided</u> lesions can be covered with clothing or watertight bandages.** May use public pools.

CUTANEOUS WARTS [VERRUCAE (COMMON, FLAT, & PLANTAR WARTS)]

- **Caused by Human papillomavirus infection (HPV) >100 types.** Skin-to-skin contact.

<u>PATHOPHYSIOLOGY</u>
- HPV infects keratinized skin, causing excessive proliferation & retention of the stratum corneum.
- <u>Types:</u> common (vulgaris), plantar (plantaris), flat (plana).

<u>CLINICAL MANIFESTATIONS</u>
- **<u>Common & plantar warts:</u> firm, hyperkeratotic papules between 1-10 mm with red brown punctations (thrombosed capillaries are pathognomonic).** Borders may be rounded or irregular. <u>Plantar:</u> HPV type 1 most common. <u>Common:</u> 2, 4 (most common), types 1, 3, 27, 29, & 57.
- **<u>Flat warts:</u> numerous, small, discrete, flesh-colored flat-topped papules measuring 1-5 mm in diameter & 1-2 mm in height.** Typically seen on the face, hands, & shins. Often HPV type 3, 10, 28.

<u>DIAGNOSIS</u>
- Clinical diagnosis, serologies. Immunofluorescence.
- <u>Histology:</u> koilocytotic squamous cells with hyperplastic hyperkeratosis.

<u>MANAGEMENT</u>
- **Most warts resolve spontaneously without treatment within 2 years if immunocompetent.**
- **<u>Common or plantar warts:</u> topical Salicylic acid first line (keratolytic agent). Cryotherapy (liquid nitrogen) is an alternative but may be painful & may lead to hypopigmentation.**
- <u>Refractory:</u> topical immunotherapy with contact allergens [dinitrochlorobenzene (DNCB) diphenylcyclopropenone (DPCP), squaric acid], intralesional Bleomycin, topical Fluorouracil.
- **<u>Flat warts:</u> Cryotherapy or topical agents** (eg, Tretinoin, Imiquimod, or Fluorouracil). Filiform warts are easily treated with cryotherapy or surgery. Excision is associated with recurrence.

CONDYLOMA ACUMINATA [CA] (ANOGENITAL WARTS)

- Etiology: caused by **Human papillomavirus (HPV) infection. HPV 6 & 11 most common causes.**
- **Transmission & risk factors**: **sexual activity.** Immunosuppression increases risk for CA.

CLINICAL MANIFESTATIONS
- **Genital warts vary from small, flat-topped painless raised papules, which can evolve into large, soft, fleshy, cauliflower-like, or dome-shaped lesions in clusters on the anogenital mucosa and surrounding skin or the oropharynx, ranging from skin-colored to pink or red.**
- Lesions persist for months & may spontaneously resolve, remain unchanged, or grow if not treated. Large lesions can interfere with toileting or sexual intercourse.
- **Complications: Squamous cell carcinoma (eg, cervix, anal, penile, vaginal, and vulvar cancers).**

DIAGNOSIS
- Condyloma acuminata is usually a clinical diagnosis, and histopathologic examination of the lesions is often unnecessary. Atypical lesions should be confirmed by histology.
- Application of dilute Acetic acid (with subsequent whitening of the lesion) may reveal areas of subclinical HPV infection, but is nonspecific, has a high false-positive rate, and is not recommended in the routine evaluation of external genital warts.
- Serologies may be performed.
- **Biopsy: rarely needed. Histology: acanthosis (overgrowth of the stratum spinosum) with overlying hyperplastic hyperkeratosis, koilocytotic squamous cells, and atypical keratinocytes with papillomatosis hyperplasia.**

MANAGEMENT
- **~80% with HPV 6 and 11 will experience spontaneous resolution of lesions within 18 months.**
- Treatment depends on location, size & number of warts. There are many treatment options, and recurrence is common. Patient preferences, available resources, cost, and clinician experience should guide treatment selection.
- **First-line patient-applied therapies include antiproliferative agents (eg, Imiquimod) and immunomodulators (eg, Podophyllotoxin and Sinecatechins).**
- **First-line clinician-administered treatments are Liquid nitrogen cryotherapy, Trichloroacetic acid, and surgical removal (Excision, Electrosurgery, or Carbon dioxide laser therapy).**
- Laser CO2 vaporization is less effective than other techniques.

PREVENTION
- Male circumcision may decrease the transmission of Human immunodeficiency virus (HIV), human papillomavirus (HPV), and herpes simplex virus (HSV) in heterosexuals.

HPV vaccine:
- **Gardasil 9: covers for HPV 6, 11, 16, 18 (16 & 18 most associated with Squamous cell carcinoma) as well as HPV types 31, 33, 45, 52, & 58.**

Indications: (ACIP): All females & males:
- Routine vaccination is recommended at 11-12 years & can be administered starting at 9 years of age.
- For adolescents and adults aged 13-26 years who have not been previously vaccinated or who have not completed the vaccine series, catch-up vaccination is recommended.
- For adults 27y-45y and older, catch-up vaccination is not routinely recommended; the ACIP notes that the decision to vaccinate people in this age group should be made on an individual basis.
- **Individuals initiating the vaccine series at 9-15 years of age — Two doses of HPV vaccine** should be given at (1) 0 and (2) at 6-12 months.
- **Individuals initiating the vaccine series at 15 years of age or older — Three doses of HPV vaccine** should be given at 0, 1-2 months (typically 2), and at 6 months. Minimum interval between first 2 doses is 4 weeks, minimum interval between the second & third is 12 weeks.

KERATOTIC DISORDERS

SEBORRHEIC KERATOSIS

- **Most common benign epidermal skin tumor** (benign proliferation of immature keratinocytes).
- Most common in fair-skinned elderly with prolonged sun exposure.

CLINICAL MANIFESTATIONS
- **Well-demarcated round or oval velvety warty lesions with a greasy or "stuck on" appearance.** Varied possible colors (eg, flesh-colored, grey, brown, & black). Hyperkeratotic; may be scaly.
- They are usually asymptomatic, but chronic irritation due to friction trauma may at times lead to pruritus, pain, or bleeding. Their appearance can mimic Melanoma.
- **The sign of Leser-Trélat**, is the **abrupt appearance of multiple Seborrheic keratoses** in association with skin tags and Acanthosis nigricans, **has been associated with a variety of malignancies, including gastrointestinal and lung cancers.**

DIAGNOSIS
- **Usually clinical.**
- **Biopsy can be performed if the diagnosis is uncertain.** Classic findings: well-demarcated proliferation of keratinocytes with characteristic small keratin-filled cysts. A dermal lymphocytic infiltrate is often present in inflamed or irritated lesions.

MANAGEMENT
- **No treatment needed** — **benign (no premalignant potential).**
- Cosmetic or symptomatic management includes **Cryotherapy (most common treatment used),** Electrodesiccation & curettage, or Laser ablation therapy.

ACTINIC KERATOSES (AK)

- **Most common premalignant skin condition (may progress to Squamous cell carcinoma).**
- Pathophysiology: proliferation of atypical epidermal keratinocytes.
- Risk factors: prolonged sun exposure, lighter skin, increasing age, & males.

CLINICAL MANIFESTATIONS
- **Dry, rough, macules or papules that feel like "sandpaper", with transparent or yellow scaling.**
- Can range from skin-colored to **erythematous or hyperkeratotic (hyperpigmented) plaques.**
- **May have a projection on the skin (cutaneous horn).**

DIAGNOSIS
- Clinical: common on scalp, face, lateral neck, dorsal forearms & hands. Dermoscopy.
Punch or shave biopsy may be performed to distinguish AK from Squamous cell carcinoma.
- Classic findings include [1] atypical epidermal keratinocytes & cells with **large hyperchromatic pleomorphic nuclei from the basal layer upwards ([2] no invasion into the dermis).**
- Indications: Lesions that are >1 cm in diameter, indurated, ulcerated, rapidly growing, and lesions that fail to respond to appropriate therapy should be considered for biopsy.

MANAGEMENT
- **Photoprotection: Avoid sun exposure. Use of sunscreen.**
- **Few localized AK: surgical — liquid nitrogen cryosurgery most commonly used treatment.** Dermabrasion; Electrodesiccation & curettage.
- **Multiple thin AK: medical "field treatment" (eg, topical 5-fluorouracil)** — most commonly used in areas with multiple thin lesions, including those of the face & scalp. Other options include topical Imiquimod, Tribanibulin, Photodynamic therapy.
- Thick lesions may need Liquid nitrogen Cryosurgery followed by topical 5-fluorouracil (5-FU).

NEOPLASMS

CUTANEOUS SQUAMOUS CELL CARCINOMA

- Malignancy of keratinocytes that invades the dermis or beyond, characterized by hyperkeratosis & ulceration.
- **Bowen's disease** = **Squamous cell carcinoma in situ** (has not invaded the dermis).
- 2nd most common skin cancer (after Basal cell carcinoma). **Slow growing** (rarely metastasizes)

RISK FACTORS
- **Sun exposure major risk factor (often preceded by Actinic keratosis).**
- Lighter-skin, Xeroderma pigmentosum, chronic wounds, old scars or burns.
- **HPV infection.** Chronic immunosuppression (eg, post-transplant).

CLINICAL MANIFESTATIONS
- **Erythematous, elevated thickened nodule** with adherent **white scaly or crusted, bloody margins**.
- **May present as a nonhealing ulceration or erosion that is slowly evolving.**
- Most commonly located on the head, lips, hands, and neck.
- **Most lower lip cancers (90%) are Squamous cell type and involve the vermillion border**, whereas upper lip cancer is usually Basal cell type and arise from the lip skin.

DIAGNOSIS
- **Biopsy (shave, punch, or excisional): atypical keratinocytes & malignant cells with large, pleomorphic, hyperchromatic nuclei in the epidermis, extending into the dermis.** May form nodules with laminated centers ("epithelial/**keratinous pearls**").

MANAGEMENT
- **Surgical excision with clear margins** (4-6 mm) **is the most frequently used treatment.**
- **Mohs micrographic surgery: recurrent/aggressive tumors and cosmetically sensitive areas.**
- Electrodesiccation & curettage: may be used for small, well-defined superficial lesions in low-risk noncritical sites. Bowen disease: surgical excision, E&C, cryosurgery, topical 5-FU.
- Cryotherapy can be used for small, well-defined, low risk lesions & Bowen's disease.
- Radiation therapy may be a nonsurgical choice in selected patients or as adjuvant therapy.

KAPOSI SARCOMA

- **Vascular cancer associated with Human herpesvirus 8 infection (HHV-8).**
- **Most commonly seen in immunosuppressed patients (eg, HIV** with CD4 count <100/mm^3 or post-transplant). Sporadic: older men of Mediterranean origin. Endemic: eastern & southern Africa.
- May affect the skin, lungs, lymph nodes and GI tract. Cutaneous KS most commonly is seen on the lower extremities, face oral mucosa & genitalia.

CLINICAL MANIFESTATIONS
- **Painless nonpruritic macular, papular, nodule(s), plaque-like dark brown, pink, red, violaceous, or black lesions.** 4 variants: classic KS, endemic KS, iatrogenic KS, and epidemic KS.

DIAGNOSIS
- Biopsy — angiogenesis, inflammation, and proliferation (whorls of spindle-shaped cells with leukocytic infiltration & neovascularization), & immunohistologic staining.

MANAGEMENT
- **HIV-associated KS: Antiretroviral therapy.**
- Radiation therapy, excision, cryotherapy, laser ablation, intralesional, topical therapy, chemotherapy.

MALIGNANT MELANOMA

- A type of cancer developing from the melanocytes most commonly affecting the skin.
- **Most common cause of skin cancer-related death. Aggressive with high malignant potential.** 3% of all skin cancer but 65% of all skin cancer-related deaths.
- Most commonly metastasizes to the regional lymph nodes, skin, liver, lungs, & brain.

RISK FACTORS

- **UV radiation associated in 80% of cases**, blistering sunburns, family history, > 3 burns before the age 20, tanning booth use, large number of nevi. Mutation in the gene that encodes BRAF (40-60%).
- Caucasians, light hair/eye color, & Xeroderma pigmentosum.
- Although it is most common on sun exposed areas, it can occur anywhere on the body.

MAJOR SUBTYPES

- **Superficial spreading: most common type (70%).** May arise de novo or from a pre-existing nevus. **Most common on the trunk in men and legs in women.**
- **Nodular: second most common type.** May be associated with rapid vertical growth phase, making it a high-risk lesion (radial growth phase may not be evident). **Found on all body surfaces, especially the trunk, especially in males.**
- **Lentigo maligna: Most commonly arises in chronically sun-damaged or sun-exposed areas of the skin in older individuals, such as the face** (usually, a lapse of many years occurs before a lentigo maligna becomes an invasive Melanoma). These lesion frequently begins as a tan or brown macule (small, flat, freckle-like lesions) that darken with marked notching of the borders.
- **Acral lentiginous: Most common type found in darker-pigmented individuals:** 60–72% in African Americans, 29-46% Asian Americans, & Hispanics. **May be seen on the palms, soles (plantar foot), nail beds beneath the nail plate**, mucous membranes, penis, and areas without sun exposure. Acral lentiginous Melanomas first appear as dark brown to black, irregularly pigmented flat macules or patches that may become raised. Subungual Melanoma arises from the nail matrix & usually presents as a longitudinal, brown or black band in the fingernail or toenail.
- **Desmoplastic: most aggressive type.**

CLINICAL MANIFESTATIONS

- **"ABCDE" A**symmetry; **B**orders: irregular; **C**olor: variation; **D**iameter: usually ≥6mm, **E**volution (suspect in a lesion with recent or rapid change in appearance).
- Lesions on the upper back, upper arm, neck, & scalp decrease the likelihood of survival.
- **The "ugly duckling" sign** in an individual with multiple nevi, MM may present as a pigmented lesion obviously different from the others in a given individual, even if it does not fulfill the ABCD criteria.

DIAGNOSIS

- **Excisional/complete (full thickness) elliptical biopsy preferred method** because prognosis is based on the measurement of the thickness of the tumor — the sample should have a 1- to 3-mm margin of healthy skin and extending to a depth including all layers of skin and some subcutaneous fat (at the thickest part of the lesion) — **atypical melanocytes and architectural disorder.**
- **Shave biopsy discouraged** because it may compromise pathologic diagnosis and complete determination of Breslow thickness.

MANAGEMENT

- **Complete local wide surgical excision mainstay of therapy for early-stage cutaneous Melanoma,** often performed with sentinel lymph node biopsy, elective node dissection, or both.
  - ≤1 mm thick (T1): a 1 cm margin of normal tissue may be performed
  - > 1–2 mm thick: 2 cm of marginal tissue recommended.
  - 2-4 mm thick (T3): 2 cm marginal tissue.
- Adjuvant therapy in some high risk: interferon-alfa, immune therapy (eg, Nivolumab, Ipilimumab), or radiotherapy. Talimogene (modified HSV). Vemurafenib (BRAF kinase inhibitor).

BASAL CELL CARCINOMA

- **Most common type of skin cancer in the US.** Most common cancer in humans.
- **<u>Slow growing</u>: locally invasive but very low incidence of metastasis.**

<u>RISK FACTORS</u>
- Lighter-skinned individuals, prolonged sun exposure (especially in childhood), Xeroderma pigmentosum (genetic disorder with inability to repair damage caused by UV light exposure).

<u>CLINICAL MANIFESTATIONS</u>
- <u>**Nodular**</u>**: small, raised (domed-shaped) papules that are pink, white, or flesh colored; translucent, waxy, or pearly quality, with raised "rolled" borders** (where the periphery is more raised than the middle)**, central depression, &/or ulceration. Overlying telangiectatic surface vessels** often become more prominent as the lesion enlarges. The ulcerative area in the center may have black-blue or brown areas within them. **Often friable (bleeds easily). 80% present on the face & head — 25-30% nose alone,** neck, or trunk (15%).
- <u>Superficial BCC</u>: (~15%) — slightly scaly, non-firm macules, patches, or thin plaques light red to pink in color resembling Eczema or Psoriasis, but often retaining the characteristic raised, pearly white borders of the nodular subtype.
- <u>Upper lip cancer</u> is usually Basal cell type and arise from the lip skin. Lower lip cancer often SCC.

<u>DIAGNOSIS</u>
- **<u>Punch or shave biopsy</u>** — clusters of basaloid cells with a palisade arrangement of the nuclei at the periphery of the clusters.
- <u>Excisional biopsy</u> may also be performed.

<u>SURGICAL MANAGEMENT</u>
- **<u>Mohs micrographic surgery</u> for facial involvement, difficult cases, high-risk cases, or recurrent cases (best long-term cure rates & tissue sparing benefit).**
- <u>Electrodesiccation & curettage</u> used most commonly on non-facial tumors with low risk of recurrence.
- <u>Surgical excision:</u> Standard excision with 4-5 mm margins and postoperative margin assessment may be used for tumors with either low or high risk of tumor recurrence (eg, primary <u>nodular</u> BCCs <20 mm on low-risk areas of the trunk or extremities).

PHOTOSENSITIVE & PHOTOTOXIC MEDICATIONS

- Most phototoxic medications are activated by ultraviolet A (UVA) vs. ultraviolet B (UVB) radiation.

<u>COMMON MEDICATIONS</u>
- **Tetracyclines (especially Doxycycline),** Fluoroquinolones, Hydrochlorothiazide, Sulfonamides
- **Psoralens, retinoids (including) Isotretinoin**
- Metformin, NSAIDs (especially Piroxicam), Phenothiazines (eg, Chlorpromazine)
- Antifungal agents (eg, Voriconazole, Griseofulvin), Amiodarone
- Tar compounds, St. John's wort.

<u>CLINICAL MANIFESTATIONS</u>
- Phototoxic reactions often appear erythema, scaling, or pruritus on patches of sun-exposed skin similar to an exaggerated sunburn. The reaction usually evolves within minutes to hours of sun exposure and is restricted to exposed skin.
- In severe cases, vesicles or bullae may be seen.
- Skin biopsy findings are identical to those of regular sunburn, with vacuolated and apoptotic keratinocytes.
Take appropriate protective measures (eg, hat, long-sleeved shirts, sunscreen).

CONTACT DERMATITIS

- Inflammation of the dermis & epidermis from direct contact between a substance & the surface of the skin. **Either irritant or allergic.**
- **Irritant: most common type.** Causes include chemicals (eg, solvents, cleaners, & detergents), alcohols, creams. Irritant contact diaper dermatitis — prolonged exposure to urine, feces (or harsh detergents from washable diapers). May develop superimposed Candida infection.
- **Allergen (ACD): nickel most common worldwide, poison ivy,** oak, or sumac; other metals, chemicals (eg, fragrances, glue, hair dyes), detergents, cleaners, acids, prolonged water exposure.

PATHOPHYSIOLOGY
- **Allergic: type IV hypersensitivity reaction** (T cell lymphocyte-mediated — **delayed by days**).
- **Irritant: non-immunologic reaction (immediate)** due to direct damage to the skin.

CLINICAL MANIFESTATIONS
- **Acute: erythematous papules or tiny vesicles (may be linear or geometric); may ooze, weep, crust, develop edema, or progress to bullae. Localized pruritus, stinging, burning, or tenderness.** Pruritic, erythematous, indurated, scaly plaques localized to the skin areas that come in contact with the allergen 12-48 hours after exposure. Irritant erythema & scales (less vesicular).
- Chronic: thickened dry skin with lichenification, fissuring, crusting, and scaling. Hyperpigmentation.

DIAGNOSIS
- Mainly a clinical diagnosis. **Patch testing** may identify potential allergens to prevent future exposures.
- Histology not usually needed but will show spongiosis (intercellular edema in the epidermis).

MANAGEMENT
- **Identification & avoidance of irritants is the most important aspect of management.**
- **Topical corticosteroids first-line medication [eg, ointments] with emollients and moisturizers. Severe or extensive reactions: Systemic (oral) corticosteroids.**
- **Topical calcineurin inhibitors (eg, Tacrolimus or Pimecrolimus) are alternatives.**

GENERAL MEASURES
- Cool saline or astringent compresses, cool baths, skin emollients.
- If oozing or weeping, drying agents (eg, aluminum acetate) can be used.
- Burrow's solution. Itching can be relieved with antihistamines or calamine lotion.
- **Prevention: protection measures (eg, gloves), barrier creams, emollients, and moisturizers.**

DIAPER RASH
- **A type of irritant Contact dermatitis, often due to prolonged exposure to urine & feces** or harsh detergents from washable diapers.

CLINICAL MANIFESTATIONS
- **Acute: erythematous papules. May develop maceration, superficial erosions most commonly involving convex areas in contact with the diaper** (eg, buttocks, genitalia, upper thighs, and lower abdomen), usually **sparing of the skin folds.**
- If severe, may be associated with extensive erythema, painful erosions, and nodules.
- **If superimposed *Candida infection* occurs, it involves the skin folds, with satellite lesions.**

MANAGEMENT
- **General skin care: first-line treatment — frequent diaper changes, topical barrier ointment, emollient, or cream (eg, petroleum or zinc oxide),** use of disposable diapers, periods of rest without a diaper; keep the affected area clean and dry.
- **Low-potency corticosteroids** if no adequate response to the above in 2-3 days.
- **Topical antifungals ± low-potency corticosteroids** in severe cases or in *Candida* superinfections.

TOXICODENDRON DERMATITIS

- **Caused by poison ivy** (most common in the east), **poison oak** (west of the Rocky Mountains), and **poison sumac** (in the southeast).

- <u>Urushiol</u>, **composed of oleoresins, initiate a type IV hypersensitivity reaction** with direct contact with the leaves.

CLINICAL MANIFESTATIONS
- **Localized intense pruritus, erythema, stinging or burning of the skin that may have come in contact with plant parts.**
- **Well-demarcated erythematous papules, vesicles, &/or bullae (<u>may be linear or geometric</u>) or plaques where a portion of the plant came in contact with the skin.**

MANAGEMENT
- <u>**Mild/limited:**</u> <u>**symptomatic treatment:**</u> **cool compresses, oatmeal baths. <u>High-potency topical corticosteroids</u> may decrease itching.**
- <u>**Severe/extensive:**</u> **systemic (oral) glucocorticoids if extensive or if involves the face or genitals.**
- <u>Prevention:</u> avoided by the use of protective barriers (eg, clothing) and washing the exposed area with detergent soap as soon as possible.

ACUTE PALMOPLANTAR (DYSHIDROTIC) ECZEMA [POMPHOLYX]

- **Recurrent pruritic vesicular rash affecting the hands &/or feet** (palms, fingers, and/or soles).
- **Most common in young adults in the third decade,** onset is <40 years of age.

TRIGGERS
- **Flares associated with sweating, emotional stress, warm & humid weather, metals (eg, nickel).**

CLINICAL MANIFESTATIONS
- **Sudden onset of the development of deep-seated pruritic small <u>tense clear vesicles</u> 1-2 mm ("tapioca-like" appearance) <u>limited to the hands &/or feet</u> [palms, & fingers (eg, lateral aspects of the digits), and soles].**
- Later, desiccation, desquamation, hyperpigmentation, papules, scaling, lichenification, fissuring, and erosions may occur after several weeks.
- Vesicles may coalesce to bullae if severe.

DIAGNOSIS
- Usually clinical, based upon the clinical appearance and location of lesions, symptoms, and history.
- In most patients, patch testing is useful to determine whether there is a component of allergic contact dermatitis. <u>Potassium hydroxide preparation</u> of unroofed vesicles to rule out bullous Tinea.

MANAGEMENT
- **Avoidance of triggers or irritants. Avoid prolonged exposure of the hands & feet to water.**
- **<u>Mild to moderate:</u> <u>Topical corticosteroid</u> ointments preferred [medium- to high-potency (group 1-3]).** Cool baths, emollients. Usually spontaneously resolves over several weeks.
- <u>Severe:</u> Oral corticosteroids. Superpotent topical corticosteroids is an alternative.
- Topical Psoralen + ultraviolet A therapy for frequent episodes not controlled with above treatment.

GENERAL MEASURES
- Cold compresses, Aluminum subacetate (Burrow's solution) or Witch hazel for weeping wet skin.
- Use of lukewarm water & soap-free cleansers to wash hands, drying hands after washing, applying emollients immediately after hand drying. <u>Prework:</u> protective clothing or accessories, using cotton gloves under nonlatex gloves when performing wet work (eg washing dishes). Moisturizers.

LICHEN PLANUS

- Acute or chronic inflammatory mucocutaneous papulosquamous dermatitis (cell-mediated immune response) — **skin, nails, mucous membranes (oral cavity), genitalia, scalp, or esophagus.**

INCREASED INCIDENCE
- **Hepatitis C infection,** medication-induced (eg, Thiazide diuretics, gold, antimalarial agents, Penicillamine, phenothiazines, sulfonamides), graft vs host, & malignant Lymphoma.
- Most commonly affects middle-aged adults. 5% of oral LP may progress to Squamous cell carcinoma.

CLINICAL MANIFESTATIONS
- Pruritic rash most common on the extremities, especially the volar surfaces of the wrists, ankles, shins, lower back, & genitalia. May involve the mouth, scalp, genitals, nails, & mucous membranes.

PHYSICAL EXAMINATION
- **Cutaneous LP: 6 Ps: purple (violaceous), polygonal, planar, pruritic, papules or plaques (flat-topped) with fine scales** & irregular borders; may have **Wickham's striae (fine gray-white lines on the skin lesions or on the oral mucosa).** May also present with hypertrophic or vesicobullous lesions. Prominent post-inflammatory hyperpigmentation is common.
- **Koebner's phenomenon — new lesions at sites of trauma (also seen in Psoriasis).**
- Nail involvement: nail dystrophy with permanent deformity or loss of fingernails and toenails.
- Scalp involvement: Lichen planopilaris affects the scalp and can lead to scarring alopecia.
- **Oral involvement: may present with only lacelike Wickham's striae or may include papular, atrophic, or erosive lesions.**
- Mucous membranes, especially the buccal mucosa, where it can present on a spectrum ranging from a mild, white, reticulate eruption of the mucosa to a severe, erosive stomatitis.
- Genital areas can also be affected by Lichen planus.

DIAGNOSIS
- Primarily a clinical diagnosis. HCV testing for Hepatitis C virus.
- Biopsy & immunofluorescence — **Hyperkeratosis, degeneration of the basal cell layer, & colloid bodies** (non-nucleated eosinophilic deposits). Saw-tooth lymphocyte infiltrate at the dermal epidermal junction. Oral LP amorphous band of **eosinophilic material** at the basement membrane.

MANAGEMENT
- **Topical corticosteroids (high or super-high potency) mainstay of treatment of LP with occlusive dressings first-line for trunk & extremity LP.** Oral Antihistamines for pruritus.
- Intralesional corticosteroids can be useful in patients with hypertrophic LP (thick lesions).
- Generalized disease or local corticosteroid-refractory disease: cutaneous LP that cannot be treated adequately with local corticosteroids may benefit from other treatments — short course of oral glucocorticoids, phototherapy [Ultraviolet B (UVB) and photosensitizing Psoralen plus ultraviolet A (PUVA) phototherapy], & oral retinoids (eg, Acitretin).
- Most patients have spontaneous remissions 6-12 months.

LICHEN SIMPLEX CHRONICUS (NEURODERMATITIS)

- **Skin thickening in patients with Atopic dermatitis** secondary to **repetitive rubbing & scratching.**

CLINICAL MANIFESTATIONS
- Scaly, well-demarcated, rough hyperkeratotic (lichenified) plaques **with exaggerated skin lines.**
- Common on the wrists, external surface of forearms, nape of neck, lower legs, and genitals.

MANAGEMENT
- **Avoid scratching the lesions & the itch-scratch cycle.**
- **Topical corticosteroids (high potency) under occlusive dressings,** antihistamines for pruritus.
- Intralesional corticosteroids.

ATOPIC DERMATITIS (ECZEMA)

- Rash due to **defective skin barrier susceptible to drying, leading to pruritus & inflammation.**
- **Atopic triad:** Atopic dermatitis (Eczema) + Allergic rhinitis + Asthma.
- Pathophysiology: disruption of the skin barrier [**filaggrin (*FLG*) gene mutation**] & disordered immune response (eg, **IgE, T cells**). Most cases manifest in infancy and almost always by age 5 years.
- Triggers: heat, perspiration, allergens, & contact irritants (eg, wool, nickel, food, synthetic fabrics).

CLINICAL MANIFESTATIONS

- **Pruritus hallmark required for diagnosis** — pruritus & dry skin are cardinal features.
- **Erythematous, ill-defined blisters, papules, or plaques with oozing.** Later the lesions dry, crust over, & scale. **Most common in flexor creases** (eg, antecubital & popliteal folds) in older children & adults. In individuals with deeply pigmented skin, lesions may appear with grayish, violaceous, or dark brown hues. **Lichenification seen with chronic lesions (Lichen simplex chronicus).**
- **Infantile AD** often face, neck, & **extensor surface involvement** (from crawling & skin rubbing).
- **Nummular eczema: sharply defined discoid or circular coin-shaped lesions,** especially on the dorsum of the hands, feet, & extensor surfaces (knees, elbows). Lesions are erythematous, edematous, vesicular, and crusted patches. Small vesicles may merge with the larger lesions.

DIAGNOSIS: clinical. Increased IgE supports the diagnosis.

CHRONIC MANAGEMENT

- **Restoration of skin barrier: maintain skin hydration** — hydration & skin emollients twice daily & within 3 minutes of exiting a lukewarm shower or tepid bath. Pat the skin instead of rubbing.
- Pruritus: oral antihistamines Cetirizine, Fexofenadine, Loratadine. Hydroxyzine, Diphenhydramine.
- **Trigger avoidance (heat, low humidity),** or irritants (eg, soaps, detergents, washcloths, frequent baths).

ACUTE (FLARE) MANAGEMENT

- **Topical corticosteroids first-line, often used with emollients. Antihistamines for itching.** Wet dressings (eg, Burrow's solution). Antibiotics if secondary infection (eg, *Staphylococcus aureus*).
- **Topical calcineurin inhibitor (Tacrolimus, Pimecrolimus) alternative to low-potency steroids on the face or skin folds (they do not cause skin atrophy).** Topical Crisaborole or Ruxolitinib.
- Moderate to severe disease: Phototherapy (narrow-band UVB, UVB, UVA). **Dupilumab,** Tralokinumab, Abrocitinib, Upadactinib Cyclosporine, Azathioprine, Mycophenolate, Methotrexate.

PITYRIASIS ROSEA

- Etiology: uncertain etiology. May be associated with **viral infections** (eg, Human herpesvirus 6 or 7).
- **Primarily seen in older children & young adults** (rare >35y). Increased incidence in spring & fall.

CLINICAL MANIFESTATIONS

- **Herald patch (solitary salmon-colored, red, or brown macule)** on the trunk 2-6 cm in diameter, followed by a general exanthem 1-2 weeks later: **smaller 1 cm round or oval, colored papules with white circular (collarette) cigarette paper scaling at the edges & central clearing, distributed in a Christmas tree pattern** (oriented along the skin cleavage lines). **Pruritus is common and often mild.**
- **Confined to the trunk & proximal extremities;** face, palms, & soles are usually spared.

DIAGNOSIS: primarily clinical. In young adults, RPR should be ordered to rule out secondary Syphilis.

MANAGEMENT

- **No management needed for most** — education, reassurance, & treatment of pruritus (if present) is the management of choice. Resolves spontaneously in 6-12 weeks.
- **Pruritus: medium-potency topical corticosteroids, oral antihistamines, or oatmeal baths.**
- Scaling: lotions or emollients.
- Severe: narrowband UVB phototherapy may be helpful if severe & started in the first week of eruption.
- Oral Acyclovir, and in some Erythromycin, may speed up healing but are not routinely used.

PSORIASIS

- Immune-mediated multisystemic disease with a genetic predisposition.

PATHOPHYSIOLOGY
- **Keratin hyperplasia & proliferating cells in the stratum basale + stratum spinosum due to T cell activation & cytokine release** (eg, IL-6, C-reactive protein, TNF-α).
- This response results in **greater epidermal thickness & accelerated epidermis turnover.**
- **Certain medications (eg, Beta-blockers, Antimalarials, Statins, Lithium, Prednisone taper), may flare or worsen Psoriasis.**

CLINICAL MANIFESTATIONS
- **Plaque: most common type — raised, well-demarcated, pink-red plaques or papules with thick silvery-white scales. Most common on the <u>extensor surfaces</u>** of the elbows, knees, scalp (most common initial spot), nape of the neck, and gluteal cleft. Usually pruritic. Arthritis in 30%.
- **Auspitz sign: punctate bleeding with removal of a plaque or scale.** Auspitz sign is not specific to Psoriasis (may also be seen in Actinic keratosis).
- **Koebner's phenomenon:** new isomorphic (similar) lesions at the sites of trauma (also seen in Eczema and Vitiligo).
- **Nail involvement: nail pitting (25%). Yellow-brown discoloration under the nail (oil spot) pathognomonic.** Separation of nail from nail bed (onycholysis).

OTHER VARIANTS
- **Guttate: small (3-10 mm), erythematous "tear drop" discrete papules with fine scales**; confluent plaques on the trunk & back (spares the palms & soles). **Often appears after Strep pharyngitis.**
- **Inverse: erythematous (lacks scale).** Most common in body folds (eg, groin, gluteal fold, axilla).
- **Pustular: widespread erythema, scaling, & deep, yellow superficial noninfected pustules** that coalesce to form large areas of pus. Fever, diarrhea, hypocalcemia, & leukocytosis may be seen. **Precipitants of Pustular psoriasis: withdrawal of oral glucocorticoids, pregnancy, & infection.**
- Erythrodermic: generalized erythematous and exfoliative (scaly) rash involving >90% of the body surface area [worst type (uncommon)].

DIAGNOSIS
- Usually a clinical diagnosis.
- **Biopsy: hyperkeratosis, parakeratosis, and acanthosis.**

MANAGEMENT
Mild-Moderate:
- **Limited disease: Topical corticosteroids mainstay of treatment (high potency);** adjunctive hydration & emollients. Maintaining proper skin hydration can help prevent irritation.
- Alternative topical agents: Vitamin D analogs (**Calcipotriene, Calcitriol**), Retinoids/Vitamin A analogs (eg, Tazarotene), Roflumilast cream, Tapinarof cream, topical coal tar, topical Anthralin.
- Topical Calcineurin inhibitors (Tacrolimus, Pimecrolimus) used for involvement of the face, penis, intertriginous, & other delicate areas, are alternatives or to low-dose corticosteroid-sparing agents.

Moderate-severe:
- **Phototherapy: Narrow-band UVB (preferred)** or PUVA (oral Psoralen followed by ultraviolet A).

Severe or >30% of body surface area:
- **Systemic treatment** — Cyclosporine, oral Retinoids (Acitretin), biologic agents (eg, TNF inhibitors Etanercept, Adalimumab, Infliximab, Certolizumab), Apremilast, Inhibitors of the IL-17 pathway (Secukinumab, Brodalumab, Ixekizumab); Inhibitors of IL-23 and related cytokines (Ustekinumab, Guselkumab, Tildrakizumab). Oral steroids <u>not</u> used (withdrawal can cause Pustular psoriasis).
- Methotrexate may be useful for Psoriatic arthritis with moderate to severe disease.
- Topical Tapinarof may also improve Psoriasis.

PITYRIASIS (TINEA) VERSICOLOR

- Fungal skin infection due to overgrowth of the yeast ***Malassezia furfur*** (part of the normal skin flora).
- Most common in adolescents & young adults.

RISK FACTORS

- Hot & humid weather (tropical climates), excessive sweating, & oily skin.

CLINICAL MANIFESTATIONS

- **Hyper- or hypopigmented or erythematous, well-demarcated round or oval macules or thin plaques with fine scaling.** Lesions often coalesce into patches **most common on the upper trunk (chest, shoulders, and back) & proximal extremities;** less often the face & intertriginous areas.
- **The involved hypopigmented skin may fail to tan with sun exposure.**

DIAGNOSIS

- **KOH prep from skin scraping: short hyphae & round spores** ("spaghetti & meatballs") appearance.
- **Wood's lamp: yellow-green fluorescence** (enhanced color variation seen with versicolor) in a minority of patients. The fine scales may not be visible but can be seen with scraping of a lesion.

MANAGEMENT

- **Topical therapy: first line — topical "azoles" (eg, Ketoconazole shampoo), topical Terbinafine, or topical Selenium sulfide shampoo.** Zinc pyrithione shampoo, Sodium sulfacetamide.
- **Systemic therapy: oral Itraconazole or Fluconazole in adults if widespread or if failed topical treatment.** Because Fluconazole is delivered to the skin via the sweat, patients must not shower a few hours after oral administration. Ketoconazole rarely used (associated with hepatotoxicity).
- Maintenance (prevention): monthly Selenium sulfide lotion or Ketoconazole shampoo.

INFANTILE SEBORRHEIC DERMATITIS

- **Common and self-limited condition most frequently involving the scalp (Cradle cap).**

PATHOPHYSIOLOGY

- Not fully understood but circulating maternal hormones in infancy may result in increased sebaceous gland overactivity + **hypersensitivity reaction to *Malassezia furfur.***

CLINICAL MANIFESTATIONS

- **Erythematous plaques with fine yellow or white greasy scales & crusts on the scalp.**

DIAGNOSIS

- Usually clinical — classic lesions in infants 3 weeks-12 months of age (peaks at 3 months).

MANAGEMENT

- **The initial management includes education, reassurance (it is benign, self-limited, peaks in 3 months, and usually resolved by 1 year of age), and conservative measures (emollients and frequent shampooing) to soften and remove the scales.**
- **Conservative measures: application of an emollient to the scalp** (eg, mineral oil, vegetable oil, baby oil, or white petrolatum) overnight or 15 minutes prior to shampooing with **baby shampoo or removal of scales with a soft brush.**
- Intertriginous areas: Ketoconazole or other azole cream can be used for Seborrheic dermatitis of the intertriginous areas. In addition, topical creams or ointments containing Zinc oxide and/or petrolatum may be applied liberally.
- **More extensive, persistent cases, or in areas other than the scalp: Ketoconazole (2% cream or shampoo) or low-potency topical Corticosteroids may be used.**

SEBORRHEIC DERMATITIS

- Chronic, relapsing form of dermatitis occurring in areas rich in sebaceous glands (scalp, face, upper trunk, or intertriginous areas).

PATHOPHYSIOLOGY
- Not fully understood but **sebaceous glands create an environment for a hypersensitivity reaction to lipid-dependent *Malassezia furfur*** (a yeast part of the normal skin flora). Most common in men.
- More severe in patients with neurologic disease (eg, **Parkinson disease**) and patients with **HIV.**
- Tends to worsen during fall & winter months (UV light helpful) & during times of stress.

CLINICAL MANIFESTATIONS
- **Erythematous plaques, patches, or dry scales covered with fine white-yellow greasy scales.**
- **Common in areas with high sebaceous gland secretion — scalp (dandruff)**, eyelids, beard mustache, nasolabial folds, chest, & groin. May be associated with burning & pruritus.

DIAGNOSIS
- Usually clinical.

MANAGEMENT
- **Scalp — antifungal shampoos (eg, Ketoconazole 2%, Ciclopirox 1%).** Alternative antifungal shampoos available over the counter include **Zinc pyrithione 1% & Selenium sulfide 2.5%.**
  Moderate to severe, inflammatory seborrheic dermatitis of the scalp: antifungal shampoos (eg, Ketoconazole 2% shampoo) in combination with a high-potency topical corticosteroid in a formulation (lotion, spray, foam).
- **Face — topical antifungal agents [eg, Ketoconazole 2% cream, other azole creams, Ciclopirox 1% cream)], low-potency topical corticosteroids (groups 6 or 7), or a combination of both. Long-term steroid use on face may cause skin atrophy, telangiectasia & pigmentation changes.**
  Steroid-sparing agents: **Topical calcineurin inhibitors (eg, Tacrolimus 0.1% ointment Pimecrolimus 1% cream),** Crisaborole 2% cream, and Roflumilast 0.3% foam are alternatives for facial SD & are not associated with skin changes (eg, atrophy, telangiectasias) with long-term use.
- **Trunk/intertriginous areas — low-potency topical corticosteroid cream (groups 6 or 7), topical antifungal agents, or a combination of the two.** Medium-potency topical corticosteroids (groups 4 or 5) can be used for Seborrheic dermatitis involving the chest or the upper back.
- Severe or resistant: oral antifungals — eg, Itraconazole, Fluconazole, Ketoconazole, Terbinafine.
- Prevention of relapse: scalp: Ketoconazole 2% shampoo or Ciclopirox 1% shampoo once per week; Face, trunk, or intertriginous areas: Ketoconazole shampoo or cream once per week. Ciclopirox.

CUTANEOUS DRUG REACTIONS

- Medication-induced changes in the skin & mucous membranes. Most are hypersensitivity reactions.
- **Most cutaneous drug reactions are self-limited if the offending drug is discontinued.**
- Triggers: antigen from foods, insect bites, drugs, environmental, exercise-induced, & infections.

PATHOPHYSIOLOGY
1. **Type I: Ig-E mediated:** eg, **Urticaria & Angioedema.** Immediate hypersensitivity reaction.
2. **Type II: cytotoxic, antibody-mediated** (drugs in combo with cytotoxic antibodies cause cell lysis).
3. **Type III: immune antibody-antigen complex** — drug-mediated vasculitis & serum sickness.
4. **Type IV: delayed (cell mediated)** — morbilliform reaction (eg, **Erythema Multiforme).**
5. Non-immunologic: cutaneous drug reactions due to genetic incapability to detoxify certain medications (eg, anticonvulsants & sulfonamides).

EXANTHEMATOUS (MACULOPAPULAR) DRUG ERUPTION

- **Morbilliform or maculopapular drug eruption characterized by macules or small papules after the initiation of drug treatment.**
- Most commonly occurs 5-14 days after initiation of the offending medication or within 1-2 days in previously sensitized individuals. Concomitant viral infection (eg, Epstein-Barr virus) increases risk.

PATHOPHYSIOLOGY
- **Type IV (delayed) T cell-mediated hypersensitivity reaction** most common reaction.
- Any drug can cause it but Penicillin, sulfa-containing medications (eg, Sulfamethoxazole), Clindamycin, NSAIDs, Carbamazepine, & Allopurinol are common causes.

CLINICAL MANIFESTATIONS
- **Generalized distribution of bright erythematous macules &/or papules that coalesce to form plaques**, primarily on the trunk & proximal extremities. Mucosal involvement is usually absent.
- Systemic symptoms are generally mild, and include low-grade fever, pruritus, & mild eosinophilia.

MANAGEMENT
- **Prompt withdrawal of the offending medication is the mainstay of treatment.** Most cutaneous drug reactions are self-limited once the offending drug is discontinued.
- **Symptomatic treatment: oral Antihistamines (H1 blockers) — Second-generation nonsedating antihistamines (eg, Cetirizine, Loratadine & Fexofenadine)** or first-generation (eg, Diphenhydramine, Hydroxyzine, Chlorpheniramine). Topical corticosteroids.
- H2 blockers (eg, Nizatidine) may be added if no response to H1 antagonists if moderate to severe.
- Oral corticosteroids (short course) usually reserved for severe cutaneous reactions.

ANGIOEDEMA

- Self-limited, localized subcutaneous (or submucosal) swelling resulting from extravasation of fluid into the interstitium.
- **Affects the mucosal tissues of the face, lips, tongue, larynx, hands, feet, genitalia, & bowel wall.**
- Onset in minutes to hours with spontaneous resolution in hours to a few days.

TYPES:
- **Mast-cell (histamine) mediated eg, allergic reactions.**
- **Bradykinin-mediated eg, Angiotensin converting enzyme inhibitor-induced** or hereditary (due to C1 esterase inhibitor deficiency).

CLINICAL MANIFESTATIONS
- Mast-cell mediated: angioedema that may be accompanied with other allergic reaction symptoms (eg, urticaria, flushing, generalized pruritus, bronchospasm, stridor, throat tightness, & hypotension).
- Bradykinin-induced: angioedema <u>without</u> allergic reaction symptoms (see above).

WORKUP
- If there is no information to suggest an external cause and the patient has isolated Angioedema (without pruritus or urticaria), then C4 levels and a C1 inhibitor antigenic level should be obtained.

IMMEDIATE MANAGEMENT
- Immediate assessment & **ongoing airway protection is paramount. IM Epinephrine if severe.**
Mast-cell mediated:
- **Glucocorticoids (IV or oral) and H1 antihistamines. IM Epinephrine if severe.**
Bradykinin-mediated:
- **Purified C1 inhibitor concentrate, Ecallantide (kallikrein inhibitor), Icatibant (bradykinin-beta2 receptor antagonist). Fresh frozen plasma** if other therapies are not available or fail.
- Danazol at lowest dose may be needed for long-term management in hereditary causes.
- ACE inhibitor: discontinuation of ACE inhibitor & monitoring for resolution.

URTICARIA (HIVES, WHEALS)

- Edema of the superficial layers of the skin due to histamine-related increased vascular permeability.
- **Type I (IgE) immediate hypersensitivity reaction leading to superficial localized edema and erythema of the dermis**, mucous membranes, & subcutaneous tissues.
- Pathophysiology: release of vasodilators (eg, **histamine,** bradykinin, kallikrein, & prostaglandins) from mast cells & basophils in the skin.

TRIGGERS: food, medications, heat or cold, stress, insect bites, environmental, & infection.
  Chronic (>6 weeks) is usually idiopathic.

CLINICAL MANIFESTATIONS
- **Sudden onset of circumscribed hives or wheals (blanchable, raised, erythematous plaques on the skin or mucous membranes) with central pallor that may coalesce.**
- **Often associated with intense pruritus.**
- **Hives are usually transient** (often disappearing within 24 hours with new crops often occurring).

DIAGNOSIS The diagnosis of urticaria is made clinically.

MANAGEMENT
- **Antihistamines (H1 blockers) initial management of choice — Non-sedating second-generation (eg, Cetirizine, Loratadine, & Fexofenadine)** often preferred over first-generation (eg, Diphenhydramine, Hydroxyzine, Chlorpheniramine) because 2nd-generation associated with less anticholinergic effects, they are minimally sedating, and they have less drug-drug interactions. Sedating H1 antihistamine at bedtime may be used in healthy patients.
- H2 blockers (eg, Nizatidine) may be added if no response to H1 antagonists in moderate-severe cases.
- Oral glucocorticoids may be needed in severe, recurrent, or persistent cases despite above treatment.
- Epinephrine if severe or concern for airway compromise. Eliminate known precipitants.

VENOUS STASIS DERMATITIS (STASIS ECZEMA)

- **Inflammatory skin changes associated with chronic venous insufficiency** (due to DVT, varicose veins, or superficial thrombophlebitis, dysfunction of the venous valves, venous flow obstruction).

CLINICAL MANIFESTATIONS
- **Dermatitis: edema, inflammatory skin changes, pruritus, and hyperpigmentation.**
- Venous insufficiency: Leg pain classically worse with prolonged standing, prolonged sitting with the feet dependent and improved with ambulation and leg elevation. Pain classically described as a burning, aching, throbbing, cramping, or "heavy leg".

PHYSICAL EXAM FINDINGS
- **Stasis Dermatitis: itchy eczematous rash** (inflammatory papules, crusts, or scales), **excoriations, weeping erosions & brownish or dark purple hyperpigmentation of the skin** (hemosiderin deposition). **Edema (medial ankle most commonly involved).**
- **Venous stasis ulcers, especially at the medial malleolus,** may be seen.
- Leg edema, increased leg circumference, varicosities, & erythema with normal pulse and temperature.
- **Atrophie blanche:** atrophic, hypopigmented areas with telangiectasias & punctate red dots.
- **Lipodermatosclerosis:** edema + circumferential narrowing of the lower leg (champagne bottle leg).

MANAGEMENT
Treatment of the underlying venous insufficiency is the mainstay of treatment.
- **Best initial steps are leg elevation, compression stockings or bandages, & exercise.**
- Skin care measures: gentle skin cleansing. Petroleum-based emollients for dry skin and pruritus.
- **Acute lesions: Topical corticosteroids for acute erythema, vesicles, oozing, and pruritus.**
- Severe or recalcitrant: short course of oral glucocorticoids (eg, Prednisone) if contact dermatitis.

SKIN INTEGRITY

BURN SIZE Rule of Nines   Not used for 1st degree burns.

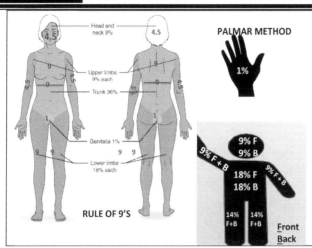

Palm size classically has been considered to represent 1% of TBSA (it accurately represents 0.4% with entire hand representing 0.8%)

Minor Burns: <10% TBSA burn in adults
<5%TBSA burn in young/old
<2% full thickness burn
- Must be isolated injury
- Must <u>not</u> involve face, hands, perineum, or feet.
- Must <u>not</u> cross major joints. Must <u>not</u> be circumferential.

MAJOR BURNS: >25% TBSA burn in adults
>20%TBSA burn in young/old
>10% full thickness burn
- <u>Burns involving</u> the face, hands, perineum, or feet
- Burns crossing major joints, circumferential burns

Lund-Browder chart is the most accurate method for estimating TBSA in both children & adults.

THERMAL BURNS
Superficial burns:
- **Involves minor damage to the <u>epidermis</u>. Manifests as erythema, pain, tenderness to palpation, & <u>dry and erythematous appearance without blistering</u>.**
- Capillary refill intact (**<u>blanches with pressure</u>**). Usually heals within 7 days without scarring.

<u>**Partial thickness burns**</u>: affects the epidermis and the dermis. Characterized by **<u>blistering</u>**.
- **<u>Superficial partial thickness:</u>** affects the epidermis and superficial portion of the dermis (papillary).
  - **Characterized by <u>blistering</u>, erythematous, pink, moist, weeping skin.**
  - **Very tender to touch, temperature, & air; intact capillary refill (<u>blanches with pressure</u>).**
  - Heals within 7-21 days. They typically heal without scarring but may leave pigment changes.

- **<u>Deep partial thickness:</u>** affects the epidermis and deeper portion of the dermis (reticular).
  - **Characterized by red, yellow, or pale waxy skin, blistering (easily unroofed), not painful (pain to pressure only), blanching absent or sluggish, decreased 2-point discrimination.**
  - Heals within 3 weeks–2 months with scarring (may require surgical management)

<u>**Full thickness burns**</u>
  - **Characterized by waxy, white, leathery, & dry, inelastic skin.**
  - **Painless, absent capillary refill, lack of blistering, & lack of sensation.**
  - Usually does not spontaneously heal well (may need skin grafting).

<u>**Deep injury (Fourth degree):**</u>
- **Burns extending beyond the skin into the underlying fat, fascia, muscle, bone, and joints.**
  - Skin is black, charred, and dry.
  - Painless, loss of capillary refill.
  - **Usually requires tissue reconstruction & debridement.**

INITIAL BURN CARE

- **Cooling: room temperature tap water or cooled, saline-soaked gauze (ice should not be directly applied to the skin),** soap and water to cleanse the burn and appropriate dressing.
- Pain and Tetanus status should be addressed.
- With all burns, 24 hour follow-up is needed if the patient is not admitted to assess burn status, assure dressing change competence, and any adjustment of analgesia as needed.

Superficial burns:
- **Superficial burns generally do not require dressings or topical antibiotics.**
- They do require follow up to monitor for progression of the burn depth.

Partial and full thickness burns:
- **Usually require dressings and topical antibiotics.**
- Application of topical antibiotic, followed by a layer of nonadherent gauze over the burn, a layer of fluffed dry gauze and an outer layer of elastic gauze.
- **Topical antibiotics:** antimicrobial ointments, silver-containing agents, Bismuth-impregnated petroleum gauze, Chlorhexidine, and Mafenide.

TOPICAL ANTIBIOTICS IN BURNS

- Antimicrobial ointments, silver-containing agents, Bismuth-impregnated petroleum gauze, Chlorhexidine, and Mafenide.

ANTIMICROBIAL OINTMENTS:

- **Bacitracin zinc-Polymyxin B sulfate, Neomycin:** single or combination agents that can be used for superficial burn wound or partial thickness burns. Compared to Silver sulfadiazine, they are easier to apply and remove and can be used on sensitive areas (eg, face, perineum, ears). Mupirocin effective against MRSA.
  Adverse effects: systemic absorption of Polymyxin B can cause nephrotoxicity or neurotoxicity (rarely systemically absorbed). Neomycin is associated with allergic reactions.

- **Silver-containing agents: Silver sulfadiazine (SSD) & Silver nitrate.** Activated silver has antimicrobial and anti-inflammatory properties. **Silver sulfadiazine is the most commonly used burn dressing.**
  Adverse effects: **SSD cannot be used on the face** (can cause yellowing of the skin), **not used in women who are pregnant, breastfeeding or infants <2 months old. Sulfa allergies, oculotoxic** (not used near the eyes), does not penetrate the eschar, may cause pseudoeschar formation, & impedes reepithelialization (should be discontinued when epithelialization is seen).

Bismuth-impregnated petroleum gauze:
- Mechanism of action: topical antimicrobial agent.
- Indications: often the preferred dressing for skin graft donor sites and for covering fresh skin grafts.
- May be useful in children as it is only applied once, so no need for wound dressing changes.

- **Mafenide acetate:** carbonic anhydrase inhibitor that is an alternative to SSD.
  Adverse effects: pain when first applied, metabolic acidosis, allergic reactions (eg, rash, pruritis, hives, erythema, eosinophilia), and respiratory complications (tachypnea).

Chlorhexidine gluconate:
- Mechanism of action: long-lasting antimicrobial cleanser that does not interfere with reepithelialization (compared to SSD).
- Indications: often used with a gauze dressing for burn wound coverage in superficial partial-thickness burns.
- A combination preparation of Silver sulfadiazine and Chlorhexidine gluconate has also been used.

MODERATE TO SEVERE BURNS

Diagnostic studies for major burns:

- CBC (hematocrit may be increased initially), electrolytes (Hyperkalemia is the most common abnormality seen early on), creatinine kinase along with UA and myoglobin to evaluate for rhabdomyolysis; carboxyhemoglobin and serum lactate for carbon monoxide and cyanide poisoning in smoke inhalation patients.

Fluid resuscitation:

- **Parkland (Modified): 4 mL/kg per percent total burn surface area** (TBSA) — counting moderate (partial thickness) and severe (full thickness) burn area only **plus** normal 24-hour maintenance fluid requirements. Add maintenance fluid with glucose for children <5 years of age.
    - **Half of the fluid is given over the first 8 hours.**
    - **The remaining half is given over the next 16 hours.**
- Isotonic crystalloid fluids — **Ringer's lactate is the resuscitation & maintenance fluid of choice for the first 24 hours.** Some experts add 5% dextrose to children < 20 kg to prevent hypoglycemia.
- Monitoring fluid status: urine output should be maintained at 1-2 mL/kg/hr in children <30 kg and 0.5–1 ml/kg/hr if ≥30 kg. Heart rate is a better monitor of circulatory status than blood pressure. Output of ≥0.5 mL/kg/hr in adults.

PRESSURE INJURY (DECUBITUS ULCER)

- Ulcers resulting from vertical pressure.
- Commonly seen on bony prominences (eg, sacrum, calcaneus, & ischium).
- Risk factors: elderly, immobilization & incontinence.

PATHOPHYSIOLOGY:

- Pressure impairs delivery of oxygen and nutrients and waste removal from the affected area. Moisture causes skin maceration, leading to skin breakdown.

ULCER STAGES:

Stage 1	**Superficial, nonblanchable redness** (does not dissipate after pressure is relieved). **The skin is intact.**
Stage 2	Epidermal damage extending into the **dermis**. Resembles a **blister or abrasion**.
Stage 3	**Full thickness (skin loss)** and may extend into the **subcutaneous layer.**
Stage 4	Deepest. Extends beyond the fascia, **extending into the muscle, tendon, or bone**.

- **Unstageable ulcer if slough or eschar obscures the extent of tissue loss.** Slough or eschar must be removed to determine if it is stage 3 or 4.

MANAGEMENT

- Wound care with a moist wound environment. Pain control (non-opioid oral medication if mild) & opioid analgesics for moderate to severe pain.
- Debridement if necrotic tissue is present. Negative pressure wound therapy. Optimize nutrition (protein and caloric intake, especially stage 3 and 4).
- **Pressure redistribution:** position and re-position and using non-powered or powered support surfaces (eg, air-fluidized beds, powered mattresses).
- Stage 1: preventive measures and wound protection with protective dressings (eg, transparent film).
- Stage 2: dressing that maintain a moist wound environment — transparent films or occlusive dressings (hydrocolloids or hydrogels) if there is no infection is present.
- Stages 3 & 4: wound cleansing (initially and during each dressing change), appropriate moist to absorbent dressing (eg, Hydrogel, Foam, Alginate), debridement of necrotic tissue (mechanical, surgical, or enzymatic), or thick eschar, and treatment of wound infection if present.
- Necrotic tissue: Stage 3 and 4 injuries may require debridement if necrotic tissue is present. A healthy granulating stage 3 or 4 wound does not require debridement.

	1ST DEGREE SUPERFICIAL	2ND DEGREE SUPERFICIAL PARTIAL THICKNESS	2ND DEGREE DEEP PARTIAL THICKNESS	3RD DEGREE FULL THICKNESS	4TH DEGREE
DEPTH	• Epidermis (Intact epidermal barrier)	• Epidermis + Superficial portion of dermis (papillary)	• Epidermis into deep portion of dermis (reticular)	• Extends through entire skin	• Entire skin into underlying fat, muscle, bone.
APPEARANCE	• Erythematous (red) • Dry	• Erythematous, pink • Moist, weeping • ⊕ *BLISTERING*	• Red, yellow, pale white • Dry • ⊕ *BLISTERING*	• Waxy, white • Leathery, Dry	• Black, charred, eschar • Dry
SENSATION	• PAINFUL • Tender to touch	• *Most PAINFUL of all burns* • *Very tender to touch*	• *Not usually painful* ±pain with pressure. • May have decreased 2 point discrimination	• PAINLESS	• PAINLESS
CAPILLARY REFILL	⊕ *refill intact:* *blanches with pressure*	⊕ *refill intact:* *blanches with pressure*	• *Absent capillary refill*	• Absent	• Absent
PROGNOSIS	• Heals within 7 days • No scarring	• Heals within 14-21 days • No scarring (but ± leave pigment changes)	• *3 weeks – 2 months* • *Scarring common* (may need skin graft or excision to prevent contractures)	• Months • Does not spontaneously heal well	• Does not heal well. • Usually needs debridement of tissues & tissue reconstruction.

SMOKE INHALATION INJURIES

Upper airway obstruction:
- Smoke inhalation injuries are usually limited to the upper airways (steam can travel to the lower airways).

PHYSICAL EXAM FINDINGS
- **Burns of the face & neck, hoarseness, stridor, dysphagia, singed nasal hairs, soot in the mouth (or nose), & black sputum.**
- Respiratory distress may not be present until hours after.

LABS
- ABG or VBG (carboxyhemoglobin level), CBC, electrolytes, UA, Chest radiographs (include soft tissue neck radiographs in children), and ECG.

MANAGEMENT
- **Early airway protection: maintain and secure the airway (low threshold for intubation) with tracheostomy if necessary.**
- Supportive: bronchodilators (Beta-2 agonists, anticholinergics).
- Carbon monoxide poisoning: high oxygen therapy — 100% Nonrebreather 10-12 L/min (goal is usually Carboxyhemoglobin levels <10%).
- Hydrogen cyanide poisoning: hydroxocobalamin, cyanide kit (Amyl nitrite for inhalation, IV sodium nitrite or thiosulfate) in select patients.

CARBON MONOXIDE POISONING
- Carbon monoxide is an odorless, tasteless, colorless, nonirritating gas that has over 200 times the affinity for hemoglobin than oxygen.

ETIOLOGIES
- **Fire-related smoke inhalation most common.** Other causes include poorly functioning or improperly vented heating systems, motor vehicles operating in poorly ventilated areas (eg, garages).

CLINICAL MANIFESTATIONS
- **Neurologic: headache most common symptom**, nausea, malaise, dizziness, altered mental status, seizures, brain hypoxia, coma; **Cardiac:** cardiac dysrhythmias, dyspnea, angina.
Physical examination:
- **Bright-red retinal vessels on funduscopy.**
- **Cherry-red skin is a classic, but not common finding** (it is usually seen postmortem).

DIAGNOSIS
- Most pulse oximeters can't differentiate between HbO_2 and carboxyhemoglobin.
- Workup for inhalation injuries: **ABG or VBG — increased carboxyhemoglobin level** (level doesn't correlate with severity), methemoglobin, CBC, CK, troponin, electrolytes, UA, chest radiograph (usually normal initially) and ECG. May need to include soft tissue neck radiographs in children.

MANAGEMENT
- **Secure airway as needed.**
- Mild: **high-flow oxygen therapy mainstay — 100% Nonrebreather 10-12 L/min. Goal is usually Carboxyhemoglobin level <10%.**
- Severe: **Hyperbaric oxygen in severe cases to reduce neurological sequalae** — eg, increased carboxyhemoglobin >25% [15% if pregnant] + acidosis (pH <7.1) + severe neurologic symptoms].

CYANIDE POISONING

CLINICAL MANIFESTATIONS
- Rapidly-developing coma, apnea (with severe lactic acidemia), cardiac derangements.

DIAGNOSIS
- Via history and physical examination. Cyanide levels

MANAGEMENT
- **Hydrogen cyanide poisoning: hydroxocobalamin is the antidote for cyanide toxicity;** cyanide kit (Amyl nitrite for inhalation, IV sodium nitrite or thiosulfate) in select patients.

HIGH VOLTAGE ELECTRIC INJURIES

- Determine current intensity (household usually ~110V), type of current – alternating current (AC) or direct current (DC), tissue resistance, duration & type of contact, area, "vertical" more dangerous than "horizontal", water immersion.
- **Electricity favors the path of least resistance (eg, nerves, muscle, and blood).** Skin has the most resistance as well as fat & bone. Tissues with the highest resistance (eg, skin, fat, and bone) tend to suffer the greatest level of damage.
- **AC currents are 3-5 times more damaging than a direct current of equal voltage and current.** AC currents can cause muscle contraction (causing patient to hold on tight to the source). DC current can often violently propel the victim from the current source (due to single, large muscle spasm) & trauma (eg, posterior shoulder dislocation).
- **In general, morbidity is often greater with low voltage** injuries than with high voltage because high-voltage injuries tend to propel the individual away from the source, reducing overall contact time. Low voltage injuries, cause muscle contracting, prolonging contact time.

CLINICAL MANIFESTATIONS
- **Cardiac:** arrhythmias — low-voltage AC may produce ventricular fibrillation. High-voltage AC/DC may produce asystole. **ECG is recommended to look for cardiac changes.**
- **Musculoskeletal: Rhabdomyolysis** (Urinalysis is performed to assess for myoglobinuria).
- Neurological: respiratory arrest, peripheral neuropathy, memory disturbances.

WORKUP
- ECG, cardiac enzymes if chest pain, UA (for Rhabdomyolysis).

MANAGEMENT
- **The first (immediate) step in management must always be scene safety and removing the patient from the source of electricity** (eg, shutting off the power source).
- Remove the patient's clothing, especially any metal that is in contact with the body (jewelry or equipment).
- Patients should be stabilized and provided both respiratory and circulatory support as needed (advanced cardiovascular life support [ACLS] & advanced trauma life support [ATLS] protocols).
- **Any patient with facial or oral burns, hypoxia, respiratory distress, loss of consciousness, or other issues resulting in difficulty protecting the airway or maintaining a patent airway should be given oxygen and airway protection** (eg, ventilation, intubation, cricothyrotomy). Patients may need to be placed on telemetry.
- Outpatient: asymptomatic patients with household burns may be discharged if normal ECG on presentation and normal physical examination.
- Admission: if >600V, admit even if asymptomatic. Keep urine output at 100ml/hr & alkalinize the urine to protect the kidney.

PEMPHIGUS VULGARIS

- **Life-threatening,** chronic autoimmune **blistering disorder** of the mucous membranes and skin.
- Acantholysis (loss of cohesion between epidermal cells & **separation of the dermis**) — **Type II hypersensitivity reaction where autoantibodies (IgG) against desmoglein, a component of the desmosome, lead to acantholysis.** Normally, desmosomes connect keratinocytes in the skin.

RISK FACTORS:
- **Adults 40-60 years.** Middle Eastern or Jewish descent. **Myasthenia gravis, thymoma, SLE.**
- Medications especially **Penicillamine, Captopril**, Cephalosporins, and Phenobarbital.

CLINICAL MANIFESTATIONS
- **[1] Mucosal membrane involvement initially (painful erosion or ulceration; intraoral most common),** followed by **[2] painful, flaccid skin bullae (blisters) that rupture easily,** leaving painful denuded skin erosions that bleed easily. **Nonpruritic.** Palms and soles are usually spared.
- Physical examination: **Positive Nikolsky sign — superficial detachment of skin under pressure/trauma** (pulls off in sheets). Because blisters rupture easily, only erosions may be seen.

DIAGNOSIS
- **Skin biopsy (eg, punch):** intraepithelial splitting with acantholysis (separation of epidermal cells). **Direct immunofluorescence: IgG throughout the epidermis,** basal keratinocytes in a pattern that resembles a "row of tombstones".
- ELISA: anti-desmoglein or anti-epithelial autoantibodies (serum IgG against Desmoglein 1 &/or 3).

MANAGEMENT
- **Systemic: Glucocorticoids mainstay of treatment, alone or in combination with immune agents** — [1] Systemic glucocorticoid therapy + Rituximab or [2] Systemic glucocorticoid therapy + adjuvant therapy (usually Mycophenolate or Azathioprine). Local wound care.

BULLOUS PEMPHIGOID

- Autoimmune disorder with blister formation & severe pruritus. **Primarily seen in the elderly (≥60y).**
- Type II hypersensitivity reaction — IgG autoantibodies against hemidesmosomes & basement membrane zone causing **SUBepidermal blistering.** Drug-induced (eg, loop diuretics, Metformin).

CLINICAL MANIFESTATIONS
- **Prodrome of pruritus with eczematous or urticarial plaques followed by multiple tense large bullae (1-3 cm) that do not rupture as easily.** Most commonly involving the groin, axilla, trunk, & flexural areas of the extremities. Blister roof contains epidermis. Mucosal disease in 10-30%.
- Physical examination: **negative Nikolsky sign (no epidermal detachment).**

DIAGNOSIS
- **Skin biopsy: with direct immunofluorescence criterion standard — linear C3 and IgG along the dermal-epidermal junction, subepidermal blisters, & eosinophilia.**
- ELISA: autoantibodies against BP antigen 230 & 180.

MANAGEMENT
- **Mild: Topical corticosteroids (high potency, such as Clobetasol propionate) first line for mild localized disease** (<20% of body surface area) **+ Doxycycline has a favorable adverse effect profile and can be used for milder presentations of Bullous pemphigoid** (eg, localized Bullous pemphigoid or development of only a few new bullae per day).
- **Severe: Systemic corticosteroids if extensive BP** (eg, widespread skin involvement or development of many new bullae per day) **who desire oral treatment or nonresponsive to topical treatment.** Alternative: Doxycycline therapy + high-potency topical corticosteroid to active lesions.

ACANTHOSIS NIGRICANS

- Common benign disorder of the skin characterized by velvety hyperpigmented plaques on the skin.

ETIOLOGIES
- Metabolic: **obesity is the most common cause**, endocrine (eg, **disorders with <u>insulin resistance</u>, such as Diabetes mellitus, Cushing syndrome, and obesity).**
- Hypothyroidism, acromegaly, Polycystic ovary disease, genetic, medications (eg, Nicotinic acid) and rarely, **malignancy** [eg, Gastric adenocarcinoma (most common), uterus, lung, breast, & ovarian].
- **Diagnostic studies** may include **fasting blood glucose, hemoglobin A1C, and postprandial blood glucose**. In older patients without obesity, underlying malignancy may be the cause.

PHYSICAL EXAMINATION
- **Poorly defined, velvety, verrucous hyperpigmented thickened plaques on the skin.**
- **Most common on skin folds** (eg, neck, forehead, groin, navel, and axillae).

MANAGEMENT
- **Treat the underlying cause**; controlling blood glucose levels via diet and exercise.
- <u>Keratolytics:</u> topical Tretinoin or topical vitamin D analog (eg, Calcipotriene) for faster resolution.

HIDRADENITIS SUPPURATIVA (ACNE INVERSA)

- Painful, chronic inflammatory suppurative condition involving the skin & subcutaneous tissue.

PATHOPHYSIOLOGY
- **Chronic infra-infundibular follicular hair follicle obstruction,** followed by secondary rupture of the sebofollicular junction of folliculopilosebaceous units, resulting in an inflammatory reaction.
- <u>Risk factors:</u> **Obesity, females, smoking,** Acne, family history, mechanical friction, & medications.

CLINICAL MANIFESTATIONS
- <u>**Recurrent, painful, & inflamed nodules:**</u> **deep-seated inflammatory nodules and abscesses, draining tracts, & fibrotic hypertrophic scars.** The nodules may rupture, discharging purulent, occasionally foul-smelling material. These nodules may coalesce into inflammatory plaques, epithelialized sinuses, "tombstone" comedones, & "rope-like" scarring.
- **Pain, chronic drainage, odor, and disfigurement are hallmark features of HS.**
- <u>**Intertriginous skin**</u> most commonly involved — most commonly affects the **axillae (most common),** perianal, groin, inframammary regions, buttocks, & apocrine gland-rich areas.

MANAGEMENT
- <u>Lifestyle:</u> dietary changes (avoid high glycemic foods), smoking cessation, local skin care, eliminate irritants (eg, synthetic & tight-fitting clothing, harsh cleaning products), reduction of skin friction.
- <u>**Hurley stage I disease (inflammatory lesions without sinus tracts or scarring)**</u> — <u>**topical Clindamycin first-line**</u>**. Oral Tetracyclines if no improvement with topical Clindamycin.** Antiandrogenic drugs and Metformin are additional treatment options that may be used alone or in conjunction with antibiotics. Refractory disease: Clindamycin & Rifampin combination therapy, Acitretin, and oral Dapsone.
- <u>Hurley stage II or III disease</u> (inflammatory lesions with sinus tracts or scarring) — for **<u>Hurley II, initial therapy with an oral Tetracycline (eg, Doxycycline) is first-line.</u>** For patients with extensive, inflammatory disease (eg, **<u>Hurley stage III HS), initial therapy is a combination of Clindamycin + Rifampin</u>**. Antiandrogenic drugs and Metformin are additional treatment options that may be used alone or in conjunction with antibiotics.
- Next-line therapies for patients who do not improve sufficiently with oral antibiotics and hormonal therapy include oral retinoids (eg, Acitretinoin) or Dapsone. Infliximab or Adalimumab.
- <u>Surgical:</u> wide excision for individuals refractory to medical therapy.

LIPOMA

- Benign subcutaneous tumors composed of mature adipocytes enclosed by a thin fibrous capsule.
- **Most common benign soft-tissue neoplasm.**
- The presence of multiple lipomas may be the presenting feature of a variety of syndromes (eg, MEN 1 syndrome, Gardner syndrome).

CLINICAL MANIFESTATIONS
- **<u>Superficial subcutaneous lesion</u>: soft, painless subcutaneous nodules ranging in size from 1 to >10 cm that with a translucent appearance. <u>Easily mobile</u>:** "slippage sign" may be elicited by gently sliding the fingers off the edge of the tumor. May be round, oval, or multilobulated.
- Most common on the trunk, neck, forearm, and proximal upper extremities.

DIAGNOSIS
- **Usually a clinical diagnosis** that may be confirmed if complete surgical excision is performed.
- Biopsy indicated if pain, rapidly enlarging, firm, or restricts movement.
- Radiologic imaging prior to surgical excision may be need if large (>10 cm), painful, fixated, or deep.

MANAGEMENT
- **No treatment needed.**
- **May perform compete surgical excision of the fat cells & fibrous capsule for cosmetic reasons or if rapidly enlarging.**

EPIDERMOID (EPIDERMAL, INCLUSION, SEBACEOUS) & PILAR CYSTS

- <u>Epidermoid cyst</u>: benign encapsulated subepidermal nodules filled with fibrous tissue and keratinous (cottage cheese like) material. Cysts result from plugging of the follicular orifices.
- **<u>Epidermoid cysts</u> originate from the epidermis, and <u>Pilar cysts</u> originate from the root sheath of hair follicles; both contain a thick, cheesy collection of keratin.** Sebaceous cyst, the name commonly used to describe **epidermoid or pilar cysts**, is a misnomer because they secrete keratin (not sebum) & do not originate from the sebaceous glands. May be seen with immunosuppressants.

EPIDEMIOLOGY
- Most commonly seen in third and fourth decades of life (rare before puberty). Male: female 2:1.
- Epidermoid cysts unusual in number & location (extremities rather than face, base of ears, and trunk) may be due to Gardner syndrome (Familial adenomatous polyposis of the colon).

CLINICAL MANIFESTATIONS
- **Asymptomatic, firm, skin-colored dermal freely mobile, compressible cyst or nodule, often with a clinically visible dark-colored central punctum** (dark comedone opening).
- **Ruptured, infected cysts become fluctuant, painful, larger, and erythematous — may lead to foul-smelling yellowish cheese-like discharge.**

DIAGNOSIS
- **Usually a clinical diagnosis.**
- <u>Histology:</u> cyst wall composed of normal stratified squamous epithelium derived from the follicular infundibulum.

MANAGEMENT
- **<u>Inflamed or not inflamed:</u> no treatment needed** — may spontaneously resolve without therapy. Intralesional injection of Kenalog in inflamed lesions can hasten resolution.
- **Complete surgical excision with the Pilar or Epidermoid cyst wall intact is the most effective treatment** if cosmetically desired by the patient or if recurrent (ideally performed once the inflammation or infection has subsided).
- **<u>Infected:</u> Incision & drainage.**

PYODERMA GANGRENOSUM

- Noninfective ulcerative skin lesion secondary to immune dysregulation (neutrophilic dermatosis).
- Misnomer as it is not infectious nor gangrenous as the name implies.

RISK FACTORS
- **Associated with inflammatory diseases** — **Inflammatory Bowel disease (Crohn, UC)**, Rheumatoid arthritis, spondyloarthropathies etc. May be associated with solid tumors or hematologic malignancies. Pathergy: may be preceded by or enlarge with trauma.
- Most commonly seen in young and middle-aged adults and women.

CLINICAL MANIFESTATIONS
- **Ulcerative**: Inflammatory, erythematous blue-red papules or pustules rapidly progress to a **painful, necrotic ulcer with irregular purple/violet raised or undermined borders & purulent base.**

DIAGNOSIS
- **Clinical or histological diagnosis of exclusion. Biopsy: neutrophilic infiltration.**

MANAGEMENT
- **Superficial or localized: topical Corticosteroids (super high or high potency).** Tacrolimus 0.1% ointment, oral Minocycline, or oral Dapsone if no response to corticosteroids. Local wound care.
- **Rapid growth, deep or refractory: systemic (oral) Corticosteroids. Cyclosporine.**
- Third line: Intravenous immunoglobulin (IVIG), Cyclophosphamide, Chlorambucil.

KELOID

- Hypertrophic benign raised scarring due to aberrant wound healing.

PATHOPHYSIOLOGY
- **Excess production of Type I & III collagen** during wound healing in response to injury.
- **Most common darker-skinned individuals.**

CLINICAL MANIFESTATIONS
- **Grossly exaggerated scar** (indurated lesions with a glossy surface) that often grows pedunculated and beyond the borders of the original scar, especially on the earlobes, face & upper extremities.

DIAGNOSIS
- Usually a clinical diagnosis; A skin biopsy should be performed if the diagnosis is uncertain.

MANAGEMENT
Linear or small hypertrophic scars resulting from surgery or trauma:
- **Silicone gel sheeting is the initial treatment.** Pressure therapy, if feasible and tolerated by the patient, may be an alternative first-line treatment.
- Second-line therapies include intralesional corticosteroids (eg, Triamcinolone), laser therapy, and surgical excision.

Keloids:
- Small/single Keloids (<20 cm²): conservative treatment with intralesional corticosteroids with or without intralesional chemotherapeutic agents (eg, Fluorouracil, Bleomycin) or corticosteroid tape/plaster. Surgical excision is an alternative.
- Large/multiple Keloids: surgical excision/volume reduction followed by postoperative radiation therapy. Postoperative radiation therapy is contraindicated in children.

DERMATITIS HERPETIFORMIS

- Pruritic autoimmune skin disorder that is a manifestation of **gluten sensitivity**, strongly <u>associated with Celiac disease</u> **(gluten sensitive enteropathy).** Increased incidence in N. European ancestry.

<u>PATHOPHYSIOLOGY</u>
- **<u>IgA immune complex deposition</u> in the dermal papillae.** Associated with autoimmune disorders.
- Almost all patients with DH carry the HLA DQ2 or HLA DQ8 haplotype.

<u>CLINICAL MANIFESTATIONS</u>
- **Intensely pruritic, papulovesicular rash most common on the extensor surfaces** (eg, forearms, elbows, knees), buttocks, back, & scalp. Excoriations and erosions often seen on examination.

<u>DIAGNOSIS</u>
- Both clinical findings and serum IgA antibodies for Celiac disease (eg, transglutaminase, epidermal transglutaminase, or endomysial antibodies).
- **<u>Definitive diagnosis:</u> direct immunofluorescence of perilesional skin — granular IgA deposition within the papillary dermis.**

<u>MANAGEMENT</u>
- **<u>Dapsone</u> first-line short-term management along with gluten-free diet.** <u>Adverse effects</u> of Dapsone include hematologic (eg, hemolysis, methemoglobinemia, and agranulocytosis), drug sensitivity reaction, peripheral neuropathy, hemolysis in patients with G6PD deficiency. Administration with Cimetidine has been shown to decrease the toxic effects of Dapsone.
- <u>Short-term potent topical corticosteroids</u> may be useful for pruritus.
- <u>Other sulfonamide drugs:</u> Sulfapyridine & Sulfasalazine can be used in patients intolerant of Dapsone.
- **<u>Gluten free diet</u> — mainstay of long-term management.**

PYOGENIC GRANULOMA (LOBULAR CAPILLARY HEMANGIOMA)

- **Benign vascular tumor of immature capillaries of the skin or mucous membranes, characterized by rapid growth & friable surface.**
- Pyogenic granuloma is a misnomer — it is neither pyogenic nor a granuloma.

<u>RISK FACTORS</u>
- **Most common in children & young adults especially after minor skin trauma,** hormonal changes **— increased incidence in pregnancy (often with oral mucosal or gingival involvement).**
- <u>Medications:</u> eg, Indinavir & chemotherapy.

<u>CLINICAL MANIFESTATIONS</u>
- **Solitary glistening, bright red (raspberry-like) nodule or papule with a characteristic epithelial hyperkeratosis collarette at the base.** Most common on the hands, fingers, arms, & legs.
- **<u>Friability:</u> The lesion is friable, often bleeds after minor trauma or ulcerates.**
- **Rapid growth** (usually evolves over a period of weeks).

<u>DIAGNOSIS</u>
- Histology — proliferation of capillary vessels with stromal edema and inflammation.

<u>MANAGEMENT</u>
- <u>Pedunculated or cosmetically sensitive areas:</u> shave excision or curettage followed by electrocautery or laser coagulation of the lesion base. Results in less evident scarring.
- <u>Nonpedunculated (sessile):</u> surgical excision followed by wound closure with sutures. Results in less postoperative bleeding & lower recurrence rate.

ERYTHEMA NODOSUM

- Form of panniculitis (inflammation of the fat layer below the skin).
- Most often occurs in women in the second to fourth decade of life but may occur at any age & in men.

ETIOLOGIES
- **Infections: most common identified etiology, especially Streptococcal infection**, Tuberculosis, sarcoidosis, fungal (eg, **Coccidioidomycosis**).
- **Inflammatory disorders: Sarcoidosis,** inflammatory bowel disease, Leukemia, Behçet disease.
- **Estrogen exposure** eg, OCPs, pregnancy.

CLINICAL MANIFESTATIONS
- **Painful, erythematous, warm, and tender subcutaneous nodules seen on the anterior shins** (range in colors from pink, red to purple). Poorly demarcated margins. Usually bilateral.
- Less often, nodules occur on the thighs, arms, calves, buttocks, or face.

DIAGNOSIS
- Usually clinical. Biopsy is useful for atypical cases — septal panniculitis without vasculitis

MANAGEMENT
- **The lesions are generally self-limited & usually resolve spontaneously within a few weeks (excellent prognosis).** Associated underlying diseases should be treated & causative drugs discontinued.
- Supportive management: leg elevation, rest, & compression may provide symptom relief.
- Nonsteroidal anti-inflammatory drug (NSAID) for pain.
- Potassium iodide usually reserved for rapid resolution.
- Persistent: short course of systemic corticosteroids (if underlying cause is not infectious in nature).

CHERRY ANGIOMA

- Cherry-red papules on the skin due to proliferation of abnormal capillaries.
- **Most commonly seen in middle-aged and older adults.**
- The somatic oncogenic mutations in *GNAQ* and *GNA11*, similar to those found in port wine stains and Sturge-Weber syndrome, have been seen with increased frequency.

CLINICAL MANIFESTATIONS
- **Cluster of cherry-red to dark red macules or papules that may be flat-topped or domed-shaped** (0.1–0.4 cm in diameter). **They do not blanch with pressure & bleed profusely if they are injured.** Most commonly seen on the trunk.

DIAGNOSIS
- Clinical.
- Examination with a dermatoscope will reveal purple, red, or blue-black lagoons.

MANAGEMENT
- **They do not generally require treatment.**

If cosmetically unappealing or subject to bleeding, options include:
- Small lesions: electrocautery after local anesthesia with 1% Lidocaine.
- Larger lesions: Shave excision and electrocauterization of the base.
- Superficial lesions: Laser therapy.
- Cryotherapy.

PORPHYRIA CUTANEA TARDA

- Hypersensitivity of the skin to abnormal porphyrins when they are exposed to light, leading to blistering skin disease of sun-exposed areas.
- Occurs due to decreased activity of the enzyme uroporphyrinogen decarboxylase.
- May be sporadic (80%) or inherited (20%).

RISK FACTORS
- **Liver disease** (eg, <u>Hepatitis C</u>, **alcoholism, Hemochromatosis**), estrogen use, smoking.

CLINICAL MANIFESTATIONS
- Chronic blistering photosensitivity of sun-exposed areas and the back of the hands, which can lead to hyper- or hypopigmentation or scarring **(bullae and vesicles leaving scars on sun-exposed areas, particularly the dorsal aspect of the hands).**
- May be complicated by a secondary infection.

DIAGNOSIS
- The diagnosis of PCT is made via the characteristic biochemical porphyrin profile — **increased plasma total porphyrins and urine porphyrins in a 24-hour collection** with a predominance of highly carboxylated porphyrins.
- Patients may have elevations in serum transaminases.

MANAGEMENT
- <u>Active skin lesions</u>: Phlebotomy (especially if iron-overloaded) or low-dose Hydroxychloroquine.
- Sun avoidance until plasma porphyrin levels have normalized. Treat underlying cause.

CHAPTER 13 – INFECTIOUS DISEASES

ANTIBIOTICS

PENICILLINS

MECHANISM OF ACTION
- **Bactericidal via <u>inhibition of cell wall synthesis</u> via beta-lactam ring.**
- Penicillin is a D-Ala-D-Ala analog that binds to penicillin-binding proteins (transpeptidases), impairing peptidoglycan cross-linking in the bacterial cell wall.

NATURAL PENICILLINS
Penicillin G benzathine-procaine (IM); Penicillin G (IM or IV); Penicillin VK (PO).
- <u>Spectrum of activity:</u> **most potent gram-positive coverage of all Penicillins. Pencillins also cover *N. meningitidis* & *Treponema pallidum*.** Covers most anaerobes (*Bacteroides* important exception).
- <u>Indications:</u> **Streptococcal pharyngitis, oral or dental infections, & Syphilis.**

PENICILLINASE-RESISTANT
Nafcillin (IV), Oxacillin (IV, IM), Dicloxacillin (PO).
- <u>Spectrum of activity</u> **gram-positive coverage,** especially ***Staphylococcal* infections (beta-lactamase producing *Staphylococcus aureus*).** Not active against Enterococcus, MRSA, or gram-negatives.

AMINOPENICILLINS
Amoxicillin, Ampicillin.
- <u>Spectrum of activity:</u> **great gram-positive & gram-negative coverage (including *H. influenzae, E.coli, Listeria, Proteus, & Salmonella*).**
- <u>Indications:</u> **UTIs in pregnancy, <u>Listeria monocytogenes</u>, Acute Otitis media, Lyme disease,** dental infections, & Enterococcal infections.

AMINOPENICILLINS WITH BETA-LACTAMASE INHIBITORS
Amoxicillin-clavulanate (oral), Ampicillin-sulbactam (IV).
- <u>Spectrum of activity:</u> gram-positive, gram-negative, and anaerobic coverage.
- <u>Indications:</u> **Acute otitis media, Acute sinusitis, animal and human bites, dental infections, skin & soft tissue infections.**

ANTI-PSEUDOMONAL PENICILLINS (EXTENDED SPECTRUM)
—**Piperacillin-tazobactam**, Ticarcillin-clavulanate, Carbenicillin.
- **Reserved for infections which may also be caused by Pseudomonal species.**

ADVERSE REACTIONS
- **<u>Gastrointestinal</u> — most common:** diarrhea (common), nausea, vomiting, abdominal pain. Increased risk of *Clostridioides difficile* infection, especially with the administration of Ampicillin.
- **<u>Hypersensitivity</u> — drug class most commonly associated with hypersensitivity reactions.**
- **<u>Neurotoxicity</u>** — may cause generalized hyperreflexia, myoclonus, and seizures at higher doses.
- **<u>Hematologic:</u>** thrombocytopenia, neutropenia, methemoglobinemia; Warm autoimmune hemolytic anemia.
- Suprainfection with yeasts, including overgrowth of yeasts.
- IV administration of Penicillin G benzathine or Penicillin procaine is associated with cardiopulmonary arrest and death. It should be given IM in the buttocks (upper outer quadrant) or thigh (anterolateral)
- <u>Hepatobiliary reactions</u> — Oxacillin and Nafcillin may cause hypersensitivity Hepatitis accompanied by fever, rash, and eosinophilia.
- <u>Acute interstitial nephritis</u> (especially Methicillin and Nafcillin).

CONTRAINDICATIONS
- Previous history of severe allergic reaction or Penicillin and its derivatives.
- History of Stevens-Johnson syndrome after administering Penicillin or a Penicillin derivative.

CEPHALOSPORINS

MECHANISM OF ACTION
- **Structurally and functionally similar to the Penicillin family with a beta-lactam ring** but are <u>**intrinsically effective against beta-lactamase producing bacteria**</u>.

SPECTRUM OF ACTIVITY
- Categorized by generations based on their spectrum of activity.
- **Increasing level of gram-negative activity & loss of gram-positive activity as you go from first to fourth generation.**
- In general, Cephalosporins are <u>not</u> effective against *Enterococci,* MRSA, *L. monocytogenes,* or *Clostridioides difficile.*

FIRST GENERATION
Cephalexin (PO), Cefazolin (IV), Cefadroxil (PO).
- <u>Spectrum of activity:</u> **great for gram-positive cocci, anaerobes, & gram-negatives rods** (eg, *E. coli, Haemophilus influenzae, Proteus mirabilus, Klebsiella pneumoniae*). Does not cover MRSA.
- <u>Indications:</u> **skin & soft tissue infections (staph, strep); UTIs, Surgical prophylaxis.**

SECOND GENERATION
Cefaclor (PO), **Cefuroxime** (IV, IM, PO), **Cefoxitin** (IV), Cefotetan (IM, IV).
- <u>Spectrum of activity:</u> broader gram-negative coverage (*Neisseria spp, M. catarrhalis*) with weaker gram-positive coverage. Cefoxitin has excellent coverage against *Bacteroides fragilis.*
- <u>Indications:</u> **skin, respiratory/ENT & urinary tract infections. Cefotetan & Cefoxitin used for anaerobic infections** (abdominal infections). <u>**Inpatient Pelvic inflammatory disease (PID)**</u> **treated with IV Doxycycline + either Cefoxitin or Cefotetan** (for their anaerobic coverage).

THIRD GENERATION
Ceftriaxone (IM/IV), **Ceftazidime** (IM, IV), Ceftibuten, Cefotaxime, Cefixime, Cefdinir, Cefpodoxime.
- <u>Spectrum of activity:</u> **broader gram-negative coverage** (including Serratia & enteric organisms). **Good CNS penetration (especially Ceftriaxone).**
- <u>Indications:</u> **bacterial meningitis, Gonorrhea, Community acquired pneumonia (hospitalized)** combined with Macrolides. Lyme disease involving the heart or brain.
- **Ceftazidime & Cefoperazone have coverage vs. *Pseudomonas*** whereas the others do not.

FOURTH GENERATION:
Cefepime (IV).
- <u>Spectrum of activity:</u> **gram-negative coverage including *Pseudomonas aeruginosa*.** Gram positive: only Methicillin-susceptible organisms. Reserved for infections due to multi-resistance organisms.

FIFTH GENERATION: **Ceftaroline (IV).**
- <u>Broad spectrum:</u> **gram-positives <u>(including MRSA)</u>** & gram-negatives including *Listeria monocytogenes* & *E. faecalis*. Does not cover Pseudomonas or anaerobes.

ADVERSE REACTIONS
- **Most common: nausea, vomiting, lack of appetite, and abdominal pain.**
- <u>**Allergic reaction:**</u> **5-15% cross reactivity with Penicillins** (therefore should not be used in any patient with an anaphylactic reaction to Penicillins, especially Cephalexin, Cefadroxil, Cefazolin). 1-2% hypersensitivity reaction in patients without a Penicillin allergy. Cephalosporins may be used in many patients with mild allergies.
- **Cefotetan & Cefoxitin can increase the risk of bleeding (hypoprothrombinemia** due to effect on vitamin K-dependent clotting factors) and Vitamin K deficiency.
- **Cefotetan causes a Disulfiram-like reaction** (due to blockage of the second step in alcohol oxidation).
- Ceftriaxone has inadequate biliary metabolism especially in neonates so **Cefotaxime preferred over Ceftriaxone in neonates** (eg, **neonatal meningitis**).

CARBAPENEMS

- **Imipenem-Cilastatin** (IV), **Meropenem** (IV), **Ertapenem** (IM, IV)

MECHANISM OF ACTION
- Synthetic beta-lactam antibiotic. **Addition of Cilastatin reduces deactivation of Carbapenems in the proximal renal tubule.** Good CSF penetration.
- Indications: **restricted use — Neutropenic fever**, severe infections.

SPECTRUM OF ACTIVITY
- **Imipenem has the broadest spectrum of all antibiotic classes.** They are not effective against MRSA, bacteria without peptidoglycan cell walls (eg, Mycoplasma) and some Pseudomonas species.
- Ertapenem does not cover any Pseudomonas species.

ADVERSE REACTIONS
- **CNS toxicity (especially with Imipenem) — includes seizures,** myoclonus, & altered mental status. **The risk of CNS toxicity is greater in patients with impaired renal function or underlying CNS disease**.
- GI: nausea, vomiting, diarrhea. Eosinophilia & neutropenia (less likely than other beta-lactams).
- Hypersensitivity: 5-10% of patients with Penicillin allergy are also allergic to Carbapenems.

MONOBACTAM

Aztreonam (IV)
MECHANISM OF ACTION
- Beta-lactam antibiotic that inhibits and disrupts cell wall synthesis, however, it is a **beta-lactam with no cross reactivity with other beta-lactam antibiotics**.

SPECTRUM OF ACTIVITY
- **Primarily gram-negative aerobes only** (including *Pseudomonas & Enterobacteriaceae*). Lacks reliable activity against gram positive organisms & anaerobes.

INDICATIONS
- Used most often clinically in patients with Penicillin allergies, renal insufficiency, those who cannot tolerate Aminoglycosides, or for synergism with Aminoglycosides.

ADVERSE REACTIONS
- Generally nontoxic but adverse reactions include: hepatitis, GI symptoms, phlebitis, & skin rashes.

POLYMYXIN

- Routes: topical, ophthalmic & otic. IM/IV.
- Mechanism of action: **alters permeability of the outer membrane** of gram-negative organisms.
- Spectrum of activity: narrow spectrum — primarily **gram-negative organisms (including *Pseudomonas aeruginosa*)**.

INDICATIONS
- **Topically for infections of the eye, ear, & skin.** May be part of triple therapy ointment, with Neomycin and Bacitracin. May be used as part of bowel prep for surgery.

ADVERSE REACTIONS
- Topical: allergic contract dermatitis.
- **IM/IV forms: nephrotoxicity & neurotoxicity so primarily used in topical forms.**

VANCOMYCIN

- **Mechanism of action:** cell wall inhibition (by inhibition of phospholipids & **peptidoglycans**). Binds to D-Ala-D-Ala to block transpeptidase, preventing elongation & cross-linking of peptidoglycan cell wall

SPECTRUM OF ACTIVITY
- **Narrow spectrum:** **gram-positive only** — *S. aureus* **[including Methicillin-Resistant *Staphylococcus Aureus* (MRSA)]**, Methicillin-Resistant *Staphylococcus epidermidis* (MRSE), *S. pneumoniae* & *Enterococcal* infections. **Vancomycin is synergistic with Aminoglycosides.**

INDICATIONS
- **IV:** **MRSA & MRSE** infections. Restricted use by the CDC.
- **Oral:** *Clostridioides difficile* colitis. Otherwise, oral Vancomycin has poor tissue penetration.

ADVERSE REACTIONS
- **Vancomycin flushing syndrome:** **flushing & pruritus due to histamine release** during rapid IV infusion. **Prevented by slow IV infusion over 1-2 hours and antihistamine administration.** Severe histamine release may lead to anaphylaxis in some patients.
- Fever and/or chills; Thrombophlebitis at the IV site.
- **Ototoxicity:** at high peak levels — **tinnitus or hearing loss.** May be reversible in some cases.
- **Nephrotoxicity at high trough levels,** especially if given with other antibiotics with similar adverse reactions (such as Aminoglycosides). **May cause Prerenal azotemia and Acute tubular necrosis.**
- Monitoring: trough levels may be needed in patients with renal impairment for renal dosing, patients on other nephrotoxic medications or in severe infections.

TETRACYCLINES

Doxycycline, Tetracycline, Minocycline
MECHANISM OF ACTION:
- **Protein synthesis inhibitor** (binds to **30S ribosomal** subunit). Bacteriostatic.

SPECTRUM OF ACTIVITY:
- **Broad spectrum of activity** — good against gram positive, gram negative, atypical organisms, and organisms other than bacteria.

INDICATIONS:
- **Doxycycline drug of choice:** *Chlamydia spp* — including *C. trachomatis* STIs, Pelvic inflammatory disease, Lymphogranuloma venereum; *Chlamydia pneumophila* pneumonia, *Chlamydia psittaci*), **Mycoplasma pneumoniae, Vibrio spp. (**eg, **V. cholerae)**, Q fever, Bubonic plague, **Cat scratch fever (Bartonella henselae). Syphilis (Treponema pallidum), S. aureus (including MRSA).**
- Tick-mediated infections: **Early Lyme disease** *(Borrelia),* **Rocky Mountain spotted fever** *(Rickettsia),* **Ehrlichiosis, Anaplasmosis.**
- **Atypical respiratory pathogens:** *Mycoplasma pneumoniae,* Legionella pneumophila, Chlamydophila.
- **Tetracycline & Minocycline used for Acne.**

ADVERSE REACTIONS
- **Poor GI tolerance:** may cause diarrhea and gastritis.
- **Deposition in calcified tissue:** deposition in teeth causes **teeth discoloration** & may affect growth (**Not usually given in children <8 years of age for >21 days**).
- **Hepatotoxic (especially in pregnancy)** — **contraindicated in pregnancy** (Doxycycline safe in some conditions).
- Photosensitivity (especially Doxycycline); Pseudotumor cerebri.
- Cation chelation: **Impaired absorption if given simultaneously with dairy products, Ca, Al, Mg, Fe.**
- Contraindicated in patients with renal impairment (except Doxycycline or Tigecycline).
- **Ototoxicity:** Minocycline and Doxycycline can cause **vestibular adverse reactions (eg, hearing loss, tinnitus).**

MACROLIDES

Azithromycin, Clarithromycin, Erythromycin

MECHANISM OF ACTION
- **Protein synthesis inhibitors: bind to the 50S ribosomal subunit, inhibiting protein synthesis.**
- Bacteriostatic at low doses, bactericidal at high doses. Azithromycin has a very long half-life (T ½ 68 hours, resulting in once daily dosing). Erythromycin has T ½ 1.5 hours, so dosed every 6 hours).

SPECTRUM OF ACTIVITY
- **Broad spectrum of activity: good against gram-positive, gram-negative, atypical organisms, and organisms other than bacteria** (eg, *Babesia microti*). No anaerobic coverage.

INDICATIONS:
- **Erythromycin:** Strep pharyngitis (PCN allergic patients), pneumonia, *C. diphtheriae*, topical use in Acne. **Safe in pregnancy.** Less gram-negative activity compared with others in the class.
- **Azithromycin:** Pneumonia — **best Macrolide for atypical coverage (*Mycoplasma, Chlamydia, & Legionella*), *Chlamydia trachomatis*.** Acute bacterial exacerbations of Chronic bronchitis (ABECB). **Anti-inflammatory in the lung.** Compared to Erythromycin, increased activity vs. *H. influenzae & M. catarrhalis* but less activity vs. *Staphylococcus* spp. & *Streptococcus* spp. Clarithromycin & Azithromycin are drugs of choice for Mycobacterium avium complex (MAC).
- **Clarithromycin:** Community-acquired pneumonia, legionella, *H. pylori*, sinusitis, bronchitis ABECB.

ADVERSE REACTIONS
- **GI upset: increased peristalsis — diarrhea and abdominal cramps, especially Erythromycin.**
- **Ototoxicity:** may cause deafness (usually reversible).
- **Prolonged QT interval: Erythromycin & Clarithromycin.**
- Cytochrome P-450 inhibition — **many drug-drug interactions (especially Erythromycin)** — may **increase levels of Warfarin, Digoxin,** Theophylline, Carbamazepine, & statins. **Azithromycin does NOT inhibit the CP450 system & NOT as prone to cytochrome P450 drug interactions** as other Macrolides.
- **Macrolides (eg, Erythromycin) increase risk of hypertrophic Pyloric stenosis in infants.**
- Contraindications: **patients on Niacin or statins (increased muscle toxicity).**
- **Acute cholestatic hepatitis (especially Erythromycin estolate).**
- **With the exception of Erythromycin (which is safe in pregnancy), avoid the other Macrolides in pregnancy** (Clarithromycin is embryotoxic).

BACITRACIN

- Routes: **topical, ophthalmic,** IM injection

MECHANISM OF ACTION
- **Cell wall synthesis inhibitor** and inhibitor of proteases and other bacterial enzymes. Mixture of cyclic peptides that are bactericidal and bacteriostatic.
- Spectrum of activity: **gram-positive only.** Little effect against anaerobes and gram-negatives.

INDICATIONS
- **Topical preparation for minor skin injuries, scrapes, cuts, and burns.**
- May be part of triple therapy ointment, with Neomycin and Polymyxin B.
- Superficial ocular infections of the cornea and conjunctiva.

ADVERSE REACTIONS
- Topical associated with allergic contract dermatitis. Patients with allergic reaction to Neomycin may also be sensitive to Bacitracin.
- **IM form is nephrotoxic so primarily used in topical form.**

CLINDAMYCIN

- Oral, IV, topical

MECHANISM OF ACTION
- **Lincosamide (binds to 50S ribosomal subunit), inhibiting protein synthesis.**
- Bacteriostatic or bactericidal depending on drug concentration and susceptibility of the bacteria.

SPECTRUM OF ACTIVITY
- **Narrow spectrum** — primarily for **gram-positive & most anaerobes, especially above the diaphragm** (little gram-negative coverage). Has **some MRSA coverage** (however there is increasing resistance). Resistance activity in general is similar to that of Erythromycin.

INDICATIONS
- Anaerobic infections (aspiration pneumonia, intra-abdominal infections), gynecologic infections (eg, bacterial vaginosis, severe PID), skin, soft tissue, bone and joint infections, streptococcal pharyngitis, acne vulgaris. Prophylaxis against infective endocarditis, babesiosis, anthrax, malaria, Toxic shock syndrome & infections due to *Bacteroides fragilis* & *Clostridium perfringens.*

ADVERSE REACTIONS
- **The most common adverse effects associated with Clindamycin are diarrhea, including *Clostridioides difficile* colitis, and allergic reactions.**
- GI symptoms most common adverse reaction: diarrhea, abdominal cramps, nausea, vomiting.
- *C. difficile* **colitis:** due to altered flora & the fact that *Clostridioides difficile* is inherently resistant to Clindamycin leads to *C. difficile* overgrowth & **Pseudomembranous colitis.**
- May be toxic in patients with renal & hepatic impairment.
- IV administration — thrombophlebitis, metallic taste.
- Topical administration can cause dermatitis, pruritus, and burning.
- Vaginal administration — vaginal candidiasis, pruritus, & vulvovaginitis.

CHLORAMPHENICOL

- Oral and IV

Mechanism of action:
- **Protein synthesis inhibitor**: binds to 50S ribosomal subunit, inhibiting bacterial protein synthesis.

Spectrum of activity:
- **Broad spectrum of activity** — good against gram-positive, gram-negative, anaerobes, & other organisms (eg, *Rickettsia rickettsii*, the causative agent of Rocky Mountain spotted fever).

Indications:
- Rocky Mountain spotted fever as the alternative to Doxycycline.
- Because of high incidence of toxicity, it is usually reserved for severe infections (eg, severe anaerobic infections or other life-threatening infections not responsive to other antibacterials).

Adverse reactions
- **Bone marrow suppression: Aplastic anemia,** reversible anemia, hemolytic anemia (especially if G6PD deficient).
- Overgrowth of *Candida albicans* common.
- **Gray baby syndrome** due to abnormal mitochondrial activity in neonates due to drug, leading to **gray skin, cyanosis, abdominal distention, & hemodynamic collapse.**
- Drug interactions: may increase levels of Phenytoin, Warfarin, and Chlorpropamide.

AMINOGLYCOSIDES

<u>Natural</u>: **Gentamicin, Amikacin;** <u>Semisynthetic</u>: **Tobramycin, Neomycin, Streptomycin**

MECHANISM OF ACTION

- **Binds irreversibly to the 30S ribosomal subunit**, inhibiting bacterial protein synthesis (bactericidal). Causes misreading of mRNA, resulting in nonfunctional protein synthesis.

SPECTRUM OF ACTIVITY

- <u>**Gram-negative aerobic bacilli only**</u> **(including** *Pseudomonas***).** There is a **synergistic effect when combined with a beta-lactam or Vancomycin.** Not good for gram-positive or anaerobic coverage (aminoglycoside entry into bacterial cells is via an oxygen-transport system).

INDICATIONS

<u>Serious gram-negative infections:</u>

- <u>Gentamicin:</u> hospital-acquired pneumonia, gram-negative bacteremia, genitourinary infections, septic shock, neonatal meningitis (used with Ampicillin), Yersinia, Tularemia, Septic shock.
- <u>Tobramycin:</u> slightly increased activity against Pseudomonas. Topical use for Keratitis.
- <u>Neomycin:</u> similar use as Tobramycin. Used as bowel prep. Topically (component of Neosporin & Corticosporin). Topical for Otitis externa (must be able to visualize the tympanic membrane).
- <u>Amikacin:</u> reserved for serious infections.
- <u>Streptomycin:</u> Tuberculosis, Tularemia, & Yersinia infections.

ADVERSE REACTIONS

- <u>**Nephrotoxicity:**</u> Acute tubular necrosis, especially if used with other nephrotoxic agents (eg, Vancomycin).
- <u>**Ototoxicity**</u>: **(vestibular & cochlear).** Cautious use of Gentamicin with other ototoxic drugs, such as Cisplatin, Furosemide, Bumetanide, Ethacrynic acid, & high-dose NSAIDs.
- <u>**Neuromuscular paralysis**</u>: **increased muscular weakness in patients with Myasthenia gravis.**
- Needs to be renally dosed in patients with renal impairment. **Monitor serum drug levels** — **peak** levels are typically evaluated **30 minutes after completion of the infusion** (monitor for toxicity). **Trough** levels should be drawn immediately before next dose is administered.
- Reduced activity in sites with acidic pH. Contact dermatitis with topical Neomycin.

LINEZOLID

- Oral & IV

MECHANISM OF ACTION

- **Linezolid binds to a unique site located on the 23S ribosomal RNA of the 50S ribosomal subunit,** and there is currently no cross resistance with other protein synthesis inhibitors.
- Synthetic oxazolidinone with bacteriostatic activity via inhibition of protein synthesis. Bacteriostatic vs. *Staphylococcus* & *Enterococci*. Bactericidal vs. *Streptococcus* & *Clostridium perfringens*.

SPECTRUM OF ACTIVITY

- **Mainly used for resistant <u>gram-positive organisms, including MRSA</u>, Vancomycin-resistant** *Enterococcus faecalis* **&** *faecium* **(VREF).** Also covers atypical organisms — Mycoplasma, Chlamydia, Legionella. Not good vs. gram negatives. Listeria monocytogenes, Corynebacterium.

ADVERSE REACTIONS

- Nausea, vomiting, diarrhea, headache. Lactic acidosis.
- <u>Hematologic:</u> anemia, thrombocytopenia (especially with treatment duration >2 weeks).
- <u>Neurologic:</u> irreversible nerve damage (peripheral neuropathy), ocular toxicity.
- <u>**MAO inhibition**</u>: avoid large amounts of foods with tyramine and sympathomimetics. **Increased risk of Serotonin syndrome when administered with serotonergic medications** [eg, selective serotonin reuptake inhibitors (SSRIs), SNRIs, MAO inhibitors, Tricyclic antidepressants].

METRONIDAZOLE & TINIDAZOLE

- Oral, IV, and topical

MECHANISM OF ACTION
- **Bactericidal: Nitroimidazole antibiotic that forms toxic metabolites and free radicals that damage DNA and inhibit bacterial DNA synthesis** (toxic to the microbe).
- Anaerobic microorganisms In anaerobic bacteria, it is activated by ferredoxin (present in anaerobic parasites, including protozoa) to form reactive cytotoxic products.

SPECTRUM OF ACTIVITY
- **Metronidazole is one of the mainstay drugs for the treatment of anaerobic bacterial infections, protozoal infections (parasites), and microaerophilic bacterial infections.**
- **Anaerobes "below the diaphragm",** including *Bacteroides fragilis*, *Clostridioides difficile*, *Gardnerella vaginalis*, *Helicobacter pylori*.
- **Protozoal infections:** *Giardia lamblia*, *Entamoeba histolytica*, & *Trichomonas spp.* (eg, *T. vaginalis*).

INDICATIONS
- Intra-abdominal infections, vaginitis, vaginosis, Pseudomembranous colitis, & Amoebic liver abscess.

ADVERSE REACTIONS
- **The primary adverse effects of Metronidazole include headache, nausea, vomiting, diarrhea, metallic taste, peripheral neuropathy, and confusion.** May potentiate the effects of Warfarin.
- **Disulfiram-like reaction if used with alcohol (acetaldehyde accumulation).** Alcohol ingestion or products containing propylene glycol should be avoided during treatment with Metronidazole and up to 48 hours after the last dose.
- Transient darkening of the urine to a deep red-brown color is common while on Metronidazole so patients should be notified it may occur.

DAPTOMYCIN

MECHANISM OF ACTION
- Cyclic lipopeptide: Binds to cell membrane via Ca^{++} dependent insertion of its lipid tail. Causes depolarization and efflux of K^+, causing inhibition of protein, DNA & RNA synthesis. IV formulation.

INDICATION:
- Empiric treatment of serious infection (eg, complicated skin & soft tissue infections) in patients known to be colonized with multi-drug resistant gram-positive organism (often alternative to Vancomycin).
- Daptomycin is not used in the treatment of Pneumonia because Daptomycin is inactivated by surfactant.

SPECTRUM OF ACTIVITY:
- **Gram-positive only including MRSA (often second-line alternative to IV Vancomycin for MRSA infections), VRE, *Enterococcus faecium* and *faecalis*.**
- Indications: **complicated skin infections** (multi-drug resistant gram-positives).

ADVERSE REACTIONS
- **The most important severe adverse effects of Daptomycin include muscle toxicity (eg, myopathy/Rhabdomyolysis) and Eosinophilic pneumonia.**
- **Muscle toxicity** (increased CPK and rhabdomyolysis). Monitor creatine phosphokinase (CPK) levels at least weekly during therapy. Concomitant use with statins increase muscle toxicity risk.
- GI symptoms, arthralgias.
- **Eosinophilic pneumonia,** hypersensitivity.

TRIMETHOPRIM-SULFAMETHOXAZOLE

- Oral and IV

MECHANISM OF ACTION

- **A reversible dihydrofolate reductase inhibitor, which impairs folate synthesis** via inhibition of the enzyme systems involved in the bacterial synthesis of tetrahydrofolic acid (THF), which inhibits thymidine synthesis, and subsequently **inhibits DNA synthesis.** Bactericidal.
- Sulfonamides compete with PABA. Trimethoprim inhibits dihydrofolate reductase (DHFR).

SPECTRUM OF ACTIVITY

- <u>**Broad spectrum**</u> — **excellent gram-negative & gram-positive coverage. Second best oral coverage against MRSA** (Linezolid is first but is not used as commonly as TMP-SMX).
- **Not active against Group A streptococcus,** so Cephalexin often added for Streptococcal coverage during empiric oral treatment for suspected MRSA cellulitis. *Pneumocystis jirovecii.*

INDICATIONS

- **Soft tissue infections with MRSA, UTIs, PCP treatment & prophylaxis,** Acute bacterial exacerbation of chronic bronchitis, Toxoplasmosis, Shigellosis, Otitis media (children), & Traveler's diarrhea.

ADVERSE REACTIONS

- **Rash, pruritus, GI symptoms, photosensitivity, & Folate deficiency are the primary adverse reactions.**
- <u>GI symptoms:</u> loss of appetite, nausea, vomiting, diarrhea. Dizziness, tinnitus, fatigue, & hyperkalemia.
- <u>Hematologic abnormalities</u> due to folic acid inhibition. May cause hemolytic anemia in patients with G6PD deficiency. May increase the levels of Warfarin & Digoxin
- **<u>Contraindications:</u>** people with increased folic acid requirements — **pregnancy (first trimester & last month), nursing mothers, & neonates <6 weeks (causes kernicterus). Sulfa allergies.**

NITROFURANTOIN

Oral

- <u>MECHANISM OF ACTION:</u> inhibits DNA, RNA, protein, and cell wall synthesis. It is excreted in the urine where the active metabolites attack multiple bacterial sites.
- <u>SPECTRUM OF ACTIVITY:</u> gram-positive & gram-negative coverage, including Enterococcus spp. **Not effective against Proteus or *Pseudomonas* spp.**
- <u>Administration:</u> **should be taken with meals to decrease adverse reactions & increase absorption.**

INDICATIONS:

- **<u>Uncomplicated acute Cystitis</u> treatment and prophylaxis only** (not used for acute Pyelonephritis or other GU infections). Nitrofurantoin is NOT used in the management of Acute pyelonephritis.
- **Safe for Cystitis in pregnancy** (except at term between 38-42 weeks' gestation or during labor).

ADVERSE REACTIONS

- **Common adverse effects of Nitrofurantoin include nausea, vomiting, loss of appetite, diarrhea, and headache.** Hepatotoxicity & peripheral neuropathy.
- **<u>Pulmonary toxicity:</u>** hypersensitivity pneumonitis & chronic pulmonary fibrosis, especially if >65 years of age.

CONTRAINDICATIONS:

- Acute or chronic renal failure. Not used in the treatment of Acute cystitis in men.
- Because of the possibility of hemolytic anemia secondary to immature erythrocyte enzyme systems, it is **contraindicated in pregnant patients at term (38-42 weeks' gestation), during labor and delivery, or in neonates <1 month of age.**

FLUOROQUINOLONES

<u>MECHANISM OF ACTION</u>
- **DNA gyrase inhibition** — removes excess positive supercoiling in the DNA helix (primary target for gram-negative bacteria).
- **Topoisomerase IV inhibition** — affects separation of interlinked daughter DNA molecules (primary target for many gram-positive bacteria).

<u>SECOND GENERATION</u> increased activity vs. aerobic gram-negative bacteria.
- **Ciprofloxacin: best gram-negative coverage of all FQs,** including *Pseudomonas,* **enteric organisms,** *H. influenzae, Neisseria.* <u>Indications:</u> **UTI, pyelonephritis, gastroenteritis,** PID, malignant Otitis externa, Sinusitis, Gonococcal arthritis, Anthrax.
- <u>Ofloxacin & Lomefloxacin:</u> enhanced coverage of *Staphylococcus* and *Streptococcus* spp. <u>Indications:</u> same as above + acute bacterial exacerbation of chronic bronchitis & community acquired pneumonia.

<u>THIRD GENERATION</u> increased activity vs. gram-positive & atypical organisms
- **Levofloxacin:** better activity vs. *S. pneumoniae.* <u>Indications:</u> **Community acquired Pneumonia,** Pyelonephritis, Prostatitis, acute Cystitis, Gastroenteritis.
- **Moxifloxacin: best gram-positive, anaerobic & atypical coverage** of the 3 generations. Poor Pseudomonas coverage. <u>Indications:</u> **intra-abdominal infections** (can be used as monotherapy), respiratory infections, Sinusitis, ophthalmic infections, & skin infections.
- Gatifloxacin ophthalmic.

<u>ADVERSE REACTIONS</u>
- **GI: — transient GI upset most common,** nausea, vomiting, diarrhea. *Clostridioides difficile* infection.
- **Serious adverse effects FQs include tendinitis, tendon rupture, disordered glucose regulation, prolonged QT interval, CNS effects (eg, seizures, peripheral neuropathy), & aortic rupture.**
- <u>CNS dysfunction:</u> headache, memory impairment, agitation, delirium, seizures, peripheral neuropathy, **may exacerbate Myasthenia gravis.**
- **Arthropathy:** may be associated with **tendinitis or tendon rupture (eg, Achilles tendon)** in adults. **Contraindicated in pregnancy & in children <18 years due to articular cartilage derangements.**
- Photosensitivity. Increased risk of hyperglycemia or hypoglycemia
- **Cardiac: May cause QT prolongation.** Aortic aneurysm, rupture, or dissection.
- Renal or hepatic dysfunction. Ciprofloxacin inhibits the CP450 system.
- **Fluoroquinolone use should be avoided for the treatment of uncomplicated infections** (eg, acute sinusitis, simple cystitis) **when the risks outweigh the benefits.**

QUINUPRISTIN/DALFOPRISTIN

<u>MECHANISM OF ACTION</u>
- **Streptogramin class.** Binds to 50S subunit to inhibit protein synthesis. Bacteriostatic but Bactericidal to some bacteria.

<u>SPECTRUM</u>
- **Mainly gram-positive,** including **MRSA & VRSA** (Vancomycin-resistant *Staphylococcus aureus*).
- Covers ***Vancomycin-resistant Enterococcus faecium*** only (*not Enterococcus faecalis*).
- Positive atypical coverage against Mycoplasma & Legionella.
- Has limited gram-negative activity.

<u>ADVERSE EFFECTS</u>
- **Thrombophlebitis** (so only given via a central line).

ADVERSE EFFECTS, ADVERSE REACTIONS, AND COMMENTS

PENICILLINS	**Hypersensitivity reaction.** Anaphylaxis in 0.05% (skin test does not predict it). Neurotoxicity. Hematologic side effects. **PCN & Cephalosporins associated** with nephrotoxicity **(Interstitial nephritis).**
AMPICILLIN	**Maculopapular rash in patients with Infectious mononucleosis** >90%, diarrhea.
CEPHALOSPORINS	**10% cross reactivity in patients allergic to PCN. Disulfiram reaction** (2nd/3rd), diarrhea. <u>Adverse effects</u>: increased LFTs, neutropenia, thrombocytopenia.
AZTREONAM	Beta-lactam that has no cross reactivity with Penicillin or Cephalosporins.
VANCOMYCIN	**"Flushing syndrome"** (Histamine release-occurs when infused too rapidly). Avoided with slow infusion over 1-2 hours. Ototoxic (reversible), nephrotoxic.
MACROLIDES	**GI upset** (less with newer ones). Cytochrome P450 inhibition. **Prolonged QT interval** **Caution if patient is on niacin or statins** (increased muscle toxicity).
FLUOROQUINOLONES	**Tendon rupture**, growth plate arrest, damage to articular cartilage **(not given if <18y or in pregnant women). May exacerbate Myasthenia Gravis.** Photosensitivity, **QT prolongation.** Ciprofloxacin inhibits the CP450 system.
CLINDAMYCIN	**May cause *C. difficile* colitis.** Does not have good CSF penetration.
TETRACYCLINES	GI upset, **deposition in teeth** causing **teeth discoloration**; hepatotoxic **(not given during pregnancy or to children <8 years of age for > 21 days). Photosensitivity.** Not given simultaneously with dairy products, Ca, Al, Mg, or iron.
SULFONAMIDES **Ex: TMP-SMX**	Rash in 3-5%; do not give after 2nd trimester: may develop **kernicterus.** **Sulfa allergy, <u>hemolysis if G6PD deficient.</u>**
METRONIDAZOLE	**Avoid alcohol during and 48 hours after last use (Disulfiram-like reaction)** **Neurotoxicity,** metallic taste, possible carcinogenic potential, pancreatitis.
PHOTOSENSITIVITY	Tetracyclines, Fluoroquinolones, Sulfonamides, Trimethoprim-sulfamethoxazole Pyrazinamide.
AUGMENTIN	Augmentin is the penicillin with the highest occurrence of diarrhea.

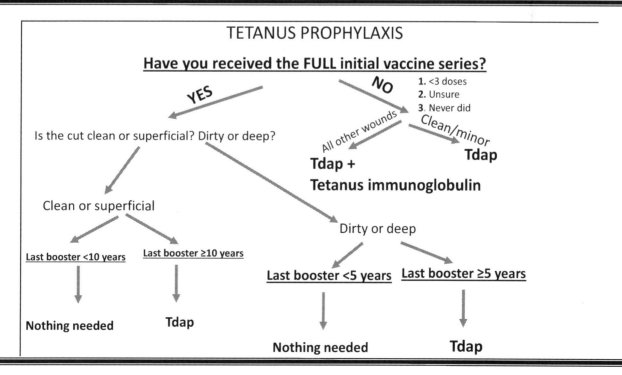

TETANUS PROPHYLAXIS

Have you received the FULL initial vaccine series?

YES

NO
1. <3 doses
2. Unsure
3. Never did

Is the cut clean or superficial? Dirty or deep?

All other wounds

Clean/minor

Tdap +
Tetanus immunoglobulin

Tdap

Clean or superficial

Dirty or deep

<u>Last booster <10 years</u>   <u>Last booster ≥10 years</u>

<u>Last booster <5 years</u>   <u>Last booster ≥5 years</u>

Nothing needed   **Tdap**

Nothing needed   **Tdap**

TETANUS

- **Muscle spasms due to autonomic disinhibition via** *Clostridium tetani,* a gram-positive rod.
- Pathophysiology: **neurotoxin (tetanospasmin) blocks neuron inhibition** by blocking the release of the inhibitory neurotransmitters GABA & glycine. This leads to **severe muscle spasm & hypertonia**.
- Transmission: ubiquitous in soil; germinates **especially in puncture & crush wounds**.

CLINICAL MANIFESTATIONS
- **Generalized:** Pain & tingling at the inoculation site followed by **spastic paralysis. Early symptoms: Muscle rigidity, most commonly, trismus (lockjaw, jaw stiffness) appears as the first symptom (>80%) with descending pattern of muscle spasms leading to stiff neck,** dysphagia, and hyperirritability, with the progression of spasms throughout the rest of the body. Autonomic overactivity may manifest as sweating and tachycardia. **Later symptoms: generalized muscle spasms, drooling,** uncontrolled urination and/or defecation. More severe autonomic symptoms (eg, profuse sweating, cardiac dysrhythmias, labile hypertension or hypotension, and fever are often present). IP: 3-21 d.
- **Neonatal:** Neonatal tetanus typically occurs in infants 5-7 days following birth (range 3-24 days). Irritability, poor feeding, difficulty opening mouth due to trismus, facial grimacing, rigidity, severe spastic contractions triggered by touch, hand clenching, dorsiflexion of the feet, increased muscle tone, muscle rigidity, and opisthotonus (spasm of spinal extensors). Occurs as a result of the failure to use aseptic techniques in managing the umbilical stump in offspring of poorly immunized mothers.
- Localized: Uncommon variant — persistent contraction of muscles localized to the site of injury (muscles around the wound) that may persist for weeks.
- Cephalic (cerebral): Limited to the muscles and nerves of the head only (eg, cranial nerve involvement).

PHYSICAL EXAMINATION
Tonic & spastic muscular contractions:
- **Generalized muscle spasms with minor stimulation** (reflex spasms occur in most patients and can be triggered by nominal external stimuli (eg, loud noise, touch, or light), **hypertonia (increased deep tendon reflexes),** tonic contraction of skeletal muscles, and intermittent intense muscular spasms that are extremely painful.
- **Trismus (lockjaw) is the presenting symptom in >80%.** Stiff neck.
- **Risus sardonicus (sardonic smile):** facial contractions with raised eyebrows and grimace facial expression with a grinning appearance.
- **Opisthotonus arched back** due to spinal extensor muscle spasm.
- Muscle rigidity in descending fashion (hands & feet usually spared).
- **These spasms may affect the respiratory and abdominal muscles, leading to abdominal board-like rigidity, tenderness, and guarding as well as respiratory distress** (eg, periods of apnea and/or upper airway obstruction). Dysphagia.
- During generalized tetanic spasms, fist clenching, back arching, arm abduction and flexion, as well as leg extension may occur, often in association with apnea.
- **Positive spatula test** — reflex spasms and involuntary jaw contraction of the masseter muscles **causing the patient to bite down instead of the normal gag reflex when the posterior pharynx is touched with a soft-tipped instrument** (eg, tongue blade or spatula).

Autonomic dysfunction
- Autonomic instability due to **disinhibition of the autonomic nervous system**: fever, labile blood pressure (tachycardia & hypertension alternating with bradycardia and hypotension), dysrhythmia, respiratory difficulties, hypothermia. **Cardiac arrest is the most common cause of death.**

DIAGNOSIS
- **Tetanus is mainly a clinical diagnosis (acute onset, trismus, dysphagia, muscle contractures with generalized muscle spasms and rigidity with no other medical cause** with a history of inadequate tetanus immunization and with or without a history of an antecedent tetanus-prone injury) as there are no particular laboratory or imaging tests to confirm the diagnosis.

MANAGEMENT
Active infection: Metronidazole, immune globulin, immunization, & a Benzodiazepine (Diazepam).
- **[1] Metronidazole** 7.5 mg/kg IV or orally every 6 hours (maximum 4 g daily) **+ [2] Human tetanus immune globulin injection [eg, a single dose of 500 units intramuscularly] to stop toxin production as well as neutralize and remove unbound circulating toxins** (HTIG does not affect toxin already bound to the CNS). Wounds should be cleaned & debrided of necrotic material. **Penicillin is an alternative to Metronidazole but is not preferred** (may exacerbate symptoms).
- **[3] Active immunization:** Because Tetanus is one of the few bacterial diseases that does not confer immunity following recovery from acute illness, **all patients with Tetanus should receive active immunization with a full series of Tetanus and Diphtheria toxoid-containing vaccines, starting immediately upon diagnosis** (eg, 3 doses in adults and children >7 years old).
- **[4] Muscles spasms: Benzodiazepines to reduce spasms (eg, Diazepam).**
  IV Magnesium has been shown to prevent muscle spasm.
- Respiratory support if needed. Debridement of the wound will control the source of toxin production.
- In addition to Benzodiazepines, autonomic hyperactivity can be treated with Labetalol or Morphine sulfate. Beta blockade without concomitant alpha blockade should be avoided.

TETANUS PROPHYLAXIS
Previously vaccinated ≥3 doses:
- **Tdap booster: tetanus toxoid containing vaccine given for clean and minor wounds if last dose was 10 years or longer** (Tdap booster now preferred over Td).
- **Tdap booster: tetanus toxoid containing vaccine given in all other wounds (eg, dirty, contaminated, deep, major) if last dose was 5 years or longer** (Tdap booster preferred vs. Td).
- Tetanus vaccine recommended for every pregnancy.

<3 doses or unknown:
- Clean and minor wounds: Tetanus-toxoid containing vaccine (eg, Tdap).
- **All other wounds: Tetanus toxoid containing vaccine (Tdap preferred or Td) given in 3 doses + Tetanus immune globulin in patients with <3 prior doses, unknown vaccination history, or if never vaccinated — first dose at initial visit,** second dose between 4-8 weeks, & third dose given between 6-12 months after the second. Tdap is now preferred over Td.

Tetanus immune globulin:
- **Tetanus immune globulin 250 units + initiation of Tetanus toxoid vaccine indicated for all wounds that are not clean or minor if (1) the individual has never been vaccinated, (2) unknown vaccination history, or (3) <3 prior doses of tetanus toxoid-containing vaccine.** DTaP used if <7 years of age.
- Tetanus immune globulin is given to induce passive immunity in individuals not fully vaccinated.

VACCINATION SCHEDULE
- **DTaP schedule in children: 5 doses** given at 2, 4, & 6 months of age, between 15-18 months, & between 4-6 years of age. Dose 5 of DTaP is not necessary if dose 4 was administered at age 4 years or older *and* at least 6 months after dose 3.
- **Adult: 3 doses: tetanus and diphtheria toxoids vaccine (Td) administered as 2 doses 4–6 weeks apart, with a third dose 6–12 months later.** For one of the three doses, Tdap (tetanus toxoid, reduced-dose diphtheria toxoid, acellular pertussis vaccine) should be substituted for Td.

Tdap booster:
- **Given at 11-12 years of age as part of the routine vaccination schedule then recommended 1 dose Tdap (preferred) or Td every 10 years.**
- If additional doses of Tetanus and Diphtheria toxoid–containing vaccines are needed in individuals not fully immunized, then patients aged 7-10 years should be vaccinated according to the catch-up schedule, with Tdap preferred as the first dose.
- **1 dose of Tdap is recommended for each pregnancy, preferably during week 27-36 of pregnancy, regardless of the last immunization** to prevent maternal tetanus and neonatal tetanus.

GAS GANGRENE (MYONECROSIS)

Clostridial myonecrosis life-threatening muscle infection characterized by rapid and severe tissue destruction with systemic toxicity that develops either:

- **[1] contiguously from an area of trauma (usually due to _Clostridium perfringens_) or**
- **[2] hematogenously from the gastrointestinal tract with muscle seeding (usually due to _Clostridium septicum_).**

RISK FACTORS
- **Anaerobic conditions local tissue hypoxia in traumatized tissues** — eg, traumatic injuries, punctures, IV drug injection.
- **Postoperative eg, recent GI or biliary surgery** (inadvertent inoculation of the surgical wound).
- **Immunocompromised patients (eg, Diabetes mellitus) & individuals with local tissue hypoxia.**

CLINICAL MANIFESTATIONS
Traumatic gas gangrene:
- **Severe muscle pain: sudden onset of edema and extreme muscle pain at the site of injury or trauma, or in an area of wound contamination** (due to toxin-mediated ischemia).
- **Cellulitis at the site of infection, fever, and chills. The infection progresses rapidly with development of edema and bullae filled with clear, cloudy, hemorrhagic, or purplish fluid** and can have a discharge with a musty odor. Symptoms are disproportionately dominant compared to physical examination.
- **Skin discoloration initially, skin pallor occurs then rapidly develops into a bronze appearance, followed by violaceous or erythematous discoloration (necrotic or dusky looking skin).**
- Bacteremia occurs in ~15% of cases and may lead to hemolysis, rapid sepsis, and death.
Spontaneous Gas gangrene:
- Abrupt onset of severe muscle pain, heaviness, numbness, malaise, confusion.

PHYSICAL EXAMINATION
- **Bullae with blood-tinged exudates** overlying the affected area with the skin surrounding the bullae having a purple hue (vascular compromise from bacterial toxins diffusing into surrounding tissues).
- **Crepitus (gas) in the soft tissues on palpation (most sensitive and specific finding).**
- **Systemic toxicity** develops rapidly — tachycardia, fever, chills, followed by shock & multiorgan failure.

DIAGNOSIS
- Radiographs: **gas within the soft tissues with muscle involvement.** CT/MRI gives more detail.
- Culture or smear of exudates: **gram-positive bacilli with few leukocytes.** Blood cultures.

MANAGEMENT
Emergent, early, and aggressive surgical debridement (may need fasciotomy) + antibiotics (eg, IV Penicillin plus Clindamycin).
- **Treatment of traumatic Gas gangrene is comprised of surgical consultation for emergent and aggressive surgical debridement, antibiotic therapy, supportive measures,** intravenous fluid resuscitation, ICU monitoring, and adjuvant hyperbaric oxygen therapy (shown to improve outcomes in some cases of severe infection).
- Tetanus status: Patients with trauma who have not received Tetanus immunization for 5 years should receive a booster vaccine against Tetanus.
- **Empiric antibiotics: broad-spectrum empiric antibiotic treatment [eg, (1) Penicillin + Clindamycin or (2) Piperacillin-tazobactam** (4.5g IV every 8 hours) **PLUS Clindamycin** (900 mg intravenously every eight hours)] **is the preferred option to cover polymicrobial infection.**
- Hyperbaric oxygen therapy can be added to improve survival in some patients.
- Antibiotic agents with excellent in vitro activity against _C. perfringens_ include Penicillin, Clindamycin, Tetracycline, Chloramphenicol, Metronidazole, and Cephalosporins.

BOTULISM

- **Flaccid paralysis** caused by ***Clostridium botulinum,*** an anaerobic, gram-positive, spore-forming rod.

PATHOPHYSIOLOGY
- **Neurotoxin inhibits acetylcholine release** at the neuromuscular junction, leading to weakness, **flaccid paralysis,** cranial nerve palsies, & possibly respiratory arrest.

TRANSMISSION
- **Infant: ingestion of honey** or dust-containing spores cause active toxin production in the gut.
- **Adult:** ingestion of preformed toxin in **canned, smoked, & vacuum-packed foods.**
- Wound: rare. Common after traumatic injury (puncture wounds, deep infections) or in **IV drug users**.

CLINICAL MANIFESTATIONS
- Symptoms occur 12-36 hours after ingestion (6-8 hours if <1 year old). **Infantile most common type.**
Muscle weakness hallmark — **descending, symmetric flaccid paralysis** (upper > lower).
- **Infantile:** "floppy baby syndrome" — neonates presenting initially with constipation followed lethargy, weakness (weak suck), feeding difficulties, flaccid paralysis, hypotonia, & weak cry.
- **Foodborne**: prodromal GI symptoms (nausea, vomiting, abdominal pain, diarrhea) followed by sudden onset of **Flaccid paralysis 8 Ds — Diplopia, Dysphagia, Dry mouth, Dilated, fixed pupils, Dysarthria, Dysphonia, Descending decreased muscle strength (descending symmetric muscle weakness and flaccid paralysis), & Decreased (or absent) deep tendon reflexes.** Descending muscle weakness usually progresses from the trunk and upper extremities to the lower extremities. **Bilateral cranial nerve (bulbar) palsies** — eg, diplopia, blurred vision, dysphagia, facial weakness. **May develop respiratory difficulty due to diaphragmatic paralysis.**
- **Wound Botulism** is similar to foodborne Botulism but differs only slightly in that [1] prodromal GI symptoms common to foodborne botulism are usually absent, [2] has a longer incubation period (5-15 days), & [3] is often associated with fever and leukocytosis, present in ~50%.

DIAGNOSIS:
- **Primary a clinical diagnosis** — Botulism should be suspected in a patient with acute onset of signs and symptoms of prodromal GI symptoms, cranial neuropathy and symmetric descending weakness, especially in the absence of fever. In infants, Botulism should be suspected when there is acute onset floppy baby syndrome (eg, weak suck, ptosis, inactivity, and constipation), especially if there is a history of honey consumption.
- Toxin assays: The diagnosis of Botulism is confirmed by identification of toxin in serum, stool, vomitus, or food sources or by isolation of *C. botulinum* from stool, wound specimens, or food sources.

MANAGEMENT OF FOODBORNE
- **Immediate treatment with antitoxin, monitoring for signs of respiratory failure, hospitalization, and supportive care.** Because respiratory failure is the primary cause of death in patients with Botulism, prompt intubation with mechanical ventilation reduce the risk of mortality.
- **Antitoxins are the mainstay of therapy for Botulism:**
    - **If >1 years of age,** use **equine-derived** heptavalent antitoxin.
    - **If <1 years of age, human-derived** botulism immune globulin.
- **No antibiotics in foodborne or infantile** (may worsen disease via toxin release from lysis of bacteria).
- Food-acquired Botulism — laxatives, enemas, or other cathartics can be given, provided no significant ileus is present.

MANAGEMENT OF WOUND
- **Antitoxin followed by extensive debridement + antibiotics, such as Penicillin G first line** (eg, 3 million units IV every 4 hours in adults).
- Metronidazole 500 mg every 8 hours is an alternative for Penicillin-allergic patients.

RESPIRATORY DIPHTHERIA

- Infectious disease caused by ***Corynebacterium diphtheriae*****, a gram-positive bacillus.**
- Vaccination has decreased incidence in the US (may still occur in children & vaccinated adults).

TRANSMISSION
- Inhalation of respiratory secretions. **Exotoxin induces an inflammatory response, primarily in the throat and pharynx,** forming a thick adherent gray pseudomembranes. Diphtheria exotoxin leads to inhibition of protein synthesis & subsequent necrosis in respiratory, cardiac, & CNS tissue.

CLINICAL MANIFESTATIONS
- **Tonsillopharyngitis or Laryngitis: classic presentation — gradual onset of sore throat, malaise, low-grade fever, and cervical lymphadenopathy.** Dysphagia, malaise, headache, Croup-like cough, and nasopharyngeal flu-like symptoms may occur. 1–7-day incubation period.
- **Myocarditis:** arrhythmias or Heart failure (exotoxin-induced inflammatory response). **Myocarditis responsible for around 50% of deaths (major cause of mortality).**
- **Neuropathy:** cranial nerves initially, producing diplopia, slurred speech, and difficulty in swallowing.
- **Myocarditis and Neuropathy are the most common & most serious complications of Diphtheria.**

Physical examination:
- **Pseudomembrane — friable, gray to white membrane on the pharynx that bleeds if scraped.** Pseudomembranes are composed of WBCs, RBCs, necrotic fibrin, dead epithelial cells, & organisms.
- **Cervical lymphadenopathy: massive swelling of the tonsils, uvula, cervical lymph nodes, submandibular region, and anterior neck ("bull neck" of toxic Diphtheria) may occur** and be complicated by respiratory stridor, respiratory compromise, and death. Aspiration of the membrane can lead to asphyxiation.

DIAGNOSIS
- **Clinical diagnosis:** presence of sore throat, cervical lymphadenopathy, fever, & pseudomembranes.
- Culture confirmation using Löffler medium or tellurite agar — definitive diagnosis. Positive toxin assay.

MANAGEMENT
- **[1] Diphtheria antitoxin (horse serum) most important + [2] either Erythromycin or Penicillin** for 2 weeks. Antitoxin reduces sequelae & increase recovery time; antibiotics prevent the spread of Diphtheria.
- **Place the patient on respiratory droplet isolation** until 2 consecutive cultures 24 hours apart are negative. Serial ECGs and cardiac enzymes to assess for Myocarditis. Airway management if needed.
- Azithromycin, Clindamycin, or Rifampin are alternatives. Endocarditis: Penicillin + Aminoglycoside.

PROPHYLAXIS FOR CLOSE CONTACTS
- **Either Erythromycin** x 7- 10 days or **Penicillin benzathine G** x 1 dose.

VACCINATION SCHEDULE
DTaP schedule:
- **5 doses** given at 2, 4, & 6 months of age, between 15-18 months, & between 4-6 years of age.
- Dose 5 of DTaP is not necessary if dose 4 was administered at age 4 years or older *and* at least 6 months after dose 3.

Tdap booster:
- **Given at 11-12 years of age as part of the routine vaccination schedule then recommended 1 dose Tdap (preferred) or Td every 10 years.**
- If additional doses of Tetanus and Diphtheria toxoid–containing vaccines are needed in individuals not fully immunized, then patients aged 7-10 years should be vaccinated according to the catch-up schedule, with Tdap preferred as the first dose.
- **1 dose of Tdap is recommended for each pregnancy, preferably during week 27-36 of pregnancy, regardless of the last immunization** to prevent maternal tetanus and neonatal tetanus.

METHICILLIN-RESISTANT STAPHYLOCCUS AUREUS (MRSA)

- **Oral agents:** Trimethoprim-Sulfamethoxazole, Doxycycline, Clindamycin. Linezolid
- **IV agents:** Vancomycin usually first line (Daptomycin alternative). Ceftaroline; Linezolid.

GONOCOCCAL INFECTIONS

- *Neisseria gonorrhoeae* **(gram-negative diplococci).** 2–8-day incubation period.

CLINICAL MANIFESTATIONS
- **Urethritis and Cervicitis:** discharge (anal, vaginal, penile, or pharyngeal).
- Pelvic inflammatory disease (PID), Epididymitis, Prostatitis.

DISSEMINATED GONOCOCCAL INFECTION (DGI)
Bacteremic spread of *Neisseria gonorrhoeae* usually presents with 1 of 2 syndromes:
- **[1] Purulent arthritis (gonococcal asymmetric septic arthritis) — especially of the knee,** wrists, ankles without any systemic symptoms. In women, it occurs more frequently during menses.
- **[2] Triad of dermatitis, polyathralgias, & tenosynovitis — [1] dermatitis** [vesicular pustules with **erythematous halos** (especially the distal extremities); may be petechia], **[2] migratory polyarthralgias** without purulent arthritis, and **[3] extensor tenosynovitis** (tenderness along a tendon sheath). Often with systemic symptoms (eg, fever, chills, & malaise).

DIAGNOSIS
- **Nucleic acid amplification (NAAT):** **Most sensitive & specific for** *C. trachomatis, N. gonorrhoeae, & M. genitalium* (recommended over culture).
    - First-void or first-catch urine is ideal to perform NAAT.
    - If disseminated, samples are taken at multiple sites (eg, urethral, rectal, pharyngeal, cervical).
- **Synovial fluid:** nucleic acid amplification testing (NAAT) or culture on chocolate agar or Thayer-Martin medium.

Point-of-care stain available: (gram stain, methylene blue, gentian violet) available:
- **Nongonococcal:** ≥2 WBCs/hpf in high-prevalence settings (≥5 in lower-prevalence settings) + **no intracellular diplococci, treat for Nongonococcal infection** (eg, Doxycycline) if low suspicion for gonococcal infection. If there is a high suspicion for gonococcal infection, treat with regimen that provides gonococcal and chlamydial coverage. Urethral swab performed in some men.
- **Gonococcal: if gram-negative intracellular diplococci present** — **treat for Gonococcal urethritis**.
- Urinalysis or dipstick: ⊕ leukocyte esterase or ≥10 WBCs/hpf (pyuria) on microscopy in men.

MANAGEMENT
Gonococcal arthritis & Disseminated gonococcal infection:
- **IV Ceftriaxone is the first-line treatment** [1 gram intravenously (or, if needed, intramuscularly) every 24 hours].
- Patients with Septic arthritis usually require Ceftriaxone for 7-14 days, along with joint drainage.
- For patients without Septic arthritis, treatment is usually continued for 7 days.

Gonococcal Urethritis or Cervicitis:
- **Ceftriaxone: single intramuscular dose of Ceftriaxone (500 mg for individuals <150 kg or 1 g for individuals ≥150 kg)** is recommended in males with symptoms of urethritis who have microscopic evidence of gonococcal urethritis (eg, gram-negative intracellular diplococci in the urethral exudate) or high clinical suspicion of gonococcal infection based on the revised CDC guidelines.
- **If testing results for** *C. trachomatis* **are not available or has not been ruled out at the time of treatment, presumptive therapy for Chlamydia coinfection is also indicated (eg, Doxycycline 100 mg twice daily for 7 days).** Azithromycin 1 gram x 1 observed dose is an alternative.

CHLAMYDIA

- *Chlamydia trachomatis* is the most common overall <u>bacterial</u> cause of STIs in the US.

CLINICAL MANIFESTATIONS
- <u>Urethritis</u>: purulent or mucopurulent discharge, pruritus, dysuria, dyspareunia (pain with intercourse), hematuria. Up to 40% asymptomatic (especially men).
- **<u>Pelvic inflammatory disease</u>: abdominal pain, ⊕ cervical motion tenderness.**
- **<u>Reactive arthritis</u>: triad of [1] urethritis, [2] uveitis, & [3] arthritis.** Reactive arthritis is an autoimmune reaction not a Septic arthritis. **⊕ HLA-B27 in many cases.**
- <u>Lymphogranuloma venereum</u>: genital/rectal lesion with softening, suppuration & lymphadenopathy.

DIAGNOSIS
- **<u>Nucleic acid amplification (NAAT)</u> most sensitive & specific for *C. trachomatis, N. gonorrhoeae*,** & *M. genitalium* (vaginal swab or first-catch urine preferred).
- **<u>Gram stain</u>: ≥2 WBCs/hpf & no organisms seen is suggestive of Nongonococcal urethritis (*Chlamydia trachomatis*).** Gram-negative intracellular diplococci = *Neisseria gonorrhoeae*.
- <u>Urinalysis or dipstick</u>: ⊕ leukocyte esterase on dipstick or ≥10 WBCs/hpf (pyuria) on microscopy suggestive.
- Genetic probe methods, culture, antigen detection.

MANAGEMENT
- **<u>Doxycycline</u> 100 mg orally twice daily for 7 days is the first-line treatment for Chlamydia.**
- **<u>Azithromycin</u> (either as 500 mg orally on day one then 250 mg orally daily for 4 days or as a single 1 g observed dose),** although the single-dose regimen is associated with lower *C. trachomatis* microbiologic cure rates than Doxycycline.
- Unless definitive diagnosis is known for Chlamydia, also treat for Gonorrhea — Ceftriaxone: single intramuscular dose of Ceftriaxone (500 mg for individuals <150 kg or 1 g for individuals ≥150 kg).

LYMPHOGRANULOMA VENEREUM (LGV)

- **Genital ulcer disease cause by <u>L1, L2 & L3 serovars of *Chlamydia trachomatis</u>*.**
- Most commonly seen in tropical & subtropical areas of the world.
- <u>Pathophysiology</u>: extension from the infection site to the draining lymph nodes.

CLINICAL MANIFESTATIONS
- **[1] <u>Primary stage</u>: <u>shallow painless genital ulcer</u> at the site of inoculation** (starts as a painless papule) **often lasting a few days (eg, 2-3 days).**
- **[2] <u>Secondary stage</u>:** appears 2-6 weeks later — inflammatory reaction with **unilateral painful/tender deep inguinal &/or femoral lymphadenopathy that is often fluctuant (buboes).** <u>Groove sign</u>: adenopathy above and below the inguinal (Poupart) ligament.
- <u>Anorectal syndrome</u>: May develop proctocolitis — bloody rectal discharge, anal pain, perianal or mucosal ulcers, constipation, fever and/or tenesmus.

DIAGNOSIS
- Often clinical presumptive diagnosis with clinical findings, risk factors & positive NAAT.
- **Nucleic acid amplification test (NAAT).** Cultures and serologic testing have low yield.

MANAGEMENT
- **<u>Doxycycline</u> treatment of choice — 100 orally twice daily for 21 days.** Test for all STIs & HIV.
- **<u>Azithromycin</u> alternative to Doxycycline & first line if pregnant** (1g orally once weekly x 3 weeks).
- Buboes may need needle aspiration or incision & drainage to avoid rupture or sinus tract formation.
- <u>Treatment of asymptomatic patients</u>: 7-day course of treatment.

GRANULOMA INGUINALE (DONOVANOSIS)

- *Klebsiella granulomatis.* Similar to Chancroid, Granuloma inguinale is exceedingly rare in the US. More common in India, New guinea, Australia, and Southern Africa.

CLINICAL MANIFESTATIONS

- **Painless genital ulcer: painless, progressive ulcerative lesion with rolled borders that is highly vascular and beefy red in appearance, without regional lymphadenopathy.**
- Visualization of **Donovan bodies** (safety-pin-shaped intracellular organisms) in monocytes on biopsy.

MANAGEMENT

- **Azithromycin 1 gram weekly until healed.** Doxycycline, Trimethoprim-sulfamethoxazole, Erythromycin. Aminoglycoside may be added. Pregnancy: Erythromycin or Azithromycin.

PAINLESS LESIONS

Lymphogranuloma venereum (LGV):
Chlamydia trachomatis **L1, L2 & L3 serovars**
- Small, shallow, **painless** ulcer or vesicle
- **Tender inguinal/femoral lymphadenopathy** (fluctuant buboes)
- **Management: Doxycycline** 100 mg PO bid x 21 days

Primary Syphilis
Treponema pallidum
- **Chancre**: painless indurated, clean-based ulcer
- **Nontender** inguinal lymphadenopathy (primary)
- **Management**: Penicillin G Benzathine; Doxycycline.

Granuloma inguinale (Donovanosis)
Klebsiella granulomatis
- **Painless ulcer**: papule that becomes a **beefy red ulcer**
- **No lymphadenopathy**
- **Azithromycin** 1g weekly until healed

Condyloma acuminata
- Painless fleshy warts

PAINFUL LESIONS

CHANCROID
Haemophilus ducreyi
- **Painful ulcer**: Multiple painful papules that ulcerate; deep undermined purulent ulcers
- **Tender** inguinal/femoral lymphadenopathy (fluctuant buboes).
- **Management**: Azithromycin 1 gram PO or Ceftriaxone 250 mg IM

GENITAL HERPES
Herpes simplex virus (HSV)
- **Multiple shallow, tender, painful lesions/ulcers that may be vesicular.** May have had prior lesions.
- **Management: Acyclovir or Valacyclovir**

CHANCROID

- **Sexually transmitted infection leading to genital ulcers, lymphadenopathy, & bubo formation.**
- Etiology: ***Haemophilus ducreyi,*** a gram-negative fastidious coccobacillus, is transmitted after a break in the skin. 10% coinfection with HSV or Syphilis in the US (rare in US and developed countries).
- Risk factors: most common in children and young adults.

CLINICAL MANIFESTATIONS
Incubation period 3-7 days.
- **[1] ≥1 painful genital ulcers** at the inoculation site (well-defined irregular borders that are sometimes undermined on an erythematous base, may be covered with a gray or yellow purulent exudate, & may bleed easily), followed by **[2] painful enlarged inguinal lymphadenopathy, which can liquefy and become [3] fluctuant (bubo formation).**

DIAGNOSIS
- Usually a clinical diagnosis (difficult to culture). PCR or immunochromatography.
- Must rule out HSV by (PCR or culture) and rule out Syphilis.

MANAGEMENT
- **Azithromycin 1g orally x 1 dose or Ceftriaxone (250 mg IM).** Alternatives include Ciprofloxacin (500 mg orally twice daily for 3 days or Erythromycin base (500 mg orally three times daily x 7 days).
- Fluctuant inguinal lymph nodes should be drained, usually by needle aspiration.

CAT SCRATCH DISEASE (CSD)

- Infectious disease caused by *Bartonella henselae,* usually characterized by [1] primary inoculation lesion, followed by [2] self-limited regional lymphadenopathy.
- *Bartonella henselae* transmitted from the scratch or bite from an infected cat, kitten, or exposure to cat fleas (2–4-week incubation period). Most common in children and young adults.

CLINICAL MANIFESTATIONS
- **[1] Erythematous or brown papule, nodule, or ulcer** at the inoculation site 3-10 days after inoculation → 1-3 weeks (7-60 days) later: **fever, headache, malaise → lymphadenopathy.**
- **[2] Lymphadenopathy often tender, with erythema of the overlying skin (especially axillary, epitrochlear,** cervical, supraclavicular, and submandibular lymph nodes). The lymphadenopathy may become suppurative. May last 1-2 months, resolving even without treatment.
- Atypical may involve various organs (neuroretinitis, neurologic, fever of unknown origin, etc.).

DIAGNOSIS
Based on clinical presentation & lab studies
- **Serologic: most common test used** — via ELISA or indirect immunofluorescence assay. **A negative test does not rule out CSD.** Empiric treatment usually given in those with a presumed diagnosis.
- Biopsy: of skin lesions or lymph node (not usually required) — PCR to detect bacterial DNA, Warthin-Starry silver staining & histology on the sample (neutrophilic infiltrate & granulomatous changes).

MANAGEMENT
- **Azithromycin first line for CSD.** Alternatives include Rifampin, Trimethoprim-sulfamethoxazole, & in adults, Ciprofloxacin. Although **some may improve without therapy,** treatment may shorten symptom duration & reduce the risk of developing systemic disease and/or long-term sequelae.
- **More serious infections:** (eg, fever of unknown origin, hepatosplenic disease) — **Rifampin plus Azithromycin.** Alternatives: Rifampin plus Gentamicin; higher doses of Azithromycin alone (adults).
- **Neurologic or ocular disease:** Doxycycline + Rifampin in adults & children ≥8 years of age. In children <8 years of age, Azithromycin or TMP-SMX may be substituted for Doxycycline.

SCARLET FEVER (SCARLATINA)

- Diffuse erythematous skin eruption due to **Group A *streptococcus* [GAS (*S. pyogenes*)]** infection.

PATHOPHYSIOLOGY
- Type IV (delayed) hypersensitivity reaction to a pyrogenic strain (**erythrogenic toxin** A, B, or C).

CLINICAL MANIFESTATIONS
- Fever, chills, **pharyngitis, dysphagia.** The rash often starts 1-2 days after the onset of pharyngitis.
- **Rash: diffuse erythema (resembles sunburn) blanches with pressure + multiple small (1-2 mm) papular elevations with a sandpaper texture.** The rash usually starts in the axillae & groin & then spreads to the trunk & extremities (usually spares the palms and soles); later it desquamates.
- **Flushed face with circumoral pallor & strawberry tongue (red tongue with enlarged papillae).**
- **Pastia's lines: linear petechial lesion** at pressure points, axillary, antecubital, abdominal, or inguinal areas.

DIAGNOSIS
- Clinical or testing for GABHS — eg, rapid strep, anti-streptolysin titer, throat culture (definitive).

MANAGEMENT
- **Penicillin G (IM) or Penicillin V potassium (PO) first line.** Amoxicillin alternative in children.
- **Penicillin allergy: Azithromycin, Clarithromycin, Clindamycin, or Cephalosporins.**
- Children may return to school or daycare 12-24 hours after antibiotic administration if afebrile.

ACUTE RHEUMATIC FEVER (ARF)

- Acute autoimmune inflammatory multi-systemic illness mainly affecting **children 5-15 years old.**

PATHOPHYSIOLOGY
- **Symptomatic or asymptomatic infection with Group A *Streptococcus* (Strep pyogenes) stimulates antibody production to host tissues & damages organs directly.**
- Symptoms usually present within 1-5 weeks (usually 2-3 weeks) of a group A streptococcal (GAS) tonsillopharyngitis (or streptococcal pyoderma in patients from tropical regions).

CLINICAL MANIFESTATIONS (5 MAJOR CRITERIA)
- **Polyarthritis: (75%) ≥2 joints affected** (simultaneous more diagnostic) **or migratory** (lower ⇨ upper joints). Medium/large joints most commonly affected (knees, hips, wrists, elbows, shoulders). **Heat, redness, swelling, & severe joint tenderness must be present.** Usually lasts 3-4 weeks. Joint pain (arthralgia) without other symptoms of arthritis doesn't classify as major.
- **Active carditis:** (40-60%) can affect the valves (especially mitral & aortic), myocardium (myocarditis) &/or pericardium (pericarditis). **Carditis confers great morbidity & mortality.**
- **Sydenham's chorea:** (<10%) "Saint Vitus dance" may occur 1-8 months after initial infection. Manifestations include sudden involuntary, jerky, non-rhythmic, purposeless movements especially involving the face, tongue, & arms. Usually resolves spontaneously. Most common in females.
- **Erythema marginatum:** often accompanies carditis. **Macular, erythematous, non-pruritic annular rash with rounded, sharply demarcated borders (may have central clearing).** Most commonly seen on the trunk & extremities (not the face). Crops last hours-days before disappearing.
- **Subcutaneous nodules** firm painless lesions over joints (extensor surfaces), scalp, & spinal column.
- Other findings not associated with Jones criteria: abdominal pain, facial tics/grimaces, epistaxis.

DIAGNOSIS

JONES CRITERIA FOR RHEUMATIC FEVER	(2 Major OR 1 major + 2 minor)
MAJOR CRITERIA	**MINOR CRITERIA**
1. **J**oint **(migratory polyarthritis)**	**CLINICAL**
2. **O**h my heart **(active carditis)**	Fever (≥101.3° F/≥ 38.5° C)
3. **N**odules (subcutaneous)	Arthralgia (joint pain)
4. **E**rythema marginatum	**LABORATORY**
5. **S**ydenham's chorea	↑acute phase reactants (↑ESR, CRP, leukocytosis)
	ECG: prolonged PR interval
PLUS	
Supporting evidence of a recent group A streptococcal infection: - Positive throat culture for GAS (definitive) or - Rapid streptococcal antigen or - Elevated/increased streptococcal Ab titers (eg, antideoxynuclease B or antistreptolysin O)	

MANAGEMENT
Treatment of ARF consists of [1] symptomatic relief of arthritis with anti-inflammatory therapy & [2] eradication of GAS infection with antibiotic therapy.
- **Anti-inflammatory:** Aspirin (2-6 weeks with taper) **or NSAIDs (eg, Naproxen, Ibuprofen).** Corticosteroids may be indicated in severe cases & in some patients who develop carditis.
- **Antibiotics: Intramuscular Penicillin G benzathine antibiotic of choice** both in acute phase & for prophylaxis to prevent worsening heart disease. All patients (even if presenting with ARF) should be treated with antibiotics. Alternatives: **Cephalosporins for mild reactions to Penicillin. Macrolides (Azithromycin, Clarithromycin) or Clindamycin for patients with anaphylaxis, other IgE-mediated reactions, or severe delayed reactions to Penicillin.**

COMPLICATIONS
- **Rheumatic valvular disease — mitral (75-80%), aortic** (30%); tricuspid & pulmonic (5%).
- PANDAS Pediatric Autoimmune Neuropsychiatric Disorders Associated with Streptococcal infection: Obsessive compulsive disorder &/or tics due to autoantibodies after streptococcal infection.

ROCKY MOUNTAIN SPOTTED FEVER (RMSF)

- Potentially fatal but usually curable tick-borne disease caused by *Rickettsia rickettsii*.
- Mortality rate is ~70% in untreated patients.

EPIDEMIOLOGY
- **Despite its name, the diagnosis is most common in the southeastern and south-central United States especially in the spring & summer**, due to more outdoor exposure.
- Most cases in the United States originate in Oklahoma, Tennessee, Arkansas, and the Carolinas.
- Seasonal variation — Most cases of RMSF occur in the spring and early summer when outdoor activity is most frequent. In Arizona, cases transmitted by the vector *R. sanguineus* may peak in July and September.

PATHOPHYSIOLOGY
- *Rickettsia rickettsii* — **gram-negative, obligate, intracellular coccobacillus with an affinity for infecting the vascular endothelial cells, leading to vascular injury, microhemorrhages, microinfarcts,** disseminated inflammation, loss of barrier function, and altered vascular permeability throughout the body.
- Transmission of *R. rickettsii* is believed to occur within several hours of feeding after a bite from an infected tick, with a rapid entry of the bacteria into human endothelial cells.
- Up to one-third of patients with proven RMSF do not recall a recent tick bite or recent tick contact.

Tick vectors:
- ***Dermacentor variabilis* (American dog tick), *Dermacentor andersoni* (Rocky Mountain wood tick)** is the primary vector in the mountain states west of the Mississippi River.
- Brown dog tick *(Rhipicephalus sanguineus)* in Arizona.

CLINICAL MANIFESTATIONS
- Incubation period of 2-14 days after tick bite. Because the tick bite may be brief (as early as 6-10 hours of tick attachment), a lack of history of a tick bite does not exclude this diagnosis.
- **Symptoms classically include the triad of [1] fever, [2] headache, and [3] a petechial or maculopapular rash** but may also include lymphadenopathy, central nervous system changes (eg, confusion or nuchal rigidity), myalgias and arthralgias, hepatitis, vomiting, and cardiovascular instability.

Early nonspecific symptoms:
- **Influenza-like symptoms** — **fever, headache (often severe), nausea, vomiting, myalgia, malaise, anorexia**, chills, arthralgias, cough, lethargy, or seizures followed by rash. Fever may be accompanied by relative bradycardia. Prominent abdominal pain may be seen in children.

Rash: 88-90%.
- Develops ~2-4 days after fever onset — **blanching, erythematous macular rash** (macules 1-4 mm in size) **first on distal extremities (eg, wrists & ankles), then spreads centripetally (extremities to trunk),** face is usually not affected. **Palms & soles involvement common** but occurs later in the disease. **The rash starts as faint macules and become papular; 50% progress to petechiae.**

Associated symptoms:
- **Bilateral periorbital or pedal edema (especially in children).**
- Conjunctivitis, & retinal abnormalities, confusion, focal neurologic signs, encephalitis, ARDS, Encephalitis, cardiac disorders, myocarditis, bradycardia, hypotension, bleeding disorders.

DIAGNOSIS
Empiric diagnosis and early initiation of therapy:
- **A presumptive clinical diagnosis of Rocky Mountain spotted fever (RMSF) is initially made** based upon clinical signs and (eg, influenza-like symptoms or the triad of fever, headache, and a petechial or maculopapular rash, with or without history of tick exposure) if they reside in or traveled to endemic areas, especially in the warmer months, **do not wait for serologies to initiate treatment.**
- **Therapy should be initiated ideally within 5 days of symptom onset.** Therefore, most patients will require empiric therapy since RMSF can rarely be confirmed or ruled out in its early phase.
- In patients without the classic rash, clinicians should **not** wait for the skin rash to develop before initiating treatment.
- The clinical diagnosis can be confirmed through serologic testing or through the use of Polymerase chain reaction (PCR) testing or special stains on a skin biopsy.

Serologies:
- Indirect immunofluorescence antibody test for IgM and IgG antibodies to *R. rickettsii.* **Serologic testing is usually not helpful during the first 5 days of symptoms (when therapy should be initiated), because the antibody response is not yet detectable**
- It is crucial to consider repeat testing after the resolution of symptoms, as serologic tests may be negative if testing occurs early in the course of illness.
- Clinically available Polymerase chain reaction testing of blood samples for RMSF may also be helpful to confirm the diagnosis, but a negative test does not rule out rickettsial infection.

Laboratory evaluation:
- **Thrombocytopenia,** pancytopenia, or mildly elevated hepatic transaminase levels.
- **Mild Hyponatremia** may occur due to release of antidiuretic hormone as an appropriate response to hypovolemia and reduced tissue perfusion. Common in patients with CNS involvement.
- CSF: normal or low glucose & pleocytosis (increased cell count). White blood count (WBC) of <100 cells per microL with either a polymorphonuclear or lymphocytic predominance.

MANAGEMENT
- **Doxycycline first-line treatment for adults and children (even if <8 years of age)** 100 mg twice daily for at least 5-7 days or for at least 3 days after fever subsides, whichever is longer. **Doxycycline is used to treat RMSF even in pregnant women,** since there is increasing evidence of the relative safety of Doxycycline in pregnancy compared with older Tetracyclines & the life-threatening potential of RMSF.
- If the diagnosis of RMSF is suspected, antimicrobial therapy should be initiated as soon as possible; delays in treatment of >5 days have been associated with an increased risk of mortality. Most patients will require empiric therapy based upon clinical judgment and the epidemiologic setting.
- **Chloramphenicol is the only known alternative agent for the treatment of RMSF.**
  Adverse effects include aplastic anemia, blood dyscrasias, and gray baby syndrome associated with third trimester usage of Chloramphenicol.

PREVENTION
- Prevention of infection requires careful attention to tick avoidance, including insect repellant, long clothing, and checking for ticks after any outdoor activities in endemic areas.
- Early detection and removal of attached ticks is the best way to prevent disease transmission.
- **Tick removal:** use fine-tipped tweezers to **pull up firmly and repeatedly on the tick's mouth part, not the tick's body, until the tick releases its hold.**
- Prophylactic therapy with Doxycycline or other antibiotic is **not** recommended following tick exposure (<2% of ticks in endemic areas are infected with *R. rickettsii).*

SPIROCHETAL DISEASES

SYPHILIS

- **Chronic infection caused by the corkscrew-shaped (spirochete) *Treponema pallidum.***
- Known as "the great imitator" because the rash & disease can present in many different ways similar to other diseases.

TRANSMISSION
- **Direct contact of a mucocutaneous lesion via sexual contact (eg, vaginal, anogenital, and orogenital).** May also be transmitted to the fetus via the placenta.

PATHOPHYSIOLOGY
- *T. pallidum* enters tissues from direct contact, forming a chancre at the inoculation site and from there, goes to the regional lymph nodes before disseminating.

CLINICAL MANIFESTATIONS
[1] Primary Syphilis (10–90-day duration)
> **Chancre: solitary painless (nontender) 1-2 cm indurated, clean based, punched out ulcer at or near the site of inoculation with a non-exudative base and raised, indurated edges/margins (usually begins as a papule that ulcerates) within 2-3 weeks after exposure.** Multiple lesions are also possible, particularly in the setting of HIV infection. Chancres heal spontaneously without scarring on average within 3-6 weeks (even without medical management). With treatment, they can resolve within days.
- **Nontender regional lymphadenopathy** (often bilateral) near the chancre site lasting 3-4 weeks.
- Neurosyphilis can occur at any time following infection.

[2] Secondary Syphilis
Symptoms may occur a few weeks to 6 months after the initial symptoms.
- **Maculopapular rash is the most characteristic finding of secondary Syphilis — painless diffuse maculopapular or papulosquamous exanthematous lesions often on the face or trunk and typically also involving the palms or soles (involvement of the palms & soles common),** with individual lesions that are discrete copper, red, or reddish-brown, measuring 0.5-2 cm in diameter.
- Systemic symptoms: fever, headache, malaise, anorexia, **alopecia.** Hepatitis (↑ alkaline phosphatase).
- **Generalized lymphadenopathy** (may be tender), arthritis, meningitis, headache,
- **Condyloma lata: wart-like, moist lesions involving the mucous membranes & other moist areas.** Especially near the chancre site. Highly contagious.

Latent (asymptomatic) Syphilis: early (<1 year); late (>1 year)
- Without diagnosis and treatment, Syphilis eventually progresses to a latent stage characterized by a (1) lack of symptoms, (2) positive serologic tests for Syphilis, and (3) normal CSF examination.

[3] Tertiary (late) Syphilis
May occur from 1-30 years after initial infection or after latent infection.
- **Cardiovascular: aortitis,** aortic regurgitation or aneurysms, coronary artery narrowing & thrombosis.
- **Gumma:** noncancerous granulomas on skin & body tissues (eg, bones).
- **Late neurosyphilis:** headache, aseptic meningitis. General paresis, a syndrome consisting of progressive dementia, seizures, and psychiatric symptoms; vision/hearing loss, incontinence; **Tabes dorsalis**: demyelination of posterior columns and spinal nerve roots, leading to areflexia, burning pain, weakness, severe unprovoked radicular pain, as well as ataxia caused by loss of proprioception. Meningovascular involvement can cause hemiplegia, aphasia, or seizures secondary to inflammation of the middle cerebral artery and its branches.
- **Argyll-Robertson pupil: bilateral, small, irregular pupils that constrict with accommodation but do not constrict (does not react) when exposed to bright light.**

DIAGNOSIS

Nontreponemal tests (screening):
- **RPR (Rapid Plasma Reagin).** These tests look at titers (eg, a positive test indicates a titer of ≥1:32). RPR is usually positive 4-6 weeks after infection. Changes in titers also help to determine therapeutic response. False positives: pregnancy, autoimmune disease.
- **VDRL:** Venereal Disease Research Laboratory.
- **Because nontreponemal tests (RPR and VDRL) are nonspecific, a positive RPR or VDRL test must be confirmed by specific treponemal testing (eg, FTA-ABS).**
- False positives can be seen with antiphospholipid syndrome, pregnancy, tuberculosis, *Rickettsial* infections (eg, Rocky Mountain spotted fever), and FTA-ABS remains elevated for life after a patient's first infection (use RPR titers instead). False negatives when serum antibodies are really high.

Treponemal testing (confirmatory):
- **Treponemal-specific tests include fluorescent treponemal antibody absorption (FTA-ABS)** [a positive titer >1:4 indicated current Syphilis], *T. pallidum* **particle agglutination**, or immunoassay.

Darkfield microscopy
- Allows for **direct visualization of *T. pallidum* from chancre, mucosal lesions, or condyloma lata.**

MANAGEMENT
- **Penicillin is the treatment of choice for all stages of Syphilis.**

Primary, secondary, & early latent (without evidence of neurosyphilis):
- **Intramuscular Penicillin G benzathine 2.4 million units (single dose).**
- **Alternatives in patients allergic to Penicillin:** Doxycycline **100 mg orally twice daily for 14 days,** Ceftriaxone 1-2 gm IM or IV daily for 10-14 days or Tetracycline or Azithromycin.

Late Syphilis: (tertiary or late latent)
- **Intramuscular Penicillin G benzathine 2.4 million units once weekly x 3 weeks.**
- **Alternative: Doxycycline (100 mg orally twice daily for 28 days)** or Ceftriaxone (2 g IV or IM daily for 10 to 14 days) if the patient cannot be desensitized.

Ocular, otic, or Neurosyphilis:
- **IV Penicillin G aqueous preferred** — 3-4 million units IV every 4 hours, or 18-24 million units per day by continuous infusion for 10 to 14 days
- **Patients with Penicillin allergy who are pregnant,** present with neurosyphilis, have cardiovascular manifestation of late syphilis, or have treatment failure **should be tested for Penicillin allergy and desensitized** (if immediate-type reaction) **or rechallenged** (if delayed reaction) with Penicillin.

MONITORING
- All patients with Syphilis should be tested for HIV and other STIs.
- All patients should be reexamined clinically & serologically at 6 months and 12 months after treatment. Patients with HIV may be monitored more frequently.
- A nontreponemal titer should be obtained prior to initiating therapy. A fourfold decline in the nontreponemal titer within 6 months is considered an acceptable response.

JARISCH-HERXHEIMER REACTION
- **An acute, self-limited febrile reaction that usually occurs within the first 24 hours after receiving therapy for a spirochetal infection** (eg, Syphilis, Lyme disease).
- It is thought to be due to the release of cytokines and immune complexes from killed organisms.
- Presentation: **fever, chills, headache, myalgias, hypotension, & worsening of the rash may occur.**

Management
- Is self-limited and usually resolves without intervention in 12 to 24 hours but NSAIDS or antipyretics may be used for symptoms.

LYME DISEASE

- Arthropod-borne disease due to *Borreliella* (previously referred to as ***Borrelia burgdorferi***), a gram-negative **spirochete**). Most common in late spring & summer (when the nymphs feed).

PATHOPHYSIOLOGY
- **Most cases are transmitted by the *Ixodes scapularis* (deer tick) in the nymphal phase** — most common sources are the white-tailed deer & white-footed mouse.
- The highest likelihood of transmission is if the tick is engorged and/or has been attached for at least 72 hours (minimum of 24 hours needed for transmission).
- **Most common in the Northeast states** (CT, NY, NJ, MA), Midwest, & Mid-Atlantic regions of the US.
- Coinfection of *B. burgdorferi* with *Babesia microti*, and/or *Anaplasma phagocytophilum* occurs in some patients since these organisms share the tick vector (*Ixodes* spp.).

CLINICAL MANIFESTATIONS
- **Early localized (stage 1): erythema chronicum migrans** (90%) — **expanding, warm, annular, slightly raised erythematous rash that may develop central clearing (bull's eye or target appearance)** or may be uniformly red, within a month of & around the area of the tick bite.
- **Constitutional (viral-like) symptoms may accompany Erythema migrans** — eg, **fatigue, headache, low-grade fever, malaise, myalgia, arthralgias, and/or lymphadenopathy.** The presence of a high-grade fever in a patient with suspected Lyme disease suggests another co-infecting tick-borne disease (eg, *Anaplasma phagocytophilum*, *Babesia spp.*) or an alternate diagnosis.

- **Early disseminated (stage 2)** (1-12 weeks): **neurologic:** cranial nerve palsies [**CN VII/Facial nerve palsy most common neurologic manifestation) and bilateral facial palsy is pathognomonic,** headache, **Aseptic meningitis,** weakness, neuropathy; **Cardiac: AV block most common cardiac manifestation,** pericarditis, & arrhythmias; **Cutaneous: Multiple erythema migrans lesions.** Ocular: conjunctivitis, keratitis, uveitis. Arthralgia or myalgia.

- **Late disease (Stage 3): intermittent or persistent arthritis** most common feature of late Lyme, especially of the large joints (**knee most common**), **persistent neurological symptoms** — eg, subtle cognitive changes, distal paresthesias, spinal radicular pain, & subacute encephalitis.

DIAGNOSIS
- **Clinical:** especially in early localized Lyme disease — **patients with the rash of erythema migrans residing in or who have recently traveled to an endemic area should be treated for Lyme (patients with the rash of EM are often seronegative in this early stage).**

- **Serologic testing: ELISA followed by Western Blot if ELISA is positive or equivocal.** IgM &/or IgG antibodies to *B. burgdorferi* are employed as an adjunct to patients with clinical symptoms suggestive of Lyme disease as it only tells if a patient has been infected with the spirochete (does not determine if the person has an active infection). Serologic testing is used in patients who fit all 3 criteria:
  - Reside in or travel to an endemic area PLUS
  - Risk factor for exposure to ticks PLUS
  - Symptoms consistent with early disseminated or late Lyme disease (arthritis, meningitis, cranial nerve palsy, carditis, radiculopathy, or mononeuritis).

  Because serologic testing takes weeks to become positive and does not distinguish acute from past infection, **serologic testing is not performed in:**
  - **patients with an erythema migrans** rash (patients with the rash of EM residing in or who have recently traveled to an endemic area should be treated for Lyme)
  - screening of asymptomatic patients living in endemic areas
  - patients with non-specific symptoms only.
- False positive ELISA: other spirochetal diseases: syphilis, yaws; viral or bacterial illnesses, & other Borrelial species.

MANAGEMENT
Early localized disease:
- **Doxycycline** first-line for nonpregnant patients & children >8 years of age **(100 mg orally twice daily for 10 days)** is also effective vs. coinfecting pathogens, such as *A. phagocytophilum.*
- **Amoxicillin or Cefuroxime axetil** for pregnant patients and children <8 years of age (14-day course).
- Macrolides (Azithromycin or Erythromycin) if Doxycycline is contraindicated & Penicillin allergic.

Early disseminated disease: multiple EM lesions, and/or neurologic or cardiac manifestations.
- **Doxycycline** for 10 days. **Amoxicillin & Cefuroxime for 14 days are alternatives**
- **Neurologic Lyme disease manifesting with meningitis, cranial neuropathy, and/or sensory or motor radiculoneuropathy: oral Doxycycline or IV Ceftriaxone are options for Meningitis.**

Late or severe:
- **IV Ceftriaxone if second/third AV heart block, syncope, dyspnea, chest pain, severe CNS disease, other than CN 7 palsy.** Ceftriaxone 2 g IV per day for 14 days (14-28 days). Cefotaxime.
- Lyme arthritis: Most patients with Lyme arthritis should receive initial therapy with an **oral regimen for 28 days — eg, Doxycycline (preferred),** Amoxicillin, or possible Cefuroxime.

PROPHYLAXIS FOR LYME DISEASE
- **Doxycycline 200 mg x 1 dose** may be given within 72 hours of tick removal & ≥20% rate of tick infection with *B. burgdorferi* in the area (eg, any location within the top 12 endemic states) for engorged ticks or ticks that have been presumed to be attached for ≥36 hours. Children >8 years [single dose of 4 mg per kg of Doxycycline (maximal dose of 200 mg)].
- If Doxycycline cannot be used (eg, allergic, contraindicated, children <8y), no prophylaxis is given.
- **Tick removal**: use fine-tipped tweezers to **pull up firmly and repeatedly on the tick's mouth part, not the tick's body, until the tick releases its hold.**

TULAREMIA

- **Zoonotic infection caused by _Francisella tularensis_ — aerobic gram-negative coccobacillus.**
- Transmission: **rabbits important reservoir, ticks, deer flies,** fleas, or handling animal tissues.

CLINICAL MANIFESTATIONS
Nonspecific symptoms: eg, fever, chills, headache, and malaise. Most are asymptomatic
- **Ulceroglandular most common type** — fever, headache, & nausea followed by a **single papule at the site of inoculation, followed by ulceration of papule with central eschar formation & tender regional lymphadenopathy.** Ulcers of the hand or arm most common after animal exposure. Ulcers of the head, trunk, or legs most common after tick exposure. Splenomegaly.
- **Glandular:** tender regional lymphadenopathy without skin lesions. Most common in children.
- **Oculoglandular:** if splashed in the eye with infected material — **conjunctivitis [eye pain, photophobia, & tearing] + regional lymphadenopathy** (preauricular, postauricular, cervical).
- Pharyngeal: fever and sore throat following ingestion of contaminated food or water.
- Typhoidal: ingestion of infected meat (eg, undercooked rabbit meat) followed by fever & GI symptoms (nausea, vomiting, diarrhea). Mesenteric adenopathy, diffuse abdominal tenderness, pharyngitis.
- Pneumonia, meningitis, pericarditis.

DIAGNOSIS
- **Serologies elevated titers.** Cultures not usually performed (they produce dangerous spores).

MANAGEMENT
- **Severe infection: Aminoglycosides (Gentamicin or Streptomycin) first line.**
Mild or moderate:
- **Adults:** oral Fluoroquinolone (eg, Ciprofloxacin). Doxycycline is an alternative.
- **Children: Gentamicin preferred.** An oral Fluoroquinolone is an acceptable alternative for children.

DISEASES WITH ESCHARS: Tularemia, Anthrax, Leishmaniasis, Coccidioidomycosis, Mucormycosis

ANTIFUNGAL MEDICATIONS

POLYENE ANTIFUNGALS Nystatin (topical, oral); Amphotericin B

MOA: binds to cell membrane sterols, increasing the permeability/fragility of the cell membrane.

AMPHOTERICIN B
- INDICATIONS: antifungal of choice for most <u>invasive or life-threatening fungal infections.</u>
- ADVERSE EFFECTS: **fever/chills during infusion,** electrolyte abnormalities ($\downarrow$K, $\downarrow$Mg), **nephrotoxicity** & hematologic toxicity (anemia), azotemia ($\uparrow$BUN/creatinine), cardiac arrhythmias.
- **Lipid-based Ampho B:** — advantages: high tissue concentrations, decreased infusion-related reactions, marked **decrease in nephrotoxicity** but VERY expensive.

NYSTATIN
- **Indications:** topically — **Cutaneous candida:** diaper rash/intertriginous Candida (eg, powder, cream, or ointment); **Oral candidiasis (Thrush) Nystatin "swish and swallow" suspension.** Vaginal.
- Because of poor oral bioavailability, there are no significant drug interactions.

"AZOLES" ANTIFUNGALS

- Imidazoles: **Clotrimazole (Lotrimin), Ketoconazole (Nizoral), Econazole, Miconazole**
- Triazoles: **Fluconazole (Diflucan), Itraconazole, Voriconazole, Posaconazole**

MOA: inhibits ergosterol synthesis (ergosterols are essential for fungal cell membrane stability). Inhibition of fungal 14-α-sterol demethylase.

INDICATIONS: Candidiasis, Cryptococcus, Histoplasmosis, Coccidioidomycosis, Tinea (topical).
- **Fluconazole – drug of choice for noninvasive Candida & Cryptococcal infections,** water soluble, **good for urine & CSF infections.** Fluconazole is eliminated by the kidney.
- **Voriconazole** EXTENDED spectrum (covers <u>Aspergillus</u>). **Voriconazole drug of choice for invasive Aspergillus.** Does not cover Mucorales species well.
- **Itraconazole:** EXTENDED spectrum (covers <u>Aspergillus</u>). **Drug of choice for noninvasive Histoplasmosis, Blastomycosis, & Coccidioidomycosis** (Adverse effect: may cause CHF).
- **Ketoconazole & Itraconazole** - lipid soluble, **poor CSF penetration,** inhibits CP450.

ADVERSE EFFECTS
- **Fluconazole:** hepatitis, nausea, rash, alopecia, headache.
- **Ketoconazole: suppression of testosterone & cortisol** (used to treat refractory Cushing's). **$\uparrow$LFTs**

ALLYLAMINES [Terbinafine; Butenafine]

MOA: inhibits ergosterol synthesis by inhibiting fungal squalene epoxidase.
INDICATIONS: **dermatophyte infections:**
- **Onychomycosis:** Terbinafine PO. **Tinea** (Corporis, Pedis, Cruris): **Terbinafine or Butenafine topical.**

GRISEOFULVIN

MOA: **inhibits fungal cell mitosis preventing proliferation & function.**
INDICATIONS: **Tinea infection: capitis (first line),** cruris, pedis, unguium.
  Give with fatty meals to increase absorption.
ADVERSE EFFECTS: **Hepatitis. Teratogenic** including males — males must avoid attempting to conceive for 6 months after treatment.

ECHINOCANDINS [CASPOFUNGIN, ANIDULAFUNGIN, MICAFUNGIN]

MOA: **Inhibits fungal cell wall glucan synthesis.** Glucan normally provides cell wall strength.
INDICATIONS: includes **azole- & AmB-resistant strains of Candidiasis & Aspergillus.**
Adverse effects: fever, thrombophlebitis, headache, $\uparrow$LFTs, rash, flushing. only IV - very expensive.

FLUCYTOSINE

Mechanism of activity:
- Metabolized by fungi (not humans) to 5-fluoruracil (5-FU).
- **The antimetabolite: 5-FU inhibits fungal DNA and RNA synthesis.**

Indications:
- **Cryptococcal meningitis** Clinical use is confined to **combination therapy with Amphotericin B for Cryptococcal meningitis.**

CHARACTERISTICS OF CLASSIC FUNGAL INFECTIONS		
ORGANISM	**MORPHOLOGY**	**CLINICAL SYNDROMES**
Candida	• **Pseudohyphae & budding yeast**	• **Mucocutaneous infections** • **Invasive infections** (eg, Candidemia due to vascular catheter) • **Mild disease: Fluconazole** • **Severe:** Amphotericin B
Blastomyces	• **Mississippi & Ohio river valley** (occupational or recreational outdoor activities) • **Histology: Round, broad-based budding yeast with thick refractile double walls.**	• Lesions involving the **lungs (Pneumonia),** • **Skin (verrucous lesions)** • **Bone (Osteomyelitis).** **Management** • **Mild disease: Itraconazole** • **Severe: Amphotericin B** then Voriconazole.
Cryptococcus	• **India ink stain: budding encapsulated yeast.** • **Cryptococcal CSF antigen**	• Pneumonia • Meningitis in immunocompromised **eg, HIV with CD4 count ≤100 cells/μL,** Management: • **Amphotericin B plus Flucytosine** for a minimum of 2 weeks, followed by **oral Fluconazole**
Coccidioides	• **Spherules with endospores** • SW United States	• Transient pulmonary syndrome followed by meninges. • **CNS disease: Fluconazole** • **Severe disease: Amphotericin B**
Histoplasma	• **Mississippi & Ohio river valley** Histology: • **Narrow-based, ovoid, budding yeast cells**; seen within macrophages.	• Mostly subclinical but may cause Pneumonia with mediastinal or hilar LAD • Dissemination Management: • **Mild: Itraconazole** • **Severe: Amphotericin**
Aspergillus	Histology • **Septate hyphae with regular branching at acute (45°) angles.**	• **Allergic Bronchopulmonary Aspergillosis:** glucocorticoids (mainstay of treatment) + antifungal **Itraconazole.** Voriconazole. • **Severe/Invasive: Voriconazole.** • **Aspergilloma: surgical resection** if symptoms; observation if no symptoms.

CANDIDIASIS

Candida albicans is part of the normal GI & GU flora but **most common opportunistic pathogen.**
- **Esophagitis:** substernal odynophagia, gastroesophageal reflux, epigastric pain, nausea, vomiting.
  - Endoscopy: white linear plaques/erosions.
  - Management: **oral Fluconazole first-line treatment.** Voriconazole, Caspofungin.

- **Oropharyngeal (Thrush): friable white plaques (may leave behind erythema if scraped).**
  Management: **Clotrimazole troches, Miconazole mucoadhesive buccal tablets, Nystatin liquid swish and swallow** are all options.

- **Intertrigo:** cutaneous infection most common in moist, macerated areas. **Pruritic rash <u>beefy red erythema</u>** with **distinct, scalloped borders & <u>satellite lesions.</u>**
  Management: **Topical azole creams (eg, Clotrimazole, Ketoconazole, Miconazole).** Keep area dry.

- **Fungemia or Endocarditis:** seen in immunocompromised patients, ± indwelling catheters.
  Management: **IV Amphotericin B. Caspofungin if severe. ± IV Fluconazole if mild.**

DIAGNOSIS
- Potassium Hydroxide (KOH) smear: **budding yeast, hyphae, & pseudohyphae.** Clinical diagnosis.

VULVOVAGINAL CANDIDIASIS

- ***Candida* is considered part of the normal vaginal flora, but overgrowth of the organism can result in vulvovaginitis.**
- Risk factors: Diabetes mellitus, HIV, recent antibiotic use, corticosteroid use, elevated estrogen levels (eg, pregnancy), & immunosuppression. Many women have no identifiable risk factors.

MICROBIOLOGY
- ***<u>Candida albicans</u>*** accounts for 80-92% of episodes of vulvovaginal candidiasis;
- *Candida glabrata* is the second most common species.

CLINICAL MANIFESTATIONS
- **Vulvovaginitis: vulvar pruritus, burning, soreness, irritation, and erythema.**
  Dysuria and dyspareunia. May be associated with a vaginal discharge.
Physical examination:
- **Vulva and/or vagina erythema**; may have vulvar excoriation and fissures.
- **Vaginal discharge may be scant or absent; when present, it is classically white, thick (clumpy, curd-like or cottage-cheese-like) & adherent to the vaginal walls with no or minimal odor.**

DIAGNOSIS
Wet mount: presence of *Candida* on wet mount (preferred).
- **Vaginal pH: normal vaginal pH <4.5.**
- **Microscopy:** adding 10% potassium hydroxide (KOH) to wet mount specimen — **budding yeast, pseudohyphae, and hyphae.**

MANAGEMENT
- **[1] Topical azoles (eg, Miconazole, Clotrimazole) or [2] single dose of oral Fluconazole 150 mg.**
- **Pregnant: topical azoles for 7 days (eg, Miconazole, Clotrimazole).** Avoid oral Fluconazole.
- Persistent vaginitis: Oral Fluconazole weekly.

CRYPTOCOCCOSIS

ETIOLOGY
- *Cryptococcus neoformans* or *C. gattii* — encapsulated budding round yeasts.

TRANSMISSION
- **Inhalation of pigeon & bird droppings;** also found in the soil.
- **Infection usually begins in the lungs** and may spread to the brain.

RISK FACTORS
- <u>**Most common in immunocompromised states:**</u> eg, **HIV with CD4 count ≤100 cells/μL**), hematologic malignancy, transplant recipients.

CLINICAL MANIFESTATIONS
[1] Pulmonary:
- **Pneumonia** (cough, pleuritic chest pain, dyspnea), nodules, abscess, or pleural effusions.

[2] Meningoencephalitis:
- **Cryptococcus most common cause of fungal meningitis** — headache, fever, malaise, & meningeal signs (neck stiffness, nausea, vomiting, photophobia).
- **Meningeal signs uncommon in patients with HIV.**

[3] Skin involvement:
- Skin lesions may be seen if disseminated.

DIAGNOSIS
Lumbar puncture:
- <u>**Fungal CSF pattern**</u> — <u>**increased WBC (lymphocytes)**</u>, <u>**decreased glucose**</u>, & increased protein. Lumbar puncture is performed even if pulmonary or dermatologic symptoms.
- <u>**CSF evaluation:**</u> **Cryptococcal antigen in CSF** (via latex agglutination or ELISA) or **visualization of budding <u>encapsulated yeast on India ink staining</u>.**
- Culture on Sabouraud agar.

Other laboratory tests:
- Cultures: may have positive blood cultures in HIV patients, respiratory cultures.
- Positive serum cryptococcal antigen.

MANAGEMENT
Meningoencephalitis:
- <u>**Induction phase**</u> **with Amphotericin B plus Flucytosine for a minimum of 2 weeks, followed by <u>consolidation phase</u> with oral Fluconazole for a minimum of 8 weeks.**
Pneumonia if immunocompetent:
- Fluconazole (400 mg daily) or Itraconazole for 6-12 months.

PROPHYLAXIS IN HIV
- Early initiation of Antiretroviral therapy best prophylaxis.
- Select patients: If positive cryptococcal antigen screening, Fluconazole may be used in adults with CD4 counts <100 cells/μL.

HISTOPLASMOSIS

- *__Histoplasma capsulatum__* — dimorphic oval yeast that is <u>not</u> encapsulated despite its name.
- <u>Transmission</u>: **inhalation of moist soil containing bird & bat feces in the Mississippi & Ohio river valleys.** Also seen with demolition, people who explore caves (spelunkers), or excavators in those areas.
- <u>Pathophysiology</u>: once inhaled, *H. capsulatum* is ingested by alveolar macrophages & grows within the phagosome, where yeast remains viable in macrophages & can disseminate via the macrophages.
- <u>Risk factors</u>: immunocompromised states — **AIDS-defining illness especially if CD4 is ≤150 cells/µL.**

CLINICAL MANIFESTATIONS

- **Asymptomatic: most patients** (flu-like symptoms if they become symptomatic).
- **Pneumonia** (atypical). Fever, nonproductive cough, myalgias. **Can mimic Tuberculosis.**
- <u>Dissemination</u>: if immunocompromised: hepatosplenomegaly, fever, headache, anorexia, weight loss, mucocutaneous lesions (eg, oropharyngeal ulcers), bloody diarrhea, adrenal insufficiency.

DIAGNOSIS

- <u>Labs:</u> increased alkaline phosphatase & LDH. Pancytopenia.
- <u>Chest radiographs:</u> pulmonary infiltrates; hilar or mediastinal lymphadenopathy.
- **PCR Antigen testing via sputum or urine — highly specific.**
- **Histology: <u>narrow-based, ovoid, budding yeast cells</u>, measuring 2-5 micrometers in diameter.**
- **Cultures most specific test** — sputum; blood culture positivity if disseminated/HIV.

MANAGEMENT

- **Asymptomatic: no treatment required (eg, pulmonary symptoms <4 weeks or nodules).**
- **Mild-moderate disease: Itraconazole first line treatment.** Posoconazole or Voriconazole.
- **Severe disease: Amphotericin B.** Also used if Itraconazole therapy is ineffective.

BLASTOMYCOSIS

- *__Blastomyces dermatitidis__* — pyogranulomatous fungal infection. It is a fungus in nature, mold in tissues.

RISK FACTORS

- Occurs **most commonly in <u>immunocompetent men</u> involved in occupational or recreational outdoor activities (around <u>soil or decaying wood</u>) in close proximity to waterways in Central & Eastern US** (eg, Mississippi & Ohio river basins or Great Lakes). HIV.

CLINICAL MANIFESTATIONS

- **[1] Pulmonary: lungs are the most common site of involvement. Many are asymptomatic.** Chronic disease: **flu-like symptoms** — cough with or without sputum production, dyspnea, headache, fever. **Pneumonia** — high fever, chest pain, productive cough.
- **[2] Cutaneous: papules progressing to <u>verrucous, crusted, or ulcerated lesions</u>** which expand (may leave a central scar when healed). Skin most common site of extrapulmonary disease.
- **[3] Disseminated: most common in the lungs, skin, bone [Osteomyelitis (eg, vertebral, pelvic, or rib pain)], & genitourinary system (Prostatitis or Epididymitis).** Brain abscess.

DIAGNOSIS

- **Urine antigen** & specimens (eg, sputum, bronchoalveolar lavage [BAL] fluid) for direct microscopy, culture, & histopathology — **<u>round broad-based budding yeast</u> with <u>thick, refractile double walls</u>.** Potassium hydroxide wet preparation or Calcofluor-white staining used on the specimens.
- <u>CXR</u>: **alveolar infiltrates or a mass lesion** (can mimic Bronchogenic carcinoma), ± Pleural effusions.

MANAGEMENT

- **Mild-moderate: Itraconazole first-line treatment.** Posaconazole, Isavuconazole, or Voriconazole.
- **Severe: lipid formulation of Amphotericin B** if rapidly progressive, AIDS-related or CNS disease (eg, meningitis). Following initial Amphotericin B therapy, transition to Voriconazole.

ASPERGILLOSIS

- Allergy, lung invasion, cutaneous infection, or extrapulmonary dissemination caused by species of _Aspergillus fumigatus_, **a fungus that most commonly affects the lungs, sinuses, & the CNS.**

TRANSMISSION
- Via inhalation. **Commonly found in garden and houseplant soil, compost, & decomposed material.**
- Immunocompromised states: eg, neutropenia, high dose glucocorticoid use, hematologic malignancy.

CLINICAL MANIFESTATIONS
- **[1] Allergic bronchopulmonary Aspergillosis: type I hypersensitivity reaction occurring almost exclusively in patients with Asthma, Bronchiectasis, or Cystic fibrosis.** Classically presents with refractory Asthma (recurrent exacerbations), fever, malaise, & **intermittent expectoration of brownish mucus plugs in the sputum.** Often associated with Eosinophilia & pulmonary infiltrates.

- **[2] Aspergilloma:** colonization of the fungus in a preexisting pulmonary cavitary lesion. **Can be an asymptomatic incidental finding on CXR or patient may complain of cough or hemoptysis.**

- **[3] Acute invasive Aspergillosis:** fever, headache, toothache, epistaxis, **invasive Chronic sinusitis. Lung involvement common — hemoptysis, pleuritic chest pain**, dyspnea, cough. Increased LDH. Often fatal. Usually occurs in severely immunocompromised patients (eg, neutropenia, leukemia).

DIAGNOSIS
- **Allergic: increased IgE, eosinophilia,** _Aspergillus_ skin test positivity or detectable IgE levels vs. _Aspergillus fumigatus._
- **Invasive: Galactomannan levels (found in the cell walls of Aspergillus - specific),** beta-D glucan assay, PCR, & culture.
- Biopsy: **tissue appears dusky & necrotic** (eg, nose).
  Histology: septate hyphae with regular branching at acute (45°) angles.

RADIOGRAPH FINDINGS
- **Allergic: Bronchiectasis,** parenchymal opacities (especially in the upper lobes), or atelectasis.
- Invasive Aspergillosis: single or multiple nodules with a halo sign (rim of ground glass opacity) with or without cavitation, patchy or segmental consolidation, peribronchial infiltrates.
- **Aspergilloma: air crescent (Monod) sign — radiopaque structure "fungal ball" that moves when the patient changes position.**

MANAGEMENT
[1] Allergic Bronchopulmonary Aspergillosis (ABPA):
- **Combination of systemic glucocorticoids as mainstay of treatment (eg, Prednisone) ± antifungal therapy (eg, Itraconazole)** to control symptoms during an exacerbation, to prevent exacerbations, & preserve lung function. **Voriconazole is an alternative to Itraconazole.**

[2] Severe/Invasive Aspergillus or Sinusitis:
- **Voriconazole first-line drug of choice. An Echinocandin (eg, Caspofungin) may be added for the first 1-2 weeks of therapy in some patients with progressive disease.** Amphotericin B may be adjunctive to Voriconazole. Surgical debridement if refractory.
- Alternatives to Voriconazole include Posaconazole or Isavuconazole.

[3] Aspergilloma:
- **Asymptomatic: observation** — in patients with stable radiographic findings, asymptomatic, or immunocompetent, a conservative management guided by close monitoring is also a feasible option. The risk of complications of intervention outweighs its benefit in asymptomatic patients.
- **Symptomatic (severe hemoptysis): surgical resection.** Patients with severe hemoptysis and good respiratory function (eg, FEV1 >1.9) can undergo surgery.

COCCIDIOIDOMYCOSIS

- Coccidioidomycosis is caused by the dimorphic fungi of the genus *Coccidioides*.
- ***Coccidioides immitis* grows in soil in arid/desert regions in <u>Southwestern US</u>** (eg, New Mexico, Southern California, Arizona, Utah, Nevada), Mexico; Central & South America. *C posadasii.*

TRANSMISSION
- Inhalation of spores when the soil is disrupted.

CLINICAL MANIFESTATIONS
- Asymptomatic in 60-65%.

[1] Primary pulmonary disease:
- **<u>Mild flu-like illness</u>** — fever, chills, nasopharyngitis, headache, cough, pleuritic chest pain, back pain.
- **<u>Pneumonia:</u>** Primary pulmonary Coccidioidomycosis is strongly suggested by the findings of rash and symmetrical arthralgias, and Pneumonia with an appropriate exposure history.

[2] Valley fever ("Desert rheumatism"):
- **<u>Classic triad</u> of [1] fever, [2] <u>arthralgias:</u> new onset of diffuse symmetric migratory arthralgias (pain &/or swelling of the ankles, knees, & wrists common)** often accompanied with periarticular swelling, **& [3] <u>skin involvement</u> eg, Erythema nodosum (desert bumps)** or maculopapular rash.

[3] Cutaneous manifestations:
- **<u>Erythema nodosum</u> — painful, erythematous nodules on the lower extremities, especially the anterior shins.** In this setting, it is known as "desert bumps" and is a nonspecific finding that indicates a favorable prognosis.
- **<u>Erythema multiforme</u>** — classically presents with target lesions on the skin with or without mucosal membrane involvement. Cutaneous manifestations are more prevalent in women than in men.

[4] Disseminated or persistent:
- **<u>CNS involvement:</u> eg, Meningitis in 50%.**
- Can affect any organ, especially the lungs, skin, soft tissue (eg, abscesses), lymph nodes, joints, or bones.
- In patients with AIDS who reside in endemic areas, Coccidioidomycosis is a common opportunistic infection.

DIAGNOSIS
- **<u>Early:</u> Enzyme-linked immunoassay (EIA) for IgM & IgG antibodies usually the first test ordered** and is usually positive 1-3 weeks after the disease onset. Negative results may warrant retesting if suspicion for Coccidioidomycosis persists.
- **<u>Immunodiffusion tests</u> usually conducted to support the diagnosis if the initial EIA is positive — eg, tube precipitin-type antibodies (reported as IgM antibodies),** immunodiffusion complement-fixing antibodies (IDCF), or complement-fixing test (CF). Immunodiffusion is more specific but less sensitive than enzyme immunoassay.
- <u>IDCF titers:</u> If the immunodiffusion test for IgG is qualitatively positive, titers are often used to monitor the response to treatment. A persistently rising IgG complement fixation titer ($\geq$1:16) is suggestive of disseminated disease.
- **<u>Cultures</u> most definitive.** PCR, skin testing.
- **<u>Histology:</u> spherules (thick-walled spherical structure containing endospores) seen in tissues.**
- <u>Meningitis:</u> CSF complement fixing antibodies, Fungal CSF pattern (lymphocytes & decreased glucose).
- **<u>Chest radiograph:</u> hilar lymphadenopathy,** cavitations, miliary pneumonia, abscesses, & nodules.

MANAGEMENT
- **Most cases are asymptomatic/mild, self-limited, & require no treatment in healthy patients.**
  Localized lung disease is treated symptomatically in most cases.
- **<u>CNS disease (eg, Meningitis), lungs, bones, soft tissues:</u> oral Fluconazole or Itraconazole.**
- Amphotericin B is reserved for severe disease (except Meningitis) or pregnancy in the first trimester.

MYCOBACTERIUM AVIUM COMPLEX (MAC)

- *M avium & Mycobacterium intracellulare* — 2 main species and are gram-positive acid-fast bacilli.
- <u>TRANSMISSION:</u> present in soil & water (not person to person).

<u>RISK FACTORS</u>
- **Underlying pulmonary disease** eg, Bronchiectasis, COPD.
- **Immunocompromised** eg, **advanced HIV (CD4 count ≤50** cells/μL), hematologic malignancy.

<u>CLINICAL MANIFESTATIONS</u>
- **[1] Pulmonary: presents similar to Tuberculosis clinically & radiographically** — eg, cough (dry or productive), chest pain, fever, weight loss, fatigue, hemoptysis, upper lobe infiltrates, & cavities.
- **[2] Disseminated: fever of unknown origin** (most common), **night sweats, weight loss, fatigue, diarrhea,** dyspnea, RUQ pain, hepatosplenomegaly. **Most commonly seen with advanced HIV.**
- **[3] Lymphadenitis: most common in children 1-4 years of age, primarily involving unilateral nontender cervical lymph nodes.** Submandibular & submaxillary lymphadenopathy also common.

<u>DIAGNOSIS</u>
- Acid fast bacillus staining. Culture — sputum; blood & urine cultures if disseminated is suspected.

<u>MANAGEMENT</u>
- **Triple therapy: [1] Macrolide (Clarithromycin) PLUS [2] Ethambutol PLUS [3] a Rifamycin (eg, Rifabutin or Rifampin) for at least 12 months first line. Azithromycin** is an alternative Macrolide.
- **IV Aminoglycosides (eg, Amikacin) may be added to the above regimen in severe or life-threatening disease.**
- <u>Second line:</u> Ethambutol PLUS a Rifamycin (eg, Rifabutin) PLUS IV Aminoglycoside may be used if the isolate is Macrolide-resistant.
- Surgical excision of infected lymph nodes is curative in 90% of patients with lymphadenitis.

<u>PROPHYLAXIS IN HIV</u>
- **Clarithromycin or Azithromycin if CD4 count ≤50** cells/μL if they are not on ART (and it will not be initiated, such as patient refusal, or if delay in initiating ART) or remain viremic despite ART.

MYCOBACTERIUM MARINUM "Fish tank Granuloma"

- *Mycobacterium marinum:* Atypical *Mycobacterium* found in freshwater & salt water.

<u>TRANSMISSION</u>
- **Inoculation of a break in the skin barrier** (laceration abrasion, puncture, etc.) **with exposure to contaminated fresh or salt water, including aquariums, marine organisms, & swimming pools.**
- **Occupational hazard** of aquarium handlers, marine workers, fisherman, & seafood handlers.

<u>CLINICAL MANIFESTATIONS</u>
- **Localized cutaneous disease: erythematous bluish papule(s) or nodule(s) at the site of trauma** that can ulcerate (history of exposure to non-chlorinated water 2–3 weeks earlier).
- **Subsequent lesions may occur along the path of lymphatic drainage** over a period of months.

<u>DIAGNOSIS:</u> culture

<u>MANAGEMENT</u>
- **Superficial papules** Monotherapy with one of the following: Clarithromycin, Minocycline, Doxycycline, Trimethoprim-sulfamethoxazole.
- **Deeper/more extensive infection:** 2 active agents — **Clarithromycin combined with EITHER Ethambutol or Rifampin.**
- <u>Duration of therapy:</u> often used for 1-2 months following resolution of symptoms (total duration is typically 3-4 months).

LEPROSY (HANSEN's DISEASE)

- Chronic disease caused by the acid-fasts rods ***Mycobacterium leprae & lepromatosis*** that primarily affects superficial tissues (especially the **skin & peripheral nerves**).
- Endemic in subtropical areas. Requires long exposure (few months to 20-50 years incubation period).

CLINICAL MANIFESTATIONS

- **[1] Lepromatous: nodular, plaque, or papular skin lesions (lepromas)** with poorly defined borders. Hypopigmented lesions can be seen especially in cooler areas of the body: face (leonine), ears, wrists, elbows, buttocks, & knees. Loss of eyebrows & eyelashes. Slowly evolving **SYMMETRIC nerve involvement (<u>sensation preserved</u>). Paresthesias in the affected peripheral nerves. Most commonly seen in immunocompromised patients.**

- **[2] Tuberculoid: limited disease: sharply demarcated hypopigmented macular lesions numb to the touch (<u>loss of sensation</u>)** with sudden onset of **<u>asymmetric</u> nerve involvement.** Most common in <u>immunocompetent patients</u> (immune system reaction in the nerves causes the loss of sensation).

- [3] <u>Mononeuritis multiplex:</u> nerve damage: posterior tibial nerve, median & ulnar involvement (clawing), common peroneal nerve (foot drop). Vibratory & proprioception usually preserved.

DIAGNOSIS

- **Acid fast bacillus smear & lepromin skin test:**
  <u>Lepromatous type</u>: abundant acid-fast bacilli in the skin lesions and a negative lepromin skin test.
  <u>Tuberculoid type</u>: few bacilli present in the lesions and a positive lepromin skin test.

MANAGEMENT

- <u>Tuberculoid disease</u>: Dapsone (100 mg daily) and Rifampicin (600 mg daily) for duration 12 months.
- <u>Lepromatous</u>: Dapsone, Rifampicin, and Clofazimine (50 mg daily) for duration 24 months.

PARASITIC DISEASES

ENTEROBIASIS (PINWORM)

- **Nematode infection caused by *<u>Enterobius vermicularis</u>* (pinworm).**

TRANSMISSION

- Via hand-mouth contact with contaminated fomites, autoinoculation, **fecal-oral contamination** (especially **school-aged children 5-10 years**). Most common helminthic infection in the US.

CLINICAL MANIFESTATIONS

- **Perianal itching, especially nocturnal** (eggs are laid at night). Perianal erythema, sleep disturbance.
- In severe cases, it may be associated with abdominal pain, nausea, & vomiting.

DIAGNOSIS

- ⊕ **Cellophane tape test** or pinworm paddle test early in AM to look for **eggs under a microscope.**

MANAGEMENT

- **Albendazole, Mebendazole, or Pyrantel.** Pyrantel avoided in children <2 years. Mebendazole and Albendazole avoided in pregnancy and Pinworm infection in children <1 year of age.
- **Pregnancy: Pyrantel is preferred if treatment is needed during pregnancy (severe symptoms).**
  Treatment in pregnancy should be reserved for patients who have significant symptoms.
<u>Reduction of spread:</u>
- Simultaneous treatment of the entire household can help to reduce reinfection.
- Hand washing, trimming of fingernails, and taking a bath early in the morning daily to reduce egg contamination is recommended.

ASCARIASIS (GIANT ROUNDWORM INFECTION)

- **_Ascaris lumbricoides_ giant roundworm infection that parasitizes the human intestine.**
- Most common intestinal helminth worldwide.
- TRANSMISSION: ingestion of food or water contaminated with _Ascaris_ eggs. Contaminated soil.

PATHOPHYSIOLOGY
- Once ingested, the eggs hatch in the small intestine and the organisms migrates hematogenously to the lungs, where the larvae mature. The larvae migrate caudally to the trachea and are then swallowed, after which they mature, mate, and produce eggs in the intestines that pass into the stool.

CLINICAL MANIFESTATIONS
- Small worm load: asymptomatic. Worms may migrate if patient is given inhaled anesthesia.
- Larger load: vague abdominal symptoms — eg, anorexia, nausea, vomiting, abdominal discomfort.
- **High load: intestinal obstruction (most common),** pancreatic or bile duct obstruction.
- **Pneumonitis in the early stage,** larvae migrating through lungs may induce an inflammatory response, especially after second infection, resulting in bronchial spasm, mucus production, and **Löeffler's syndrome (fever, cough, wheezing, dyspnea, lung infiltrates, eosinophilia, & ↑IgE).**

DIAGNOSIS
- **Stool ova and parasite:** examination for ova or visual examination of adult worms. Eosinophilia

MANAGEMENT
- **Albendazole (single dose) or Mebendazole. Pyrantel given if pregnant** (given after first trimester)

TRICHINOSIS (TRICHINELLOSIS)

- Parasitic nematode (roundworm) infection cause by **_Trichinella_ species (especially _T. spiralis_).**

TRANSMISSION
- **Raw or undercooked meat (especially pork, wild boar, bear, or game).**

PATHOPHYSIOLOGY
- Larvae cysts are ingested then go to the duodenum and jejunum to grow into adults & replicate.
- Adults are excreted in the stool & larva penetrate intestinal wall & **encapsulate (form cysts) in striated muscle tissue.** Severity of disease correlates with the number of ingested larvae.

CLINICAL MANIFESTATIONS
- **[1] GI phase:** abdominal pain, nausea, diarrhea, & vomiting, followed by progression to muscle phase.
- **[2] Muscle phase: myositis: muscle pain (myalgias),** tenderness, swelling, and weakness **with high fever.** Eye: **palpebral or circumorbital edema,** retinal hemorrhages, conjunctival hemorrhages. **Subungual splinter hemorrhages;** macular or urticarial rash, dyspnea, dysphagia.
- Cardiac: **myocarditis** (due to eosinophilia). CNS: encephalitis or meningitis. Pulmonary: pneumonia.

DIAGNOSIS
- Usually a clinical diagnosis confirmed with serologies (anti-Trichinella IgG antibodies, ELISA confirmed with Western blot). Consider in any patient with **periorbital edema, myositis, & eosinophilia.**
- **Eosinophilia** hallmark; muscle involvement: **increased muscle enzymes (creatine kinase & LDH).**
- Muscle biopsy: if the diagnosis is uncertain — encapsulated larvae seen in affected muscle tissue.

MANAGEMENT
- Mild cases: **most are mild & self-limited; symptomatic treatment (analgesia and antipyretics).**
- **CNS, cardiac, or pulmonary: Anti-helminthics: Albendazole preferred (or Mebendazole) plus supportive therapy.** Albendazole & Mebendazole contraindicated in children ≤2 years & during pregnancy.
- Glucocorticoids (eg, Prednisone) added to severe disease or if Albendazole is given during pregnancy.

HOOKWORM

- **_Ancylostoma duodenale_ (human hookworm)** in the tropics or subtropics *or **_Necator americanus_*** (N. or S. America, Central Africa, South Pacific, and India). Occasional cases occur in the United States (Southeast). *Ancylostoma ceylanicum* (India & SE Asia). 25% of the world is infected.
- **Common in countries with poor access to adequate water, sanitation, and hygiene.**

TRANSMISSION
- 3 conditions needed — **[1] human fecal contamination of soil, [2]** favorable soil conditions for larvae growth (**moisture, warmth, shade**), and **[3] contact of human skin with contaminated soil** (eg, barefoot or open footwear).

PATHOPHYSIOLOGY
- The larvae penetrate the skin & migrate to the pulmonary capillaries. They are carried to the mouth via the mucociliary escalator & swallowed, where they enter the small bowel and suck blood (whole cycle about ~4 weeks).

CLINICAL MANIFESTATIONS: 4 phases:
- **Phase 1 (dermal penetration):** **focal very pruritic erythematous maculopapular dermatitis (ground itch) at the site of larvae entry (eg, feet, between toes, & ankles)** in previously sensitized hosts that usually resolves within a few days. Less often, **pruritic serpiginous tracks of intracutaneous migration** (similar to cutaneous larva migrans).
- **Phase 2 (transpulmonary):** **usually asymptomatic.** Transpulmonary passage of larval migration through the lungs may lead to a **transient pneumonitis** — mild dry cough, wheezing, low-grade fever, or pharyngeal irritation. **Löeffler's syndrome low-grade fever, & pulmonary symptoms (cough, wheezing, dyspnea, lung infiltrates), eosinophilia, & ↑IgE.**
- **Phase 3 (GI):** **GI symptoms usually occur after 1 month of infection** — **nausea, diarrhea, vomiting, mid epigastric pain** (usually with postprandial exacerbation, mimicking gastric ulcers), and increased flatulence. GI bleeding is rare.
- **Phase 4 (chronic nutritional impairment):** **major impact of Hookworm infection.** Hookworms cause blood loss by lacerating capillaries and ingesting blood, leading to **daily loss of blood, iron, and albumin. Iron deficiency is the major consequence of chronic Hookworm infection.** Loss of iron, blood, and albumin may be accompanied by impairment in growth and cognitive development in children.

DIAGNOSIS
- **Stool examination via microscopy for stool ova and parasites using the Kato-Katz technique** (eggs in fresh stool, larvae in old stool). Not helpful for skin or pulmonary phase. Serial exams may be necessary if negative.
- **Eosinophilia,** increased IgE.
- Chronic blood loss: **iron deficiency anemia** (hypochromic microcytic anemia) and positive guaiac.

MANAGEMENT
- **Albendazole is the preferred treatment for Hookworm infections (single 400 mg dose on empty stomach). Supportive: iron supplementation, multivitamins.**
- Second line: Mebendazole (100 mg orally twice daily for 3 days) and Pyrantel pamoate (11 mg/kg per day for 3 days, not to exceed 1 g/day) are acceptable but less effective alternative therapies.

PREVENTION
- Improved hygiene, such as drinking safe water, properly cleaning and cooking food, hand washing, and wearing shoes.
- Mass administration of Anthelminthic drugs may sometimes be used in populations at risk with the intention of maintaining low individual worm burdens.

NEUROCYSTICERCOSIS (PORK TAPEWORM)

- ***Taenia solium,*** **the pork tapeworm, is transmitted to humans by ingestion of food or water contaminated with the eggs.**

EPIDEMIOLOGY
- Found in tropical areas & resource-limited countries.
- Consumption of undercooked pork produces an intestinal infection that is caused by the adult worm.
- Individuals infected with an adult worm can infect themselves or others with the eggs via fecal-oral route.

PATHOPHYSIOLOGY
- If humans ingest *T. solium* eggs, larvae can encyst (cysticerci) in different human tissues, including the skin, muscle, kidney, heart, liver, and brain.
- In the small intestine, the egg releases an oncosphere that crosses the gut wall and spreads hematogenously to the brain leading to neurocysticercosis.

CLINICAL MANIFESTATIONS
- Most are asymptomatic; may develop abdominal pain or diarrhea.
- **Neurocysticercosis should be suspected in any child with new onset seizures and/or headache with a history of living in an endemic area or exposed to someone from an endemic area.** Increased intracranial pressure: nausea, vomiting, focal neurological signs, & altered mental status.

DIAGNOSIS
- **MRI of the brain most useful test; MRI provides information about cyst viability and associated inflammation** — cystic lesions, ring enhancing lesions (degenerating phase), and/or calcifications (nonviable phase). More than 1 phase can be seen in the same individual. CT scan of the brain.
- Antibody tests: enzyme-linked immunoelectrotransfer blot (EITB) using parasite glycoproteins performed on serum. All patients should undergo an eye exam to rule out ocular involvement.

MANAGEMENT
- Untreated hydrocephalus, cysticercal encephalitis, or calcified lesions only: antiparasitic therapy is not indicated. Most cysts resolve spontaneously with time.
- **1-2 parenchymal cysts that are viable and/or degenerating: Albendazole.**
- **>2 parenchymal cysts that are viable and/or degenerating: Albendazole plus Praziquantel.**
- Adjunctive administration of corticosteroids with antiparasitic therapy usually recommended.

BEEF TAPEWORM

- ***Taenia saginata*** **occurs worldwide but is most common in areas where consumption of undercooked beef is customary (eg, Europe and parts of Asia).**
- Most human carriers of adult tapeworms are asymptomatic. *T. saginata* is motile so carriers may sense movement of proglottids through the anus. Associated symptoms include nausea, anorexia, or epigastric pain. Anxiety, headache, dizziness, and urticaria can also occur.
- A peripheral eosinophilia (≤15%) may occur.
- Occasionally, segments can enter the appendix, common bile duct, or pancreatic duct and cause obstruction.

DIAGNOSIS
- Identification of eggs or proglottids in the stool.

MANAGEMENT
- Praziquantel oral: 5-10 mg/kg as a single dose.

CHAGAS DISEASE

- Disease caused by ***Trypanosoma cruzi***, a protozoan parasite, that is characterized by **dilated cardiomyopathy and GI disease. Leading cause of CHF in Latin America.**
- TRANSMISSION: vector is the **assassin (kissing) bug** that bites in the evening. Prevalent in Latin America northward to Texas. Congenital. Consumption of contaminated food or drink.

ACUTE
- Most are asymptomatic. Symptoms are more common in children & are nonspecific (eg, malaise, fever anorexia). Acute illness can last 8-12 weeks. *T. cruzi* infection rarely detected during the acute phase.
- **Chagoma: swelling or inflammation of the skin at the bite site. Romaña sign: unilateral periorbital swelling & conjunctivitis.** Fever, lymphadenopathy, hepatosplenomegaly.

CHRONIC
- Indeterminate form is associated with positive serologies but no GI or cardiac disease & normal ECG.
- Determinate form associated with destruction of nerve cell ganglia, cardiac, and/or GI complications.
- Cardiac: **dilated cardiomyopathy, decompensated heart failure,** arrhythmias, thromboembolism.
- GI complications: **Megacolon** — progressive constipation, colicky abdominal pain & bloating. **Megaesophagus** — progressive dysphagia & regurgitation of food.

DIAGNOSIS
- Acute phase: peripheral blood smear: trypomastigote (flagellated motile form) seen on microscopy of fresh preparations of anticoagulated blood or buffy coat. PCR.
- Chronic phase: serology (ELISA).
- ECG: may show arrhythmias (eg, AV blocks).
- Echocardiogram: **cardiomegaly with apical atrophy or aneurysm.**

MANAGEMENT
- **Benznidazole (preferred) or Nifurtimox** for 90-120 days depending on age (obtained from CDC). Indications include **acute phase and patients without significant cardiac and/or GI disease.**

HUMAN AFRICAN TRYPANOSOMIASIS (SLEEPING SICKNESS)

- Protozoa ***Trypanosoma brucei*** *(rhodesiense & gambiense).* **"African sleeping sickness".**
- Transmission: vector is the **Tsetse fly.** Prevalent in Sub-Saharan Africa as well as South & Central America.

CLINICAL MANIFESTATIONS: 2 stages:
- Early hemolymphatic stage: **painless chancre at the bite site** 2-3 days after bite, increasing in size, resolving in 2-3 weeks. Intermittent ever, general malaise, headaches, joint pains, & itching. **Generalized or regional lymphadenopathy (often extremely large). Winterbottom sign — posterior cervical lymphadenopathy.** Transient serpiginous rash.
- Late CNS stage: **persistent headache, daytime sleepiness followed by nighttime insomnia** (tryptophol released by *T. brucei* induces sleep), behavioral changes, wasting syndrome, seizures in children.

DIAGNOSIS: Peripheral blood smear or aspiration of an affected lymph node. Anemia, thrombocytopenia.

MANAGEMENT
Infectious disease consult.
- *T. brucei gambiense:* Early stage: Fexinidazole PO. Pentamidine. Late stage: Eflornithine & Nifurtimox.
- *T. brucei rhodesiense:* Early stage: Suramin IV. Pentamidine isethionate IM or IV. Late stage: Melarsoprol (may add Nifurtimox).

MALARIA

- **Mosquito-borne red blood cell disease caused by *Plasmodium spp.* (*falciparum, vivax, ovale, malariae*). Falciparum most dangerous type.**
- Distribution: throughout most of the tropics, especially in Sub-Saharan Africa.
- Sickle cell trait & thalassemia trait are protective vs. Malaria.
- Pathophysiology: *Plasmodium spp.* infects red blood cells causing RBC lysis, leading to cyclical fever.

TRANSMISSION
- **Protozoa are transmitted via the female *Anopheles* mosquito,** especially at dusk & dawn.

CLINICAL MANIFESTATIONS
- Prodrome: Acute manifestations of Malaria are characterized by a prodrome of headache, myalgias, fatigue, and GI symptoms, followed by fever, tachycardia, tachypnea, chills, diaphoresis (sweating), cough, anorexia, nausea, vomiting, abdominal pain, diarrhea, arthralgias, and myalgias.
- **Cyclical fever** (cold stage/chills followed by hot stage/fever followed by diaphoretic stage every other or third day), headache, fatigue, myalgias, GI symptoms. Splenomegaly. **Cyclical fever every 48 hours (*P. vivax* & *P. ovale*) & 72 hours (*P. malariae*); irregular fever pattern with *P. falciparum.***
- ***P. falciparum* severe symptoms: cerebral malaria** — AMS, delirium, seizures, coma. **blackwater fever** — severe hemolysis + hemoglobinuria (dark urine) + renal failure.

DIAGNOSIS
- Clinical diagnosis — suspect in patients with fever who traveled to endemic area + parasitic diagnosis.
- **Giemsa-stained blood smear: (thin & thick)** — parasites (trophozoites & schizonts) in RBCs with light microscopy. **Thick smear for detection, thin smear for speciation.** Schuffner's dots (small brick-red granules throughout the erythrocyte cytoplasm) seen with *P. vivax* & *ovale.*
- Rapid diagnostic tests: antigen or antibody testing able to detect very low parasitemia.
- Routine laboratory findings: **Leukopenia, hemolytic anemia, thrombocytopenia.**

MANAGEMENT
Chloroquine sensitive *P. falciparum:*
- **Artemisinin combination therapy (ACTs).** When ACT is not readily available, Chloroquine or Hydroxychloroquine is an alternative. Chloroquine disrupts the erythrocytic stage of infection.
- **Primaquine is an add-on agent used to kill latent hypnozoites in *P. vivax* & *P. ovale* infections in the liver to prevent recurrence (test for G6PD prior to use).**
- *P. falciparum* is resistant to Chloroquine and Sulfadoxine-pyrimethamine in most areas, with the exceptions of Central America west of the Panama Canal and Hispaniola.
Chloroquine resistant *P. falciparum*:
- **Artemisinin combination therapy** (ACTs) include a short-acting Artemisinin and longer-acting partner drug. First line therapies in nearly all endemic countries (eg, Artemether-Lumefantrine or Artesunate combinations). Atovaquone-proguanil is an alternative to ACTs.
- Second line: Quinine sulfate plus either Doxycycline, Tetracycline, or Clindamycin. Quinine must be taken for 7 days and is poorly tolerated, so it is often reserved for the treatment of severe Malaria and for treatment after another regimen has failed.
Chloroquine-resistant *P. vivax*:
- Artemisinin combination therapy (ACTs) may be used.
- Quinine sulfate plus Doxycycline or Tetracycline + Primaquine
- Atovaquone-proguanil plus Primaquine. Mefloquine plus Primaquine.
Life threatening infection:
- **IV or IM Artesunate children and adults with severe Malaria, including pregnant women in all trimesters, and lactating women, should receive intravenous or intramuscular Artesunate for at least 24 hours** (2.4 mg/kg intravenously every 12 hours for 1 day, then daily).

BABESIOSIS

- Infectious disease caused by Malaria-like protozoa of the *Babesia spp.* (eg, **_Babesia microti_**) in the US.

TRANSMISSION
- **Tick vector** (eg, *Ixodes scapularis*, **the same tick for Lyme disease**). 1–4-week incubation period.
- Rarely, transmission can occur via blood transfusion, congenitally, or via organ transplantation.
- **Similar to Malaria, the *Babesia* protozoa infect and lyse red blood cells, leading to hemolysis.**

RISK FACTORS
- Location: endemic to upper Midwest & **coastal Northeast US** (same geography as Lyme disease).
- **Elderly (age >50 years), asplenia, immunocompromised, neonatal prematurity.**

CLINICAL MANIFESTATIONS
- Many individuals have asymptomatic infection.
- **Malaria & flu-like symptoms** — gradual onset of **fatigue, malaise, fever**, chills, sweats, headache, **weakness, & myalgias.** Arthralgia, anorexia, nausea, dry cough, emotional lability, dark urine.
- Physical examination: jaundice, hepatomegaly, splenomegaly, petechiae, ecchymosis.

DIAGNOSIS
- CBC: **mild to severe hemolytic anemia hallmark feature** — decreased haptoglobin, increased reticulocytes. Lymphopenia, thrombocytopenia. Increased transaminases (LFTs).
- **Peripheral blood thin smear for identification of organisms best initial test** (with Giemsa or Wright stain) — **parasites (merezoites) within RBCs, especially in pathognomonic tetrads (Maltese cross appearance). Intraerythrocytic ring forms with central pallor.**
- **PCR: for detection of *Babesia* DNA most accurate test.** Serologies (4-fold rise in *Babesia* IgG titers).

MANAGEMENT
- For individuals with asymptomatic *B. microti* infection, no antimicrobial therapy is needed.
- Mild-moderate: **oral Atovaquone + oral Azithromycin first-line.** Quinine + Clindamycin alternative.
- **Severe: oral Atovaquone + IV Azithromycin.** High-grade parasitemia: may add exchange transfusion.

LEISHMANIASIS

- **Caused by *Leishmania* protozoan transmitted via the female Sand fly.**
- Prevalent in Mediterranean, Central & South America, Africa, & Asia.

CLINICAL MANIFESTATIONS
- **Localized cutaneous: ❶ small erythematous papule** that enlarges into a nodule, leading to **painless ulceration with an indurated border OR ❷ dry, indurated plaque with satellite pustules** that develops at the bite site weeks to months after infection. May crust over in the center, **leaving a raised bordered scar. May become painful later but not painful initially.** May be multiple lesions if diffuse. **Regional lymphadenopathy.**
- **Mucocutaneous: ulcers of the skin, mouth, and nose,** especially cartilaginous areas.
- **Visceral:** fulminant disease with migration to the liver, spleen, & bone marrow (**hepatosplenomegaly**).

DIAGNOSIS
- Evidence of the parasite in a clinical specimen (often the skin) via culture, histology, or PCR.
- Disseminated: direct visualization of aspirates from the liver, spleen, or marrow if visceral (*Leishmania donovani* has a higher incidence of causing visceral infection).

MANAGEMENT
- Infectious disease consult. Sores usually heal spontaneously. Topical Paromomycin cream may be used for ulcerative lesions. Oral systemic agents include azoles and Miltefosine.

TOXOPLASMOSIS

- **Infection due to _Toxoplasma gondii_, an obligate intracellular protozoan**.
- Most common CNS infection in patients with AIDS not receiving appropriate prophylaxis or not on ART.

TRANSMISSION
- **Ingestion of infectious oocysts, usually from soil or cat litter;** food or water contaminated with feline feces (eg, **unwashed produce**); or **undercooked or raw meat from an infected animal**.

CLINICAL MANIFESTATIONS
[1] Primary infection:
- Usually asymptomatic infection in immunocompetent patients. **May develop a Mono-like illness with** (**fever**, chills, sweats, malaise, fatigue, headache, sore throat) + **bilateral, symmetrical, nontender cervical lymphadenopathy.** ⊕ IgG & IgM serologic tests or increased titers during acute infection.
[2] Reactivation associated with Encephalitis, Chorioretinitis, Pneumonitis, and Myocarditis.
- **Encephalitis: most common presentation in AIDS, especially with CD4 count ≤100 cells/microL** — headache, neurologic symptoms, fever, AMS, focal neurologic deficits.
- **Chorioretinitis:** posterior uveitis — ocular pain, floaters, and decreased visual acuity.
- Pneumonitis: fever, dyspnea, & nonproductive cough (similar to PCP pneumonia).

DIAGNOSIS
- Clinical diagnosis: presumptive diagnosis if CD4 ≤100 cells/microL not on prophylaxis, compatible symptoms, ⊕ _T. gondii_ IgG antibody, MRI imaging that is consistent (ring-enhancing lesions).
- Serologies: **anti-toxoplasma IgG antibodies** via ELISA (distant infection if immunocompromised).
- Neuroimaging: **multiple necrotizing ring-enhancing lesions** (nonspecific as they may also be seen with CNS lymphoma). MRI preferred > head CT.
- CSF: mononuclear pleocytosis, increased protein, may have reduced CSF glucose. CSF PCR.

MANAGEMENT
- **Therapy is generally not necessary for most immunocompetent, nonpregnant individuals** who only have lymphadenopathy or Mono-like illness since primary illness is self-limited.
- **Immunocompromised: Sulfadiazine (or Clindamycin) + Pyrimethamine (with Folinic acid/Leucovorin to prevent folic acid depletion** from Pyrimethamine). Glucocorticoids are added to the standard regimen with cerebral edema & ocular Toxoplasmosis. IV Trimethoprim-sulfamethoxazole.
- **Toxoplasma Encephalitis, pregnancy ≥14 weeks':** Pyrimethamine-Sulfadiazine for 10-14 days.
- **Spiramycin in pregnancy if <14 weeks'** to reduce frequency transmission to the fetus by ~60%.

PROPHYLAXIS
- **Trimethoprim-sulfamethoxazole is first-line prophylaxis when CD4 count is ≤100** cells/microL.
- Second line: Dapsone + Pyrimethamine + Leucovorin. Atovaquone with or without Pyrimethamine and Leucovorin.

CONGENITAL TOXOPLASMA INFECTION
Triad of [1] chorioretinitis, [2] hydrocephalus, & [3] intracranial calcifications (diffuse).
- These infants may be asymptomatic and appear normal at birth but develop a wide range of signs and symptoms later in life, including chorioretinitis, strabismus, epilepsy, psychomotor retardation, seizures. Physical examination: jaundice, hepatomegaly, lymphadenopathy.
- **Congenital Toxoplasma infection is part of ToRCH syndrome: Toxoplasmosis, Other (Syphilis), Rubella, CMV, HSV.**

DIAGNOSIS
- Serologies: **anti-toxoplasma IgM antibodies** best initial test. PCR for Toxoplasmosis most accurate.

MANAGEMENT
- **Sulfadiazine + Pyrimethamine + Folinic acid**

PRENATAL TRANSMISSION OF DISEASES

CONGENITAL VARICELLA SYNDROME

- Occurs in infants whose mothers develop Varicella (chickenpox) <u>8-20 weeks' gestation</u>.

<u>CLINICAL MANIFESTATIONS</u>

- <u>Intrauterine growth restriction</u> — **most common manifestation.**
- <u>Scarring skin lesions</u>, which may be depressed or pigmented
- <u>Ocular abnormalities</u>: eg, **cataracts, chorioretinitis**, microphthalmos, Horner syndrome, nystagmus.
- <u>Limb abnormalities</u>: **eg, hypoplasia of bone and muscle**.
- <u>CNS abnormalities:</u> seizures, cognitive deficits, cortical atrophy, intellectual disability.

NEONATAL VARICELLA

- **Neonates born to mothers with VZV infection, or who were exposed <u>within 2-3 weeks of delivery</u>** are at risk for Neonatal varicella during the first 4-6 weeks of life.
- **Neonates may be infected (1) in utero by transplacental viremia, (2) at birth by ascending infection, or (3) after birth by respiratory droplets or direct contact with infectious lesions.**
- **The risk of mortality is increased when the mother develops symptoms of varicella infection from 5 days before to 2 days after delivery because there is insufficient time for the development and transfer of maternal antibody.** Mortality rate as high as 30%.

<u>CLINICAL MANIFESTATIONS</u>

- Variable presentation — mild illness resembling chickenpox in older children to a disseminated infection similar to manifestations seen in immunocompromised hosts.
- Neonatal chickenpox within the first 4 days is usually mild.
- **<u>Mild illness resembling Chickenpox</u>: fever often within the first days (5-10) after birth, followed by a generalized vesicular eruption.** The rash starts as macules & rapidly progresses to papules and then to the classic vesicular lesions before crusting. It usually appears first on the head and then generalizes. **The lesions characteristically are in various stages of development and healing**. The generalized involvement and appearance of lesions in different stages of development distinguish Varicella from the vesicular rash seen in Neonatal herpes simplex virus (HSV), which classically appears in localized groups (clusters). In mild cases, the lesions heal within 7 to 10 days.
- **<u>Disseminated disease</u>:** May follow the initial mild illness, with progression to different organs — eg, varicella Pneumonia, Hepatitis, and Meningoencephalitis.

<u>DIAGNOSIS</u>: clinical: classic rash in different stages. If testing is needed, PCR is the diagnostic test of choice.

<u>MANAGEMENT</u>

- **<u>Varicella-zoster immune globulin</u> (VZIG) prompt administration to infants born to women with active varicella infection at delivery may improve neonatal disease.**
- **<u>IV Acyclovir</u> is given to neonates with active disease** (rash, pneumonia, encephalitis, severe hepatitis, thrombocytopenia). Breastfeeding is encouraged in newborns exposed to or infected with varicella because antibody in breast milk may be protective.

<u>PREVENTION</u>

<u>Varicella Immune globulin</u> (VZIG) reduces the severity of infection after exposure to Varicella virus in patients at high risk for severe infection and complications including:

- **Newborns of mothers with Varicella 5 days before to 2 days after delivery. Varicella immunoglobulin is <u>not</u> needed if maternal infection >5 days before birth** (because maternal antibodies are formed & transferred to the neonate, conferring protection).
- Preterm infants ≥28 weeks' gestation who are exposed and whose mother has no evidence of immunity. Premature infants <28 weeks' gestation or who weigh <1,000 g at birth and were exposed during hospitalization.
- Pregnant women who lack evidence of immunity to VZV.

NEONATAL HERPES SIMPLEX VIRUS (HSV)

- Neonatal HSV may be acquired in utero (congenital HSV), perinatally from contact with infected vaginal secretions (~85% of cases), or postnatally (~10% of cases).

PERINATALLY-ACQUIRED HSV INFECTION

- **Majority of Neonatal HSV infection are acquired perinatally (85%), via an infected maternal genital tract** (eg, exposure to infected vaginal secretions).

CLINICAL MANIFESTATIONS

- **3 main categories of Neonatal HSV therapeutic & prognostic significance — [1] localized skin, eye, and mouth (SEM); [2] CNS disease with or without SEM; and [3] disseminated disease involving multiple organs.**
- **[1] Localized to the skin, mouth, and eyes** — skin: classic vesicular lesions in clusters that coalesce; mouth: localized ulcerations of the mouth, tongue, and palate; eyes: conjunctivitis, excessive tearing, eye pain.
- **[2] CNS disease:** seizures (focal or generalized), irritability, tremors, lethargy, poor feeding, temperature instability (fever or hypothermia), and full anterior fontanel.
- **[3] Disseminated disease:** involves multiple organs (including skin & CNS involvement) — nonspecific signs and symptoms of neonatal sepsis (eg, temperature dysregulation, apnea, irritability, lethargy, respiratory distress, abdominal distension, hepatomegaly, ascites), which can lead to jaundice, hypotension, respiratory distress, DIC, & septic shock. The mortality of untreated disseminated neonatal HSV is >80%.

DIAGNOSIS

- Neonatal HSV infection is determined through isolation of HSV in culture, detection of HSV DNA using qualitative or quantitative Polymerase chain reaction (PCR) assays, and detection of HSV antigens using direct immunofluorescence assays (DFA). Serologies are not helpful.

All of the following tests should be performed:

- Viral culture or HSV PCR on surface swabs of the conjunctivae, mouth, nasopharynx, and rectum.
- Viral culture or HSV PCR (with or without DFA) of swabs/scrapings of any skin and mucous membrane lesions; CSF HSV PCR.
- Whole blood or plasma HSV PCR.
- Viral culture or HSV PCR of tracheal aspirate, if intubated.
- **Most infected infants have positive viral culture and/or PCR in one or more of the specimens listed above.**

MANAGEMENT

- **High-dose IV Acyclovir for 14 days, followed by oral suppressive Acyclovir for 6-12 months.** Topical ophthalmic solution (eg, Trifluridine, Idoxuridine, Ganciclovir) added if ocular involvement.

CONGENITAL (IN UTERO) HSV INFECTION Rare.

- Intrauterine infection due to maternal viremia: occurs due to primary HSV infection during pregnancy.
  - **Clinical manifestations: triad of [1] skin vesicles, [2] ulcerations, or [3] scarring + severe CNS involvement (eg, hydranencephaly, microcephaly) + ocular damage.**

- Intrauterine infection due to ascending infection: occurs in mothers with active HSV infection after prolonged rupture of membranes.
  - Clinical manifestations: cutaneous skin lesions, cutaneous scarring, signs of disseminated disease, or fatal neonatal pneumonitis.

ZIKA VIRUS

- Arthropod-borne flavivirus transmitted by *Aedes* mosquito (eg, *A. aegypti*).

TRANSMISSION
- **Bite of an infected mosquito, sex** (oral, vaginal, and anal), **maternal-fetal,** blood product transfusion, organ transplantation, and laboratory exposure.

RISK FACTORS
- Residence in or travel to an area where mosquito-borne transmission of Zika virus infection has been reported or unprotected sexual intercourse with a person who meets these criteria (common in Central & South America, the Caribbean, & the Pacific).

ASSOCIATED CONDITIONS
- Guillain-Barré syndrome or permanent neurological damage.
- **Congenital Zika syndrome: microcephaly, intracranial cerebral malformation,** ocular lesions, congenital contractures, and hypertonia.

CLINICAL MANIFESTATIONS
- **Most are asymptomatic**.
- Self-limited symptoms in 20% include low-grade fever, maculopapular pruritic rash (trunk followed by extremities), arthralgias (especially small joints of hands and feet), or conjunctivitis (nonpurulent).
- Hematospermia in males.

DIAGNOSIS
- **Serum or urine Zika virus IgM initial test of choice**.
- Reverse-transcriptase PCR for Zika viral RNA (in the serum, urine, or whole blood). Can be used as screening in pregnant women (in the first & second trimester) with risk factors.

MANAGEMENT
- **Supportive care:** hydration, acetaminophen for fever and arthritis. There is no specific treatment.
- Aspirin should not be used until Dengue fever has been ruled out and not used in children (increased risk of Reye syndrome).

PREVENTION
- CDC recommendation — **men with relevant history should wait at least 3 months** after symptom onset of Zika virus (if symptomatic) or last possible exposure (if asymptomatic) before having unprotected sex.
- **Women (whether symptomatic or not) should wait at least 8 weeks** after symptom onset (if symptomatic) or last possible exposure (if asymptomatic) before having unprotected sex.
- Relevant exposure = residence in or travel to an area where mosquito-borne transmission of Zika virus infection has been reported or unprotected sexual intercourse with a person who meets these criteria.
- Pregnant women should avoid or consider postponing travel to areas below 6,500 feet where mosquito transmission is ongoing.

CONGENITAL ZIKA SYNDROME
Characterized by 5 main features:
- **[1] severe microcephaly**
- **[2] decreased brain tissue:** including subcortical calcifications
- **[3] ocular damage:** macular and retinal changes
- **[4] congenital contractures:** eg, clubfoot or arthrogryposis
- **[5] hypertonia** restricting body movement after birth.

PERINATAL OR PRENATAL HPV INFECTION

- Perinatal or prenatal Human papillomavirus (HPV) infection can occur via ascension of the infection into the uterus and via hematogenous spread. May present as perianal or genital warts.

CONGENITAL RUBELLA SYNDROME

- **Rubella infection is teratogenic, <u>especially in the first trimester.</u>** Part of the ToRCH syndrome

CLINICAL MANIFESTATIONS

- Most are asymptomatic at birth. Neonates may have growth retardation, radiolucent bone disease, hepatosplenomegaly, purpuric skin lesions **"<u>blueberry muffin" rash</u>** (due to Thrombotic thrombocytopenic purpura and extramedullary hematopoiesis).
- **Triad of [1] <u>auditory defects</u> (eg, sensorineural deafness), [2] <u>cardiovascular defects</u> (eg, Patent ductus arteriosus), [3] <u>ocular defects</u> (eg, cataracts). Of all the manifestations, hearing loss is the most common finding and may the only defect observed**, followed by intellectual disability, cardiovascular defects, and ocular defects.
- **[1] <u>Auditory defects</u>: sensorineural deafness (most common finding).**
- **[2] <u>Cardiac defects</u>: Patent ductus arteriosus (most common),** branch pulmonary artery stenosis.
- **[3] <u>Ocular defects</u>: cataracts,** cloudy cornea, glaucoma, retinopathy, microphthalmia, retinopathy.
- <u>Neurologic</u>: meningoencephalitis, microcephaly, mental and motor delay, autism.
- <u>Endocrine</u>: Diabetes mellitus, thyroid dysfunction, liver dysfunction, hyperbilirubinemia.

DIAGNOSIS

- **<u>Rubella-specific IgM</u>: Elevated Rubella-specific IgM antibody via enzyme immunoassay.** In case of a negative result for IgM in specimens taken earlier than day 5 after rash onset, serologic testing should be repeated. Rubella-specific IgG in infants after 6 to 12 months of age.
- <u>RTPCR</u>: Real-time reverse transcriptase-Polymerase chain reaction detection of viral RNA is an alternative modality when false-negative or false-positive IgM results are of concern.

MANAGEMENT: Supportive care only (organ specific) as there is no specific treatment for CRS.

PREVENTION

- <u>Maternal screening</u> with anti-Rubella IgG antibody titers in early pregnancy. Laboratory diagnosis if symptoms consistent with Rubella (RV-IgG and IgM titers).

CONGENITAL SYPHILIS

- Congenital infection can lead to stillbirth, prematurity, & hydrops fetalis. Part of the ToRCH syndrome.
- Adequate treatment of the mother before the 16th week of pregnancy should prevent fetal damage.

CLINICAL MANIFESTATIONS

- ~60–90% of live-born neonates with Congenital syphilis are asymptomatic at birth .
- **<u>Early <2 years of age</u>: mucocutaneous [eg, syphilitic rhinitis with nasal discharge ("snuffles'), rash],** bone changes (periostitis of long bones on imaging), generalized lymphadenopathy, hematologic (thrombocytopenia, anemia, jaundice) CNS, pulmonary complications, hepatomegaly,
- **<u>Late >2 years of age</u>: facial abnormalities — saddle nose deformity, Hutchinson teeth (notched, spaced upper incisors).** Interstitial keratitis, sensorineural hearing loss, & developmental delays.

DIAGNOSIS

- Symptoms consistent with congenital Syphilis + VDRL or RPR titer ≥fourfold the maternal titer; Positive Darkfield microscopy or fluorescent antibody testing of the umbilical cord, placenta, or body fluids.

MANAGEMENT

- <u><1 month of age</u>: **Penicillin G Benzathine IM x 1 or IV Penicillin x 10 days.** <u>>1 month</u>: **IV Penicillin.**

BRUCELLOSIS

- **Zoonotic infection** due to **Brucella spp.** are gram-negative coccobacilli (*B. melitensis* most common).
- **Endemic in Mediterranean, Mexico & South America.** Rare in US.

TRANSMISSION

- **Ingestion of infected dairy products (eg, unpasteurized milk or cheese), consumption of undercooked meat,** or by contact with infected tissue or fluids.
- **Occupational exposure, such as Veterinarian or farmer or contact with livestock** (eg, goat, sheep, cattle, hogs) or those handling infected tissues. 2–4-week incubation period.

CLINICAL MANIFESTATIONS

- **Triad of [1] <u>undulant fever</u> (most common) + [2] <u>profuse sweating</u> (often with a <u>moldy, wet hay smell</u>) + [3] <u>migratory arthralgia or myalgia</u> (muscle pain).**
- <u>Nonspecific symptoms</u> — weakness, headache, low back pain, dizziness, anorexia, weight loss, malaise, easy exhaustion, abdominal pain, dyspepsia, cough.
- <u>Physical examination:</u> fever, hepatomegaly, splenomegaly, or lymphadenopathy may be seen.

<u>Complications:</u>
- Endocarditis most lethal. Meningoencephalitis.
- <u>Osteoarticular disease:</u> 20% develop Osteomyelitis (especially of the lumbar spine), peripheral arthritis, sacroiliitis, spondylitis.
- <u>Genitourinary involvement:</u> orchitis and/or epididymitis, tubo-ovarian abscess, cystitis.
- <u>Neurologic involvement:</u> meningitis (acute or chronic), encephalitis, brain abscess, myelitis, radiculitis, and/or neuritis (with involvement of cranial or peripheral nerves).
- <u>Pulmonary involvement:</u> bronchitis, interstitial pneumonitis, lobar pneumonia, lung nodules.

DIAGNOSIS

- Blood culture, bone marrow culture (higher yield), serologies (IgM or IgG). Thrombocytopenia.
- Elevated transaminases; <u>CBC</u>: leukopenia or leukocytosis (relative lymphocytosis), anemia.

MANAGEMENT

- **<u>Combination therapy</u>: Doxycycline + aminoglycoside (Streptomycin or Gentamicin) for 6 weeks.**
- **<u>Children ≥8 years</u>: Rifampin plus Doxycycline.**
- **<u>Children <8 years</u>: Rifampin + Trimethoprim-sulfamethoxazole** (substituted for Doxycycline).

<u>Spondylitis, Neurobrucellosis, or Endocarditis:</u>
- <u>Nonpregnant adults & children ≥8 years</u>: Doxycycline plus Rifampin plus Aminoglycoside (Streptomycin or Gentamicin). TMP-SMX is substituted for Doxycycline if <8 years..
- <u>For nonpregnant adults and children ≥8 years</u>: Ceftriaxone, Rifampin, & Doxycycline.

HOT TUB FOLLICULITIS

- Benign self-limited skin lesions caused by **Pseudomonas aeruginosa.**
- Commonly seen 8-48 hours after exposure to water in a **contaminated spa, whirlpool, swimming pool, or hot tub (especially if it is made of wood).**

CLINICAL MANIFESTATIONS

- **Small** (2–10 mm), **tender, pruritic, pink to red papules, papulopustules or nodules** around the hair follicles within 1-4 days after exposure. May have flu-like symptoms (eg, malaise, low grade fever).

MANAGEMENT

- **No treatment needed in most cases** — usually spontaneously resolves within 7–14 days without treatment.
- **Oral Ciprofloxacin if persistent.**

Q FEVER

- Zoonotic infection caused by ***Coxiella burnetii.*** Gram-negative.

TRANSMISSION
- **Contact with farm animals**: inhalation of spores or ingestion. **Exposure to farm animals (eg, sheep, goats, cattle), cats, & their products** (eg, **wool, unpasteurized milk, animal hides,** urine, feces). Individuals living downwind from farms & contaminated manure, straw, or dust. Acquired in the lab.

CLINICAL MANIFESTATIONS
Acute Q fever (<6 months) 3 classic presentations:
- **[1] Atypical pneumonia main manifestation of acute Q fever** — non-productive cough and fever.
- **[2] Influenza-like illness** 2-3 weeks after exposure: eg, **abrupt onset of high-grade fever (often with a relative bradycardia), severe headache (often retro-orbital), and fatigue most common symptoms.** Cough, fatigue, myalgia, abdominal pain. <u>CNS involvement</u> — eg, Encephalopathy.
- **[3] Hepatitis** — hepatomegaly, acute febrile episode, or prolonged fever of unknown origin with granulomatous hepatitis seen on liver biopsy.

Chronic Q fever:
- **Culture-negative Endocarditis is the main manifestation of chronic Q fever.**

DIAGNOSIS
- <u>Acute</u>: **immunofluorescence IFA most common** — Coxiella anti-phase II ≥200 for IgG & ≥50 for IgM.
- <u>Chronic</u>: Phase I IgG immunoglobulin titer >800 associated with persistent localized infection.
- Leukopenia, increased LFTs (Hepatitis). Weil-Felix testing was used prior to IFA.
- <u>Chest radiography</u> lobar opacities or patchy infiltrates
- **All patients with Q fever should have a transthoracic echocardiogram to assess for Endocarditis.**

MANAGEMENT
- **Doxycycline initial treatment of choice.** Quinolones. <u>Pregnancy</u>: Trimethoprim-sulfamethoxazole.
- **Severe disease & endocarditis: Doxycycline plus Hydroxychloroquine.**

ERYSIPELOID

- ***Erysipelothrix rhusiopathiae*** (gram-positive bacillus) causes a self-limited soft tissue infection. May lead to systemic infection. *Erysipelothrix* has 3 major clinical manifestations.

TRANSMISSION
- **Occupational exposure follows skin abrasion or puncture wound from raw fish, shellfish, raw meat or poultry** (eg, butchers, slaughterhouse workers, fisherman, farmers, & veterinarians).

CLINICAL MANIFESTATIONS
- **[1] Localized cutaneous:** subacute Cellulitis limited to hands, fingers, or web spaces at the ports of entry — **red macule at inoculation site followed by non-pitting edema, <u>purplish (violaceous)</u> lesion with sharp irregular raised borders extending peripherally but <u>clearing centrally</u>.**
- [2] <u>Diffuse cutaneous</u>: proximal progression from initial site + involvement of other areas, fever, arthralgia.
- [3] <u>Systemic infection with bacteremia</u>: low grade fever + skin lesions. Endocarditis may occur.

DIAGNOSIS
- Usually clinical. Culture from material obtained during biopsy or blood culture if bacteremic.

MANAGEMENT
- **Localized cutaneous: Penicillin first line** (eg, **Penicillin V or Amoxicillin**) for 5-7 days. <u>Penicillin allergy</u>: Cephalexin, Ciprofloxacin, or Clindamycin are alternatives (5-7 days).
- **Diffuse cutaneous disease: IV Penicillin G.** Ceftriaxone, Fluoroquinolone, Daptomycin, or Imipenem.
- <u>Systemic & bacteremia</u>: IV Penicillin G. Ceftriaxone, Cefazolin, Fluoroquinolone, Daptomycin, Imipenem.

PLAGUE

- *Yersinia pestis* **(gram-negative rod).** Incubation period 2-10 days.
- Rare in US (10-15 cases/year in US in SW states like Arizona, New Mexico, California, Colorado, Utah).

TRANSMISSION
- **Flea bites (eg, rodent fleas).** Respiratory droplets from untreated person with pulmonic form.

CLINICAL MANIFESTATIONS
- Rapid onset of fever, chills, weakness, malaise, myalgias, tachycardia, severe headache, & altered mental status (delirium), followed by one of **3 main forms:**
- **[1] Bubonic: most common form (80-95%) — acute extremely swollen, warm, red, & painful lymph nodes (buboes) 2-10 cm in diameter in the groin, axilla, & cervical regions.** Lymphatic spread may lead to hematogenous spread (can become septicemic or pulmonic).
- **[2] Septicemic (10-20%): subsequent, advanced disease characterized by DIC & gangrene.** Plague without the presence of buboes. **DIC: extensive purpura 'black death".** **Acral gangrene:** distal extremities, nose, or penis. Patients often die from pneumonia or meningitis.
- **[3] Pneumonic:** pneumonia, tachypnea, productive cough, frothy **blood-tinged sputum "red death",** cyanosis. **Most lethal form** (nearly 100% mortality if not treated within 24 hours of symptom onset).

DIAGNOSIS
- Gram stain from tissue/buboes: **bipolar staining (safety pin appearance).** Cultures. Serologic tests.

MANAGEMENT
- **Aminoglycosides (Gentamicin or Streptomycin) first line treatment or a Fluoroquinolone** (eg, Levofloxacin, Ciprofloxacin, Moxifloxacin) **or Doxycycline** for 10-14 days.
- Combination therapy if septicemic or pneumonic.
- Place on strict respiratory isolation for at least 48 hours after initiating antibiotic therapy.
- Post exposure prophylaxis: Doxycycline, Levofloxacin, Ciprofloxacin, or Moxifloxacin for individuals with unprotected face-to-face contact (within 2 meters) of patients with known or suspected disease.

NECROTIZING SOFT TISSUE INFECTIONS (FASCIITIS, MYOSITIS, CELLULITIS)

- Necrotizing soft tissue infection leading to rapid tissue destruction, systemic toxicity, & high mortality.
- Etiologies: **usually a polymicrobial infection. Group A *Streptococcus* (GAS) most common isolate.** ***Clostridium perfringens* is an important cause of Gas Gangrene.**
- Risk factors: **Diabetes mellitus,** chronic corticosteroid use, alcohol use disorder, IV drug use.

CLINICAL MANIFESTATIONS
- **Rapid progression of erythema, edema extending beyond the visible erythema & extreme pain out of proportion to physical exam,** development of **blue, hemorrhagic bullae (blisters at site),** followed by **gangrene & necrosis,** followed by septic shock. Crepitus may be elicited.
- **Fournier gangrene: necrotizing fasciitis of the perineum, often with scrotal involvement** especially seen with **impaired immunity (eg, Diabetes Mellitus)** or after trauma to the area.

DIAGNOSIS
- **Diagnosis is established via surgical exploration** of the soft tissues in the operating room.
- Although imaging is often obtained, *imaging should never delay antibiotics & surgical exploration.*

MANAGEMENT
- **Immediate, early, & aggressive surgical exploration with debridement of necrotic material mainstay of treatment + broad spectrum empiric antibiotics** + hemodynamic support.
  - **Broad-spectrum antibiotics: either [1] Carbapenem** (eg, Imipenem, Meropenem, Ertapenem) **OR Piperacillin-Tazobactam PLUS [2] MRSA coverage (Vancomycin or Daptomycin) PLUS [3] Clindamycin** (Clindamycin has antitoxin effects on streptococci and staphylococci).

LISTERIOSIS

- **_Listeria monocytogenes_** non-spore forming, <u>endotoxin-producing</u>, gram-positive bacilli.
- <u>Transmission:</u> most commonly found in contaminated food (eg, **cold deli meats, hot dogs, & unpasteurized dairy products, such as soft cheese & milk, refrigerated seafood & meats).**

RISK FACTORS
- <u>Highest in 4 populations</u>: neonates (<30 days), the elderly, immunocompromised, & during pregnancy.

CLINICAL MANIFESTATIONS
- **<u>Listerial febrile gastroenteritis:</u>** fever, "flu-like" symptoms, & diarrhea. Self-limited (lasts 48 hours).
- **<u>Listeriosis:</u> bacteremia and/or meningitis in infants <2 months, immunocompromised, & elderly.** Third most common cause of neonatal bacterial Meningitis.
- **<u>Pregnancy:</u> third trimester** — febrile illness (diarrhea or bacteremia) **associated with preterm labor, intrauterine fetal demise, or infected newborns** (brown or cloudy amniotic fluid).

DIAGNOSIS: <u>Cultures:</u> blood or CSF — gram-positive facultative intracellular bacilli.

MANAGEMENT
- **<u>CNS or bloodstream infection</u>: <u>IV Ampicillin</u> initial management of choice or IV Penicillin G.**
- **<u>Gentamicin</u> often added for synergy** in meningitis, endocarditis, & infections in patients that are immunocompromised. _Listeria is resistant to all Cephalosporins._
- **<u>Penicillin allergy</u>: desensitization or treatment with Trimethoprim-sulfamethoxazole.**
- <u>Empiric management of Meningitis (Listeria coverage):</u> **<1 month old**: Ampicillin + Cefotaxime + Gentamicin if <1 month old. **>50 years of age**: Vancomycin + Ceftriaxone + Ampicillin.
- **<u>Listerial febrile gastroenteritis</u>: oral Amoxicillin in immunocompromised, pregnancy, and older adult patients.** Trimethoprim-sulfamethoxazole is an alternative in non-pregnant patients. **In all other immunocompetent patients, antibiotics are <u>not</u> usually given since it is self-limited.**

AMEBIASIS

- **_Entamoeba histolytica_** — protozoan most commonly transmitted by ingestion of cysts from fecally contaminated food and/or water, institutionalized patients, and men who have sex with men.
- Not common in the US. Usually occurs in migrants from or travelers to endemic tropical areas.
- **May develop an <u>amebic liver abscess.</u>**

CLINICAL MANIFESTATIONS
- Most infections are asymptomatic.
- <u>GI symptoms:</u> 1–3-week subacute onset, varying from **mild diarrhea to severe dysentery** (abdominal pain, diarrhea, bloody stools, mucus in stools weight loss, fever). **Recurrent diarrhea.**
- **<u>Amebic liver abscess:</u> fever, RUQ pain, anorexia, weight loss, tender hepatomegaly.**

DIAGNOSIS
- **_E histolytica_-<u>specific antigen</u> in the stool (eg, ELISA) sensitive, easy to perform, and rapid.**
- <u>Stool microscopy O&P</u> (ova & parasites) — cysts with ingested RBCs. Because cysts are not constantly shed, at least 3 stool samples on different days should be examined. Not as sensitive as stool antigen.
- <u>Stool PCR</u> — detects parasitic DNA or RNA in the stool. Leukocytosis.
- <u>Liver abscess:</u> ultrasound, CT, or MRI. Increased LFTs with amebic liver abscess.

MANAGEMENT
- **<u>Colitis:</u> Metronidazole (first line) or Tinidazole, followed by an intraluminal agent (eg, Paromomycin,** Diloxanide furoate, or Diiodohydroxyquinoline).
- **<u>Liver abscess:</u>** Metronidazole or Tinidazole + intraluminal amebicide followed by Chloroquine. May need drainage (eg, needle aspiration) if no response to medications after 3 days.
- <u>Asymptomatic infections</u> should be treated with an intraluminal agent alone.

ANTHRAX

- *Bacillus anthracis* (gram-positive, spore-forming rod) **is naturally found in livestock (eg, cattle, horses, goats, sheep, swine).**

TRANSMISSION
- Direct contact (eg, **wool, handling animal hide or hair**). Inhalation or ingestion of spores.

CLINICAL MANIFESTATIONS
- **[1] Cutaneous:** 5-14 days after exposure — erythematous papule at the inoculation site that ulcerates followed by a **painless black depressed eschar with edematous borders & vesicles.** Regional lymphadenopathy, and lymphangitis. **Cutaneous most common type of Anthrax.**
- **[2] Gastrointestinal:** rare in the US. Ingestion of meat with spores lead to ulcerative lesions in the GI tract (eg, GI bleeding, abdominal pain, nausea, vomiting), oropharyngeal ulcers, cervical adenopathy.
- **[3] Inhalation:** inhalation of spores — nonspecific flu-like symptoms rapidly progressing to dyspnea (pleural effusions), hypoxia & shock. Rapidly fatal. Inhalation <5%. Called "woolsorter's disease".

DIAGNOSIS
- Clinical diagnosis confirmed with positive PCR, serology, culture, or immunochemistry.
- Cultures: **boxcar-shaped, encapsulated gram-positive rods with a "Medusa head" appearance** on microscopy.
- Chest radiograph (inhalation): **widening of the mediastinum (due to hemorrhagic lymphadenitis).**

MANAGEMENT
- **Cutaneous Anthrax without systemic involvement:** not involving the head or neck without systemic involvement or extensive edema — **oral antimicrobial therapy with a single agent: Fluoroquinolones (eg, Ciprofloxacin,** Levofloxacin, Moxifloxacin) **or Doxycycline.**
- **Systemic: IV bactericidal (eg, Ciprofloxacin) PLUS a protein synthesis inhibitor (eg, Clindamycin or Linezolid) + an antitoxin (eg, Raxibacumab, Obiltoxaximab, or anthrax immunoglobulin) + supportive care** (eg, pleural effusion drainage) + consideration of adjunctive glucocorticoids.
- Suspected Meningitis: Ciprofloxacin plus Meropenem plus Linezolid + an antitoxin.

ACANTHAMOEBA KERATITIS

- Infection of the cornea due to *Acanthamoeba,* a free-living amoeba.
- Present in tap water and swimming pools.
- Risk factors: **most common in contact lens wearers with poor contact lens hygiene** (eg, **wearing lens for long periods of time,** swimming or showering with contact lens).
- Transmission: use of nonsterile tap water in preparation of contact lens solution, or use of infected contact lens solution.

CLINICAL MANIFESTATIONS
- **Keratitis:** ocular pain, photophobia, tearing, blurred vision, conjunctival injection. Physical exam: **partial or complete ring infiltrate of the corneal stroma,** hypopyon, pseudo-dendritic lesions.
- Encephalitis & granulomatous disease may be seen in immunocompromised patients.

DIAGNOSIS
- Staining of cornea scrapings: trophozoites can visualized using the fluorescent dye calcofluor.
- Corneal cultures of scrapings. PCR.

MANAGEMENT
- Combination treatment: Polyhexamethylene biguanide or Biguanide-Chlorhexidine digluconate (0.02%) in combination with topical Propamidine isethionate or Hexamidine. Miconazole.
- Chronic refractory: corneal transplantation. Oral Itraconazole or Ketoconazole added if deep keratitis.

EHRLICHIOSIS (HME) & ANAPLASMOSIS (HGA)

- **Tick-borne illnesses caused by gram-negative obligate intracellular coccobacilli that destroy white blood cells.** HME common in men 60–69 years of age; HMA common in men >40 years of age.

ETIOLOGIES: **2 diseases with similar presentations:**
- **[1] Human granulocytic Anaplasmosis (HGA):** due to *Anaplasma phagocytophilum* transmitted by the *Ixodes scapularis* blacklegged tick (the same tick associated with Lyme disease & Babesiosis).
- **[2] Human monocytic Ehrlichiosis (HME):** *Ehrlichia chaffeensis* & *canis* transmitted by the **Lone star tick** (*Amblyomma americanum*). Endemic to SE, SC, & mid-Atlantic US.

CLINICAL MANIFESTATIONS
- Symptoms usually begin 7-10 days after a tick bite with a **prodrome of rigors, malaise, nausea, vomiting, followed by high fever, chills, myalgia, headache.** Splenomegaly may occur.
- Rash is uncommon but if it develops, it can be macular or maculopapular. If a rash is present, coinfection with other tick-borne diseases or an alternative diagnosis should be suspected.
- Petechial rash reflects thrombocytopenia.

DIAGNOSIS
- Serologies: **Indirect fluorescent antibody test most useful test to support the diagnosis** performed on acute and convalescent sera. ELISA. **PCR** most sensitive during the first week of the illness.
- **Peripheral blood smear or Buffy coat: morulae in WBCs** (granulocytes in HGA; monocytes in HME). **Morulae = clusters in the cell vacuoles, forming large mulberry-shaped aggregates**, especially with HGA (less often with HME).
- Supportive laboratory findings: **Leukopenia** (reflects the WBC destruction associated with infection), **increased LFTs (transaminitis), & thrombocytopenia are commonly seen.**

MANAGEMENT
- **Doxycycline first-line treatment in children & adults as soon as HME or HGA suspected** [treatment for at least 3 days after defervescence or a minimum of 10 days (7-14 days in children)]. **Doxycycline is also first line in pregnancy.** Although most Tetracyclines are contraindicated in pregnancy because of the risk of hepatotoxicity in the mother and adverse effects on fetal bone and teeth, these are extremely rare with Doxycycline and the benefits outweigh the potential risks.
- **Severe allergy: Rifampin is an alternative for individuals who cannot take Doxycycline.**
- Preventive measures include the use of tick repellants, protective clothing, and early examination and removal of ticks after exposure to tick-infested environments.

TYPE OF PRECAUTIONS	COMMON DISEASES
AIRBORNE	• Tuberculosis (including N95 mask) • Chickenpox (contact & airborne) • Disseminated Herpes zoster • Measles
DROPLET	• Influenza • Neisseria meningitidis • Respiratory Diphtheria • Pertussis • Mumps • Rubella • RSV (droplet and contact)
CONTACT	• Clostridioides difficile • MRSA, VRE • RSV (droplet and contact) • Adenovirus • Cutaneous Diphtheria • Chickenpox (until all lesions are crusted & healed). Contact and airborne.

HERPES SIMPLEX VIRUS 1 (HSV-1)

TRANSMISSION
- Direct contact with contaminated saliva or other infected bodily secretions (eg, mouth to mouth contact, shared drinkware).
- Pathophysiology: Direct contact at mucosal or skin sites cause viral entry into the epidermis until it reaches the sensory & autonomic nerve endings. Triggers: stress, illness, and UV light exposure.

Oral lesions:
- **[1] Primary infection**: Most primary infections are asymptomatic but may cause **tonsillopharyngitis** in adults or **gingivostomatitis** in children.
- **[2] Recurrent infection: Herpes labialis (cold sore): reactivation of latent infection** in ganglion neurons — **prodromal symptoms** (pruritus, burning, tingling, pain) within 24 hours followed by the development of **grouped vesicles on an erythematous base that crust over prior to healing.**

Cutaneous lesions:
- **Herpetic whitlow of the finger** seen in dentists & healthcare workers exposed to infected secretions.
- Herpes gladiatorum — vesiculopustular rash on the face, neck, & arms of wrestlers or rugby players.
- Eczema herpeticum — patients with Atopic dermatitis are at risk for developing an HSV-related skin rash characterized by cutaneous pain and new vesicular new skin lesions secondary to HSV-1.

DIAGNOSIS
- **PCR: test of choice (most sensitive & specific).** HSV-1 serology (antibody detection via Western blot).
- Viral cultures, direct fluorescent antibody; Tzanck smear (nonspecific finding of multinucleated giant cells).

MANAGEMENT
- Orolabial: **oral Valacyclovir** (2 g twice daily x 1 day). **Acyclovir** is an alternative. Docosanol cream.
- Chronic suppression may be needed for recurrent outbreaks.

GENITAL HERPES

- **Most recurrent genital lesions caused by Herpes simplex 2 (HSV-2).** ~25% of population in the US.

TRANSMISSION
- Sexually transmitted via direct close contact with infected lesions. HSV-1 less common cause.
- The virus can enter and stay dormant in the sensory nerve ganglion where it can become activated.

CLINICAL MANIFESTATIONS
- **Painful fluid-filled vesicles that progress to shallow-based genital ulcers; often preceded by prodromal symptoms** (eg, burning, paresthesias, numbness).
- Primary infection: systemic symptoms, dysuria, fever, headache, malaise, & tender lymphadenopathy.

PHYSICAL EXAMINATION
- **Multiple, shallow, tender grouped 2-4 mm vesicles on an erythematous base that progress to vesicopustules, erosions, and ulcerations** with scalloped borders.
- Primary infection: skin lesions and painful (tender) inguinal lymphadenopathy.

DIAGNOSIS
- **PCR is the test of choice (most sensitive and specific).**
- HSV-1 serology not as sensitive or specific as PCR. Viral cultures, direct fluorescent antibody.
- Tzanck smear: **multinucleated giant cells** (intranuclear eosinophilic Cowdry A inclusions) is classic but not specific (can be seen with HSV-1, HSV-2, and Varicella zoster virus).

MANAGEMENT
- **Valacyclovir** (often preferred because it is dosed less frequently) **or Acyclovir or Famciclovir**

HSV ENCEPHALITIS

- **Severe infection of the brain parenchyma caused by HSV-1. Most common cause of Encephalitis.**
- **Associated with high mortality** (>70% if untreated, 20-30% with treatment).
- Pathophysiology: virus gains access to the brain along axons of the trigeminal ganglia, leading to **temporal lobe necrosis.**

CLINICAL MANIFESTATIONS

- **Focal neurologic findings: rapid onset of fever, headache, seizures, mental status & alertness changes & focal neurologic signs & deficits** (eg, hemiparesis, cranial nerve deficits, dysphasia, aphasia, ataxia). Primarily affects the **temporal lobe,** leading to bizarre behavior & focal deficits.

DIAGNOSIS

- **Lumbar puncture: classic viral CSF pattern — increased lymphocytes + normal CSF glucose, elevated CSF red blood cells,** & increased protein. **PCR detection of HSV DNA in CSF criterion standard.** Brain biopsy may be indicated in cases refractory to treatment.
- **Neuroimaging: temporal lobe involvement** characteristic of HSV-1 Encephalitis; ± frontal lobe.

MANAGEMENT

- **IV Acyclovir** initiated empirically as soon as the diagnosis is considered.
- Do not delay treatment while waiting for laboratory confirmation. Even with early administration of therapy, many patients have significant residual neurologic deficits.

EPSTEIN-BARR VIRUS [EBV] (INFECTIOUS MONONUCLEOSIS) – HHV-4

- **Infection due to Epstein-Barr virus characterized by fever, lymphadenopathy, and tonsillar pharyngitis, most common in adolescents & young adults (especially 15-25 years of age).**
- Pathophysiology: EBV, part of the Human herpesvirus family (HHV-4), infects B cells.
- Transmission: **saliva** (known as the "kissing disease"). 80% of adults are seropositive.

CLINICAL MANIFESTATIONS

- **Pharyngitis sore throat; may have exudative tonsils &/or petechiae on the hard palate.**
- **Systemic symptoms eg, fever, fatigue (often marked), pharyngitis,** headache, malaise, myalgia.
- **Lymphadenopathy posterior cervical > anterior;** lymphadenopathy may be generalized.
- May develop **splenomegaly (>50%)** or hepatomegaly. Transient upper lid edema (Hoagland sign).
- **Generalized maculopapular rash** seen in ~5%, **especially if given Ampicillin or Amoxicillin.**

DIAGNOSIS

- **Heterophile antibody (eg, Monospot) — test of choice** (positive within 4 weeks).
- **EBV-specific antibodies** IgM & IgG antibodies directed against viral capsid antigen. Increased LFTs.
- **Peripheral smear: lymphocytosis (>50%) with >10% atypical lymphocytes** (Downey cells).
- In patients with negative Mono testing, consider acute CMV & acute HIV in the differential diagnosis.

MANAGEMENT

- **Supportive mainstay of treatment** — rest, analgesics (eg, Acetaminophen, NSAIDs), antipyretics, warm gargles. Symptoms, especially fatigue, may last for months.
- Corticosteroids administered ONLY if airway obstruction due to enlarging lymphadenopathy, hemolytic anemia, or severe thrombocytopenia. Group A streptococcus & EBV can coexist.
- **Avoid trauma & contact sports at least 3 weeks from symptom onset (noncontact sports) or 4 weeks (contact sports) if splenomegaly is present to prevent splenic rupture.**

COMPLICATIONS

- **Rare complications: splenic rupture, airway obstruction, hemolytic anemia, thrombocytopenia.**
- Lymphoma (Hodgkin, Burkitt, CNS), Nasopharyngeal carcinoma, Gastric carcinoma, hairy leukoplakia.

VARICELLA ZOSTER VIRUS [VZV] (HHV-3)

- **Varicella zoster virus** is part of the Human herpes virus family (HHV-3).
- VZV causes 2 clinically distinct diseases: **[1] Primary — varicella (chickenpox) & [2] reactivation of latent VZV infection [Herpes zoster (Shingles)],** most common after the sixth decade of life.

CHICKENPOX (VARICELLA)

TRANSMISSION

- **[1] <u>aerosolized droplets</u>** from nasopharyngeal secretions or **[2] <u>direct contact</u>** with skin lesions.
- 10–20-day incubation period (often within 15 days).

CLINICAL MANIFESTATIONS

- <u>Prodrome</u>: low-grade fever, malaise, myalgia, anorexia, oral enanthem (pharyngitis with oral cavity lesions) followed by generalized exanthem (vesicular rash), usually within 24-48 hours.
- **<u>Vesicular rash:</u> classic evolution — usually pruritic, erythematous macules that become papules then vesicles and pustules, and then crust over.** The rash begins on the face, then goes to the trunk before rapidly spreading to the extremities and other areas. **The rash of Chickenpox occurs in successive crops over a 2–5-day period, resulting in <u>different stages of evolution simultaneously</u>.**

PHYSICAL EXAMINATION

- **<u>Asynchronous rash in different stages of evolution,</u>** including, macules, papules, clusters of **vesicles on an erythematous base ("dew drops on a rose petal"),** & crusted lesions. More severe in adults.

DIAGNOSIS

- **Usually a clinical diagnosis.**
- **<u>Polymerase chain reaction (PCR)</u> has the highest yield when testing is needed.** Can be performed on fluid from lesions, skin scrapings or CSF.
- <u>Direct fluorescent antibody staining</u> has largely replaced Tzanck smear.
- <u>Tzanck smear</u> — multinucleated giant cells (can also be seen with HSV).
- <u>Serologies</u>: anti-VZV IgM in response to an acute infection (not used often). IgG denotes immunity.

MANAGEMENT

- **<u>Previously healthy child 12 years or younger</u> — supportive & symptomatic treatment, often without antiviral therapy — symptomatic management of rash and fever;** Pruritus can be treated with antihistamines, topical dressings (eg, Calamine lotion), daily bathing with tepid water may be soothing and prevent infection, wet compresses, and soaks (eg, Aluminum acetate). **Avoid Acetylsalicylic acid (increased risk of Reye syndrome).** NSAIDs increase risk of superinfection.
- **<u>Acyclovir</u> should be given to adolescents (unvaccinated children ≥13 years old), adults, pregnant women, & immunocompromised patients** because they are susceptible to complications (eg, pneumonia, encephalitis, & hemorrhagic complications). When given within 72 hours of onset, Acyclovir can reduce both the severity & duration of Varicella. **Valacyclovir.**
- Hospitalized patients should be placed on BOTH **contact and airborne precautions.**
- **Chickenpox can be spread from 48 hours prior to the onset of the rash up until all the lesions have crusted over.** During that time frame, patients should avoid contact with pregnant women and unvaccinated individuals.

COMPLICATIONS

- **<u>Bacterial superinfection</u> most common complication in in children** (eg, Group A streptococcus and *Staphylococcus aureus*) including Cellulitis, Erysipelas, Scarlet fever. Bullous impetigo is uncommon.
- **<u>Varicella pneumonia</u> is the leading cause of mortality & morbidity in adults** (may develop within 3-7 days following the rash). Cigarette smokers, HIV, and pregnancy are risk factors.
- Encephalitis. Reye syndrome (fatty liver with encephalopathy) rare. Aseptic meningitis.

PREVENTION VIA ROUTINE CHILDHOOD VACCINATION: Live attenuated vaccine

- <u>Single antigen vaccine</u>: **administered at 12–15 months of age & second at 4–6 years.** Alternatively, the MMRV vaccine: first dose at 12–15 months of age & second dose before elementary school entry.

POST EXPOSURE TO VARICELLA

Varicella zoster immune globulin within 96 hours of exposure is recommended in susceptible individuals with high risk of developing Varicella (ideally as soon as possible) if there has been exposure within 10 days.

A second full dose is administered to high-risk patients with additional exposures to Varicella >3 weeks after the first dose.

VZIG reduces the severity of infection after exposure to Varicella virus in patients at high risk for severe infection and complications including:

- **Immunocompromised children & adults who lack evidence of immunity to VZV** (unvaccinated or seronegative).
- **Newborns of mothers with Varicella 5 days before to 2 days after delivery**.
- Premature infants ≥28 weeks' gestation who are exposed and whose mother has no evidence of immunity.
- Premature infants <28 weeks' gestation or who weigh <1,000 g at birth and were exposed during hospitalization.
- Pregnant women who lack evidence of immunity to VZV.

POST HERPETIC NEURALGIA (PHN)

- **Persistent pain or sensory symptoms >90 days (3 months) after onset of Herpes zoster (shingles).** The pain is often prolonged and can be debilitating. Once it occurs, it is difficult to treat.
- <u>Epidemiology</u>: Most commonly seen in the elderly.

<u>RISK FACTORS FOR PHN</u>:
- **Increasing age** ~10-15% of patients with Herpes zoster will develop PHN; **individuals >60 years of age account for 50% of cases.**
- Female gender
- Moderate to severe pain with preceding acute Herpes zoster episode.
- Ophthalmic involvement.

<u>CLINICAL MANIFESTATIONS</u>
- **Significant pain** (eg, burning, stabbing or sharp) **and/or alteration in skin sensation persisting for >90 days (3 months) after the onset and resolution of the rash. Located along a dermatome —** most commonly affects the thoracic, cervical, and trigeminal nerve dermatomes.
- <u>Sensory symptoms</u> can also include intermittent or persistent pain (eg, burning, stabbing, or sharp pain), numbness, dysesthesias, pruritus, and allodynia (hypersensitivity) in the affected dermatome.
- Changes in sensation in the dermatome, resulting in either hypo or hyperesthesia, are common. The pain may be prolonged and debilitating.

<u>MANAGEMENT</u>
- **Gabapentinoid: Gabapentin or Pregabalin initial management of choice in most patients**.
- **Topical Capsaicin** in milder disease in patients who prefer topical therapy.
- **Tricyclic antidepressants (eg, Amitriptyline, Nortriptyline, Desipramine)** may be used as an alternative to Gabapentinoids if unable to tolerate the first-line agents.
- <u>Alternative therapies</u> include other **antiseizure medications (eg, Valproic acid, Carbamazepine) & Serotonin-norepinephrine reuptake inhibitors [SNRIs (eg, Duloxetine, Venlafaxine)].**

<u>Additional therapies</u>:
- Options include oral or transdermal opioid analgesics and intrathecal glucocorticoid injections.
- Interventional and surgical approaches usually reserved for patients with refractory disease not responsive to other therapies. They include Botulinum toxin injections, Neuromodulation, and Cryotherapy.

HERPES ZOSTER (SHINGLES)

- VZV causes 2 clinically distinct diseases: [1] Primary — varicella (chickenpox) & **[2] reactivation of latent VZV infection [Herpes zoster (Shingles)], most common after the sixth decade of life.**
- Pathophysiology: after initial infection, the virus becomes latent in the dorsal root ganglia or trigeminal ganglia, where it can reactivate.
- Risk factors: **age >50 years, immunocompromised** (eg, chemotherapy, HIV, post-transplant, etc.).

CLINICAL MANIFESTATIONS

- **Prodrome** of fever, malaise, sensory changes (pain, burning, paresthesias), followed by painful rash.
- **[1] Unilateral dermatomal vesicular rash**: erythematous papules, followed by **painful eruption of grouped vesicles, bullae, and pustules on an erythematous base within a single dermatome** (or several continuous dermatomes) **that does not usually cross the midline. Thoracic & lumbar roots most common** [T3 to L3], lumbosacral, cervical, trigeminal, & facial nerve roots common.
- **[2] Acute neuritis**: pain often described as a deep "stabbing," "burning," or "throbbing," sensation.

COMPLICATIONS

- Cranial neuropathies, CNS involvement. Dissemination: ≥3 dermatomes, far outside of the dermatome, or organ involvement. Dissemination is most common in immunocompromised individuals.
- Post-herpetic neuralgia: persistent pain or sensory symptoms >90 days after the onset of Herpes zoster.

DIAGNOSIS

- **Usually a clinical diagnosis. PCR has the highest yield when testing is needed.** Viral cultures.
- Direct fluorescent antibody staining has largely replaced Tzanck smear.
- Tzanck smear — multinucleated giant cells (can also be seen with HSV).

MANAGEMENT

- **Antivirals: Valacyclovir, Famciclovir, or Acyclovir in patients who present within 72 hours of clinical symptoms with uncrusted lesions (or after 72 hours if new lesions are appearing at the time of presentation,** immunocompromised lesions along V1 dermatome, & patients age >65 years). Antivirals promote healing of skin lesions, reduce the severity and duration of acute neuritis, and reduce the incidence or severity of chronic pain (Postherpetic neuralgia).
- Analgesics for pain — eg, oral (NSAIDs &/or Acetaminophen), topical Lidocaine, or nerve blocks.
- **The patient is no longer infectious once all the lesions crust over** (on average about 7-10 days). During the infectious stage, they should avoid pregnant patients, immunocompromised people, and those who are not immunized against VZV.

POST-EXPOSURE PROPHYLAXIS

Varicella zoster immune globulin is given to people exposed to shingles who are at risk of infection within 72 hours of exposure. Passive immunization via the VZIG is recommended in:
- **Immunocompromised patients** (primary or acquired).
- Persons taking immunosuppressive therapies
- Persons with neoplastic diseases
- Neonates

PREVENTION [VARICELLA (HERPES ZOSTER) VACCINATION]

Vaccination with a live attenuated zoster vaccine reduces incidence & severity of zoster and PHN.
- **Recombinant zoster vaccine: adults aged ≥50 years; 2 dose series 2-6 months apart.** In immunocompromised individuals ≥19 years who already received the live attenuated vaccine, the 2-dose series should also be given (≥8 weeks after live vaccination) due to waning immunity.
- The vaccine has an efficacy of 97.2% in patients ≥50 years of age and **helps to reduce the incidence of Herpes zoster & Postherpetic neuralgia (PHN).**
- Also effective in older patients (efficacy 90% for 70–79 years of age and 89.1% for ≥80 years of age).

HERPES ZOSTER OPHTHALMICUS (KERATITIS)

- Potentially sight-threatening disorder that is a variant of reactivation, **Varicella zoster (shingles).**
- Pathophysiology: after initial infection, Varicella zoster virus becomes latent in the dorsal root ganglia or trigeminal ganglia, where it can reactivate, involving the **ophthalmic division of the Trigeminal (cranial nerve V).**

CLINICAL MANIFESTATIONS

- **Prodrome:** Herpes zoster ophthalmicus (HZO) begins with a prodrome of headache, malaise, and fever. Unilateral pain or hypesthesia in the affected eye, forehead, and top of the head may precede or follow the prodrome.
- **Vesicular rash: grouped vesicles on an erythematous base on the face.**
- Ocular involvement: with the onset of the rash, hyperemic **conjunctivitis, uveitis, episcleritis, and keratitis may develop.** Acute keratitis typically involves the epithelial, stromal, or endothelial layers of the cornea and may lead to vision loss.

PHYSICAL EXAMINATION

- **Hutchinson sign: Vesicular lesions on the tip of the nose, inner corner of the eye, root and side of the nose indicate involvement of the trigeminal nerve and correlate highly with eye involvement.** Lesions in this area of the face signify involvement of the nasociliary branch of the trigeminal nerve (CN 5), which also innervates the globe.
- Slit lamp examination: **pseudodendrites (branching) uptake of fluorescein** in keratoconjunctivitis.

DIAGNOSIS

- **Mainly a clinical diagnosis.**
- **Polymerase chain reaction viral DNA analysis via PCR has the highest yield when testing is needed (eg, atypical cases)** as it is 95% sensitive. Can be performed on fluid from blisters, skin scrapings, and non-skin samples, such as BAL fluid or CSF.

MANAGEMENT

- **Immediately ophthalmologist referral, analgesics for severe pain, Atropine, and antivirals (eg, Acyclovir, Valacyclovir, or Famciclovir).**
- The use of glucocorticoids should be made by the ophthalmologist.
- IV Acyclovir if immunocompromised or in cases requiring hospitalization for sight-threatening cases.

HERPES ZOSTER OTICUS (RAMSAY-HUNT SYNDROME)

- **Reactivation of Varicella zoster virus in the geniculate ganglion of the sensory branch of cranial nerve 7 (facial nerve)** with or without subsequent spread to cranial nerve (CN) 8.

CLINICAL MANIFESTATIONS

- **Triad: ipsilateral [1] ear pain, [2] vesicles in the external auditory canal &/or on the auricle, and [3] ipsilateral facial paralysis (palsy).**
- In addition, other ipsilateral findings of facial nerve palsy (eg, loss of sense of taste in the anterior two-thirds of the tongue), decreased hearing tinnitus, hyperacusis, & decreased lacrimation) may occur.

DIAGNOSIS

- **Mainly a clinical diagnosis.** Direct fluorescent antibody (DFA) testing. Viral culture
- **Polymerase chain reaction viral DNA analysis via PCR has the highest yield if testing needed.**

MANAGEMENT

- **Valacyclovir and adjunctive glucocorticoids (eg, Prednisone).**
- In severe cases, IV therapy may be initiated with transition to oral antivirals as the condition improves.

CYTOMEGALOVIRUS [CMV] (HHV-5)

- **CMV — Human herpesvirus 5 (HHV-5)** transmitted via body fluids or vertical transmission.
- CMV is present in most people (70% in the US) with **clinical disease seen primarily in immunocompromised patients.**

CLINICAL MANIFESTATIONS
[1] Primary CMV infection:
- Most cases of primary CMV infection in immunocompetent individuals are *usually asymptomatic.*
- **CMV Mononucleosis: if symptomatic, symptoms are similar to EBV Mononucleosis** (fever, cough, myalgia, arthralgias, rash) **except in CMV Mononucleosis, exudate tonsillopharyngitis, cervical lymphadenopathy, & the presence of Heterophile antibodies characteristic of EBV are rare.**
[2] Secondary CMV reactivation:
Most common in immunocompromised: eg, HIV, long-term steroid, chemotherapy, post-transplant.
- **CMV colitis: most common reactivation manifestation** — diarrhea, fever, abdominal pain, bloody stools. Increased risk in advanced HIV with CD4 ≤100 cells/μL.
- **CMV retinitis:** decreased visual acuity & floaters. Funduscopy — **fluffy, yellow-white retinal lesions with indistinct margins, sometimes with a granular appearance, with or without intraretinal hemorrhage** ("scrambled eggs/ketchup" or "pizza pie" appearance). **CD4 count often ≤50** cells/μL.
- **CMV Esophagitis:** odynophagia & dysphagia. **Upper endoscopy: large superficial ulcers.**
- CMV Pneumonitis especially post-transplant. Neurologic: Encephalitis, Guillain-Barré syndrome.

DIAGNOSIS
- **Acute CMV: Serologies: CMV Mononucleosis can be confirmed by the detection of CMV-specific IgM antibodies** (suggesting recent seroconversion) **OR a ≥four-fold increase in CMV-specific IgG titers** in paired specimens obtained at least 2-4 weeks apart. **Negative Heterophile test.**
- **Reactivation CMV: Serologies: (eg, CMV-specific IgG antibody) helpful in determining past exposure to CMV infection,** Quantitative PCR assays.
- Labs: lymphocytes with atypical lymphocytosis similar to EBV mononucleosis.
- Biopsy of tissues: **owl's eye appearance (epithelial cells with enlarged nuclei surrounded by clear zone & cytoplasmic inclusions).**

MANAGEMENT
- Primary disease in immunocompetent patients is mainly supportive therapy.
- Primary CMV infection during early pregnancy high-dose Valacyclovir to prevent fetal problems.
- **Severe or reactivation: Antiviral therapy (eg, Ganciclovir) may be used in immunocompromised patients, severe disease, or organ damage.** Second line: Valganciclovir, Foscarnet, Cidofovir.

CONGENITAL CMV
- **Most common congenital viral infection.** Part of the ToRCH syndrome. Can lead to stillbirth, prematurity, & hydrops fetalis. Most common nonhereditary cause of sensorineural hearing loss.

CLINICAL MANIFESTATIONS
- Most are asymptomatic at birth. Neonates may develop petechiae, **blueberry muffin–like hemorrhagic purpuric eruptions,** jaundice, hepatosplenomegaly, & hepatitis.
- **[1] Neurologic: sensorineural hearing loss most common sequelae, periventricular calcifications,** cerebral palsy, microcephaly, & seizures. Intrauterine growth restriction.
- **[2] Eye involvement: congenital cataracts** or glaucoma, pigmentary retinopathy, **chorioretinitis.**
- **[3] Heart defects** eg, PDA, branch pulmonary artery stenosis (valvular & pulmonary artery).

DIAGNOSIS
- Viral culture or Polymerase chain reaction (PCR) tests for CMV DNA on urine &/or saliva samples.

MANAGEMENT
- **Life-threatening disease IV Ganciclovir; Non-life-threatening disease: Valganciclovir.**

RABIES

- **Life-threatening Rhabdovirus infection of the CNS (encephalitis of gray matter).**
- Rhabdovirus goes through axons from the peripheral to central nervous system via **cellular uptake of the virus via acetylcholine receptors.** Incubation period ~1-3 months (can occur after years).

TRANSMISSION

- **Infected saliva from rabid animal bites. The 4 major animal reservoirs in the US are bats (most common), raccoons, skunks, & foxes. Dogs cause ≥90% in developing countries.**
- **If a person was asleep in a room with a bat, they should be given prophylaxis <u>even if no visible bat bite</u> is seen.**
- **Rodents & lagomorphs (eg, rabbits) have not been known to transmit Rabies to humans.** The only rodent that will survive long enough to transmit it is a woodchuck.

CLINICAL MANIFESTATIONS

- <u>Prodromal syndrome</u> **pain, paresthesias, or pruritus at or near the initial site of the bite (earliest specific symptom);** <u>nonspecific symptoms:</u> fever, malaise, headache, nausea, and vomiting. The skin is sensitive to changes of temperature, **especially air currents (aerophobia).** Percussion myoedema (mounding of muscles after a light pressure stimulus).
- <u>**The CNS stage**</u> begins ~10 days after the prodrome and may be either <u>**[1] encephalitic (80%)**</u>: delirium (rabid rage) alternating with periods of calm, extremely **painful laryngeal spasms on after drinking, seeing, or hearing water (hydrophobia), autonomic stimulation (hypersalivation),** and seizures; or <u>**[2] paralytic**</u> (20%) an acute ascending paralysis similar to Guillain-Barré syndrome. **Both forms progress to coma, autonomic nervous system dysfunction, & death.**

DIAGNOSIS

- Isolation of virus or detection of viral RNA via polymerase chain reaction (PCR) testing from the saliva, virus-specific immunofluorescent staining (skin biopsy), or CSF or serum anti-rabies antibodies.

Animal evaluation:

- **A normally behaving domestic dog, cat, or ferret may be observed for 7-10 days to see if signs or symptoms of Rabies occur.** Sick or dead animals should be tested for Rabies.
- A wild animal, if captured, should be sacrificed and the head shipped on ice to the nearest laboratory qualified to examine the brain for evidence of rabies virus. <u>Immunofluorescence:</u> **Negri bodies** in the brain of euthanized animals (especially in the hippocampus).
- When the animal cannot be examined, raccoons, skunks, bats, & foxes should be presumed to be rabid.

MANAGEMENT

- **There is no established management of Rabies once symptoms occur (the vast majority of cases are fatal), so prevention via post exposure prophylaxis is the mainstay of management.**

POST EXPOSURE PROPHYLAXIS

Post exposure first episode:

- **The wound should be washed with soap and water and treatment should be instituted with Rabies immune globulin and Rabies vaccine** [human diploid cell vaccine (HDCV)].
- <u>**Wound care is the first step in the treatment of feared Rabies exposure.**</u> Appropriate wound care alone has been noted to be ~100% effective if initiated within 3 hours of inoculation.
- <u>**HDCV (Rabies Vaccine)**</u> **days 0, 3, 7, 14 + Rabies Immune Globulin (HRIG) 20 IU/kg administered once on day 0. If immunocompromised, include a fifth dose at day 28 in the HDCV vaccine schedule.** As much as possible of the full dose of HRIG should be infiltrated around the wound, with any remaining injected intramuscularly at a site distant from the wound). Ideally should be administered as promptly as possible when indicated and within 6 days of the exposure.
- Rabies vaccines and HRIG should never be given in the same syringe or at the same site of HDCV.

Subsequent exposures:

- **Rabies vaccine only on days 0 & 3.** No immunoglobulin.

HANTAVIRUS (HEMORRHAGIC FEVER)

- **Hantavirus** associated with 2 syndromes: **[1] hemorrhagic fever with renal syndrome & [2] hemorrhagic fever with pulmonary syndrome** (Sin Nombre virus) **due vascular leakage.**
- Transmission: **inhalation of aerosolized wild rodents (eg, Deer mouse) feces, saliva, or urine.**
- **Most common in the SW United States (rural areas).** 3-week incubation period.
- Risk factors: affects primarily young, healthy adults, especially males.

CLINICAL MANIFESTATIONS

- **Prodromal febrile phase:** the aerosolized virus enters the lung causing a febrile flu-like syndrome (**fever, chills, severe myalgias especially involving the back & legs**) followed by nausea, vomiting, diarrhea, headache, weakness, cough. Lasts 2-8 days. This is followed by 1 of 2 syndromes:
- **[1] Renal syndrome:** flu-like prodrome followed by **hemorrhage** (petechiae, subconjunctival hemorrhage), **hypotension, & oliguric acute kidney injury (3-7 days);** followed by diuretic phase.
- **[2] Cardiopulmonary syndrome:** flu-like prodrome 2-8 days, with abrupt onset of **noncardiogenic pulmonary edema & shock** (dry cough followed by tachypnea, hypoxia, diffuse rales that may progress to cardiovascular collapse). Generally, lasts 2-7 days and recovery is rapid in survivors.

DIAGNOSIS

- Mainly a clinical diagnosis. Reverse transcriptase PCR. **Thrombocytopenia. Increased LDH & LFTs.**
- **Serologies:** ELISA for antiviral IgM & IgG (four-fold IgG rise distinguishes acute from past infection).
- **HRS: increased BUN & creatinine,** decreased complement 3; UA: hematuria, proteinuria.
- **HCPS:** increased creatine kinase, decreased serum albumin. **Chest radiograph: pleural effusion, central pulmonary infiltrates**, pericardial haziness (shaggy heart sign).

MANAGEMENT: **supportive**: IV hydration, hemodynamic & respiratory support, ICU admission.

DENGUE FEVER

- Febrile infection caused by 1 of 4 dengue viruses transmitted by **Aedes** mosquito (*aegypti or albopictus*).
- Seen mainly in the tropical & subtropical climates. 7-10 day incubation period.
- Virus replication destroys bone marrow & causes plasma leakage (increased capillary permeability).

CLINICAL MANIFESTATIONS

- **Biphasic fever phase: sudden onset of chills, initial high fever** ($\geq$38.5°C) for 3-7 days, followed by remission hours to 2 days followed by **second fever phase** (1-2 days). **Severe myalgias ("break bone" pain), headache, retro-orbital or ocular pain**, sore throat, nausea, vomiting, arthralgia, rash.
- **Biphasic rash:** erythematous skin mottling, **flushed skin (sensitive & specific)** followed by defervescence & onset of a **maculopapular rash** (spares palms & soles), then **petechiae** on extensor surface of limbs.
- **Hemorrhagic fever:** ecchymosis, petechiae, gastrointestinal bleeding, menorrhagia, epistaxis. Hemorrhagic fever usually occurs in children in endemic areas. **Positive "tourniquet test":** purpura from the pressure of the tourniquet placed on the arm. **Hepatitis,** pleural effusion, ascites.
- **Critical phase: at defervescence, some patients (often children & young adults) develop plasma leakage, hemorrhagic shock** (rapid weak pulse, narrow pulse pressure, hypotension, cold clammy skin). This phase usually lasts 1-2 days.

DIAGNOSIS

- Leukopenia, thrombocytopenia, elevated LFTs (hepatitis is common in the febrile phase).
- Reverse transcriptase PCR: detection of viral nucleic acid or viral nonstructural protein. Most helpful during the first week. Serologies: IgM, IgG.

MANAGEMENT

- **Supportive care mainstay: Acetaminophen, volume support (eg, IV crystalloids).** Pressors may be needed in shock. Avoid NSAIDS to reduce bleeding complications and avoid Aspirin to reduce bleeding complications and Reye syndrome).

MUMPS

- Acute onset of unilateral or bilateral **Parotid gland or other salivary gland enlargement.**
- **Mumps is caused by Paramyxovirus**, an enveloped, helical, single-stranded, negative-sensed RNA, part of the Paramyxoviridae family.
- Mumps infection is observed to occur most frequently in the 5-15 year age group & frequently occurs in older age groups, primarily college students.

TRANSMISSION
- Respiratory droplets, saliva, and household fomites.
- ~12-14 day incubation period. Increased incidence in the spring.
- Patients are most infectious 48 hours prior to the onset of parotitis and are infectious around 9 days after the onset of parotitis.

CLINICAL MANIFESTATIONS
- **Parotitis:** Prodrome of low-grade fever, fatigue, myalgia, malaise, headache, and earache followed within 48 hours by **parotitis (parotid gland pain and swelling) usually bilateral.**
- Physical examination: parotid swelling and tenderness. Erythema and edema of Stensen's duct.

COMPLICATIONS
- **Epididymo-orchitis is the most common complication of Mumps,** especially in postpubertal males (15-30%). May occur 5-10 days after the onset of parotitis. Unilateral in 60-80%.
- Neurologic — aseptic meningitis (most common), encephalitis, deafness.
- Oophoritis, arthritis, infertility.
- Mumps is the most common infectious cause of acute Pancreatitis in children.

DIAGNOSIS
- Clinical. Serologies. Increased amylase, leukopenia with a relative lymphocytosis.

MANAGEMENT
- **Supportive therapy mainstay of treatment because it is self-limited illness lasting 7-10 days —** **antipyretics (eg, Acetaminophen, Ibuprofen), analgesics, and** application of warm or cold compresses to the parotid area may be helpful.
- If hospitalized, the patient should be placed on droplet precautions and the CDC recommends isolation for at least 5 days after the onset of parotid swelling.

Epididymo-orchitis:
- Testicular pain may be minimized by the local application of cold compresses and gentle support for the scrotum. Anesthetic blocks also may be used.

Meningitis:
- Lumbar puncture is occasionally performed to relieve headache associated with meningitis.

PREVENTION
Dosing:
- **MMR vaccine (2 doses):** [1] given at 12-15 months of age with [2] a second dose at age 4-6 years of age. If vaccinated as an adult, 2 doses separated by at least 28 days.
- In 2018, the CDC recommended individuals vaccinated prior with 2 doses of MMR are at increased risk for population outbreak and should receive a third dose (eg, college students).

Contraindications:
- **MMR is a live attenuated vaccine so it is contraindicated in pregnant women and significant immunosuppression** (eg, AIDS, leukemia, lymphoma, chemotherapy). **However, patients with HIV without severe immunosuppression may receive the vaccine.**
- Women should wait 4 weeks after MMR vaccination to become pregnant.

ROSEOLA INFANTUM [(EXANTHEM SUBITUM) SIXTH DISEASE]

- **Most commonly caused by <u>human herpesvirus 6 (HHV-6)</u>;** sometimes HHV-7.
- <u>Transmission:</u> respiratory droplets. ~10-day incubation period. 90% occur in children <2 years of age

CLINICAL MANIFESTATIONS

- **<u>Fever prodrome (3-5 days):</u> abrupt onset of high fever [often reaching >40°C (104°F)] & lymphadenopathy in an otherwise mildly ill child** (child appears well & active during the febrile phase but may be irritable). Mild accompanying symptoms may include cough, coryza, anorexia, and abdominal discomfort. Lymphadenopathy may be present. The fever resolves abruptly before the onset of the classic rash.
- **<u>Rash</u>: rose-pink, blanchable macular or maculopapular rash <u>beginning on the trunk, buttocks, and neck</u>** before spreading to the face. Macules 2-5 mm & rash lasts hours up to 2 days. **Roseola is the <u>only childhood viral exanthem that starts on the trunk.</u>**
- **<u>Nagayama spots</u>: erythematous papules, macules, or ulcers on the soft palate and uvula.**
- Erythematous tympanic membranes, respiratory symptoms, anorexia. 15% risk of febrile seizures.

DIAGNOSIS

- **<u>Clinical diagnosis</u> — high fever in a child aged 6-36 months associated with minimal toxicity (relative well-being) and a rose-pink maculopapular rash that appears when fever subsides.**
- Detection of HHV-6 and HHV-7 by PCR is available but rarely influences clinical management.
- Labs may show neutropenia, atypical lymphocytosis, thrombocytopenia, or sterile pyuria.

MANAGEMENT

- **<u>Supportive:</u> mainstay of treatment (self-limited)** — rest, hydration, antipyretics (eg, Acetaminophen, Ibuprofen). Besides febrile seizures, RI is otherwise benign and self-limited.
- Adequate handwashing is important to prevent spread of infection.

RUBELLA (GERMAN MEASLES)

- Caused by the Rubella virus, part of the Togavirus family.
- <u>TRANSMISSION:</u> respiratory droplet inhalation. 2–3-week incubation period.

CLINICAL MANIFESTATIONS

- Rubella is typically characterized by rash, fever, and lymphadenopathy.
- <u>Prodrome:</u> **low-grade fever**, cough, anorexia, **<u>lymphadenopathy (posterior cervical and posterior auricular lymphadenopathy</u> most prominent; suboccipital lymphadenopathy).**
- **<u>Exanthem</u>: irregular pink or light red nonconfluent maculopapular rash** starts on the face and spreads to the trunk and extremities (centrifugal distribution), sparing the palms & soles. **Rash <u>lasts 3 days</u>.** Compared to Rubeola, Rubella spreads more rapidly and does not coalesce or darken.
- **<u>Forchheimer spots</u>: small red macules or petechiae on the soft palate** (may also be seen with Scarlet fever).
- **<u>Arthralgias & arthritis</u> occur among as many as 70% of teenagers and adult women** (rare in children and adult males). Transient photosensitivity.

DIAGNOSIS

- Mainly a clinical diagnosis. Rubella-specific IgM antibody via enzyme immunoassay.

MANAGEMENT

- **<u>Supportive</u> mainstay of treatment** — eg, Acetaminophen, Ibuprofen, oral hydration.
<u>Prognosis:</u>
- **Generally, not associated with complications in children** (compared to Rubeola).
- **Teratogenic especially in the first trimester** (may cause Congenital rubella syndrome).

	PRODROME	RASH	MISCELLANEOUS
VARICELLA Chicken Pox	• Flu-like sx: fever, headache, malaise	• *Rash in DIFFERENT stages simultaneously** (macules, papules, vesicles, crusted lesions) • Face initially ➪ extremities.	• *Vesicles on erythematous base dew drops on a rose petal"*. • Usually does not involve palms/soles
VARIOLA Smallpox	• Flu-like sx: fever, headache, malaise	• *Lesions appear in the SAME stage simultaneously** • Vesicles ➪ pustules ➪ scarring	• *Classically involves palms/soles*
RUBEOLA Measles	• URI prodrome: *3 C's:* - *Cough, Coryza, Conjunctivitis*	• *Maculopapular BRICK-RED* rash beginning @ hair line/face ➪ extremities. Lasts 7 days.*	• *KOPLIK SPOTS on buccal mucosa** • *Otitis Media MC long term cx*,* encephalitis, pneumonia in children
RUBELLA German Measles	• URI prodrome. • *Post cervical & postauricular lymphadenopathy*	• *Maculopapular pink-light red* spotted rash on face ➪ extremities. Lasts 3 days**	• *Photosensitivity & arthralgias (joint pains) especially in young women* • Not long term sequelae in children • *TERATOGENIC in 1st trimester:* (ToRCH)
ROSEOLA Sixth's disease	• 3 days of *high fevers* • *Child appears well during febrile phase.**	• *Pink maculopapular blanchable rash.* • *Only childhood viral exanthema that STARTS ON TRUNK/EXTREMITIES* then goes to face*	• Lasts 1-3 days. • Associated with HHV-6 & HHV-7
ERYTHEMA INFECTIOSUM 5th's disease	• Coryza, fever	• *Red flushed face "SLAPPED CHEEK APPEARANCE" with CIRCUMORAL PALLOR ➪ LACY RETICULAR RASH on the body*	• *Arthropathy in older adults* • *Aplastic crisis in Sickle Cell disease** • *Increased fetal loss in pregnancy* • *Parvovirus B-19*
COXSACKIE A VIRUS Hand Foot Mouth	• Fever, URI symptoms	• *Vesicular lesions on a reddened base with an erythematous halo in oral cavity ➪ vesicles on the hands/feet (includes palms & soles)*	• *Seen especially in summer* • Affects hands, feet, mouth & genitals
ENDEMIC TYPHUS	• Flu-like sx: fevers, chills, severe headache.	• Maculopapular rash trunk & axilla ➪ extremities (spares the face, palms & soles)	• *Flushed face, hearing loss (CN 8 involvement), conjunctivitis*
SCALDED SKIN SYNDROME	• Local S. aureus infection	• Fluid filled blisters with *positive Nikolsky sign: (sloughing of skin with gentle pressure)* • *Painful diffuse red rash begins centrally*	• *Seen in children <6y* • *Due to S. aureus exotoxin*
TOXIC SHOCK SYNDROME	• High fever, watery diarrhea • Sore throat, headache • *Staph aureus exotoxin*	• *Red rash (diffuse, maculopapular) with desquamation of palms & soles*	• *Seen in adults (ex tampon use, nasal packing left in too long) due to* • Management: IV Antibiotics
ROCKY MOUNTAIN SPOTTED FEVER	• Triad: fever, headache, rash	• *Red maculopapular rash first on wrists/ankles** ➪ *central (eventually palms & soles). Petechiae*	• *Fever with relative bradycardia*
KAWASAKI	• Fever, conjunctivitis, cervical lymphadenopathy	• *Strawberry tongue, edema/desquamation of palms & soles. Rash can present in different ways*	• *Rare but dreaded complication is myocardial infarction & coronary artery involvement*
SCARLET FEVER		• *Strawberry tongue, sandpaper rash*, facial flushing with circumoral pallor.* Desquamation can occur	• *Forchheimer spots:* small red spots on the soft palate (resolves quickly)

HUMAN IMMUNODEFICIENCY VIRUS (HIV)

- <u>HIV</u>: retrovirus (changes viral RNA into DNA via **reverse transcriptase**).
- HIV-1 (most common) & HIV-2.
- <u>Early HIV infection</u>: the approximate six-month period following HIV acquisition.
- <u>Acute HIV infection (Acute retroviral syndrome)</u>: refers to symptomatic early infection.

CLINICAL MANIFESTATIONS

- Patients may present at any stage and have varied presentations.
- 10-60% of individuals with early HIV do not experience symptoms.

Acute HIV seroconversion (Acute retroviral syndrome):

Classically presents 2-4 weeks after primary exposure.

- **The most common findings are lymphadenopathy & <u>Mononucleosis-like syndrome</u> (fever, sore throat, generalized macular rash, diarrhea, myalgia/arthralgia, headache, weight loss).**
- <u>Flu-like symptoms</u>: fever, fatigue, sore throat (pharyngitis), arthralgia. Aseptic meningitis.
- <u>Nontender lymphadenopathy</u> primarily involving the axillary, cervical, occipital nodes also common.
- **Rash** — **maculopapular rash** of the upper thorax, collar region, and face are most often involved.
- **Painful mucocutaneous ulceration distinctive manifestation of acute HIV — shallow, sharply demarcated ulcers with white bases surrounded by a thin area of erythema may be found on the oral mucosa, anus, penis, or esophagus.**
- Pharyngeal edema and hyperemia, usually without tonsillar enlargement or exudate.
- <u>Gastrointestinal symptoms</u>: diarrhea, nausea, vomiting, cramps.
- During this stage of early HIV infection, they are highly infectious to others (due to the transient high viral loads).

<u>Opportunistic infections</u>:

- Oral and esophageal Candidiasis is the opportunistic infection most commonly seen in these patients. CMV infection (proctitis, colitis, and hepatitis), PCP pneumonia, cryptosporidiosis.

AIDS:

- **Defined as CD4 count <200** cells/μL. Recurrent severe & potentially life-threatening infections or opportunistic malignancies. AIDS-associated dementia/encephalopathy, HIV wasting syndrome (chronic diarrhea & weight loss idiopathic in nature).

LABS ASSOCIATED WITH EARLY HIV INFECTION

- **Viral RNA levels are usually high** (> 100,000 copies/mL) often in the millions and CD4+ count may decrease transiently.
- Leukocyte count and lymphocytes vary during the acute illness. CD4 counts tend to be lower than CD8 counts.
- Elevation of liver enzymes, mild anemia, and thrombocytopenia.

DIAGNOSIS OF SUSPECTED EARLY HIV INFECTION

If there is a possibility of acute or early HIV infection, an HIV virologic RNA (viral load) [eg, RT-PCR] is the most sensitive diagnostic test, performed with a combination antigen/antibody test.

- **[1]** <u>HIV RNA (viral load) and CD4 count</u>: In early HIV infection, the viral RNA level is typically very high (eg, >100,000 copies/mL) and the CD4 cell count can drop transiently (but may be normal). HIV viral load also used to monitor infectivity & treatment effectiveness in patients diagnosed with HIV.
- **[2]** <u>Combination antigen/antibody test</u> **in addition to an HIV viral load test**
  - **Fourth generation (HIV IgM and IgG antibody/p24 antigen).** Reactive tests are followed by HIV-1/HIV-2 differentiation immunoassay or Western blot to confirm the diagnosis.
    - If reactive HIV antigen/antibody immunoassay but a negative HIV-1/HIV-2 differentiation Immunoassay, an HIV viral load test (nucleic acid test) should be performed.

  - **<u>Negative screening antigen/antibody test + positive detectable HIV RNA (viral load)</u> strongly suggests early HIV infection** (HIV viral load may be positive in the window period). A second positive virologic test suggests HIV infection.
  - **<u>Positive HIV screening antigen/antibody test + positive HIV RNA</u>** = early or established infection. **Confirm with a second test (eg, repeat HIV RNA or serologic test) several weeks later.** A positive screening immunoassay should prompt a second antibody-only immunoassay (preferably the HIV-1/HIV-2 differentiation immunoassay).
  - A very low viral RNA (eg, <100 copies/mL) may represent a false positive test; repeat test.

ROUTINE SCREENING FOR HIV INFECTION

4th generation antigen/antibody combination HIV-1/2 immunoassay (screening test)

- It detects both HIV-1 and HIV-2 antibodies as well as HIV P24 antigen.
- **The combination test is better than the antibody only tests because it can detect the HIV P24 antigen** when antibody testing may be negative (eg, window period).
- P24 antigen, a viral core protein, appears in the blood as the viral RNA level rises following HIV infection.
- Rapid combination antigen/antibody tests are not as sensitive as the standard combination test. Antibody only test can pick up HIV infection as early as 3 weeks.
  - **[1] If 4th generation assay is negative,** the person is not considered to be infected with HIV and **no further testing needs to be done.**
  - **[2] If 4th generation assay is positive,** a confirmatory HIV-1/HIV-2 antibody differentiation immunoassay or Western blot is performed.
    - **If confirmatory HIV-1/HIV-2 antibody differentiation immunoassay is positive, a plasma HIV RNA (viral load) should be obtained** to evaluate for acute infection.
    - **If confirmatory is indeterminate or negative, a plasma HIV RNA should be performed.**

HIV MANAGEMENT

- <u>Guidelines for ART initiation:</u> Antiretroviral therapy (ART) should be offered to all HIV-infected patients, including asymptomatic individuals regardless of their immune status (eg, CD4 count).
- Drug resistance testing should be performed after the initial diagnosis of HIV infection.
- **For most treatment-naïve patients, an <u>INSTI-containing regimen is preferred</u>:**
  - **INSTIs (eg, Bictegravir, Dolutegravir)** have equivalent and, in some cases, superior efficacy when compared with both boosted PIs and Efavirenz, and they appear to be better tolerated.

In most otherwise healthy patients, options include:
  - **[1] <u>Bictegravir-Emtricitabine-Tenofovir alafenamide</u>** (Biktarvy) [INSTi + NRTI + NRTI] OR
  - **[2] <u>Dolutegravir plus Tenofovir alafenamide-Emtricitabine</u> as the nucleoside combination.** Tenofovir alafenamide-Emtricitabine is associated with less kidney & bone toxicity compared with Tenofovir disoproxil fumarate-Emtricitabine. Lamivudine is an alternative to Emtricitabine.
  - **[3] Ritonavir-boosted Darunavir plus Tenofovir and either Emtricitabine or Lamivudine.**

Benefits of INSTI-containing regimens:
  - high barrier to resistance (combination treatment used to prevent resistance).
  - do not require a boosting agent (which increases the risk of drug interactions).
  - can be started pending the results of the initial evaluation.

NRTIs
  Zidovudine
  Emtricitabine
  Tenofovir
  Abacavir
  Lamivudine
  Didanosine
  Zalcitabine
  Stavudine
  Emtricitabine-Tenofovir
    (Truvada)
	NUCLEOSIDE & NUCLEOTIDE REVERSE TRANSCRIPTASE INHIBITORS (NRTIs)
	Mechanism of action:
	• **Inhibits viral replication** by interfering with **HIV viral RNA-dependent DNA polymerase** (polymerase normally turns viral RNA to viral DNA).
	Adverse effects:
	• All NRTI agents carry the risk of lactic acidosis with hepatic steatosis.
	• **Tenofovir alafenamide: GI symptoms, headache, increased creatinine, proteinuria, bone loss.**
	• **Zidovudine: bone marrow suppression** (eg, macrocytic anemia, neutropenia); peripheral neuropathy, pancreatitis. Insomnia, myopathy.
	• Abacavir is contraindicated if the patient is positive for HLA-B*5701 allele, because of the increased risk of hypersensitivity reaction.
	  Abacavir associated with increased risk of Myocardial infarction.
	• Emtricitabine: headache, nausea, vomiting, rash, hyperpigmentation.

NNRTI'S
  Efavirenz
  Delavirdine
  Etravirine
  Nevirapine
  Rilpivirine
	NON-NUCLEOSIDE REVERSE TRANSCRIPTASE INHIBITORS (NNRTIs)
	• **Allosteric inhibition of reverse transcriptase** inhibits viral replication by interfering with HIV viral RNA-dependent DNA polymerase (DNA polymerase normally turns viral RNA to viral DNA).
	Adverse effects:
	• **CNS toxicity: Efavirenz causes vivid dreams and neuropsychiatric problems.**
	• Baseline genotype testing to determine resistance recommended. Rash.
	• Moderate hepatic enzyme inducer; Many CYP450-3A4,2D6,2C9,2C19 drug interactions.

PROTEASE INHIBITORS
  Atazanavir
  Darunavir
  Lopinavir (boosted with
    Ritonavir)
  Nelfinavir
  Indinavir
  Ritonavir
  Fosamprenavir
  Saquinavir
	PROTEASE INHIBITORS (PIs)
	Mechanism of action:
	• **Inhibits HIV protease,** leading to **production of noninfectious, immature HIV particles** (block the maturation because it **inhibits cleavage of viral polyprotein into final structural proteins).**
	• Ritonavir used only as a PK boosting agent with other PIs (eg, Lopinavir).
	• Atazanavir: may require PK boosting with Ritonavir or Cobicstat.
	Adverse effects:
	• **Metabolic: All PI agents carry the risk of hyperlipidemia, fat maldistribution (lipodystrophy), hyperglycemia, and insulin resistance.** Rash.
	• **Gastrointestinal**: nausea, vomiting, diarrhea, dyspepsia.
	• **All are CYP3A4 substates/inhibitors,** resulting in drug interactions, **leading to increased levels of other medications.**
	• Atazanavir: may cause unconjugated hyperbilirubinemia.

INSTI
  Raltegravir
  Dolutegravir
  Bictegravir
	INTEGRASE STRAND TRANSFER INHIBITOR (INSTi)
	Mechanism of action:
	• Prevents integration: prevents insertion of a DNA copy of the viral genome into the host DNA.
	• **Well tolerated, not prone to resistance, therefore frequent choices as part of first-line regimens.**
	Adverse effects:
	• Hyperlipidemia, GI symptoms, insomnia, headache, increased LFTs.

FUSION INHIBITORS Enfuvirtide	Mechanism of action: • Disrupts the virus from fusing with healthy T cells. Adverse effects: • Hyperlipidemia, GI symptoms. Twice-daily injections, which often lead to local cutaneous reactions.

CCR5 ANTAGONISTS
  Maraviroc (Selzentry)
  Ibalizumab
	Mechanism of action:
	• **Blocks viral entry into WBCs.** The chemokine receptor 5 (CCR5) is found on the cell surface & promotes cellular migration (used by HIV to infect cells).
	• Use in patients with multidrug-resistant HIV who are failing ART.

PREVENTION OF OPPORTUNISTIC INFECTIONS IN HIV

INFECTION	RISK FACTORS	PROPHYLAXIS
Pneumocystis jirovecii	• **CD4 count ≤200**/mm³ • Oropharyngeal candidiasis	• **Trimethoprim-sulfamethoxazole** Alternatives: • Dapsone, Atovaquone suspension, or aerosolized Pentamidine. Discontinue when the CD4 count is >200 cells/microL for at least 3 months.
Toxoplasmosis	• **CD4 count ≤100**/mm³ • Positive *Toxoplasma* IgG antibody	• **Trimethoprim-sulfamethoxazole** Alternatives: • Dapsone plus Pyrimethamine and Leucovorin • Atovaquone with or without Pyrimethamine and Leucovorin.
Mycobacterium avium complex [MAC] (*M. avium & M. intracellulare)*	• **CD4 count ≤50**/mm³	• **Azithromycin** • For patients who are initiating ART, antimicrobial prophylaxis to prevent infection may not be needed.
Coccidioidomycosis	<u>Select patients with</u> • **CD4 counts ≤250**/mm³	• Annual IgG & IgM serologic screening in asymptomatic patients with CD4 ≤250 cells/microL who live in endemic areas (eg, Arizona or California). • **Fluconazole** if they have a newly positive serologic test. Therapy is discontinued in patients receiving ART when their CD4 is >250 for ≥6 months.

PRE-EXPOSURE PROPHYLAXIS (PrEP)

Pre-exposure prophylaxis (PrEP) can reduce the risk of HIV acquisition by >90% and is generally offered to those at substantial risk for new HIV infection due to:

- **Sexual behaviors**: **HIV-positive partner with detectable viral load**; men who have sex with men and individuals from high prevalence areas (eg, sub-Saharan Africa) with recent bacterial sexually transmitted infection, sex exchange for money, **inconsistent condom use, or high number of partners.**
- **Injection drug use**: HIV-positive injecting partner; sharing of injecting equipment.

Treatment includes:
- **Once-daily 2-drug antiretroviral therapy with Tenofovir plus Emtricitabine.**
- Because 2-drug regiments incompletely treat active HIV infections, which can lead to drug resistance; to qualify for PrEP, patients must have negative fourth-generation HIV testing and no manifestations of acute HIV.
- Normal renal function and documented hepatitis B infection/vaccination status is also required.

Monitoring:
- Patients on PrEP require:
  - follow-up every 3 months for HIV testing
  - risk-reduction counseling, and
  - medication adherence/side-effect assessment.
  - Regular creatinine levels and screening for sexually transmitted infections is also recommended.

CHAPTER 14 – HEMATOLOGY

ROULEAUX FORMATION

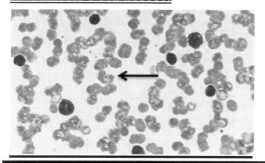

- RBCs stick together like a **"stack of coins"** due to ↑plasma proteins (such as immunoglobulins or fibrinogen).
- The increased density of the RBCs stuck together cause them to settle in the tube faster = ↑**ESR** (Erythrocyte Sedimentation Rate).
- <u>Diseases:</u> high protein (**Multiple Myeloma**). disorders with ↑fibrinogen:
      Infections (acute/chronic).

AUTO AGGLUTINATION

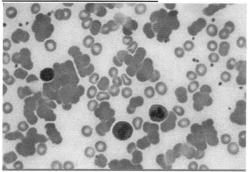

- **Clumping of RBCs** due to IgM autoantibodies coating the surface of RBCs, leading to ↑RBC destruction by macrophages.
- Cold IgM Ab agglutinins are reactive at colder temperatures (ex 28-31°C).

DISEASES
- **Cold agglutinin autoimmune hemolytic anemia** (eg, *Mycoplasma pneumoniae*, **Epstein-Barr virus**)
- Cryoglobulinemia
- Ag-Ab reaction if blood not typed & cross-matched.

HOWELL-JOLLY BODIES

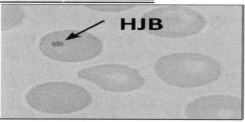

- Small dense basophilic RBC inclusions (usually removed by the spleen).

DISEASES
- <u>Decreased splenic function:</u> autosplenectomy (eg, **Sickle cell disease**), post splenectomy
- Severe hemolytic anemia, megaloblastic anemia

HEMOLYTIC CELLS

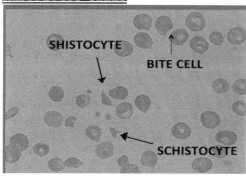

- <u>BITE CELLS</u> (degmacyte) = bite-like deformity due to phagocyte removal of denatured Hgb.
   - Thalassemia, G6PD deficiency

- <u>SCHISTOCYTES:</u> Fragmented RBCs.
   - Hemolytic anemias, Microangiopathic diseases

- <u>KERATOCYTES</u> "Helmet-shaped" RBCs.
   - Mechanical RBC damage in small vessels (microangiopathic diseases - eg, TTP, HUS, DIC, prosthetic valves)

BASOPHILIC STIPPLING

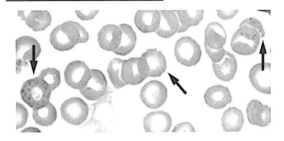

- Coarse blue granules in RBCs (residual RNA in RBCs – looks similar to reticulocytes but **basophilic stippling is evenly distributed throughout the RBC.**

Most commonly acquired:
- **Sideroblastic anemia,** heavy metal poisoning (eg, **lead,** arsenic), TTP
- Hemoglobinopathies: eg, **Thalassemias**
- Myelodysplasia, chronic alcohol use

ECHINOCYTES "Burr cells"

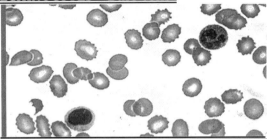

- RBCs with numerous, small, evenly spaced projections due to abnormal cell membrane.

DISEASES
- **Uremia**
- Pyruvate kinase deficiency
- Hypophosphatemia

ACANTHOCYTES "Spur cells"

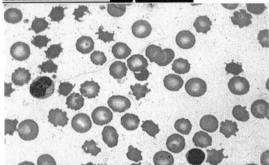

- Few large spiny, irregular projections on the RBC membrane.

DISEASES
- Liver disease (eg, alcoholic cirrhosis)
- Post splenectomy
- Thalassemia
- Autoimmune Hemolytic Anemia
- Renal disease

TARGET CELLS (Codocytes) & SPHEROCYTES

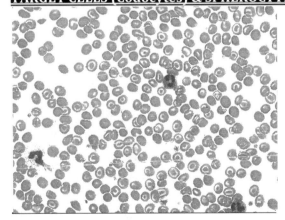

TARGET CELL: hypochromic RBC with round area of central pigment "target shaped." Seen if there is excess cell membrane in relation to the hemoglobin content.

DISEASES
- **Hemoglobinopathies:** sickle cell, **Thalassemia,** severe iron deficiency, asplenia, liver disease.

SPHEROCYTES: usually associated with hyperchromia (often with microcytosis).

DISEASES
- **Hereditary Spherocytosis**
- **Warm Autoimmune Hemolytic Anemia**

HYPERSEGMENTED NEUTROPHILS

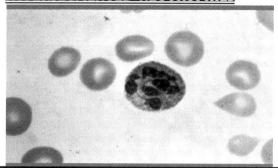

- Neutrophils with >5 lobes

DISEASES
- **B$_{12}$ & Folate deficiencies**
  (especially if macrocytosis is present)

AUER RODS

Acute Myelogenous Leukemia:
Seen in promyelocytic variant
Myeloperoxidase positive

REED-STERNBERG CELL

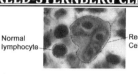

Hodgkin
Lymphoma

Echinocyte, Acanthocyte, Hypersegmented Neutrophil & Reticulocyte Images reproduced with permission from: Rosenthal DS. Evaluation of the peripheral blood smear. In: UpToDate, Post TW (Ed), UpToDate, Waltham MA. (Accessed on 2/1/2014.) Copyright ©2014 UpToDate, Inc. For more information visit www.uptodate.com

APPROACH TO ANEMIA

MORPHOLOGIC APPROACH

Anemia with a low reticulocyte count can be separated (via Mean Corpuscular Volume [MCV]) into Normocytic (80 – 100 fL), Microcytic (<80 fL), or Macrocytic (>100 fL).

Hemolytic anemia:
- **Jaundice, splenomegaly**
- ↑ Reticulocyte count
- ↑ LDH
- ↑ Indirect bilirubin
- ↓ Haptoglobin
- Schistocytes (if intravascular)
- Hemoglobinuria (dark urine) if intravascular

APPROACH TO ANEMIA

High reticulocyte count Signifies ↑ blood loss or ↑ RBC destruction

Low reticulocyte count Signifies ↓ RBC production

MCV

<80 fL   80-100 fL   >100 fL

↑ blood loss
- Tissue losses
- Occult losses

↑ RBC destruction
Intrinsic, hereditary hemolysis:
- **G6PD deficiency**
- **Sickle cell disease**
- **Thalassemia**
- **Hereditary spherocytosis**
Extrinsic, acquired hemolysis:
- Autoimmune hemolytic anemia (cold agglutinin disease, warm AIHA)
- Hypersplenism
- DIC, TTP, HUS
- Paroxysmal nocturnal hemoglobinuria

Microcytic anemia
- **Iron deficiency anemia (IDA)**
- **Thalassemia**
- **Lead toxicity**
- Early ACD
- Sideroblastic anemia

Normocytic anemia
- **Anemia of chronic disease (ACD)**
- **Renal disease**
- Early IDA
- Endocrine
- Mixed anemia
- Dilutional

Macrocytic anemia
- **B12 deficiency**
- **Folate deficiency**
- Liver disease
- Alcohol use
- Hypothyroidism

MICROCYTIC ANEMIAS

ETIOLOGIES: 3 most common clinically are **iron deficiency, alpha/beta thalassemia, early anemia of chronic disease (ACD). Lead toxicity is also in the differential.**

❶ **↓iron availability:** severe iron deficiency, anemia of chronic disease, copper disease

❷ **↓heme production**: lead poisoning, sideroblastic anemia

❸ **↓globin production**: thalassemia & hemoglobinopathies (eg, sickle cell, Hgb SC).

They all present with a **hypochromic, microcytic anemia.**

IRON DEFICIENCY ANEMIA (IDA)

- **Most common cause of anemia worldwide**, especially in women of childbearing age, children, and individuals living in under-resourced & middle-income countries (~12% of the world population).

ETIOLOGIES
- **Chronic blood loss: most common cause in the US** — menstruation, occult GI blood loss (eg, Colon cancer). In older adults, workup of for occult malignancy is recommended.
  Parasitic hookworms most common cause of blood loss-related IDA in resource-poor countries.
- Decreased absorption: **diet (most common cause worldwide),** Celiac, bariatric surgery, *H. pylori*.

RISK FACTORS
- Increased metabolic requirements: **children, pregnant, and lactating women.**
- **Cow milk ingestion in young children:** infants <1 year of age fed cow's milk; toddlers fed large volumes of cow's milk.

PATHOPHYSIOLOGY
- Decreased RBC production due to lack of iron & decreased iron stores (decreased ferritin). Normally, iron is stored in ferritin primarily in the bone marrow, liver, and spleen.
- **The first step is depletion of iron stores (↓ferritin)** without anemia, followed by anemia with a normal RBC size (normal MCV), followed by anemia with reduced red blood cell size (low MCV).

CLINICAL MANIFESTATIONS
- Classic symptoms of anemia: easy fatigability, weakness, exercise intolerance, exertional dyspnea.
- CNS: poor concentration, apathy, headache, irritability, cognitive disturbances. Restless legs syndrome. **Plummer-Vinson syndrome: dysphagia, atrophic glossitis + esophageal webs + IDA.**
- **Pagophagia: craving for ice (specific). Pica:** appetite for non-food substances (eg, clay, starch).
- Physical examination: **koilonychia (spooning of the nails)**, angular cheilitis (inflammation of one or both corners of the mouth), tachycardia, glossitis (smooth tongue), signs of anemia (eg, pallor).

DIAGNOSIS
- CBC: **microcytic hypochromic anemia classic** (may be normocytic, normochromic early on). **Increased RDW** (red cell distribution width), anisocytosis. Decreased reticulocytes (decreased RBC production), decreased red blood cell count, target cells. May have thrombocytosis & poikilocytosis.
- **Iron studies: decreased ferritin <30 ng/mL if anemic (pathognomonic due to ↓iron stores)** [some sources use a cutoff level of <12-15 ng/mL], **increased TIBC (transferrin), decreased transferrin saturation** <20-15% (due to increased transferrin), **decreased serum iron.**
- **Bone marrow iron stain: absent iron stores is the criterion standard (rarely performed).**

MANAGEMENT
- **Iron replacement** results in symptom resolution, increased reticulocytes (peaks within 5-10 days), correction of anemia (6-8 weeks), & repletion of iron stores (1-3 months). Lack of response may be due to nonadherence to oral iron (most common), continuing blood loss, misdiagnosis, or the presence of additional diagnoses.
- Preparations: oral (eg, Ferrous sulfate, 325 mg once daily or every other day on an empty stomach), iron-containing formulas in bottle-fed infants. Iron-enriched food and red meats. Parenteral iron.
- Increased absorption: **take iron replacement with vitamin C (ascorbic acid), with water or orange juice, & on an empty stomach.** Iron should be taken 2 hours before or 4 hours after ingestion of antacids (reduced acidity impairs absorption).
- Adverse effects: **GI most common** (eg, nausea, vomiting, constipation, flatulence, diarrhea, dark stool). Strategies to reduce these effects include reducing the dose, reducing the frequency to every other day, dietary modifications, and switching to a liquid formulation.
- Severe life-threatening anemia: red blood cell transfusion (eg, myocardial ischemia).

LEAD POISONING ANEMIA (PLUMBISM)

PATHOPHYSIOLOGY
- Lead poisons enzymes, causing cell death; it shortens the life span of RBCs; it inhibits multiple enzymes needed for heme synthesis, causing an **acquired sideroblastic anemia.**

RISK FACTORS
- **Most common in children** (especially in children <6 years of age) due to increased permeability of the blood-brain barrier as well as iron deficiency (may increase lead absorption).

SOURCES
- **Ingestion or inhalation of environmental lead (eg, paint chips or lead dust) is the primary source of childhood lead poisoning in the US** (lead was used in household paints prior to the 1970s).
- Lead in gasoline and industrialized use of lead.

CLINICAL MANIFESTATIONS
- Children with lead poisoning usually are asymptomatic or have nonspecific symptoms.
- **Neurologic symptoms: ataxia, fatigue, learning disabilities, difficulty concentrating,** developmental delays, hearing loss. **Peripheral neuropathy (eg, wrist or foot drop).** Encephalopathy: mental status changes, vomiting, seizures, cerebral edema, SIADH.
- **GI: lead colic — intermittent abdominal pain, constipation, vomiting, loss of appetite.**
- Anemia: pallor, shock, coma.
- Renal: glycosuria, proteinuria, chronic interstitial nephritis.
- Burton lines: thin, blue-black lines at the base of the gums near the teeth (seen primarily in adults).

DIAGNOSIS
- **Elevated blood lead levels**: For children <6 years of age in the US, elevated blood level is ≥3.5 mcg/L. **Capillary fingerstick sample often the initial test performed.** **Venous sampling is most accurate**, with repeat venous blood lead level to confirm the diagnosis.
- Peripheral smear: **microcytic hypochromic anemia with basophilic stippling (dots of denatured RNA seen in RBCs). Ringed sideroblasts in the bone marrow** (biopsy not usually performed).
- Screening for iron levels should be done — Normal or increased serum iron & decreased TIBC are classically seen in Lead poisoning if Iron deficiency anemia is not present.
- Increased Free erythrocyte protoporphyrin (↑FEP): elevations can be seen in both Iron deficiency & Lead poisoning but tend to be worse in Lead poisoning.
- Radiographs: **"lead lines" — linear hyperdensities at the metaphyseal plates in children.**

MANAGEMENT
- **Removal of the source of lead is the most important component of treatment in all cases of elevated blood levels.**

Mild <45 mcg/dL:
- Outpatient follow-up and changes in the home; **No chelation therapy.**

Moderate (45-69 mcg/dL):
- **Chelation therapy — Succimer first line as inpatient (oral chelation).** Calcium disodium edetate (CaNa2EDTA) if oral therapy not tolerated. D-Penicillamine third line.

Severe (≥70 mcg/dL):
- Severe without encephalopathy — chelation with Succimer + CaNa2EDTA.
- Severe with Encephalopathy — chelation with Dimercaprol (IM), followed by CaNa2EDTA (IM or IV).

GI decontamination:
- **Children with lead flecks or leaded foreign bodies demonstrated on abdominal radiographs should receive gastrointestinal decontamination with whole bowel irrigation.**

	IRON DEFICIENCY ANEMIA (IDA)	THALASSEMIA	ANEMIA OF CHRONIC DISEASE
MCV	Low/normal	Low/normal	Low/normal
RDW	High*	Normal/low	Normal
Iron	Low	Normal/High*	Low
Ferritin	Low*	Normal	Normal/high*
TIBC/transferrin	High	Normal	Low/normal*
Transferrin saturation	Low	Normal	Low/normal
RBC count	Low	Normal or High*	
Reticulocyte count	Low	Normal or high*	Low

THALASSEMIA OVERVIEW

THALASSEMIA: **decreased production of globin chains.** Distribution of Thalassemia follows *Plasmodium falciparum* — thought to be genetic benefit vs. Malaria. Most affected adults are heterozygotes.

- **Normally after 6-9 months of age, adult hemoglobin (Hb A) is the predominant Hb produced:**

Hgb A (Adult Hb):	2 alphas, 2 betas $(\alpha\alpha\beta\beta)$	**95-99%**
Hgb A$_2$:	2 alphas, 2 deltas $(\alpha\alpha/\delta\delta)$	1.5-3%
Hgb F (Fetal Hb):	2 alphas, 2 gammas $(\alpha\alpha\gamma\gamma)$	trace amounts

Suspect Thalassemia if **[1] microcytic anemia** [microcytosis disproportionate to the degree of anemia (eg, 55-75 fL)] **with [2] normal/↑ serum iron or [3] no response to iron replacement therapy.**

Alpha thalassemia # of deletions (# of normal alleles/4)	**SYNDROME**	**MCV**	**Hemoglobin (Hb) Electrophoresis**
4/4	Normal	Normal	Normal ratios
1 deletion (3/4)	**Alpha thal minima (silent carrier):** **No symptoms & no anemia.** Diagnosed during reproductive testing counseling (DNA analysis).	Normal	**Normal ratios** of Hb A, A2, & F.
2 deletions (2/4)	**Alpha thal minor (trait):** **Mild microcytic anemia** Often an incidental finding on CBC.	**Decreased** (60–75 fL)	**Normal ratios** of Hb A, A2, & F.
3 deletions (1/4)	**Alpha thal Intermedia (Hb H):** **Moderate microcytic anemia** **Symptoms often begin at birth** (eg, neonatal jaundice, anemia).	**Decreased** (60–77 fL)	**Hemoglobin H (10-40%)** **(beta globin tetramers)*** Hb A2 (≤4%)
4 deletions (0/4) **Complete lack of alpha chains**	**Alpha thal major (Hb Barts):** Death in utero or stillborn Not compatible with life.	**Decreased** (<60 fL)	**Hemoglobin Barts** **(gamma globin tetramers)**
Beta thalassemia Point mutation	**SYNDROME**	**MCV**	**Hemoglobin (Hb) Electrophoresis**
No mutation	Normal	Normal	Normal
1 mutation (1/2) Heterozygous beta+ or beta⁰	**Beta thal minor (trait):** **Asymptomatic in most or** **mild to moderate anemia**	**Decreased** (55-75 fL)	**Increased Hb A2 (≥4-8%)** **Increased Hb F (up to 5%)**
2 mutations (2/2) Homozygous beta⁰/beta⁰, beta+/beta⁰, or beta+/beta+	**Transfusion-dependent thal (TDT)** **Beta thal major (Cooley anemia):** **Severe anemia occurring initially** **during late infancy (6-12** **months at initial presentation).** **No symptoms at birth.**	**Decreased**	**Increased Hb A2 (≥5%) &** **Increased Hb F (up to 95%)** **Little to no Hb A** (minimal to no beta globin chain production).
Milder homozygous form	**Non-transfusion-dependent thal:** **(Beta thal Intermedia)** Usually presents at 2-4 years of age.	**Decreased** (55-75 fL)	**Increased Hb A2 (≥4-10%)** **Increased Hb F (up to 50%)** **Decreased Hb A (≤30%)**

ALPHA THALASSEMIA

- **Decreased α-globin chain production.** 4 genes determine it.
- **Most common in Southeast Asians** (68%), Africans (30%), Mediterranean (5-10%).

Disease	Normal Alleles	CLINICAL MANIFESTATIONS
Silent carrier state (minima)	3/4	Clinically normal — **usually asymptomatic & no anemia.**
Alpha Thalassemia minor (trait)	2/4	**Mild microcytic anemia — no treatment needed.**
Alpha Thalassemia Intermedia (Hemoglobin H disease)	1/4	**Presents similar to β-Thalassemia major but usually symptomatic at birth (eg, neonatal jaundice).**
Hydrops Fetalis (Hb Barts)	0/4	Associated with stillbirth or death shortly after birth.

<u>Thalassemia</u> should be suspected in any patient with:
- **Microcytic hypochromic anemia** (microcytosis disproportionate to the degree of anemia)
- **Normal or increased serum iron**
- **Normal or increased ferritin**

<u>Hemoglobin electrophoresis in Beta thalassemia:</u> **increases in Hb A2 &/or Hb F.**
<u>Hemoglobin electrophoresis in Alpha Thalassemia:</u>
- <u>1 & 2 gene deletions:</u> **normal Hb ratios in adults** (distinguishes alpha from beta Thalassemia).
- <u>3 gene deletion:</u> presence of **Hb H (beta chain tetramers)** 10-40%; **Heinz bodies.**
- <u>4 gene deletion:</u> presence of Hb Bart [gamma tetramers (γγγγ)].
DNA analysis provides definitive diagnosis.
<u>Alpha-thalassemia minima and trait</u> **require no treatment.** Folic acid may be used if mild anemia.

HEMOGLOBIN H DISEASE (ALPHA THALASSEMIA INTERMEDIA)
PATHOPHYSIOLOGY
- **3/4 gene deletions (--/a-) cause decreased alpha chain production. Excess beta chains pair together to form insoluble <u>beta chain tetramers</u> (Hb H/Heinz bodies)** with no oxygen-carrying capacity in the RBCs. The presence of Heinz bodies in RBCs lead to their destruction by the spleen (hemolytic anemia). Associated with **moderate to severe anemia** (hemoglobin levels of 7-11 g/dL).

CLINICAL MANIFESTATIONS
- **Usually symptomatic at birth (neonatal jaundice & anemia)** but do not require transfusions.
- **Symptoms of anemia, hepatosplenomegaly** (due to chronic hemolysis), pigmented gallstones.
- **Increased bone marrow hematopoiesis: frontal bossing,** maxilla overgrowth, Osteopenia.

DIAGNOSIS
- **CBC: Microcytosis** (MCV 60-77 fL), **hypochromia, hemolytic anemia (schistocytes,** tear drop cells, **increased reticulocytes), target cells (codocytes), <u>normal or ↑RBC count,</u>** ↓hemoglobin (7-11 g/dL). Acanthocytes (cells with irregularly spaced spiked projections). ⊕ **Heinz bodies.**
- <u>Hemolysis:</u> increased indirect bilirubin, increased lactate dehydrogenase (LDH), decreased haptoglobin.
- <u>Iron overload:</u> **normal or increased serum iron.** Causes include ineffective erythropoiesis, which promotes increased intestinal iron uptake, and transfusional iron overload.
- **Hemoglobin electrophoresis: presence of Hb H (beta globin tetramers) comprising 10-40% of hemoglobin.**

MANAGEMENT
- **Vitamin C & folate supplementation** (Folate 1 mg/day orally) are substrates for RBC production.
- **Hb H disease is usually not transfusion dependent.** Some individuals with Hb H disease may have severe anemia & become transfusion-dependent [eg, **episodic blood transfusions during periods of increased hemolysis or severe anemia** (eg, infection, pregnancy)].
- **Iron chelation Deferoxamine (preferred)** or Deferasirox **prevent iron overload & remove excess iron from chronic transfusions.** Avoid iron supplementation (patients are iron-overloaded).
- <u>Splenectomy,</u> in some cases, stops RBC destruction; may be needed by the second or third decade.
- <u>Bone marrow transplantation</u> definitive treatment in Hb H disease.

BETA THALASSEMIA

- Genetic hemoglobinopathy characterized by **decreased production of beta-globin chains**, leading to excess alpha chains.
- Risk factors: **most common in Mediterranean** (eg, Greek, Italian), Africans, & Indians.

Disease	Point mutations
β-Thalassemia trait (minor)	1/2 (heterozygous)
TDT [β-Thalassemia Major (Cooley's Anemia)]	2/2 (homozygous)
β-Thalassemia Intermedia	Milder homozygous form

CLINICAL MANIFESTATIONS
- **Beta thalassemia minor (trait): most common type.** Only one point mutation (heterozygous). **Usually asymptomatic but may have mild to moderate anemia.**
- Beta thalassemia intermedia: milder homozygous form (anemia, hepatosplenomegaly, bony disease).
- **Transfusion-dependent [Beta thalassemia major (Cooley's anemia)]:** both beta genes are mutated (homozygous). Deficient beta-chain production leads to excess alpha chains that are not able to form tetramers. This leads to ineffective erythropoiesis & shortened RBC life span.

CLINICAL MANIFESTATIONS OF TRANSFUSION-DEPENDENT THAL (BETA-THAL MAJOR):
- **Symptoms occur in late infancy (after 6-9 months of life)** when the switch from fetal hemoglobin (HbF-containing gamma globin), to adult hemoglobin (HbA containing beta globin) normally occurs. **Neonates with TDT (Beta thalassemia major) are asymptomatic at birth.**
- **Severe chronic anemia:** pallor, irritability, dyspnea, developmental delays.
- **Hemolysis: jaundice, pigmented gallstones** (Ca^{+2} bilirubinate), **hepatosplenomegaly, dark urine**.
- **Extramedullary hematopoiesis:** marked overgrowth of the sinuses, abnormal, delayed skeletal development, increased prominence of the malar eminences, producing the characteristic **"chipmunk facies" & dental malocclusion. Extramedullary expansion (frontal bossing,** "hair on end" appearance of the skull, Osteoporosis, abnormal ribs).
- Osteoporosis: by age 10, haematopoietically active red marrow is replaced by inactive yellow marrow, leading to Osteoporosis, fractures, cord compression, scoliosis, & disc degeneration.
- Endocrine abnormalities: (due to iron overload) — hypogonadism, diabetes, growth failure, hypothyroidism. Enlarged kidneys (due to increased hematopoiesis in the kidney).
- Cardiac dysfunction: heart failure (high output), arrhythmias.

HEMOGLOBIN ELECTROPHORESIS

	Hb F	Hb A₂	Hb A
β-Thal trait (minor):	↑ (up to 5%)	↑ (≥4-8%)	↓ to >90% (due to ↓beta chain production)
β-Thal Major (Cooley's):	↑ (up to 95%)	↑ (≥5%)	Little to no Hb A

- **CBC in TDT (Beta thalassemia major): hypochromic, microcytic anemia (↓MCV), normal or ↑RBC count, normal or ↑serum iron.** ↓ hemoglobin (usually ~6 g/dL).
  Peripheral smear: **microcytosis, target cells (codocytes),** teardrop cells, basophilic stippling, nucleated RBCs.
Skull radiographs: bossing with "hair on end appearance" (due to extramedullary hematopoiesis).

MANAGEMENT
- **Beta thalassemia minor (trait) requires no treatment.** Genetic counseling.
- Moderate disease: folate (if increased reticulocyte count), avoid oxidative stress (eg, Sulfa drugs).

Management of Transfusion-dependent Thalassemia [Beta thalassemia major (Cooley anemia)]:
- **Often require frequent transfusions** during periods of increased hemolysis or severe anemia.
- **Iron chelating agents** [eg, **Deferasirox (preferred),** Deferoxamine] prevent iron overload & remove **excess iron** due to chronic transfusions. Patients may develop endocrine deficiencies as a result of iron overload (eg, hypothyroidism, hypoparathyroidism, gonadal failure, diabetes mellitus) or CHF.
- **Vitamin C & folate supplementation** if increased reticulocyte count (substrates for RBC production).
- Splenectomy in some cases (stops RBC destruction). Allogeneic stem cell transplantation (curative).
- Luspatercept promotes erythroid maturation, reducing transfusion needs in Beta-thalassemia major.

B12 (COBALAMIN) DEFICIENCY

- <u>Sources of B12</u>: **natural sources mainly animal in origin** (eg, fish, meats, eggs, dairy products).
- <u>Absorption</u>: **B12 is released by the acidity of the stomach and combines with intrinsic factor** (produced by the parietal cells) in an acidic environment, **later absorbed mainly via distal ileum.**
- <u>Function of B12</u>: Vitamin B12 is essential for neurologic function, red blood cell production, and DNA synthesis; it is a cofactor for 3 major reactions: **conversion of methylmalonic acid** to succinyl coenzyme A; conversion of homocysteine to methionine; & conversion of 5-MTH to tetrahydrofolate.
- Substantial hepatic B12 stores may delay manifestations for 5-10 years after the onset of deficiency.

<u>ETIOLOGIES</u>
Decreased B12 absorption:
- **Decreased intrinsic factor: Pernicious anemia most common cause of B12 deficiency** (lack of intrinsic factor due to parietal cell antibodies, leading to gastric atrophy), gastric bypass, post gastrectomy, gastritis, achlorhydria, tropical sprue, Gastrinoma (Zollinger-Ellison syndrome).
- **Ileal disease: Crohn disease** (affects the terminal ileum), Ileal resection, Fish tapeworm (rare).
- <u>Medications</u>: **H2 blockers & Proton pump inhibitors** (decrease acid), decreased nucleic acid synthesis (**Metformin**, Zidovudine, Hydroxyurea), anticonvulsants. **Chronic alcohol use.**
<u>Decreased intake</u>: **Vegans** (due to lack of consumption of meat and meat products).

<u>CLINICAL MANIFESTATIONS</u>
- **Anemia symptoms similar to Folate deficiency but associated with spinal cord involvement.**
- <u>Hematologic</u>: fatigue, exercise intolerance, pallor. <u>Epithelial</u>: glossitis, diarrhea, malabsorption.
- **Neuropsychiatric symptoms: symmetric paresthesias & numbness most common initial symptoms** (especially involving the legs). Later, **lateral and <u>posterior spinal cord demyelination & degeneration</u> — gait ataxia, weakness, vibratory, sensory, & proprioception deficits**, including difficulty with balance. May develop dementia, psychosis, or seizures. On examination, **decreased deep tendon reflexes** (hypotonia) or ⊕ Babinski may be seen.

<u>DIAGNOSIS</u>
- **CBC with peripheral smear: increased MCV (macrocytic anemia) + megaloblastic anemia (macro-ovalocytes & <u>hypersegmented neutrophils</u> with >5 lobes). Mild pancytopenia** may be seen [leukopenia, reticulocytes, and/or thrombocytopenia (B12 deficiency affects all cell lines)].
- Increased serum LDH & indirect bilirubin due to intramedullary destruction of developing abnormal erythroid cells.
- **Decreased serum B12 levels**: <200 pg/mL; symptomatic patients are often <100 pg/mL.
- **Increased homocysteine nonspecific (can be seen in both B12 and Folate deficiencies).**
- **Increased methylmalonic acid [MMA] distinguishes B12 from Folate deficiency**, (FD is associated with increased homocysteine & normal MMA). ↑MMA in B12 deficiency occurs because B12 is a cofactor in conversion of methylmalonyl-CoA to succinyl-CoA.

<u>MANAGEMENT</u>
<u>B12 replacement</u>: oral, sublingual, nasal and intramuscular/deep subcutaneous injection.
Symptomatic anemia or neurological findings:
- **Start with intramuscular (IM) Cyanocobalamin** injection weekly until the deficiency is corrected & then once monthly. Patients can be switched to oral therapy after resolution of symptoms. **Patients with Pernicious anemia need lifelong monthly IM therapy (or high-dose oral therapy).**
- With adequate treatment, a brisk reticulocytosis occurs in 5–7 days, and the hematologic picture normalizes in 2 months.
- Hypokalemia may complicate the first several days of therapy, particularly if the anemia is severe (due to placement of potassium into the newly formed cells).
<u>Dietary deficiency:</u> Oral B12 replacement.

FOLATE [VITAMIN B9] DEFICIENCY

- <u>Functions of Folate:</u> folate required for DNA synthesis. Folate deficiency causes **abnormal synthesis of DNA**, nucleic acids, & metabolism of erythroid precursors. Folate stores only last for 2–4 months.

EPIDEMIOLOGY
- Most common vitamin deficiency in the US.
- If it occurs during pregnancy, there is an increased risk of neural tube defects in neonates.

ETIOLOGIES
- **<u>Inadequate dietary intake:</u> most common cause** — eg, **alcohol use, unbalanced diet, anorexia.**
- **Increased requirements: pregnancy, lactation, chronic hemolytic anemia,** infancy, malignancy. Exfoliative skin disease (eg, Psoriasis or Eczema) due to increased skin turnover. Hemodialysis.
- Impaired absorption: Celiac disease, Inflammatory bowel disease, chronic diarrhea, bariatric surgery. anticonvulsants (eg, **Phenytoin**, Phenobarbital, Carbamazepine), malnutrition, chronic alcohol use.
- Impaired metabolism: **Methotrexate, Trimethoprim, Pyrimethamine (sometimes given with Folinic acid to prevent Folate deficiency),** Pentamidine, antiseizure agents (eg, Phenytoin, Valproate, Carbamazepine), ethanol.

CLINICAL MANIFESTATIONS
- **Anemia symptoms similar to B12 deficiency but <u>without</u> neurologic abnormalities** [eg, no subacute degeneration of the cord (no progressive weakness, ataxia, paresthesias, paraplegia)].
- <u>Hematologic:</u> Anemia: fatigue, exercise intolerance, pallor.
- <u>Epithelial:</u> glossitis, aphthous ulcer, diarrhea, malabsorption.
- <u>Chlorosis:</u> pale, faintly green complexion – extremely rare.

DIAGNOSIS
- **<u>CBC with peripheral smear:</u> increased MCV (macrocytic anemia) >100 fL + megaloblastic anemia (hypersegmented neutrophils, macro-ovalocytes),** decreased reticulocytes. May develop pancytopenia.
- **Decreased serum folate levels <2 ng/mL.** <u>Decreased RBC folate levels</u> <150 ng/mL.
- **Increased homocysteine, <u>normal methylmalonic acid</u>** (distinguishes Folate from B12 deficiency). Patients should also be evaluated for B12 deficiency as both can coexist. Increased LDH.

MANAGEMENT
- **Oral folic acid first line** (eg, 1–5 mg/day) 1-4 months or until there is lab evidence of hematologic recovery. Diet rich in fruits and vegetables. Overconsumption of folate may be associated with increased risk of malignancy. Lack of correction of folate may be due to Magnesium deficiency.
- <u>Parenteral folic acid</u> in severe Folic acid deficiency.
- **Replacing folic acid in patients with B12 deficiency may correct the anemia but neurologic symptoms will worsen and may cause permanent neurological damage.**
- In patients on chronic folic antagonist therapy (eg, Methotrexate, Pyrimethamine), Folic acid or Folinic acid supplementation may be given to reduce the incidence of Folate deficiency.

- **EXAM TIP**
- <u>B12 & folate (in common):</u> anemia, macrocytosis, macro-ovalocytes, decreased reticulocytes, hypersegmented neutrophils, and increased homocysteine.
- **B12 only: neurologic symptoms (posterior cord symptoms) + increased methylmalonic acid.**
- **Folate only: no neurologic (posterior cord) symptoms + normal methylmalonic acid.**

CAUSES OF MACROCYTIC ANEMIA
- **B12 (Cobalamin) deficiency. Folate deficiency**
- Chronic liver disease, Alcoholism, Hypothyroidism
- Myelodysplastic syndrome and acute leukemia

NORMOCYTIC ANEMIAS

ETIOLOGIES
Anemia of chronic disease (most common), renal, mixed disorders (eg, iron + B_{12} deficiency); endocrine, early iron deficiency, asplenia, dilutional, sickle cell, G6PD deficiency.

ANEMIA OF CHRONIC DISEASE

- Anemia due to decreased red blood cell production in the setting of chronic disease.

ETIOLOGIES
- **Chronic inflammatory conditions** — chronic infection, inflammation, autoimmune disorders, malignancy.

PATHOPHYSIOLOGY
3 main factors decrease serum iron:
- **Increased hepcidin:** hepcidin is an acute phase reactant that blocks the release of iron from macrophages (iron sequestration) & reduces GI absorption of iron.
- **Increased ferritin:** ferritin is an acute phase reactant that sequesters iron into storage.
- Erythropoietin inhibition due to cytokines.

DIAGNOSIS
Complete blood count (CBC):
- **Mild normocytic normochromic anemia classic;** may present with microcytic hypochromic anemia early on.
- Hemoglobin usually not <9-10 mg/dL if isolated Anemia of chronic disease.
- Decreased reticulocytes due to decreased RBC production.
- Normal to increased Red cell distribution width (RDW).

Iron studies:
- **Normal or increased ferritin + normal or decreased TIBC (transferrin) + decreased serum iron.**
- Normal or low transferrin saturation.
- Iron studies should be performed in all patients because Iron deficiency anemia (IDA) can be concurrent with Anemia of chronic disease, and IDA is the most common cause of anemia (early IDA may be normocytic normochromic early on).

MANAGEMENT
- **Treating the underlying disease will help to correct the anemia.**
- **Erythropoietin-alpha if renal disease** or low erythropoietin levels.
- If hemoglobin is <7 g/dL or if a patent is profoundly symptomatic, transfusion of packed red blood cells (PRBC) may be indicated.

- **EXAM TIP**
- **Iron deficiency anemia**: microcytic hypochromic anemia, **decreased ferritin** (depleted iron stores), decreased serum iron, **increased TIBC.**
- **Anemia of chronic disease:** normocytic, normochromic anemia (may be microcytic early on), normal or **increased ferritin, decreased TIBC**, decreased serum iron.
- **Thalassemia**: microcytic hypochromic anemia, **normal or increased ferritin, normal or increased serum iron. Increased RBC count.**

	SERUM FE	TIBC	FERRITIN
FE DEFICIENCY	↓(<30µg/dL)	↑	↓ (<20 µg/dL)
ANEMIA OF CHRONIC DISEASE	↓(<50µg/dL)	↓	↑ or normal

UNDERSTANDING HEMOLYTIC ANEMIAS

- Hemolytic anemia: anemia caused by ↑RBC destruction when the rate of destruction exceeds the bone marrow's ability to replace the destroyed cells. There are two types: (1) intrinsic & (2) extrinsic.
  - Intrinsic (inherited disorders):
    - Sickle cell anemia, Thalassemia, G6PD deficiency, Hereditary spherocytosis.
  - Extrinsic (acquired disorders): Autoimmune hemolytic anemia (AIHA), DIC, TTP, HUS, Paroxysmal nocturnal hemoglobinuria (PNH), Hypersplenism.

DIAGNOSIS

- **Jaundice, hepatomegaly, and/or splenomegaly** from hemolysis (spleen/liver), indirect bilirubin.
- **Intravascular hemolysis: dark urine (due to hemoglobinuria); schistocytes on peripheral smear.**

- Peripheral smear: **increased reticulocytes** (immature RBCs). **Schistocytes (bite cells) if intravascular hemolysis is present.**

- **Haptoglobin is decreased:** haptoglobin becomes depleted when haptoglobin binds the free hemoglobin in the setting of continued RBC destruction.

- **Indirect bilirubin is increased** due to increased RBC destruction, which overwhelms the liver's ability to convert indirect bilirubin to direct bilirubin.

- **Reticulocyte count increases** in response to increased RBC destruction. The immature RBCs (reticulocytes) are sent into circulation to replace the mature RBCs that are being destroyed.

- **LDH increases** because LDH is an enzyme that is released from the destroyed RBCs.

LOOK FOR THE FOLLOWING TO HELP DISTINGUISH BETWEEN THE HEMOLYTIC ANEMIAS:

- Sickle cell anemia: **sickled cells on peripheral smear, Hgb S** on hemoglobin electrophoresis.

- Thalassemia: **microcytic anemia with normal/↑ serum Fe or no response to Iron treatment.** Thalassemias are also associated with severe anemia & abnormal peripheral smear for a given hematocrit level.
  - **Alpha Thalassemia:** hemoglobin electrophoresis with **normal Hb ratios** of Hb A, A_2, & F (Alpha thalassemia minima & minor); the presence of **Hemoglobin H** in Alpha thalassemia intermedia (Hemoglobin H disease). Hb Bart (gamma tetramers).
    - Alpha thalassemia is a diagnosis of exclusion (since the peripheral smear is normal).
  - **Beta Thalassemia:** hemoglobin electrophoresis: **↑Hb A_2 &/or ↑Hb F; ↓**Hb A.

- G6PD deficiency: **EPISODIC hemolytic anemia due to medications, fava beans, or infections.**

- Hereditary spherocytosis: **microspherocytes, Coombs NEGATIVE, ⊕ osmotic fragility or EMA test.**

- Autoimmune hemolytic anemia: **microspherocytes, Coombs POSITIVE,** RBC agglutination.

- TTP & HUS: **normal coags** (PT & aPTT; unable to distinguish between TTP & HUS via labs).
  - **TTP: Pentad:** Thrombocytopenia, hemolytic anemia, kidney damage, <u>neurologic symptoms, fever</u>.
  - **HUS: Triad:** Thrombocytopenia, hemolytic anemia, & <u>kidney damage.</u> HUS is most commonly seen in children (especially with diarrhea prodrome). HUS has a higher association with kidney involvement than TTP & without fever or neurologic symptoms.

- Disseminated intravascular coagulation: abnormal coags (prolonged PT & PTT), decreased fibrinogen.

- Paroxysmal nocturnal hemoglobinuria: dark urine (worse in the morning).

AUTOIMMUNE DISORDERS

HEREDITARY SPHEROCYTOSIS (HS)

- Chronic hemolytic anemia due to a genetic red cell membrane defect. HS is a result of heterogeneous alterations in 1 of 5 genes that encode red blood cell (RBC) membrane proteins and cytoskeleton, most commonly spectrin (*SPTA1* & *SPTB* genes) & ankyrin (*ANK1* gene). Often autosomal dominant.
- Most common in Northern Europeans, with a 1 in 5,000 incidence in this population.

PATHOPHYSIOLOGY
- Normally, spectrin & ankyrin are proteins that strengthen the linkage between the RBC & underlying cytoskeleton, allowing for the elastic deformability of the RBC and its normal biconcave disc shape.
- **In HS, deficiency in red cell membrane & cytoskeleton proteins (eg, spectrin, ankyrin, & actin), leads to increased RBC fragility, & sphere-shaped RBCs** due to decreased RBC surface.
- **The abnormal spherocytic red cells are detected, destroyed, & removed by the spleen (splenic macrophages) as they pass through the splenic microcirculation (<u>extravascular hemolysis</u>).**

CLINICAL MANIFESTATIONS
- **[1] <u>Mild or moderate hemolytic anemia</u>: splenomegaly, jaundice,** pigmented gallstones (Calcium bilirubinate). Mild cases may not present until adulthood. <u>Aplastic crisis</u> in severe cases.
- **[2] <u>Neonates</u>: severe cases may present in infancy (neonatal jaundice & hyperbilirubinemia);** the serum bilirubin level may not peak until several days after birth. May have normal hemoglobin at birth with severe anemia particularly in the first 3 weeks. **May have a family history of anemia.**
- **[3] <u>Incidental finding</u>** of hemolytic anemia or spherocytes on blood smear in mild cases.
- <u>Anemia</u>: fatigue, pallor, and delayed capillary refill time. Medial malleolar ulcers (chronic hemolysis).
- **<u>Hemolysis</u>: intermittent episodes of Coombs-negative (eg, non-immune) hemolytic anemia (anemia, dark-colored urine, & splenomegaly) hallmark,** often associated with infections (eg, viral such as Parvovirus B19), stress, fatigue, pregnancy; Pigmented gallstones (calcium bilirubinate). Aplastic crisis with Parvovirus B19 infection is a possible complication.
- <u>Nutrient deficiencies:</u> due to high RBC turnover, patients may develop folate, iron, or B12 deficiency.

DIAGNOSIS
- **<u>Peripheral smear:</u>**
  - **<u>HypERchromic microcytosis</u>, ≥80% spherocytes (round RBCs that lack central pallor).**
  - **<u>Increased MCHC*</u> most reliable** (Mean corpuscular hemoglobin concentration MCHC >36). Increased RDW (>14%). **<u>Suspect HS in patients with microcytosis + increased MCHC</u>.**
  - May have a hemolytic smear — eg, increased reticulocytes.
- <u>Hemolysis:</u> increased indirect bilirubin, increased reticulocyte count, decreased haptoglobin.
- **<u>Negative Coombs testing [DAT]:</u> Coombs negativity distinguishes Hereditary spherocytosis from Autoimmune hemolytic anemia** (which also has spherocytes but is Coombs positive).
Confirmatory tests:
- **⊕ <u>Osmotic fragility test:</u>** RBCs placed in a relatively hypotonic solution rupture easily due to the **increased permeability of the RBC membrane** (can be used if EMA not available or is equivocal).
- **<u>EMA binding</u>: preferred confirmatory test (most accurate; most sensitive & specific test).** Flow cytometric analysis of eosin-5'-maleimide (EMA)-labeled intact red blood cells — decreased fluorescence in patients with HS.
- Osmotic gradient ektacytometry, Glycerol lysis (regular or acidified). Cryohemolysis.
- <u>Definitive diagnosis:</u> Genetic testing may also be used for confirmation of HS.

MANAGEMENT
- **<u>Mild to moderate:</u> Folic acid** not curative but helpful to sustain RBC production & DNA synthesis.
- **<u>Splenectomy</u> curative in severe or refractory disease (stops splenic RBC destruction by eliminating the site of destruction).** When possible, it should be delayed in children until ≥4-6 years of age (reduces risk of severe sepsis from asplenia). Pneumococcal vaccine prior to removal.

AUTOIMMUNE HEMOLYTIC ANEMIA (AIHA) [WARM AIHA & CAD]

- Acquired hemolytic anemia due to autoantibody production against RBCs.

PATHOPHYSIOLOGY
- **[1] Warm AIHA: IgG antibodies activated by protein antigens on self RBC surface at body temperatures,** leading to **RBC destruction by splenic macrophages** &/or complement 3 (C3) activation-mediated RBC destruction by hepatic Kupffer cells (hemolysis is mostly <u>extravascular</u>).

- **[2] Cold agglutinin disease (CAD): IgM antibodies** against polysaccharides bind to the RBC surface especially at **colder temperatures** (<39F). When the RBCs return to a warmer temperature, the IgM dissociates, leaving complement (C3b) on the cell, causing hepatic RBC destruction by hepatic Kupffer cells **(extravascular hemolysis).** Intravascular complement-mediated RBC hemolysis.

ETIOLOGIES
- **Warm AIHA: idiopathic most common (50%);** <u>Medications</u> eg, **Penicillin, Cephalosporins,** Methyldopa, Rifampin, Phenytoin; <u>Autoimmune:</u> eg, **Systemic lupus erythematosus, RA**; **Malignancy: eg, CLL,** non-Hodgkin lymphoma; <u>Viral infections</u> especially in children, HIV.

- **Cold agglutinin disease (CAD):** idiopathic (most common); <u>infection:</u> eg, ***Mycoplasma pneumoniae,* Epstein-Barr virus,** HIV; **lymphoid malignancy: CLL, lymphoma,** Waldenström macroglobulinemia.

CLINICAL MANIFESTATIONS
- <u>Anemia:</u> pallor, fatigue, weakness, dyspnea. **Hemolysis: splenomegaly, hemoglobinuria (dark urine), jaundice.** Warm AIHA has rapid onset (may be life-threatening); slower onset with CAD.
- **Cold-induced vascular phenomenon in CAD: acrocyanosis numbness or mottling of the fingers, toes, nose, or ears when exposed to cold temperatures that resolve with warming up of the affected body parts.** Raynaud phenomenon, livedo reticularis (mottling).
- ~10% of patients with **warm AIHA have coincident immune thrombocytopenia (Evans syndrome).**

DIAGNOSIS
- **CBC + peripheral smear:** decreased hemoglobin, **hemolysis (reticulocytosis), microspherocytes (especially warm),** may have increased MCHC. Polychromasia. **RBC agglutination only in CAD.**
- <u>Labs:</u> **hemolysis**: increased indirect bilirubin, increased LDH, decreased haptoglobin, ↑reticulocytes.
- ⊕ **Direct Coombs [Direct antiglobulin test (DAT)] test:**
    - **Warm AIHA: IgG &/or C3 positivity** (most accurate test).
    - **Cold agglutinin disease (CAD): positive for complement only (C3b, C3d).** IgG negative.
- <u>Cold agglutinin titer</u> most accurate laboratory test for CAD (>1:64).

MANAGEMENT
Warm AIHA:
- <u>First line:</u> **Glucocorticoids first-line if symptomatic (± Rituximab) + Folic acid 1 mg daily.**
- **Second line: Rituximab** (anti CD20) can be added if no response & it wasn't given previously &/or **Mycophenolate mofetil.** IV Cyclophosphamide may be used if severe intravascular hemolysis. Azathioprine, Cyclosporine. Sirolimus if coexisting autoimmune lymphoproliferative syndrome.
- **Splenectomy is an option if 1 or 2 other immunosuppressive agents have been tried.**
- Transfusion if severe (eg, Hb <7 g/dL). Treat the underlying cause.

Cold agglutinin disease (CAD):
- **Avoidance of cold temperatures & exposure mainstay of treatment;** warm fluids if hospitalized.
- <u>Secondary CAD:</u> Treat the underlying etiology if secondary CAD is suspected.
- <u>Need for rapid-acting agent:</u> RBC transfusion (use blood warmer), Sutimlimab, or Plasmapheresis.
- <u>Treatment needed but not urgently:</u> **options include Rituximab ± Bendamustine;** Sutimlimab, <u>B-cell receptor inhibitors</u> Venetoclax or Ibrutinib; or <u>Proteasome inhibitor:</u> Bortezomib.

SICKLE CELL TRAIT & DISEASE

- **Group of inherited disorders affecting the beta-globin gene, leading to the production of RBCs that sickle, causing hemolysis (hemolytic anemia) & vaso-occlusive disease.**
- Disorders include Sickle cell disease (homozygous sickle mutation), sickle beta thalassemia, Hemoglobin SC disease, etc.

PATHOPHYSIOLOGY
- **Point mutation where <u>valine substitutes for glutamic acid on the beta chain</u>. Sickle hemoglobin (Hb S) has decreased solubility under hypoxic conditions,** leading to conformational change of the RBC shape (sickling) with subsequent **vaso-occlusion** (microthrombosis) & hypoxia.
- **Sickled cells are destroyed by the spleen (hemolytic anemia).**

SICKLE CELL TRAIT
- **<u>Heterozygous (AS).</u>** 8% of African Americans. Patients with Sickle cell trait are usually asymptomatic & are not anemic unless exposed to severe hypoxia, extreme physical stress, high altitudes, or dehydration. **May develop episodic hematuria or isosthenuria** (due to papillary necrosis).

SICKLE CELL DISEASE
- **<u>Homozygous sickle mutation (SS)</u>. 0.2% of African Americans.** The main clinical manifestations are due to **hemolytic anemia and vaso-occlusion** (eg, acute or chronic pain, tissue ischemia or infarction).

SICKLE CELL TRAIT
<u>Sickle cell trait</u>: heterozygous (AS).
- <u>Epidemiology</u>: **8% of African Americans**. Increased in populations where Malaria is endemic.
- <u>Pathophysiology:</u> In Sickle cell trait, about 35-45% of their hemoglobin is Hb S.

CLINICAL MANIFESTATIONS
- **Patients with Sickle cell trait are usually asymptomatic and are not anemic** unless exposed to severe hypoxia, extreme physical stress, low temperatures, high altitudes, or dehydration.
- **<u>Kidney involvement</u>: May develop episodic hematuria or isosthenuria** (concentrating defects) due to infarction & necrosis of the papillae of the renal medulla from the sickled cells in the kidney.
- Small increased risk for Rhabdomyolysis & venous thromboembolism (eg, DVT, PE).
- <u>Splenic infarction</u> may occur at high altitude; sudden death with prolonged exercise or extreme exertion.

DIAGNOSIS
- <u>Peripheral smear</u>: usually normal hemoglobin, hematocrit, reticulocyte count, and peripheral smear.

Hemoglobin electrophoresis:
<u>Sickle cell trait</u>:
- **<u>Hb S, decreased Hb A</u> — presence of both hemoglobin A (Hb A) and Hemoglobin S (Hb S) [~35-45% Hb S] with the <u>amount of Hb A greater than Hb S</u>.**
- FAS pattern in neonates.
- The presence of <35% Hb S suggests the co-presence of Alpha thalassemia.

MANAGEMENT
- **Sickle cell trait usually does not require treatment but genetic counseling is recommended.**
- <u>Papillary necrosis</u>: conservative (eg, IV fluids, bed rest, and pain management).
<u>Genetic counseling:</u>
- **<u>If both parents have the trait</u>: 25% of offspring will have normal hemoglobin; 50% will have the trait; & 25% will have Sickle cell disease** due to the autosomal recessive inheritance.

SICKLE CELL DISEASE

- Group of inherited <u>autosomal recessive disorders affecting the beta globin gene</u>, leading to production of RBCs that sickle, causing hemolysis, vaso-occlusive disease, & recurrent pain episodes.
- Point mutation where <u>valine substitutes for glutamic acid on the beta chain.</u> Sickle hemoglobin (Hb S) has decreased solubility with dehydration, acidosis, or hypoxic conditions, leading to conformational change of the RBC shape (sickling) with subsequent vaso-occlusion (microthrombosis) & hypoxia. Sickle cell disease is a homozygous condition (Hb SS).

CLINICAL MANIFESTATIONS
Symptoms begin as early as 6-9 months when Hb S replaces fetal hemoglobin (Hb F).
- Dactylitis most common initial presentation of Sickle cell disease in infancy.
- Delayed growth & development, fever, infections. Bone infarction.

- Infections:
  - Functional asplenia & autosplenectomy (from repeated splenic infarctions) often by 1.5–3 years of age lead to increased risk of infection with encapsulated organisms (eg, *S. pneumoniae, H. influenzae, N. meningitidis*, Group B *Streptococcus, Klebsiella, Salmonella*).
  - *S. pneumoniae* is the most common cause for sepsis and meningitis.
  - Osteomyelitis: *Salmonella spp.* common organism in patients with Sickle cell disease.
  - Parvovirus B19 infection may result in Aplastic crisis.

- Splenic sequestration crisis: vaso-occlusion in the spleen & RBC pooling in the spleen leads to [1] acute splenomegaly (often tender), [2] rapid decrease in hemoglobin concentration ≥2 g/dL, [3] thrombocytopenia, and [4] reticulocytosis. Hypovolemic shock. Often occurs in children.
- Hemolytic anemia: jaundice, pigmented gallstones (calcium bilirubinate).

- Acute pain episodes (vaso-occlusive "crisis"): triggered by hypoxia, cold weather, infection, dehydration, alcohol, & pregnancy. Abrupt onset of pain (Acute chest syndrome, back, abdominal, bone pain). Renal or hepatic dysfunction. Priapism common. Myocardial infarction, DVT, PE.

- Acute chest syndrome: fever, cough, tachypnea, acute chest pain, oxygen desaturation, and pulmonary infiltrates on chest radiographs. Must be distinguished from an infectious Pneumonia.

- Bony vaso-occlusion: Avascular (ischemic) necrosis of bones (eg, femoral or humeral head), "H"-shaped vertebrae central endplate depression with normal anterior & posterior margins.

- Skin ulcers: especially on the tibia.

- Chronic hypoxia: Pulmonary hypertension, Congestive heart failure, symptoms of fatigue, dyspnea.

- Stroke (25% have one by age 45y, 25% children have silent episodes). Myocardial infarction.
- Renal infarction or medication toxicity. Retinopathy.

DIAGNOSIS
CBC + peripheral smear: best initial test:
- Sickled erythrocytes (5-50% of RBCs), target cells (codocytes), decreased hemoglobin (baseline 8-10 g/dL but decreased in an acute crisis), decreased hematocrit, reticulocytosis, nucleated RBCs.
- Howell-jolly bodies indicates functional asplenia.

Hemoglobin electrophoresis:
- Sickle cell disease: Hb S majority (85-98%), no Hb A; increased Hb F, normal amounts of Hb A2.

DNA analysis definitive diagnosis of Sickle cell disease.

916

MANAGEMENT

__Acute pain (vaso-occlusive) episodes:__
- **Pain control: IV hydration & oxygen first step in the management of pain episodes** (reverses & prevents sickling). Fast-acting oral or intravenous opiate for pain. Meperidine is not recommended in patients with SCD (may lead to seizures & renal failure at high doses).
- RBC transfusion therapy may be needed in some crises (eg, Acute chest syndrome, splenic sequestration, preoperative transfusion). **Broad spectrum antibiotics for Acute chest syndrome.**
- **Exchange transfusion therapy used if there is severe or intractable vaso-occlusive crisis (eg, Acute chest syndrome, Stroke, Priapism, or retinal infarction leading to visual changes).**

__Reduction of episodes:__
- **Hydroxyurea is first line.** Options for individuals who cannot tolerate Hydroxyurea or who have continued pain despite Hydroxyurea include L-glutamine, Crizanlizumab-tmca, & Voxelotor.

__Long-term management:__
- Folic acid supplementation needed for RBC production & DNA synthesis <u>without</u> iron supplements.
- Stroke prevention: **Children with SS who are aged 2–16 years should have annual transcranial ultrasounds** and, if the Doppler velocity is abnormal (≥200 cm/s), beginning transfusions to prevent stroke should be considered. Iron chelation needed if on chronic transfusion therapy.
- **Allogeneic stem cell transplant: potentially curative treatment for Sickle cell disease** but has significant adverse effects. Ideally performed in childhood before end-organ damage.
- CRISPR (Clustered regularly interspaced short palindromic repeats).

INFECTION PREVENTION IN CHILDREN
- In patients with Sickle cell disease, functional asplenia & autosplenectomy (from repeated splenic infarctions often by 1.5–3 years of age), lead to increased risk of infection with encapsulated organisms (eg, *S. pneumoniae, H. influenzae, N. meningitidis*, Group B Streptococcus, Klebsiella, Salmonella). **Salmonella Osteomyelitis is usually associated with Sickle cell disease.**
- **Prophylactic Penicillin (Erythromycin if Penicillin-allergic) is given as early as 2-3 months of age until at least 5 years of age to prevent infectious complications.**
- Pneumococcal and Influenza vaccines also help to reduce mortality.

HYDROXYUREA
Mechanism of action:
- **Increases production of Hb F** (which does not sickle and has a higher affinity for oxygen), increases RBC water, **reduces RBC sickling**, alters RBC adhesion to the endothelium. Inhibits ribonucleotide reductase.

Indications:
- **Mainstay of long-term treatment in Sickle cell disease — reduces the frequency and severity of pain episodes, decreases hospitalization rates, and prolongs survival.**
- Because it takes weeks to months to take full effect, it is not used for acute episodes.

Uses:
- Sickle cell disease, Polycythemia vera, Essential thrombocythemia.
- The combination of Hydroxyurea and L-glutamine can have additive benefits.

Adverse effects:
- Myelosuppression, GI symptoms (eg, anorexia, nausea). Contraindicated in pregnancy.

- **EXAM TIP**
- **Aplastic crisis vs. Splenic sequestration:**
- <u>Seen in both:</u> **rapid drop in hemoglobin, thrombocytopenia.** Both may be caused by Parvovirus B19 infections.
- **Aplastic crisis: drop in reticulocytes, mild neutropenia.**
- **Splenic sequestration crisis: 4 features: [1] reticulocytosis, [2] rapidly enlarging spleen (often tender),** [3] drop in hemoglobin, & [4] thrombocytopenia. Hypovolemia may also be seen.

G6PD DEFICIENCY

- X-linked recessive RBC enzyme disorder that may cause [1] neonatal hyperbilirubinemia, [2] **episodic acute hemolytic anemia,** or [3] chronic hemolysis.

EPIDEMIOLOGY
- **Primarily males** (X-linked recessive). **Black males most commonly affected in the US — 10-15%.**
- Common in areas where Malaria is endemic: most commonly affects persons of African, Southeast Asian, Mediterranean, Middle Eastern descent (G6PDD thought to decrease risk of severe Malaria).

PATHOPHYSIOLOGY
- Glucose-6-phosphate dehydrogenase (G6PD) is an enzyme that normally catalyzes NADP to generate nicotinamide dinucleotide phosphate (NADPH), which protects erythrocytes from oxidative injury.
- **In G6PD deficiency, decreased G6PD activity during oxidative stress results in rapid depletion of reduced glutathione, resulting in an oxidative denatured form of hemoglobin (methemoglobin) that precipitates as Heinz bodies.**
- Hemolysis: RBC membrane damage & fragility cause both **extravascular & intravascular hemolysis.** Extravascular RBC destruction by reticuloendothelial macrophages in the spleen, marrow & liver.

EXACERBATING FACTORS
- **Infection most common cause** (eg, DKA). **Fava beans (broad beans) ingestion.**
- **Oxidative medications: Dapsone, Primaquine, Nitrofurantoin, Phenazopyridine, Rasburicase, Methylene blue,** Naphthalene mothball, henna, Amyl nitrate (RUSH). **"Sulfa" drugs at high doses.**

CLINICAL MANIFESTATIONS
- **[1] Most are clinically asymptomatic with no anemia or hemolysis** throughout their lifetime. Some patients may develop episodic acute hemolytic anemia during an oxidative challenge (stress).
- **[2] Episodic acute hemolytic anemia: symptoms 2-4 days after exposure of precipitants — anemia (eg, fatigue, pallor), dark urine (hemoglobinuria), jaundice (indirect bilirubinemia), back or abdominal pain, splenomegaly.** Acute kidney injury may occur in severe cases.
- **[3] Neonatal jaundice:** G6PD deficiency should be considered in **neonates who develop hyperbilirubinemia 2-3 days after birth** or within the first 24 hours of life.
- Physical examination: during hemolytic episodes ± jaundice, scleral icterus, & transient splenomegaly.

DIAGNOSIS
- **Peripheral smear: Normocytic hemolytic anemia only during crises — schistocytes (intravascular hemolysis), degmacytes [("bite" cells) punched out cells], blister cells.**
  ⊕ **Heinz bodies hallmark (denatured globin).** Smear is usually normal when not in acute stage.
- **Hemolytic anemia:** increased reticulocytes, increased indirect bilirubin, increased lactate dehydrogenase (LDH), and decreased haptoglobin. Direct antiglobulin test (Coombs) negative.
Screening tests:
- **G6PD activity enzyme assays: Rapid fluorescent spot test most sensitive in detecting the generation of NADPH from NADP.** The test is positive if the blood spot fails to fluoresce under ultraviolet light. Timing of testing: Performed after episodes because in acute hemolysis, testing for G6PD deficiency may be falsely negative (older erythrocytes with higher enzyme deficiency have been hemolyzed). If initial testing is negative + suspicion remains, repeat testing in ~3 months.
- Confirmatory tests: Quantitative G6PD assays. Molecular, genetic, or DNA testing not used routinely.

MANAGEMENT
- **Conservative: avoidance of oxidative stressors is the mainstay of treatment, such as avoiding offending food & medications,** treating underlying infection. Acute hemolysis usually self-limited.
- **Severe anemia: iron and folic acid supplementation.** Rarely, blood transfusions are indicated if severe (eg, hemoglobin <7 g/dL without hemolysis if hemoglobin <9 g/dL with hemolysis).
- Neonatal jaundice: Phototherapy first-line. Exchange transfusion if refractory to Phototherapy.

PAROXYSMAL NOCTURNAL HEMOGLOBINURIA (PNH)

- **Rare, <u>acquired</u> hematopoietic stem cell mutation — <u>RBCs become deficient in GPI anchor surface proteins (CD55 & CD59)</u>, resulting in <u>complement-mediated hemolytic anemia</u>.**

PATHOPHYSIOLOGY

- **<u>Loss of complement inhibitor proteins</u>**: CD55 & CD59 proteins normally protect RBCs from complement destruction. Deficiency in these proteins due to a mutation in the PIGA gene leads to **increased complement activation, leading to formation of the membrane attack complex-mediated intravascular RBC destruction (<u>intravascular hemolysis</u>).**
- Hemolysis is dramatically increased during viral or bacterial infections (antigen-antibody reactions).
- PNH may appear de novo or arise in the setting of Aplastic anemia or Myelodysplasia with possible progression to Acute myeloid leukemia (AML).

CLINICAL MANIFESTATIONS

- **Triad of [1] <u>hemolytic anemia</u> (hemoglobinuria due to intravascular hemolysis) + [2] <u>pancytopenia</u> + [3] <u>unexplained thrombosis</u> in atypical veins** (clotting despite low platelets).
- **[1] Hemolytic anemia: dark, cola-colored urine during the night or early in the morning with partial clearing during the day.** <u>Anemia</u>: fatigue, weakness, dyspnea, tachycardia.
- **[2] Pancytopenia:** protein deficiency seen in RBCs, WBCs, & platelets derived from stem cells, causing bone marrow failure. Often occur after bone marrow injury. **Hypercoagulability despite thrombocytopenia & pancytopenia is hallmark of PHN.**
- **[3] Venous thrombosis of large vessels:** due to haptoglobin and nitric oxide depletion. **Thrombosis in unusual veins** [eg, hepatic vein thrombosis (Budd-Chiari syndrome), cerebral, abdominal, subdermal vein thrombosis (leading to painful skin ulcers)]. Abdominal or back pain, erectile dysfunction, chest pain. **Thrombosis is usually the cause of death.**

DIAGNOSIS

- <u>CBC:</u> anemia of variable severity may be seen. The white blood cell count and platelet count may be decreased in the setting of Aplastic anemia. **Negative Direct antiglobulin test (Coombs).**
- <u>Hemolysis:</u> increased indirect bilirubin, increased LDH, increased reticulocytes, & decreased haptoglobin. Hemosiderinuria (due to increased intravascular hemolysis).
- Iron deficiency is commonly present, due to chronic iron loss from hemoglobinuria — low serum iron, increased transferrin, low ferritin, absent bone marrow iron.

Screening tests:

- **<u>Flow cytometry test:</u> best screening test to look for PNH — discrete population of CD55/CD59-deficient erythrocytes (RBCs)** and granulocytes. FLAER assay by flow cytometry more sensitive.
- <u>RBC fragility:</u> sucrose test (cells lyse in hypotonic sucrose solution) & Osmotic fragility test.
- Increased RDW & Direct antiglobulin test (Coombs) negativity.
- <u>Bone marrow morphology</u> is variable and may show either generalized hypoplasia or erythroid hyperplasia or both. Not required for diagnosis but can rule out marrow failure or myelodysplasia.

MANAGEMENT

- **<u>No substantial PNH-associated symptoms</u> watchful waiting with no intervention is an option.**
- **<u>Complement (C5) inhibitors [C5i]:</u>**
  - **Ravulizumab** derivative of Eculizumab with longer half-life, lower expense, & lower adverse effects.
  - **Eculizumab — anti-complement antibody targeting & binding human complement protein C5, inhibiting the terminal complement activation & the membrane attack complex formation.** <u>Indications:</u> in patients with severe hemolysis (usually requiring red cell transfusions) or thrombosis (or both), organ dysfunction, or pain.
- <u>Supportive therapy:</u> Folic acid supplementation 1 mg orally daily. <u>Thrombosis:</u> anticoagulation + C5i.
- <u>Complement 3 inhibitor:</u> Pegcetacoplan if refractory to Complement 5 inhibitors.
- <u>Allogeneic hematopoietic cell transplantation</u> only potential for cure in the setting of Myelodysplasia or previous Aplastic anemia.

HEMOSTASIS

The process to stop bleeding (prevents exsanguination during injuries). 2 phases:

PRIMARY HEMOSTASIS: **PLATELETS** form a plug at the site of vascular injury: **platelet adhesion, activation, & aggregation**. Platelets adhere to site of the injury becoming activated, sending out ADP & Thromboxane A2, which attract other platelets to aggregate, **forming a platelet plug.**
- **Disorders that affect platelets will affect primary hemostasis & bleeding time** (eg, immediate bleeding after surgery) but **PT & aPTT are usually unaffected** (clotting factors are unaffected), with the exception of Von Willebrand disease, where the aPTT may be prolonged.
- **Thrombocytopenia classically causes <u>mucocutaneous bleeding</u>** — oral (eg, bleeding after brushing teeth), petechiae, epistaxis, bruising, or menorrhagia. GI bleeding is uncommon.
- <u>**Disease examples**</u>**: thrombocytopenia (ITP, TTP, HUS, DIC) and von Willebrand disease.**

SECONDARY HEMOSTASIS: **CLOTTING FACTORS** (proteins) respond in a cascade to form **fibrin strands which <u>strengthens the platelet plug</u>** that was formed during primary hemostasis.
- Disorders that affect the extrinsic pathway may prolong the PT (DIC); disorders that affect the intrinsic pathway may prolong the aPTT (Hemophilia, DIC, & von Willebrand disease).
- **Hemophilias classically cause deep delayed bleeding (eg, hemarthrosis = bleeding into the joints, soft tissues, & muscles) or delayed bleeding after surgery.**
- <u>**Disease examples**</u>**: Hemophilia, DIC, & von Willebrand disease.**

PRIMARY HEMOSTASIS
PLATELET adhesion, activation, aggregation.

SECONDARY HEMOSTASIS
<u>CLOTTING FACTORS</u> leading to fibrin formation.

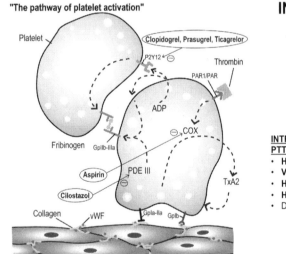

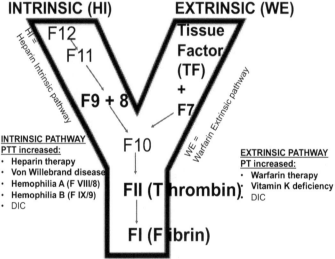

TxA2 = thromboxane A2
COX = cyclooxygenase

PTT (Partial Thromboplastin Time) measures efficacy of the **INTRINSIC** & common coagulation pathway. Normal PTT times require the presence of Factors 1, 2, 5, **8, 9**, **11, & 12.**
  <u>Prolonged PTT</u>: Heparin, DIC, vWD, Hemophilia A & B, & Antiphospholipid antibody syndrome (which paradoxically increases thrombogenicity).
  <u>Heparin overdose antidote</u>: Protamine sulfate.

PT (Prothrombin Time):
  Measures the **EXTRINSIC (tissue factor) pathway** & common pathway.
  Normal PT times primarily require the presence of Factors 1, 2, 5, **7 & 10 and Tissue factor**.
    <u>Prolonged PT</u>: Warfarin therapy, Vitamin K deficiency, DIC.
    <u>Warfarin overdose antidote</u>: Vitamin K.

THROMBOTIC THROMBOCYTOPENIC PURPURA (TTP)

- **Thrombotic microangiopathic hemolytic anemia resulting from deficiency of and/or inhibitory autoantibodies to ADAMTS13 (severely reduced ADAMTS13 activity ≤10%).**
- More common in females, pregnancy, & Black individuals. Can be any age (median age is 40 years).

PATHOPHYSIOLOGY
- Von Willebrand factor is normally secreted as ultra-large multimers, which are then cleaved by ADAMTS13 (ADAMTS13 is a von Willebrand factor-cleaving protease).
- **ADAMTS 13 deficiency leads to large vWF multimers that cause small vessel thrombosis** via pathogenic platelet adhesion & aggregation — **Microangiopathic hemolytic anemia (MAHA) & thrombocytopenia.**

ETIOLOGIES
- **Primary: idiopathic (autoimmune) — autoantibodies against ADAMTS13.**
- Secondary: malignancy, bone marrow transplantation, **Systemic lupus erythematosus,** estrogen, pregnancy, HIV-1; Medications: **Quinidine, Ticlopidine, Clopidogrel, Cyclosporine, Tacrolimus.**

CLINICAL MANIFESTATIONS: **pentad:**
Only ~25% of patients with TMA manifest all components of the pentad. Since Plasma exchange therapy, it is rare for patients to present with all 5 simultaneously.
- **[1] Thrombocytopenia: mucocutaneous bleeding** — epistaxis, bleeding gums, petechiae, purpura, easy bruising, menorrhagia.

- **[2] Microangiopathic hemolytic anemia:** anemia, jaundice, fragmented RBCs (schistocytes on peripheral smear). **Splenomegaly.** Gastrointestinal: abdominal pain, nausea, vomiting, diarrhea.

- **[3] Neurologic symptoms**: headache, visual changes, confusion, somnolence, delirium, seizures, CVA.

- **[4] Fever** (rare).

- **[5] Kidney dysfunction**: Acute kidney injury uncommon (less so than Hemolytic uremic syndrome).

DIAGNOSIS
- Labs: **thrombocytopenia with normal coagulation studies (PT, aPTT, fibrinogen)** are seen in both TTP & HUS. Normal coagulation studies (PT & aPTT) help to distinguish TTP & HUS from DIC.
- **Hemolysis:** peripheral smear — schistocytes (helmet cells), bite or fragmented cells, reticulocytosis. Increased lactate dehydrogenase [LDH], increased bilirubin, decreased haptoglobin.
- **Decreased ADAMTS13 levels (especially if ≤10%). ⊕ autoantibodies against ADAMTS13.**
- Direct antiglobulin (Coombs) test negative. Increased bleeding time due to thrombocytopenia.

MANAGEMENT
- **Plasmapheresis: Therapeutic plasma exchange mainstay of treatment of TTP.** Plasmapheresis removes autoantibodies against ADAMTS13 & adds ADAMTS13 to serum. Monitor & continue plasma exchange until LDH & platelets normalize for at least 2 days. **Glucocorticoids often added.**
Immunosuppression:
- **Glucocorticoids &/or Rituximab added if no response to Plasmapheresis.** Cyclophosphamide.
- Caplacizumab is an anti-VWF nanobody, decreases mortality when used in patients with ADAMTS13 <10% + severe features (critical illness, neurologic findings, high troponin).
Other management:
- Platelet transfusions not usually indicated (may potentiate thrombi formation).
- Splenectomy an option in TTP refractory to Plasma exchange and immunosuppressants.

HEMOLYTIC UREMIC SYNDROME (HUS)

- **Thrombotic microangiopathy due to platelet activation by exotoxins** leads to microvascular thrombosis.

- <u>Triad:</u> **[1] thrombocytopenia, [2] microangiopathic hemolytic anemia, & [3] renal dysfunction (uremia).** Fever and neurologic symptoms seen in TTP are often absent in HUS.

RISK FACTORS

- **Predominantly seen in children (especially <5 years) with a recent history of gastroenteritis.**
- In adults, it is often associated with HIV, SLE, antiphospholipid syndrome, or chemotherapy (eg, Mitomycin, Bleomycin, Cisplatin Gemcitabine).

PATHOPHYSIOLOGY

- **D+ HUS (classic): associated with diarrhea prodrome (>90% in children). Exotoxins [eg, Shigella toxin & Shiga-like toxin of *Enterohemorrhagic E. coli* O157:H7 (STEC)]** enter the blood, where they **damage the vascular endothelium, activating platelets (microthrombi formation),** eventually depleting platelets. The toxins preferentially damage the kidney, leading to **uremia.**

- <u>P-HUS:</u> *Streptococcus pneumoniae* releases neuraminidase, which initiates an inflammatory reaction. Occurs mainly in young children and infants. Usually present with Pneumonia.

- <u>Complement-mediated [D- HUS (atypical)]:</u> not associated with diarrhea (not related to Shiga toxin). Not common. Genetic defects in proteins that regulate complement activity.

CLINICAL MANIFESTATIONS

- **Children may have a prodromal diarrheal illness (abdominal pain, diarrhea which is usually bloody, nausea, vomiting) 5-10 days prior to renal manifestations (eg, oliguria & hematuria).**
- <u>Anemia:</u> fatigue, dyspnea, tachycardia; <u>Acute kidney injury:</u> oliguria, anuria, hematuria.
- <u>Physical examination:</u> pallor (anemia), jaundice (hemolysis), **hepatosplenomegaly.** Petechiae & purpura are uncommon. Fever and neurologic symptoms seen in TTP are often absent in HUS.

DIAGNOSIS

Labs are similar in TTP and HUS except ADAMTS13 is low in TTP & is usually normal in HUS.
- <u>Labs:</u> **thrombocytopenia with normal coagulation studies (PT, aPTT, fibrinogen)** are seen in both TTP & HUS. Normal coagulation studies (PT & aPTT) help to distinguish TTP & HUS from DIC.
- Increased bleeding time (due to thrombocytopenia). Direct antiglobulin test (Coombs) negative.

- **Hemolysis:** peripheral smear — schistocytes (helmet cells), bite or fragmented cells, reticulocytosis. Increased lactate dehydrogenase [LDH], increased bilirubin, decreased haptoglobin.

- **Acute kidney injury: increased BUN and creatinine.**

- <u>Positive stool culture</u> for E coli O157:H7 or detectable antibody to Shiga toxin in D+ HUS.

MANAGEMENT OF HUS CAUSED BY STEC:

- **Supportive therapy mainstay of treatment — eg, fluid & electrolyte replacement, dialysis, discontinuation of any nephrotoxic medications.** RBC transfusion if severe anemia (eg, hemoglobin level ≤7 g/dL or hematocrit <18%). Eculizumab if severe CNS involvement.
- <u>Plasma exchange therapy [Plasmapheresis],</u> with or without fresh frozen plasma, if severe, neurologic complications (eg, stroke), & non-renal complications.
- **Antibiotics and anti-motility agents are usually avoided because they may worsen the condition** (may lead to increased release of the harmful toxins).

DISSEMINATED INTRAVASCULAR COAGULATION (DIC)

- **Pathological intravascular activation of the coagulation system (coagulation & fibrinolysis).**

PATHOPHYSIOLOGY:

- Uncontrolled fibrin production due to tissue factor activation leads to **widespread microthrombi,** which consumes coagulation proteins (V, VIII, fibrinogen) & platelets. Consumption then leads to **severe thrombocytopenia,** manifested by **diffuse bleeding** & organ ischemia from microthrombi.

ETIOLOGIES

- Usually occurs as an acute complication of underlying life-threatening illnesses.
- **Infections (eg, bacterial sepsis most common), Rocky Mountain spotted fever,** viral.
- **Malignancies:** Acute myelogenous leukemia (AML); Lung, GI, or prostate malignancies.
- **Obstetric:** Pre-eclampsia; ~50% of patients with Abruptio placentae or amniotic fluid embolism have evidence of DIC, septic abortion; Hemolysis, Elevated liver enzymes, and low platelet count (HELLP syndrome).
- **Massive tissue injury & trauma,** complications after surgery, burns, liver disease. Acute pancreatitis.
- Aortic aneurysm, Acute respiratory distress syndrome (ARDS).

CLINICAL MANIFESTATIONS

- **Bleeding: oozing from venipuncture sites, catheters, drains,** extensive bruising, bleeding from multiple sites (eg, gingiva, areas of trauma or surgery, the rectum, the vagina, etc.), ecchymoses.
- **Thrombosis:** arterial and/or venous — **gangrene or multi-organ dysfunction** (eg, renal, hepatic).

Physical examination:

- Bleeding: ecchymosis, purpura, petechiae, hematomas, obvious bleeding, frank hemorrhage in various areas of the body may be noted. Clotting: mottling, cyanosis, gangrene.

DIAGNOSIS

- **Increased thrombin formation: decreased fibrinogen** (widespread activation of the clotting cascade). Reduced levels of coagulation inhibitors (eg, antithrombin, protein C, and protein S).
- **Coagulation factor consumption: prolonged prothrombin time (PT) and activated partial thromboplastin time (aPTT), increased International normalized ratio (INR).** Decreased levels of procoagulant factors [eg, factors 7, 10, 5, and 2 (prothrombin)]. Increased bleeding time.
- **Increased fibrinolysis: elevated fibrin degradation products and D-dimer.** D-dimer is a fibrin degradation product that has a high sensitivity but low specificity for the presence of DIC.
- **CBC with peripheral smear: thrombocytopenia, fragmented RBCs, & schistocytes.**

MANAGEMENT

- **Treating the underlying cause that led to DIC is the mainstay of treatment.**
- Platelet transfusion if platelet count <20,000/microL (some use <10,000) if not actively bleeding.
- Fresh frozen plasma if severe bleeding (replaces coagulation factors)
- Cryoprecipitate replaces fibrinogen in patients with severely low levels.
- Heparin for thrombosis in some patients.

DISORDERS	PT	PTT	BLEEDING TIME	PLATELET count
THROMBOCYTOPENIA (ITP, TTP, HUS)	Unaffected	Unaffected	**Prolonged**	**Decreased**
HEMOPHILIA	Unaffected	**Prolonged**	Unaffected (normal platelets)	Unaffected
VON WILLEBRAND DISEASE	Unaffected	**Normal** or **prolonged**	**Prolonged** (especially with **Aspirin challenge**).	Unaffected
VITAMIN K DEFICIENCY (EG, WARFARIN)	**Prolonged**	Normal or minor prolongation.	Unaffected	Unaffected
DIC	**Prolonged**	**Prolonged**	**Prolonged**	**Decreased**

IMMUNE THROMBOCYTOPENIC PURPURA (ITP)

- Acquired, immune-mediated **isolated thrombocytopenia** (low platelet count) due to a combination of **[1] increased platelet destruction & [2] reduced platelet production as well as release from megakaryocytes caused principally by** **antiplatelet autoantibodies.**

PATHOPHYSIOLOGY
- **Autoantibodies against platelets lead to splenic destruction of platelets.** The autoantibodies develop against the GP IIb/IIIa receptor on platelets. ITP is often a chronic disease in adults.

TYPES
- **Primary ITP:** idiopathic. **~60% of children with newly diagnosed ITP have a history of a preceding viral illness within the past month (self-limited).** Most common type in adults.
- **Secondary ITP:** immune-mediated but **associated with underlying disorders** (eg, SLE, **HIV, HCV,** Antiphospholipid syndrome). More commonly seen in adults & is usually recurrent.

CLINICAL MANIFESTATIONS
- Often asymptomatic. Fatigue may be seen.
- **Mucocutaneous bleeding:** eg, epistaxis, bleeding gums, petechiae, purpura, bruising, menorrhagia.
- Severe bleeding: intracranial hemorrhage, GI bleeding, hematuria.
- **Not associated with splenomegaly** because ITP is not associated with hemolytic anemia.

DIAGNOSIS
- **Isolated thrombocytopenia** with otherwise normal CBC (normal WBC count, normal hematocrit, & peripheral smear is usually normal). Megakaryocytes or large immature platelets may be seen.
- **Normal coagulation studies: normal aPTT, PT, and INR.**
- Bleeding time may be increased as with other causes of thrombocytopenia.
- **Bone marrow: Megakaryocytes (large-sized platelets)** may be seen.
   Marrow testing usually reserved for older patients or non-responsive patients.
- Evans syndrome: ITP associated with coincident warm Autoimmune hemolytic anemia (AIHA).

MANAGEMENT IN ADULTS
Minor bleeding (platelet count usually <50,000):
- **Glucocorticoids first-line therapy & preferred** (blunts the immune response) **or IVIG or anti-D.**
- **Intravenous immunoglobulin (IVIG) second-line** therapy or may be used if rapid rise in platelet count is required. Anti-D immune globulin use is reserved only for Rh+ patients without hemolysis.
- Refractory: **Rituximab or TPO receptor agonist** (eg, Eltrombopag, Romiplostim) **or Splenectomy.**

Severe (critical) bleeding (GI/CNS) + platelets <30,000:
- Platelet transfusion + IVIG + high-dose Glucocorticoids.

No bleeding + platelet ≥30,000:
- **Observation and monitor the platelet count.**

No bleeding + platelet <20,000-30,000:
- **Glucocorticoids (preferred)** or IVIG or anti-D immune globulin (if Rh+ & no evidence of hemolysis).

MANAGEMENT IN CHILDREN
- **No bleeding or mild bleeding not at risk:** observation. Restrict physical activity with risk of trauma.
- **When treatment is indicated, options include [1] Intravenous immune globulin (IVIG), [2] Glucocorticoids, or [3] anti-D immune globulin (anti-D)** limited to Rh+ patients with a spleen.
- **Intravenous immunoglobulin (IVIG)** if rapid rise in platelet counts required.
- **Glucocorticoids** if increased risk of bleeding but rapid rise in platelets not needed.
- **Life-threatening bleeding: IV Glucocorticoids plus IVIG;** platelets may be added if needed.

	ITP	TTP	HUS	DIC
Pathophysiology	• *Autoimmune-Antibody reaction vs. platelets** with splenic platelet destruction ⇨ consumptive thrombocytopenia	• *Auto-Ab vs. ADAMTS13** (vWF-cleaving protease) ⇨ unusual large vWF multimers ⇨ micro thrombosis of small vessels ⇨ *thrombocytopenia (consumptive) & hemolytic anemia.*	• *Exotoxins* (Shiga-like & Shiga toxins) damages vascular endothelium*, activating platelets ⇨ *microthrombosis of small vessels* ⇨ consumptive *thrombocytopenia* **and** *hemolytic anemia.* • *ADAMTS13 normal*	• *Pathologic clotting cascade activation ⇨ widespread thrombi ⇨* consumption of platelets ⇨ *diffuse bleeding*
Incidence	• *Predominantly young children 2-4y. Often 1-3 weeks following acute viral infection.** Often self-limited in children. • **Adult:** young women <40y idiopathic. Often recurrent	• *Young adults 20-50y* • *MC women*	• *Predominantly seen in children with diarrhea prodrome*: Enterohem. E coli O157:H7 (80%). Shigella, Salmonella,* • Adults: seen with HIV, SLE, Anti phospholipid syndrome.	• *MC in young or elderly* • *MC gram negative sepsis** • *OB emergencies* • *Malignancy* • *Massive tissue trauma.*
Clinical Manifestations	• Often asymptomatic. • ↑*mucocutaneous bleeding: petechiae, bruising, purpura, bullae,* bleeding of tooth & gums, menorrhagia. • *NO SPLENOMEGALY**	**PENTAD*:** 1. *Thrombocytopenia:* bruising, purpura, bleeding. 2. *Microangiopathic hemolytic anemia:* anemia, jaundice. 3. *Kidney failure/uremia:* (not as common as in HUS. 4. *Neuro sx:** headache, CVA, AMS 5. *Fever*	**TRIAD*:** 1. *Thrombocytopenia:* bruising, purpura, bleeding 2. *Microangiopathic hemolytic anemia:* anemia, jaundice 3. *Kidney failure/uremia: predominant feature.** *Suspect HUS if renal failure in children with diarrhea prodrome*.*	• *Diffuse hemorrhage: venipuncture sites, mouth, nose; extensive bruising.* • *Thrombosis: renal failure, gangrene* (as clots block circulation). • Patients usually acutely ill
Diagnosis	• *ISOLATED THROMBOCYTOPENIA** • Normal coag tests (PT, PTT)	• *Thrombocytopenia* **Hemolytic anemia:** • Peripheral smear: ↑*reticulocytes, schistocytes* ("bite or fragmented cells) • LFTs: ↑*Ind bili;* ↓*haptoglobin* • Normal coag tests (PT, PTT)	• *Thrombocytopenia* **Hemolytic anemia:** • Peripheral smear: ↑*reticulocytes, schistocytes* ("bite or fragmented cells) • LFTs: ↑*Ind bili;* ↓*haptoglobin* • ↑*BUN/Creatinine** (Renal failure) • Normal coags (PT, PTT) distinguish TTP & HUS from DIC*	**Hemolytic anemia:** • Peripheral smear: ↑*reticulocytes, schistocytes* ("bite or fragmented cells) • LFTs: ↑*Ind bili;* ↓*haptoglobin* • *ABNORMAL COAG TESTS*:* ↓*fibrinogen,* ↑*D-dimer,* ↑*PT, PTT. severe thrombocytopenia.*
Management	• **CHILDREN:** *observation ~80% resolve without tx within 6 months.* ±*Intravenous immunoglobulin.* • **ADULTS:** *CORTICOSTEROIDS** (blunts the immune response) ⇨ *IVIG* ⇨ *SPLENECTOMY IN REFRACTORY CASES.**	• *PLASMAPHERESIS mainstay** (↓es mortality). Removes Ab & adds ADAMTS13 • *Immunosuppression: steroids,* Cyclophosphamides etc.	• *Observation in most children (usually self-limited).* • *Plasmapheresis* • ±FFP if severe, • *NO antibiotics** - may worsen the disease (↑toxin release).	• *Reversal of the underlying cause mainstay of tx** • ±Platelet transfusion (if <20,000) • ±Fresh frozen plasma • ±Heparin in select cases.

VON WILLEBRAND DISEASE (VWD)

- Autosomal dominant disorder associated with **ineffective platelet adhesion** due to deficient (types **1 & 3) or defective function (type 2) of von Willebrand Factor.**
- **Most common hereditary bleeding disorder** (1% of population). May also be acquired.

FUNCTION OF VWF:
- Von Willebrand factor (VWF) promotes platelet adhesion by crosslinking the GP1b receptor on platelets with exposed collagen on damaged epithelium. VWF also prevents Factor VIII degradation.

CLINICAL MANIFESTATIONS
- **"Platelet-like" mucocutaneous bleeding:** eg, **prolonged bleeding from mucosal surfaces (oral, uterine, gastrointestinal) & skin** — epistaxis, bleeding from gums & oral cavity, easy bruising, petechiae, purpura, prolonged bleeding after minor cuts, dental extractions or procedures, trauma, or other forms of surgery, heavy menstrual bleeding, postpartum hemorrhage, gastrointestinal.
- Incisional bleeding less common in VWD than in Hemophilia (except in severe types 2N & type 3).

INITIAL LABS
- **Platelet count usually normal** (except in type 2B, which is associated with mild thrombocytopenia).
- Coagulation studies: **normal or prolonged PTT that corrects with mixing study**. PT is _not_ affected by VWD. **Increased bleeding time. PTT & bleeding time prolongation worse with Aspirin.**

Screening tests:
- Plasma VWF antigen **decreased VWF:Ag ≤30% or VWF activity ≤30% (≤30 IU) is diagnostic.**
- Plasma VWF activity **VWF activity ≤30% (≤30 IU)** via Ristocetin cofactor activity and VWF collagen binding. No platelet aggregation with Ristocetin in VWD. Factor VIII activity: may be decreased.

Specialized assays helps to determine the type of VWD.
- VWF multimer distribution analysis using gel electrophoresis. Factor VIII activity to VWF antigen.
- **Ristocetin-induced platelet aggregation (RIPA) criterion standard.**

MANAGEMENT (TYPE 1): Quantitative deficiency (most common type — 75%)
- **Mild to moderate bleeding: DDAVP (Desmopressin) first line.** VWF concentrates alternatives. Antifibrinolytics: Tranexamic acid (TXA) or ε-aminocaproic acid used in some as add-on therapy.
- **Severe: VWF-containing product** (plasma-derived or recombinant) — **eg, factor VIII concentrates, purified VWF concentrates, or recombinant VWF.**
- **Minor procedures: Desmopressin used in type 1 and 2A** for minor trauma, dental and minor surgical procedures.
- **Major procedures: VWF containing products** — eg, human derived Factor VIII concentrates.

MANAGEMENT OF TYPE 2 [qualitative deficiency (VWF dysfunction)]:
- **Desmopressin (DDAVP) for most.** VWF-containing product or DDAVP prior to procedures.
- Patients with Type 2B may also require platelet transfusion prior to some procedures.

MANAGEMENT OF TYPE 3 (severe, absent VWF):
- **VWF-containing product** eg, human-derived factor VIII concentrates, purified VWF concentrates, Recombinant VWF. Desmopressin not used because Type 3 is associated with undetectable VWF.

Desmopressin (DDAVP)
- Mechanism of action: **transiently increases plasma concentration of VWF & Factor VIII (8) levels by releasing them from endogenous VWF storage pools in platelet granules and vascular endothelial cells.** Synthetic analog of Arginine vasopressin [Antidiuretic hormone (ADH)].
- Indications: **used in Type 1 and Type 2A VWD.** Desmopressin increases plasma von Willebrand factor and factor VIII (8) levels from twofold to more than fivefold over baseline levels.
- Administration: Desmopressin is generally administered for short periods (48 to 72 hours), and no more often than at 24- to 48-hour intervals because of tachyphylaxis and adverse effects.
- Monitoring: if a longer duration or shorter intervals are required, the patient should be monitored for fluid and electrolyte abnormalities because **Desmopressin is synthetic ADH & may lead to ADH-induced symptomatic Hyponatremia (eg, neurological symptoms & seizure).**

HEMOPHILIA A [Factor VIII (8) Deficiency]

- **X-linked recessive** disorder **occurring predominantly in males** (rarely in homozygous females). Can also be caused by spontaneous mutation.
- **Most common type of Hemophilia.** First episode usually <18 years of age.
- **Lack of Factor VIII (8)** affects the clotting cascade, leading to **failure of hematoma formation.**

CLINICAL MANIFESTATIONS
- **Deep tissue bleeding (joints, muscles) or soft tissue hematomas: Hemarthrosis: swelling in weight-bearing joints** (eg, **ankles,** knees, elbows), arthropathy. Delayed bleeding after trauma.
- **Excessive hemorrhage in response to trauma & surgery or incisional bleeding** (eg, tooth extraction). Epistaxis, bruising (large ecchymosis). GI or urinary tract hemorrhage (hematuria).
- Hemophilias less commonly present with purpura & petechiae (because platelet function is normal) or spontaneous hemorrhage [except in the severe form (Factor 8 level <1% of normal)].

DIAGNOSIS
- **Low Factor VIII (8) <40% — most sensitive test.** Mild disease >5%; moderate: 1-5%; severe <1%.
- CBC & coagulation studies: **Prolonged aPTT.** Normal PT, fibrinogen, platelet levels (bleeding time).
- Mixing studies: **PTT corrects with mixing studies with normal plasma** (indicating a factor deficiency).

MANAGEMENT
- **Factor VIII infusion first-line therapy** to increase levels 25-100% (depending on severity). Can be given in response to an **acute bleeding episode or prophylaxis** (eg, prior to surgery, after trauma).
- **Desmopressin (DDAVP): transiently increases Factor VIII & VWF** release from endothelial stores. **May be used prior to procedures to prevent bleeding in mild disease.**
- Emicizumab is a humanized bispecific monoclonal antibody that binds to both factor IXa and factor X, substituting for the role of factor VIII in hemostasis.
- Significant arthropathy can be minimized by long-term regular prophylaxis with factor concentrate.

HEMOPHILIA B [(Factor IX/9 Deficiency) Christmas Disease]

- **X-linked recessive** disorder **occurring almost exclusively in males** (rarely in homozygous females).
- **Lack of Factor IX (9)** affects the clotting cascade, leading to **failure of hematoma formation.**

CLINICAL MANIFESTATIONS
Clinically indistinguishable from Hemophilia A.
- **Deep tissue bleeding (joints, muscles) or soft tissue hematomas: Hemarthrosis: swelling in weight-bearing joints** (eg, **ankles,** knees, elbows), arthropathy. Delayed bleeding after trauma.
- **Excessive hemorrhage in response to trauma & surgery or incisional bleeding** (eg, tooth extraction). Epistaxis, bruising (large ecchymosis). GI or urinary tract hemorrhage (hematuria).
- Hemophilias less commonly present with purpura & petechiae (because platelet function is normal) or spontaneous hemorrhage [except in the severe form (Factor 9 level <1% of normal)].

DIAGNOSIS
- **Low Factor IX (9) <40% — most sensitive test.** Mild disease >5%; moderate: 1-5%; severe <1%.
- CBC & coagulation studies: **Prolonged aPTT.** Normal PT, fibrinogen, & platelets (bleeding time).
- Mixing studies: **PTT corrects with mixing studies with normal plasma** (indicating a factor deficiency).

MANAGEMENT
- **Factor IX (9) infusion first-line therapy** to increase levels 25-100% (depending on severity). Can be given in response to an **acute bleeding episode or prophylaxis** (eg, prior to surgery).
- **Unlike Hemophilia A, Desmopressin is not useful in Hemophilia B.**
- Significant arthropathy can be minimized by long-term regular prophylaxis with factor concentrate.

FACTOR V LEIDEN MUTATION (ACTIVATED PROTEIN C RESISTANCE)

- **Most common inherited cause of hypercoagulability (thrombophilia), especially in Whites.**
- 5% of the US population of European descent is heterozygous for this mutation (autosomal dominant).

PATHOPHYSIOLOGY
- **Mutated activated factor V is resistant to normal breakdown (inactivation) by activated protein C**, resulting in increased hypercoagulability & conversion of prothrombin to thrombin.

CLINICAL MANIFESTATIONS
- **Venous thromboembolism (VTE): increased incidence of DVT, PE; thrombosis in unusual veins (eg, hepatic vein, portal vein, or cerebral vein thrombosis).** Recurrent VTE.
- Pregnancy complications: ↑ risk of miscarriage, Preeclampsia, Placental abruption, & stillbirth.
- Not associated with increased risk of arterial thrombosis (eg, Myocardial infarctions or CVA).

DIAGNOSIS
- **Activated protein C resistance assay. If positive, confirm with DNA testing.** Normal PT & aPTT.
- DNA testing mutation analysis. Used in patients with a family history of Factor V Leiden mutation or for members of a thrombophilic family. Homozygous → higher risk of thrombosis.

MANAGEMENT
- **Asymptomatic heterozygous for FVL: not treated routinely with anticoagulation.**
- **High-risk: indefinite anticoagulation (Direct oral anticoagulant or Warfarin).** May need thrombophylaxis with Low molecular weight heparin during pregnancy to prevent miscarriages.
- Moderate-risk: (eg, 1 thrombotic event with a prothrombotic stimulus or asymptomatic) prophylaxis during high-risk procedures.

PROTEIN C or S DEFICIENCY

PATHOPHYSIOLOGY
- **Proteins C & S are vitamin K-dependent anticoagulant proteins** produced by the liver that stimulate fibrinolysis and inactivate factors Va and VIIIa, which are needed for thrombin formation.
- **Decreased protein C or S levels lead to hypercoagulability.**

ETIOLOGIES
- Inherited: both are autosomal-dominant inherited hypercoagulable disorders (C more common).
- Acquired: end-stage liver disease, severe liver disease with synthetic dysfunction, early Warfarin administration (vitamin K antagonist), Disseminated intravascular coagulation (DIC).

CLINICAL MANIFESTATIONS
- **Venous thromboembolism Increased incidence of DVT & PE.** Thrombosis in an unusual vein (eg, portal, hepatic, mesenteric, cerebral).
- **Warfarin-induced skin necrosis** any patient presenting with this should be tested for deficiency.
- Purpura fulminans in newborns — red purpuric lesions at pressure points, progresses to painful black eschars.

DIAGNOSIS
- Protein C and S functional assay, plasma protein C and S antigen levels. Genetic testing (rarely done).

MANAGEMENT
- Thrombosis protein C concentrate. Indefinite anticoagulation (Direct oral anticoagulant or Warfarin).
- Warfarin-induced necrosis: immediately discontinue Warfarin, administer IV Vitamin K, therapeutic Heparin, protein C concentrate or fresh frozen plasma.

ANTITHROMBIN III DEFICIENCY

- **Decreased levels of antithrombin III, leading to hypercoagulability**.

PATHOPHYSIOLOGY
- Antithrombin III is a natural anticoagulant that inhibits coagulation by neutralizing the activity of factors 2a (thrombin), 9a, & 10a. Decreased levels or dysfunction lead to increased risk of clotting.

ETIOLOGIES
- Inherited: autosomal-dominant.
- Acquired: liver disease, Nephrotic syndrome, DIC, chemotherapy.

CLINICAL MANIFESTATIONS
- **Increased incidence of venous thromboembolism — DVT & PE.**
- **Suspect if no significant change in aPTT with Heparin administration**.

DIAGNOSIS
- Antithrombin III assays [eg, plasma AT activity (AT-heparin cofactor assay)] is the best first test.

MANAGEMENT
- Asymptomatic: anticoagulation only before surgical procedures or high-risk surgery.
- Thrombosis: high-dose IV Heparin followed by oral anticoagulation therapy indefinitely.

HEPARIN INDUCED THROMBOCYTOPENIA [(HIT) type II]

- **Acquired thrombocytopenia especially within the first 5-10 days of the initiation of Heparin.**
- In HIT, [1] the thrombocytopenia is not usually severe, with nadir counts rarely <20,000/μL. [2] Heparin-induced thrombocytopenia (HIT) is not associated with bleeding and, in actuality, **markedly increases the risk of thrombosis despite thrombocytopenia**.

RISK FACTORS
- Unfractionated Heparin > Low molecular weight Heparin; surgical > medical; female > male.

PATHOPHYSIOLOGY
- **Autoantibody formation to the hapten complex of Heparin + platelet factor 4** causes platelet activation & consumption, leading to simultaneous **thrombocytopenia & thrombosis**.

CLINICAL MANIFESTATIONS
- Thrombocytopenia most common but bleeding is uncommon (due to prothrombotic nature of HIT).
- Thrombosis: venous thrombosis, gangrene, organ infarction and skin necrosis.

DIAGNOSIS
- **4 Ts**: **T**hrombocytopenia, **T**iming of platelet drop, **T**hrombosis, absence of o**t**her causes.
- HIT antibody testing: **Enzyme-linked immunoassay (ELISA) with PF4/polyanion complex as the antigen (screening)**. If positive, confirm with functional assays (**14-C-serotonin release assay**).
- Patients with overt HIT should be screened with lower extremity US to assess for asymptomatic DVT.

MANAGEMENT
- **Immediate discontinuation of all Heparin + initiation of non-Heparin anticoagulants.**
- Non-Heparin anticoagulants: **Direct thrombin inhibitor** (eg, **Argatroban, Lepirudin, Bivalirudin**), **Fondaparinux, direct oral anticoagulant** (eg, **Apixaban, Edoxaban, Rivaroxaban, Dabigatran**).
- Long-term anticoagulation with Warfarin can only be started [1] after other non-Heparin anticoagulation has been started & [2] the thrombosis has decreased because of the initial prothrombotic state normally associated with the first 5 days of the initiation of Warfarin therapy.

APLASTIC ANEMIA (AA)

- **Immune-mediated suppression of, or injury to, the hematopoietic stem cell characterized by bone marrow failure leading to varying degrees of [1] peripheral blood <u>pancytopenia</u> and [2] bone marrow hypocellularity** (decreased or absent hematopoietic precursors in bone marrow).

PATHOPHYSIOLOGY
- **<u>Loss of hematopoietic stem cells (HSCs):</u> bone marrow hypoplasia or aplasia, most often due to autoimmune injury to multipotent hematopoietic stem cells (T cells attack hematopoietic stem cells)** or direct stem cell damage leads to bone marrow failure, including replacement of marrow with fat. Other causes include viral suppression of stem cells.
- Loss of HSCs result in a decrease in peripheral mature blood cells and pancytopenia.

ETIOLOGIES
- **<u>Idiopathic</u> most common cause (65%) — T-cell mediated autoimmune response.**
- <u>Ionizing radiation</u> exposure (predictable, dose-related response). Chemicals (eg, Benzene).
- **<u>Viral infections</u>: seronegative viral hepatitis** (non-A through G) seen in 5-10% and most often affecting boys and young men, HIV. **Parvovirus B19 in patients with baseline hemolytic anemias (eg, Sickle cell disease, G6PD deficiency).** Other viruses.
- <u>Medications:</u> antibiotics **(eg, Chloramphenicol, Sulfa drugs)**, cytotoxic chemotherapy (anticipated dose-related effect), **anti-epileptics (Carbamazepine**, Phenytoin, Valproic acid), Quinine, NSAIDs, anti-thyroid medications (eg, PTU), immunosuppressive agents (eg, Azathioprine, Methotrexate).
- <u>B12 & Folate deficiency</u> can cause pancytopenia.
- <u>Acquired clonal abnormalities</u> — **Paroxysmal nocturnal hemoglobinuria** (PNH), Myelodysplastic syndromes (MDS), or Acute myelogenous leukemia (AML).
- **<u>Fanconi anemia</u>: most common hereditary cause — pancytopenia, organ hypoplasia (short stature, thumb & arm abnormalities, small head circumference), bone defects, & café-au-lait spots.**

CLINICAL MANIFESTATIONS
<u>Symptoms of pancytopenia</u> — bleeding, easy bruising, frequent infections, & fatigue.
- <u>Thrombocytopenia:</u> **mucocutaneous bleeding** — eg, epistaxis, bleeding gums, petechiae, purpura, easy bruising, menorrhagia.
- <u>Anemia:</u> weakness, fatigue, dyspnea, pallor. <u>Leukopenia:</u> recurrent or frequent infections, fever.
- Hepatosplenomegaly, lymphadenopathy, or bone tenderness should NOT be present.

DIAGNOSIS
- **<u>CBC/peripheral smear:</u> ≥2 cytopenias** — reticulocytopenia <1% or <40,000/microL, neutropenia <500/microL, thrombocytopenia <20,000/microL, and/or anemia. No abnormal hematopoietic cells.
- **<u>Bone marrow biopsy:</u>** hypocellular/aplastic bone marrow — **<u>marked hypocellularity</u> with normal cell morphology, <u>fatty bone marrow</u>** (replacement of normal marrow elements with fat cells & marrow stroma). **No infiltration of the bone marrow with fibrosis or malignant cells.**
- Diagnosis of exclusion in the setting of bone marrow failure (r/o PNH & Myelodysplastic syndrome).

MANAGEMENT
- **<u>Supportive management</u> initial treatment of choice** — eg, infection prophylaxis with broad-spectrum antibiotics, PRBC transfusion for hemoglobin <7 mg/dL, platelet transfusion for counts <10,000 or active bleeding.
- <u>Moderate AA:</u> — For most medically-fit or less-fit patients with moderate AA, initial treatment with either [1] lower-intensity Immunosuppressive therapy (IST) or [2] single-agent Eltrombopag, rather than intensive IST or allogeneic HCT may be used.
- <u>Severe AA in otherwise healthy patients <40 years:</u> **Allogeneic hematopoietic stem cell transplantation treatment of choice** with HLA-matched donor rather than immunosuppressants.
- **<u>Immunosuppressive therapy:</u> severe or very severe AA in patients ≥40 years of age (some experts advise >50 years) or in younger patients without a matched donor. Triple therapy used if medically fit (eg, horse anti-thymocyte globulin + Cyclosporine + Eltrombopag).**

HEREDITARY HEMOCHROMATOSIS (HH)

- Autosomal recessive disorder characterized by **excess deposition of iron as hemosiderin in the parenchymal cells of the heart, liver, pancreas, & endocrine organs.**
- **The associated <u>C282Y HFE</u> genotype on chromosome 6** (6p21.3) **is increased in N. Europeans.**

PATHOPHYSIOLOGY
- *HFE* protein (C282Y or H632) mutation leads to decreased hepcidin, the iron regulatory hormone**.**
- **Decreased hepcidin leads to <u>increased intestinal iron absorption</u>** despite normal iron intake. **Iron accumulation leads to organ dysfunction** from iron deposition in the parenchymal cells as hemosiderin.

CLINICAL MANIFESTATIONS
- Symptoms usually begin after 40 years of age in men & after menopause in women (women lose iron through menstruation). Early manifestations include fatigue, weakness, arthralgias, and lethargy.
- Liver: abdominal pain, **cirrhosis,** fatigue, weakness, hepatomegaly, spider angiomata, jaundice.
- Endocrine: **Diabetes mellitus** from pancreatic beta cell damage. Hypothyroidism.
- Heart: **restrictive or dilated cardiomyopathy, arrhythmias**, heart failure, heart blocks.
- Reproductive: **hypogonadism, erectile dysfunction,** testicular atrophy.
- Joints: arthralgias, arthritis, synovitis, **symmetric arthropathy**.
- Skin: **skin hyperpigmentation** with metallic or bronze skin color (from both iron and melanin deposition) **"<u>bronze Diabetes</u>"** (due to the color of the skin and pancreatic involvement).
- **Increased susceptibility to bacteria that feed on iron (eg, *Yersinia enterocolitica, Vibrio vulnificus., Listeria monocytogenes*).** Increased risk of Porphyria cutanea tarda.

DIAGNOSIS
- **Iron studies: initial test to assess for iron overload — increased serum iron, ↑ <u>ferritin</u>** (>300 mcg/L in men or postmenopausal women and >200 in premenopausal women), ↑ **<u>transferrin saturation</u>** (>55% for women or >45% for men); **normal or decreased TIBC (transferrin).**
- Liver enzymes: LFTs are usually elevated but not usually higher than twice the normal levels.
- **Genetic testing for *HFE* variants (C282Y and H63D) followed by Abdominal MRI performed if iron studies are abnormal.** Homozygosity for C282Y (C282Y/C282Y) accounts for ~90% of cases.
- **<u>MRI of the liver</u> is the best non-invasive way to measure liver iron content.**
- **Liver biopsy: most accurate test — increased hemosiderin in the liver parenchyma** with Prussian blue staining. Not usually required for diagnosis but may be performed if genetic testing & MRI are negative or to rule out hepatic fibrosis or Cirrhosis.
- Other testing: fasting blood glucose levels need to be checked for Diabetes mellitus, echocardiogram for cardiomyopathy, hormone levels to evaluate hypogonadism, and bone densitometry to evaluate for Osteoporosis. Genetic testing in first degree relatives of patients with Hemochromatosis.

MANAGEMENT
- **<u>Regular phlebotomy</u> mainstay of treatment** — by removing red blood cells, the major mobilizer of iron in the body, iron toxicity, can be minimized. May be performed once or twice weekly to obtain a ferritin in the normal or iron-deficient range (50-100 mcg/L), a decrease in transferrin saturation, or until a mild anemia occurs. May need maintenance phlebotomy therapy (eg, 3-4 times a year for life).
- **<u>Iron chelating agents</u> in patients who are unable to undergo phlebotomy** (oral Deferasirox or Deferiprone; IV Deferoxamine). More effective in patients with erythropoietic hemochromatosis.
- **Avoid iron supplementation** & excess consumption of iron-rich foods (red meat). Avoid Vitamin C (increased iron absorption), alcohol intake (alcohol can accelerate hepatic and pancreatic toxicity), & raw shellfish consumption (to prevent *Vibrio vulnificus* infection).
- Treat the underlying cause. End-stage liver disease is an indication for liver transplantation.
- Because Hepatocellular carcinoma accounts for ~30% of mortality in HH, all patients with Hemochromatosis should undergo surveillance, with ultrasound and alpha-fetoprotein levels performed every 6 months.

WALDENSTRÖM MACROGLOBULINEMIA (LYMPHOPLASMACYTIC LYMPHOMA)

- **Lymphoplasmacytic B-cell lymphoma** that <u>produces excess IgM paraprotein.</u>
- Considered an indolent type of B-cell non-Hodgkin Lymphoma (incurable but treatable).
- <u>Pathophysiology:</u> **Proliferation of IgM-producing plasmacytoid lymphocytes** (hybrid of plasma cells & lymphocytes) **in the bone marrow with monoclonal B cell immunoglobulin M (IgM) production** (postgerminal center IgM memory B cell that has failed to switch isotype class).

CLINICAL MANIFESTATIONS

- **Often asymptomatic (smoldering) in ~25% of patients. <u>No</u> lytic bones lesions of Myeloma.**
- <u>Triad:</u> If symptomatic, associated with **"OVA" [1] <u>O</u>rganomegaly, [2] <u>V</u>iscosity, & [3] <u>A</u>nemia.**
- **[1] <u>O</u>rganomegaly:** lymphadenopathy, splenomegaly, hepatomegaly (30-40%).
- **[2] <u>Hyperviscosity syndrome:</u>** large IgM molecules increase serum viscosity, slowing the passage of blood through the capillaries, leading to blurred vision, **engorged tortuous retinal veins (venous "sausaging"), papilledema, headache, vertigo,** nystagmus, dizziness, tinnitus, ataxia, coma. **<u>Chronic, oozing of blood from nose & gums:</u>** IgM interaction with platelets & inhibition of fibrin.
- **[3] <u>A</u>nemia:** (bone marrow failure) — weakness, fatigue, pallor. <u>Systemic:</u> weight loss, fever, chills.
- **Peripheral neuropathy** (10%) especially due to IgM acting as an autoantibody vs. myelin-associated glycoproteins in nerves & other nerve components — paresthesias, weakness, motor deficits.
- **Cryoglobulinemia: Raynaud phenomenon,** urticaria. **IgM autoantibodies against RBCs can lead to a Coombs-positive autoimmune Cold hemolytic anemia,** acral cyanosis, &/or tissue necrosis.

DIAGNOSIS

- **Serum protein electrophoresis:** IgM monoclonal protein spike (macroglobulinemia) hallmark.
- <u>Cytopenia:</u> anemia, thrombocytopenia, neutropenia. Rouleaux formation. ↑ beta-2 microglobulin level.
- **Bone marrow biopsy: ≥10% lymphoplasmacytic infiltrate** (r/o CLL). MYD88 L265P mutations. **<u>Dutcher bodies:</u>** plasma cells with IgM filled cytoplasm appearing as intranuclear inclusions.

MANAGEMENT

- <u>Asymptomatic:</u> Observation with 4-6 month follow up. Responsive to chemotherapy (rarely curative).
- <u>Symptomatic:</u> **Rituximab + Bendamustine first-line medical management.** <u>BKI:</u> Ibrutinib.
- <u>Failure or relapse:</u> Repeat regimen, BTK inhibitor (eg, Ibrutinib), or Bortezomib, combination therapy.
- **Severe <u>Hyperviscosity syndrome</u>: with complications — Plasmapheresis** (removes IgM).

MONOCLONAL GAMMOPATHY OF UNDERTERMINED SIGNIFICANCE (MGUS)

- **Clinically asymptomatic** premalignant clonal lymphoplasmacytic or plasma cell proliferative disease, leading to **increased immunoglobulins.**
- 1% of adults, 3% of adults >70y. 1% yearly risk of developing Multiple myeloma or Lymphoma
- **IgG most common** (69%), IgM (17%), IgA (11%), IgD, kappa light chain (62%), lambda light chain (38%).
- May be associated with other diseases, infection, autoimmune disorders (eg, SLE, ITP).

CLINICAL MANIFESTATIONS

- **Usually asymptomatic; no end-organ damage from the paraprotein** — often an incidental finding.

DIAGNOSIS

<u>Workup:</u> SPEP, serum FLC assay, complete blood count, creatinine, and serum calcium.
- **Serum protein electrophoresis (SPEP):** IgG monoclonal spike **(elevated but usually <3g/dL).** Monoclonal spike is usually stable over time (usually does not progress).
- <u>Urine protein electrophoresis:</u> none (or stable) amounts of Bence-Jones proteins.
- **Absence of symptoms of Multiple myeloma:** hypercalcemia, anemia, renal failure, lytic bone lesions.
- **<u>Bone marrow:</u> <10% clonal plasmacytoid or plasma cells.** Biopsy obtained if abnormal workup.

MANAGEMENT

- **Conservative or observation: low malignant potential risk.** Repeat testing after 6 months.

PLASMA CELL MYELOMA (MULTIPLE MYELOMA, PLASMACYTOMA)

- **Cancer associated with proliferation of a single clone of immunoglobulin-producing plasma cells,** leading to ↑ production of ineffective monoclonal antibodies: **IgG (60%)**; IgA (20%); IgM.
- **Most common primary bone malignancy in adults.**
- Risk factors: **older adults (median age 65 years), Black individuals, men,** Benzene exposure.
- Pathophysiology: plasma cells accumulate in the bone marrow, interrupting bone marrow's normal cell production. Protein accumulation causes end-organ damage (eg, kidney injury, bone lesions).

CLINICAL MANIFESTATIONS: Bones "BREAK" in Multiple Myeloma.
- **B**one pain: most common symptom. Vertebral involvement most common & ribs.** Due to **osteolytic lesions (skeletal destruction)**, pathogenic osteopenic fractures, spinal cord compression, radiculopathy (plasma cells can form soft tissue tumors). Neurologic involvement.
- **R**ecurrent infections: due to leukopenia & ineffective Ig production. Hyperviscosity (esp. with IgM).
- **E**levated calcium: due to osteoclast activating factor from plasma cells, leading to bone destruction.
- **A**nemia: fatigue, pallor, weakness, weight loss, hepatosplenomegaly.
- **K**idney injury: due to light chain antibody protein deposition in tubules. Increased BUN & creatinine.

DIAGNOSIS
- CBC: **Rouleaux formation — RBCs with a "stack of coins" appearance** due to increased plasma protein (**increased ESR**). Normochromic normocytic anemia. **Hypercalcemia**. ↑ BUN & creatinine.
- Serum protein electrophoresis: **monoclonal protein spike — IgG most common** 60%, IgA (20%).
- Urine protein electrophoresis: **Bence-Jones proteins** (composed of **kappa or lambda light chains**). 15% of MM is light chains only. Serum free light chain assay. Whole body CT or MRI. PET scan.
- Radiographs: **"punched-out" lytic lesions.** Bone scans NOT helpful (little osteoblast activity in MM).
- Bone marrow aspiration: **plasmacytosis (clonal plasma cells) ≥10% — definitive diagnosis.**

MANAGEMENT
- **Autologous stem cell transplant (HCT) most effective therapy** — may be preceded by induction chemotherapy (eg, Dexamethasone with Lenalidomide & Bortezomib) prior to stem cell collection.
- **Ineligible for HCT: Bortezomib quadruple or triple therapy:** Bortezomib, Lenalidomide, Dexamethasone (VRd) ± Daratumumab (DVRd).

SECONDARY ERYTHROCYTOSIS

- Major cause of ↑RBC mass. Most common in obesity or history of cigarette smoking.
- **Secondary erythrocytosis = ↑hematocrit as a response to another process.**

ETIOLOGIES 3 major causes:
- **[1] Reactive (physiologic): due to hypoxia** — eg, **pulmonary disease (COPD),** high altitude, tobacco smokers, cyanotic heart disease. **Reactive most common type. Increased erythropoietin.**
- [2] Pathologic: no underlying tissue hypoxia. Renal disease (eg, renal cell CA), fibroids, hepatoma.
- [3] Relative polycythemia: normal RBC mass in the setting of ↓plasma volume or dehydration.

CLINICAL MANIFESTATIONS
- Symptoms related to the underlying precipitating cause (eg, COPD, renal disease, cyanosis etc).
- Physical Exam: cyanosis, clubbing, hypertension, hepatosplenomegaly, ± heart murmur.

DIAGNOSIS
- **↑RBCs/hematocrit with normal WBC & platelets.**
- **Increased erythropoietin levels & RBC mass if reactive or pathologic.** Relative polycythemia: Normal erythropoietin levels & normal RBC mass because the polycythemia is relative (due to ↓ plasma volume).

MANAGEMENT: treat underlying disorder. Smoking cessation.

POLYCYTHEMIA RUBRA VERA (PRIMARY ERYTHROCYTOSIS)

- Acquired myeloproliferative disorder with **autonomous bone marrow overproduction of all 3 hematopoietic myeloid stem cell lines [primarily increased RBC mass]** but also associated with increased granulocytic WBCs (neutrophils, basophils, eosinophils) and platelets.

- PATHOPHYSIOLOGY: **JAK2 mutation leads to Primary erythrocytosis** (increased hematocrit in the absence of hypoxia & ↓EPO). Risk factors: **peaks 50-60 years of age. Most common in men** (60%).

CLINICAL MANIFESTATIONS
- **Symptoms due to increased RBC mass (hyperviscosity &/or thrombosis).** Gout (↑ uric acid)
- **Hyperviscosity:** headache, dizziness, tinnitus, blurred vision, weakness, fatigue, **pruritus, especially after a hot bath or shower** (due to histamine release from basophils), **epistaxis, bleeding.**
- **Thrombosis:** Thrombotic complications (eg, hepatic vein thrombosis, DVT, TIA). **Erythromelalgia** (episodic burning or throbbing of hands & feet with edema, cyanosis, or pallor) is rare but classic.
- Physical examination: **hepatosplenomegaly, facial plethora (flushing), & engorged retinal veins.**

LABS:
- **CBC/peripheral smear:** in pre-polycythemia & overt polycythemia, excess of normochromic & normocytic red blood cells are seen — **increased hemoglobin & hematocrit** (a **hypochromic & microcytic pattern** can accompany concomitant iron deficiency). **Thrombocytosis is common. Granulated white blood cell leukocytosis (predominantly with neutrophils)** in the absence of fever or infection (lymphocytes & monocytes are not usually significantly increased in PV & blasts are not a characteristic feature). In contrast, the post-polycythemic stage (spent phase), myelofibrosis — teardrop red blood cells, elliptical RBCs, poikilocytosis, & nucleated red cells.
- **Normal O2 saturation:** arterial oxygen saturation usually ≥92%. **Increased uric acid levels.**
- **Increased leukocyte alkaline phosphatase (LAP)** often >100 U/L due to increased functioning WBCs. Helps to distinguish PV (high LAP) from Chronic myelogenous leukemia (low LAP).
- **Increased serum B12** levels >900 pg/mL in ~30% of because of increased transcobalamin-III, a binding protein found in WBCs (↑ total WBC counts in the peripheral blood & bone marrow).
- **Iron deficiency** despite polycythemia due to disordered iron metabolism, defects in iron absorption, aberrant hypoxia sensing and signaling, and increased frequency of bleeding.

DIAGNOSIS: All 3 major OR first 2 major + 1 minor
Major criteria:
- **[1] Increased RBC mass: increased hemoglobin & hematocrit*** — Hg ≥16.5 g/dL or Hct ≥49% in men; Hg ≥16.0 g/dL or Hct ≥48% in women; or red blood cell mass >25% above mean normal predicted.
- **[2] Bone marrow biopsy:** hypercellularity with **trilineage** growth (panmyelosis with erythroid, granulocytic, & megakaryocytic proliferation) with pleomorphic, mature megakaryocytes.
- **[3] *JAK2* mutation presence (most accurate)** — *JAK2 V617F* exon 14 or *JAK2* exon 12 mutation.
Minor criterion:
- **Low or subnormal serum erythropoietin (EPO) level** increased RBCs despite low EPO level due to negative feedback. Increased EPO levels usually suggest Secondary erythrocytosis.

MANAGEMENT
- **Low-risk (<60 years & no thrombosis): Phlebotomy first-line until hematocrit <45% + low-dose Aspirin to reduce vasomotor symptoms and to prevent thrombosis** (not used if aVWS).
- **High-risk (≥60 years &/or thrombosis): all the above + cytoreduction [eg, Hydroxyurea** or Pegylated Interferon-alfa (second line)]. **Ruxolitinib (JAK inhibitor)** if no response to Hydroxyurea.
- Symptomatic: Antihistamines (H1 blockers) for pruritus. Allopurinol if hyperuricemia.
- Avoid iron supplementation. Avoid alkylating agents (increased risk of myelofibrosis & progression to AML). PV can evolve into Myelofibrosis of Acute myelogenous leukemia (AML).

ESSENTIAL THROMBOCYTHEMIA [ET (ESSENTIAL THROMBOCYTOSIS)]

- Rare **myeloproliferative neoplasm** characterized by **excessive, clonal platelet production** with a **tendency for thrombosis &/or hemorrhage.** Increased granulocytes & RBCs may also be seen.
- May progress to Myelofibrosis or Acute myeloid leukemia.
- ET usually presents in middle aged and older adults (50-60 years median age at diagnosis).

PATHOPHYSIOLOGY
- **JAK2, CALR, or MPL mutation:** (90%) — driver mutation in *JAK2*, *CALR*, or *MPL*. These mutations result in the upregulation of genes in the JAK-STAT pathway (increased production of myeloid lines).

CLINICAL PRESENTATION
- **Increased platelets may lead to microvascular occlusions (usually reversible), large vessel thrombosis, or (paradoxically & less commonly) bleeding.** Splenomegaly may be seen. HTN.
- **Asymptomatic in 50%** — incidental finding of high platelet count seen on CBC (nonreactive). Fatigue.
- **Vasomotor symptoms:** eg, headache, dizziness, vision changes, **Erythromelalgia** (burning of hands & feet), acrocyanosis, cutaneous ulcers. Pruritus is not a feature of ET because basophils are minimal or absent. **Complications of thrombosis:** DVT, PE, hepatic thrombi, CRVO, first-trimester fetal loss.
- **Bleeding typically mucosal (eg, easy bruisability, petechiae, epistaxis, & GI bleeding) due to a qualitative platelet defect or acquired Von Willebrand syndrome.** May be seen in some patients with platelet counts >1 million/microL (↑ platelets use up free Von Willebrand factor).

LABORATORY STUDIES
- CBC: **Elevated platelets >450,000/microL (large platelets with normal morphology), normal red cell mass (hemoglobin & hematocrit) unlike PV.** Normal WBC (may be slightly elevated). Normal basophils. Elevated platelet count is not reactive (reactive thrombocytosis is more common).
- **Patients with bleeding or platelets >1,000,000/microL (>1000 x10⁹/L) should be tested for acquired von Willebrand syndrome (aVWS)** — Ristocetin cofactor (RCo) activity <30% if aVWS.

DIAGNOSIS
Diagnostic criteria requires all 4 of major criteria or the first 3 major criteria plus the minor criterion:
Major criteria:
- [1] **Elevated platelet count*** ≥450,000/microL. **Large platelets with normal morphology.**
- [2] **Bone marrow biopsy proliferation mainly of the megakaryocyte lineage** with increased numbers of enlarged, mature megakaryocytes with hyperlobulated nuclei. No significant increase or left shift neutrophil granulopoiesis or erythropoiesis & rarely minor (grade 1) ↑ in reticulin fibers.
- [3] **Exclude other conditions** not meeting WHO criteria for *BCR::ABL1* Chronic myeloid leukemia, Polycythemia vera, Primary myelofibrosis, Myelodysplastic syndromes, or other myeloid neoplasm.
- [4] **Presence of *JAK2*, *CALR*, or *MPL* mutation** on molecular testing. **JAK2V617F most common.**
Minor criterion:
- Presence of a clonal marker or absence of evidence for reactive thrombocytosis.

MANAGEMENT
- **High risk (>60y or prior thrombosis; +JAK2): cytoreductive agent (eg, Hydroxyurea) plus low-dose Aspirin if ≥40 years and not pregnant.** Age <40 years &/or potential for malignancy: Aspirin + Interferon alfa. Anegralide (reduces megakaryocytes) if patients do not tolerate Hydroxyurea.
- Pregnant: Low-dose Aspirin + LMWH with or without Interferon alfa (Hydroxyurea contraindicated).
- **Prior arterial thrombosis: twice-daily low-dose Aspirin.**
- **Prior venous thrombosis: Systemic anticoagulation is added to cytoreduction.**
- Intermediate-risk ET: either low-dose Aspirin alone or low-dose Aspirin plus Hydroxyurea.
- Low risk ET (≤60 years + no h/o thrombosis + no JAK2): **low-dose Aspirin** preferred rather than cytoreduction. **Very low-risk ET: either observation or low-dose Aspirin.**
- **Aspirin should be used with caution in patients with acquired von Willebrand disease (aVWS)** or extreme thrombocytosis due to the likelihood of aVWS. **aVWS responds to cytoreduction.**

PRIMARY MYELOFIBROSIS (PMF)

- Rare **myeloproliferative neoplasm** characterized by leukoerythroblastic blood smear, proliferation of **abnormal bone marrow megakaryocytes and granulocytes, & variable marrow fibrosis.**
- *JAK2* **mutation is present in 60-65%,** *CALR* mutation (20-25%), *MPL* mutation (5%), & "triple negative" disease (eg, no *JAK2, CALR,* or *MPL* mutation) in 8-10%.
- PMF usually presents in middle-aged and older adults (mean age 67 years).

PATHOPHYSIOLOGY
- **[1] Atypical megakaryocytes: megakaryocyte hyperplasia and dysplasia** — Janus kinase 2 activity may lead to hyperplasia of atypical megakaryocytes crowding the marrow, resulting in
- **[2] proliferation of fibroblasts (fibrosis)** fibrotic obliteration of the bone marrow resulting from increased collagen production due to elevated platelet-derived growth factor (PDGF).

CLINICAL PRESENTATION
- **Patients most commonly present with <u>severe fatigue</u> due to anemia (50-70%) or abdominal fullness (25-50%) due to splenomegaly or hepatomegaly.** Few patients are asymptomatic.
- <u>Other findings</u>: constitutional symptoms (eg, loss of appetite, weight loss, fatigue), Pulmonary hypertension, pruritus, Gout (high uric acid levels), or thrombotic events. Bone pain (upper legs).
- **Marked splenomegaly (>90%)** &/or hepatomegaly (50%) due to extramedullary hematopoiesis to compensate for bone marrow fibrosis — **abdominal fullness, early satiety** (spleen compresses the stomach), heavy sensation in left upper abdomen.

DIAGNOSIS
CBC with peripheral smear:
- Anemia (50%). White blood cell and platelet counts are variable (normal, high, or low).
- <u>Peripheral blood smear (Leukoerythroblastic)</u>: **[1] <u>teardrop-shaped RBCs (dacrocytes)</u>* in peripheral blood,** nucleated red blood cells (RBCs), anisocytosis (RBCs of varying sizes), poikilocytosis (RBCs of varying shapes), & variable degrees of polychromasia; **[2] <u>circulating granulocyte precursors</u>** (myelocytes, metamyelocytes, and blasts); **[3] <u>giant abnormal (bizarre looking) platelets</u> due to hyperplasia of atypical megakaryocytes.**

Bone marrow biopsy:
- <u>Often difficult to aspirate ("dry" tap)</u> — **variable marrow fibrosis & proliferation of <u>abnormal bone marrow megakaryocytes</u>** (megakaryocyte hyperplasia & dysplasia) & granulocytes.

Diagnostic criteria: PMF diagnosis requires all of the following:
- **[1] <u>Bone marrow</u>: <u>megakaryocyte proliferation & atypia</u>**; reticulin and/or collagen fibrosis.
- **[2] <u>Exclude other MPNs</u>**: Criteria for Polycythemia vera (PV), Chronic myeloid leukemia (CML), Myelodysplastic syndrome (MDS), or other myeloid neoplasm are not met.
- **[3] <u>Clonality</u>** – presence of *JAK2, CALR,* or *MPL* mutation or another clonal marker

Minor criteria: at least one of the following:
- WBC ≥11 x 10^9/L, palpable splenomegaly, Anemia not attributable to another condition, increased serum lactate dehydrogenase (LDH), Leukoerythroblastosis.

MANAGEMENT
- <u>Anemic patients</u> are supported with transfusion. Anemia can also be controlled with androgens (eg, Danazol); Erythropoiesis-stimulating agent. Prednisone + either Thalidomide or Lenalidomide.
- <u>Asymptomatic</u>: observation with monitoring is recommended.

Higher-risk, HCT-eligible:
- **Allogeneic hematopoietic stem cell transplant** recommended for certain patients with intermediate-risk and those with high- or very high-risk disease, as HCT is the only potentially curative treatment modality for Primary myelofibrosis. Limited to patients ≤70 years.
- **<u>Splenomegaly without anemia</u>**: Hydroxyurea. **Splenomegaly with anemia & good platelets** (≥50,000/microL): **JAK2 inhibitors reduce spleen size (eg, Ruxolitinib,** Fedratinib, Pacritinib) or Momelotinib. <u>Splenomegaly with anemia and low platelets <50,000/microL</u>: Pacritinib.

MYELODYSPLASTIC SYNDROMES (MDS)

- Heterogenous group of preleukemic disorders characterized by **[1] clonal hematopoiesis**, **[2] abnormal maturation of cells of the myeloid cell line**, resulting in ineffective hematopoiesis in the bone marrow & **[3] ≥1 cytopenias** eg, anemia, neutropenia, &/or thrombocytopenia.

RISK FACTORS
- **>65 years**, radiation or chemotherapy, Benzene exposure, tobacco smoke, mercury or lead exposure.

CLINICAL MANIFESTATIONS
- May be asymptomatic detected by pancytopenia on routine CBC due to bone marrow failure.
- **Symptoms of pancytopenia — easy bruising, bleeding, frequent infections, fatigue, dyspnea.**

DIAGNOSIS
- CBC with peripheral smear:
  - **Decreased number of ≥1 myeloid cell lines** — platelets, neutrophils, or RBCs (may be nucleated). Normocytic or macrocytic anemia (macro-ovalocytes common). WBC count normal or reduced.
  - **Hyposegmented granulocytes: reduced segmentation often accompanied by decreased or absent granulation &/or bilobed nuclei (pseudo Pelger-Huet abnormality).**

DIAGNOSTIC CRITERIA
- **Cytopenia:** — **≥1** of the following: hemoglobin <10 g/dL (100 g/L); absolute neutrophil count <1.8 x 10^9/L (<1800/microL); &/or platelets <100 x 10^9/L (<100,000/microL). Low reticulocytes.
- **Dysplasia** — **Morphologic or immunophenotypic evidence of significant dysplasia in ≥10% of erythroid precursors, granulocytes, or megakaryocytes on the blood smear or bone marrow examination**, in the absence of other causes of dysplasia. **Increased myeloblasts** in the blood and/or bone marrow **(but <20%)**.
- **Cytogenetic abnormalities** chromosomal abnormalities characteristic of MDS and not a component of Acute myelogenous leukemia [AML abnormalities include t(8;21)(q22;q22); inv(16)(p13.1q22) or t(16;16)(p13.1;q22); & t(15;17)(q22;q21.1)].

MANAGEMENT
Goals to improve symptoms & survival & to **decrease progression to Acute myelogenous leukemia** (especially monosomy 5 & 7). **Deletion 5q alone associated with good prognosis (use Lenalidomide).**
Lower-risk MDS management:
- **Asymptomatic patients: monitoring rather than immediate treatment is often used** because early treatment of asymptomatic patients does not improve long-term survival and deferral management reduces treatment-related adverse occurrences.
- **Symptomatic patients are treated according to the severity of cytopenias and symptoms** (eg, ongoing transfusion requirements, progressive cytopenias, or a reduced quality of life). **Most patients are treated with a lower-intensity therapy** — eg, intermittent transfusions, Erythropoietin alfa, Luspatercept (hematopoietic growth factor), Hypomethylating agent (eg, Azacytidine, Decitabine), or **Lenalidomide (if 5q deletion present).**

Higher-risk MDS management:
- **Medically-fit** — therapy choice is influenced by adverse pathologic features (eg, *TP53* mutation, adverse cytogenetic abnormalities), targetable mutations, availability of a stem cell donor, and individual values and preferences. **Treatment may include intensive (eg, intensive remission induction chemotherapy, with or without Allogeneic hematopoietic stem cell transplant) or lower-intensity therapies.**
- **Medically-unfit, but not frail** — **lower-intensity therapy for most patients**, with the choice of therapy based on pathologic features, drug availability, and patient preference.
- **Frail** — patients are unlikely to tolerate treatment besides supportive care.

ACUTE LYMPHOBLASTIC LEUKEMIA (ALL) & LYMPHOBLASTIC LYMPHOMA (LBL)

- **Malignancy arising from precursor (immature) lymphoid stem cells in the bone marrow.**
- B cell (most common), T cell, or null type (non-B or non-T cell). Also seen in patients >65 years of age.
- **Most common childhood malignancy** (25%) **peak 2-5 years of age**, boys, Down syndrome >5y.
- PATHOPHYSIOLOGY: overpopulation of immature nonfunctioning WBCs (blasts) overtake normal hematopoiesis (bone marrow infiltration), resulting in pancytopenia.

CLINICAL MANIFESTATIONS
Pancytopenia: fever, bruising, pallor, palpable liver, palpable spleen. Mediastinal mass common.
- **Pancytopenia: fever & infections** (leukopenia), **bleeding** from thrombocytopenia (eg, petechiae, purpura), & **anemia** eg, **persistent pallor, fatigue. Bone pain or musculoskeletal pain.**
- CNS symptoms: headache, stiff neck, visual changes, vomiting. **METS most common to CNS & testes.**
- Physical examination: **hepatomegaly or splenomegaly most common** — may manifest as anorexia, weight loss, abdominal distention, or abdominal pain. **Lymphadenopathy.**

DIAGNOSIS
- CBC & peripheral smear: WBC 5,000-100,000, cytopenia anemia, thrombocytopenia.
  Lymphoblasts: small, uniform blasts with scant cytoplasm (high nuclei to cytoplasm ratio).
- **Bone marrow aspiration: hypercellular with >20% lymphoblasts (definitive diagnosis).**
- **Flow cytometry test:** most accurate test to distinguish subtypes. **Terminal deoxynucleotidyl transferase (TdT) positive lymphoblasts hallmark of ALL.*** CD10+; CD2+, CD8+, and CD3+.

MANAGEMENT
- **Highly responsive to combination chemotherapy** (remission >85%). **Induction chemotherapy: Anthracyclines, Vincristine, Asparaginase, & Corticosteroids.** Maintenance therapy: 6-MP and Methotrexate. Imatinib used if Philadelphia chromosome positive. **Relapsing: stem cell transplant.**
- **CNS disease or CNS preventative: intrathecal Methotrexate. Perform LP on all patients with ALL.**

TUMOR LYSIS SYNDROME

- Oncologic emergency occurring with the treatment of neoplastic disorders due to **rapid tumor cell lysis after initiation of chemotherapy,** releasing massive amounts of potassium, phosphate, and nucleic acids into the circulation. Calcium & uric acid deposition can lead to Acute kidney injury.

RISK FACTORS
- High tumor burden (eg, initial WBC count > 20,000/microL), dehydration, & volume depletion.
- Large proliferation rate (eg, Acute lymphoblastic leukemia) and high-grade Lymphomas (eg, Burkitt).

CLINICAL MANIFESTATIONS
- Related to the metabolic derangements — muscle cramps, tetany, nausea, vomiting, diarrhea, anorexia, lethargy, syncope, hematuria, heart failure, kidney injury, & cardiac dysrhythmias.

LABORATORY FINDINGS:
- **Hyperphosphatemia, hypocalcemia, hyperuricemia, hyperkalemia, and Acute kidney injury** (including uric acid nephropathy).

MANAGEMENT
- **Treatment of electrolyte abnormalities, IV fluids (may add loop diuretic)** to promote excretion & wash out of the obstructing uric acid crystals, & a hypouricemic agent (**Rasburicase preferred**).
- **Hemodialysis (renal replacement therapy) if severe.**

PROPHYLAXIS
- **Rasburicase (or Allopurinol) PLUS aggressive IV fluid hydration.**
- Rasburicase: recombinant uricase that catalyzes oxidation of uric acid to a stable compound. May be more effective than Allopurinol. **Rasburicase contraindicated if G6PD deficient.**
- Allopurinol: xanthine oxidase inhibitor, resulting in decreased uric acid production.

CHRONIC LYMPHOCYTIC LEUKEMIA (CLL)/SMALL LYMPHOCYTIC LYMPHOMA (SLL)

- Indolent malignancy characterized by **clonal proliferation of morphologically mature but immunologically & functionally incompetent B cells** (considered the dame disease as Small cell lymphoma) **[SLL].** CLL = primarily in the blood; SLL = primarily in the lymph nodes.
- **Most common form of Leukemia in adults.** Risk factors: **increasing age** (mean age 70y), men.

CLINICAL MANIFESTATIONS
- **Usually asymptomatic, often an incidental finding of lymphocytosis on routine CBC testing.**
- **Pancytopenia:** anemia (eg, **fatigue most common**, dyspnea), increased infections (neutropenia), mucocutaneous bleeding (thrombocytopenia). Typical "B" symptoms of lymphoma (10%).
- Physical examination: **lymphadenopathy* most common physical exam finding** (cervical, supraclavicular axillary or generalized). The lymph nodes are usually firm, round, nontender and freely mobile. **Splenomegaly second most common finding** (25-55%) and is usually painless and nontender to palpation. Hepatomegaly. Skin lesions (leukemia cutis).

DIAGNOSIS
- **CBC/peripheral smear: initial diagnostic test. Isolated lymphocytosis** hallmark: increased WBC (>20,000/mcL) with >80% lymphocytes, **absolute lymphocytosis ≥5,000/mcL — small, well-differentiated, normal & mature-appearing lymphocytes** with a darkly stained nucleus, partially condensed (clumped) chromatin, and indiscernible nucleoli. **Scattered "smudge cells"** (lab artifact when the fragile B cells become crushed by the cover slip during slide preparation). Neutropenia,
- **Hypogammaglobulinemia:** decreased IgG, IgA, and IgM in ~25% of patients at the time of initial diagnosis. Increased incidence of Autoimmune hemolytic anemia. May have evidence of ITP.
- **Flow cytometry: most accurate test** — immunophenotypic analysis: **clone of mature B cells** with expression of B cell-associated antigens **CD19 + CD5 marks B cell maturity**; CD 23, low CD20.
- Bone marrow aspirate and biopsy not required for CLL. Excisional or core biopsy used for SLL.

MANAGEMENT
Indolent, asymptomatic, early stages (I and II):
- **No management (observation).** During this observation period, the clinical examination of the patient and blood counts should occur every 3 months. Radiation in some.
Chemotherapy:
- **Indications: symptomatic, progressive, stages III and IV** for symptomatic relief, cytopenia reversal, prolonged remission, & prolonged survival in patients. Despite treatment, CLL remains an incurable disease.
- **Very High risk (17p deletion &/or *TP53* mutation)** — high risk of either not responding to initial chemoimmunotherapy or relapsing soon after remission. **Initial treatment with targeted therapy** rather than chemoimmunotherapy, regardless of patient age — eg, continuous Acalabrutinib or Zanabrutinib. Continuous Ibrutinib. Venetoclax + Obinutuzumab. Ibrutinib ± Venetoclax.
- **High risk [IGHV unmutated (without 17p deletion or *TP53* mutation)]** — **targeted therapy** Acalabrutinib (Bruton tyrosine kinase inhibitor) ± Obinutuzumab, Zanabrutinib. Venetoclax (bcl2 inhibitor that induces apoptosis) + Ibrutinib; Venetoclax + Obinutuzumab. Ibrutinib as a single agent (all ages) or with either Rituximab (anti-CD20 antibody) or Obinutuzumab; Chemoimmunotherapy.
- **IGHV mutated (without 17p deletion or *TP53* mutation)** – chemoimmunotherapy or targeted therapy is used. If chemoimmunotherapy is chosen, the preferred regimen depends on clinical fitness – FCR: **Fludarabine,** Cyclophosphamide, and Rituximab for 6 cycles (younger patients); BR: Bendamustine plus Rituximab for 6 cycles (older patients); Targeted therapy: Venetoclax + Obinutuzumab, Venetoclax plus Ibrutinib. Acalabrutinib ± Obinutuzumab; Ibrutinib.
Curative therapy: Allogeneic stem cell transplant.
Acute blast crisis: treat similar to Acute myelogenous leukemia.

Poorer prognosis: ZAP-70+, del(11q), deletion of chromosome del(17p), *TP53* mutation.
- Richter transformation: CLL transforms into Large-cell lymphoma (poor prognosis)

ACUTE MYELOID LEUKEMIA (AML)

- Group of hematopoietic neoplasms characterized by clonal proliferation of myeloid precursors with decreased ability to differentiate into more mature cells & blood, bone marrow, & tissue infiltration.
- **Most common <u>acute</u> leukemia in adults (80% of cases).** Median onset 65 years of age.
- <u>PATHOPHYSIOLOGY</u>: **accumulation of leukemic blasts (immature WBCs)** in the bone marrow, peripheral blood, or occasionally other tissues. Increased production leads to pancytopenia.

<u>3 MAJOR SUBTYPES</u>
- **[1] Acute promyelocytic leukemia (APL or M3): t(15;17). Associated with DIC, presence of Auer rods (myeloperoxidase-positive cytoplasmic inclusions), & myeloperoxidase positivity.**
- **[2] Acute megakaryoblastic leukemia:** common in **children <5y of age with Down syndrome**.
- **[3] Acute monocytic leukemia:** associated with **infiltration of the gums (gingival hyperplasia).**

<u>CLINICAL MANIFESTATIONS</u>
- **Pancytopenia: <u>anemia</u>:** eg, **general fatigue most common presenting symptom,** dyspnea, weakness; **thrombocytopenia:** mucocutaneous bleeding; **& <u>neutropenia</u>:** increased infections & fever. Leukostasis. Uncommon symptoms include lymphadenopathy and hepatosplenomegaly.

<u>DIAGNOSIS</u>
- **CBC with peripheral smear: best initial test** — normocytic normochromic anemia with normal or decreased reticulocyte count. Thrombocytopenia. May have circulating **myeloblasts.** The median presenting leukocyte count is ~15,000/µL (but they are dysfunctional).
- <u>Bone marrow biopsy</u>: **gold standard: ≥20% myeloblasts** (immature cells with prominent nucleoli). **Auer rods pink/red rod-like granular structures in the cytoplasm with APL.**
- **Immunophenotyping: flow cytometry** helps to characterize the types with **FISH analysis — most accurate test. Myeloperoxidase positivity with APL.** 11q23 abnormalities with Monocytic.

<u>MANAGEMENT</u>
- **Combination chemotherapy: The most commonly used induction regimen includes Cytarabine PLUS an anthracycline (Doxorubicin, Daunorubicin, Idarubicin)** alone or with other agents.
- **All-trans-retinoic acid can be added to M3/APL (Promyelocytic leukemia)** because it induces the differentiation of leukemic cells bearing the t(15;17) [t(15;17) disrupts of retinoic acid receptor (RAR) required for myeloblast maturation; All-trans-retinoic acid reverses that].
- **Hematopoietic stem cell transplant curative in some after remission.**

LEUKOSTASIS REACTION [HYPERLEUKOCYTOSIS]

- Symptomatic hyperleukocytosis most commonly seen in Acute myeloid leukemia or Chronic myeloid leukemia in blast crisis. **Medical emergency** due to decreased tissue perfusion from leukostasis.
- <u>Pathophysiology</u>: leukostasis leads to increased blood viscosity and **white cell plugs in the microvasculature,** impeding blood flow in addition to causing local hypoxemia due to high metabolic activity of the rapidly dividing blasts.

<u>CLINICAL MANIFESTATIONS</u>
- **Pulmonary:** dyspnea, hypoxemia with or without diffuse alveolar or interstitial infiltrate formation.
- **Neurologic:** headache, dizziness, visual changes, tinnitus, gait instability, confusion, somnolence, coma. <u>Other:</u> priapism, bowel infarction, myocardial ischemia.

<u>DIAGNOSIS</u>
- **Hyperleukocytosis: WBC >100,000/microL (50-100 x 10^9/L) + symptoms due to tissue hypoxia (eg, lung, CNS).**

<u>MANAGEMENT</u>
- **Cytoreduction: leukapheresis (associated with rapid improvement), cytoreduction therapy (eg, Hydroxyurea), or induction chemotherapy.** Prophylaxis for Tumor lysis syndrome initiated.

CHRONIC MYELOID LEUKEMIA (CML)

- Myeloproliferative disorder of **uncontrolled production of mature and maturing granulocytes** with fairly normal differentiation (**predominately neutrophils** but also basophils & eosinophils).

PATHOPHYSIOLOGY
- Fusion of 2 genes: BCR (on chromosome 22) & ABL1 (on chromosome 9), result in **BCR-ABL1 fusion gene**. **Translocation between chromosomes 9 & 22 [t(9;22]** = Philadelphia chromosome (abnormal chromosome 22 harbors BCR-ABL1 gene) causes **hyperactive tyrosine kinase activity**. This cause excessive accumulation of maturing granulocytic cells in blood, marrow, liver, & spleen.

CLINICAL MANIFESTATIONS
- **Chronic phase: 70% asymptomatic** — usually detected incidentally on CBC (well-differentiated WBCs — granulocyte proliferation). **Pruritus after hot baths/showers (histamine release from Basophils).** Fatigue, night sweats, malaise, weight loss, fever, early satiety. **Splenomegaly most common physical examination finding in CML.** Tenderness over the lower sternum.
- **Accelerated phase:** neutrophil differentiation becomes progressively impaired and leukocyte counts are more difficult to control with chemotherapy. **Fatigue, weight loss, excessive sweating, bleeding from thrombocytopenia, infections, & abdominal pain (enlarging splenomegaly).**
- Blastic crisis: presents as acute leukemia and extramedullary tissue involvement (eg, lymph nodes, skin, and soft tissues). May be associated with rapidly enlarging spleen.

DIAGNOSIS
- CBC with peripheral smear: **leukocytosis** (may be strikingly elevated) with **granulocytic cells** (eg, **basophilia, neutrophilia, & eosinophilia).** The cells look morphologically normal but are cytochemically abnormal on immunochemistry. **Normal or increased platelets.*** Anemia (1/3).
- **Leukocyte alkaline phosphatase score**: decreased LAP score due to dysfunctional WBCs (LAP only found in functioning WBCs (eg, Polycythemia vera) not the leukemic cells of CML.
- Bone marrow biopsy: granulocytic hyperplasia (hypercellular with elevated basophils & eosinophils). Chronic: <5% blasts, Accelerated: 10-19% blasts; Acute blast crisis: ≥20% blasts.

Genetic testing:
- **Cytogenic analysis and fluorescence *in situ* hybridization (FISH) most accurate** - genetic testing for the **Philadelphia chromosome (BCR-ABL1 fusion gene)** or the fusion *BCR-ABL1* fusion mRNA via conventional cytogenetic analysis (karyotyping) or via reverse transcription polymerase chain reaction (RT-PCR) performed on peripheral blood or bone marrow aspirate. **90-95% have the t(9;22)(q34;q11.2) reciprocal translocation that results in the Philadelphia chromosome.**

MANAGEMENT:
- **Tyrosine kinase inhibitors: first-line therapy for most newly diagnosed CML: First-generation TKI (Imatinib) or second-generation TKI (Dasatinib, Nilotinib, or Bosutinib). TKIs inhibit Philadelphia chromosome tyrosine kinase activity & myeloid leukemic cell proliferation implicated in the pathogenesis of CML.** Most patients achieve long-term control (especially in the chronic phase). Accelerated phase CML & blastic crisis much more difficult to control & initial response to TKI therapy is often of short duration. For chronic phase, CML with **intermediate- or high-risk score, second-generation tyrosine kinase inhibitors (Bosutinib, Dasatinib, Nilotinib)** have an additional benefit over Imatinib. **Ponatinib (3rd generation TKI) for resistant to second line TKIs.**
- **Omacetaxine** is a selective inhibitor of the synthesis of the BCR-ABL1 oncoprotein used as a treatment option in cases refractory to Tyrosine kinase inhibitor (TKI) therapy that advanced from chronic phase CML.
- Allogeneic hematopoietic stem cell transplant is a curative treatment option but not often used as first-line therapy because it is associated with potential increase in toxicity and early mortality. Indications include treatment of advanced CML (accelerated phase & blast crisis), and chronic phase in patients with a suitable donor who are resistant to TKI therapy.
- Palliative therapy (cytotoxic agents) — Hydroxyurea, Interferon alfa ± Cytarabine, and Busulfan.

	HODGKINS DISEASE (HD) LYMPHOMA	NON HODGKINS LYMPHOMA (NHL)
AGE	• Bimodal* peaks in 20s then in 50s	• >50y, Increased risk with immunosuppression: ex HIV, viral infection
CELL TYPE	• REED STERNBERG CELLS pathognomonic* B cell proliferation with bilobed or multilobar nucleus "owl eye."	• B CELL: Diffuse large B cell MC (more aggressive). Follicular (indolent but less curable); Mantle Cell, Burkitt's, Marginal zone MALT lymphoma is an extranodal type of marginal zone lymphoma), small cell lymphoma (SCL) & CLL thought to be same disease with different presentations (SCL primarily in the lymph nodes, CLL in the bone marrow/peripheral blood). • T cell: (T cell, T lymphoblastic), Natural Killer Cells.
LYMPH NODE INVOLVEMENT	• UPPER LYMPH NODE INVOLVEMENT*: neck, axilla, shoulder, chest (mediastinum). ± painful lymph nodes c ETOH ingestion* Usually painless lymph nodes. • CONTIGUOUS spread to LOCAL LYMPH NODES. Usually Localized, single group of nodes (extranodal rare).	• PERIPHERAL MULTIPLE NODE INVOLVEMENT*: axillary, abdominal, pelvic, inguinal, femoral. Waldeyer's ring (tonsils, base of tongue, nasopharynx) • NONCONTIGUOUS EXTRANODAL SPREAD*: GI MC, Skin 2nd MC (especially T cell), testes, bone marrow, GU, liver, spleen, thyroid, kidney, spine, CNS (headache, lethargy, spinal cord compression, focal neurologic symptoms).
ASSOCIATED SYMPTOMS	• B sx: fever, weight loss, anorexia, night sweats. Associated with a poorer prognosis. • PEL EBSTEIN FEVER: intermittent cyclical fevers x1-2 weeks* (40%)	• B symptoms not as common on presentation (but may be seen with advanced disease or aggressive disease). • Leukemic phase can be seen at times with NHL.
EBV ASSOCIATION (EPSTEIN-BARR VIRUS)	• ↑associated with Epstein-Barr Virus*	• Rare in most types of NHL. • EBV common in Burkitt's lymphoma – ❶ Endemic (Africa): associated with jaw involvement, ❷ Immunodeficient: ex. post transplant lymphoma & AIDS-associated lymphoma. ❸Sporadic (not associated with EBV).
MANAGEMENT	• Excellent 5y cure rate (60%)	• Variable.

	AML	CML	ALL	CLL
EPIDEMIOLOGY	• MC acute form of leukemia. >50y	• Older males	• MC children* (peaks 3-7y)	• MC Leukemia in adults
DIAGNOSIS	>20% blasts (immature WBCs). • PROMYELOCYTIC - ⊕AUER RODS* - Sudan Black & Myeloperoxidase ⊕ • ACUTE MONOCYTIC: - Gingival infiltration/hyperplasia • MEGAKARYOCYTIC: ↑Down syndrome	• PHILADELPHIA CHROMOSOME* • Striking ↑WBC: >100,00 • Chronic <5% blasts • Accelerated 5-30% blasts • Acute >30% blasts	• >30% blasts. PAS ⊕ • Precursor B-cell ALL (~85%) associated with CNS sx. • Precursor T cell MC associated with adolescents with mediastinal mass & CNS sx	• SMUDGE (SMEAR) CELLS* • Well differentiated lymphocytes • ZAP-70 ⊕ ⇨ 8y survival. ZAP-70 negative ⇨ >25y.
MANAGEMENT	• Chemotherapy • Stem cell Transplant. • Tumor Lysis syndrome c chemotx: ↑K, ↓Ca, ↑Phos, Hyperuricemia & renal failure. Tx: Allopurinol, IV fluids.	• PO Chemotherapy (ex. Hydroxyurea, Imatinib). • Imatinib BCR-ABL tyrosine kinase inhibitor (Philadelphia ⊕).	• PO Chemotx in Philadelphia ⊕ • Induction: kills detectable disease for complete remission. • Consolidation: short term intensive therapy to sustain remission. • Maintenance: low dose to eradicate any remaining undetectable cells.	• Indolent: observation. • Symptomatic or progressive: Chemotherapy. • Allogeneic stem cell transplant is curative

	Bleeding Syndrome	Petechiae	Ecchymosis	Bleed after minor cuts	Bleeding after surgery
THROMBOCYTOPENIA (Quantitative/Qualitative)	Mucocutaneous bleeding*, petechiae (oral, nasal, GI, GU), petechiae	Common*	Small superficial	Yes	Immediate
FACTOR DEFICIENCY: Hemophilias	Deep bleeding* (joint, muscles)	Uncommon	Large hematomas	Not usually	Delayed*

NON-HODGKIN LYMPHOMAS

- Heterogenous group of lymphocyte neoplasms with proliferation in the lymph nodes & spleen.

RISK FACTORS
- **Increased age,** history of radiation therapy, family history. Chromosomal translocations.
- **Immunosuppression: HIV,** HCV, viral infection, organ transplantation. Autoimmune disorders.
- **Infections**: EBV, HHV-8, HIV. *H. pylori* **associated with gastric lymphoma. HCV with splenic.**

MAJOR TYPES
- **[1] Diffuse large B-cell: most common type of NHL. Fast growing, aggressive form (rapidly enlarging lymph nodes** of the neck, abdomen, & groin). Most common in the middle aged & elderly (average age 70 years). Extranodal in 40%. Large size B cell proliferation. CD 20+. Bcl-2 & Bcl-6.
- **[2] Follicular:** second most common. Small cell proliferation in follicles (circular pattern) CD20+. Most common in adults. Presents with painless lymphadenopathy (especially neck, groin, & axilla). **Follicular is usually indolent (slow growing) but hard to cure.** Sometimes not treated until symptomatic. Associated with **t(14;18) mutation [BCL-2].** May progress to large B cell lymphoma.
- **[3] Mantle cell:** small cell proliferation surrounding the follicular zone (mantle). 5-15%. CD 20+, CD5+ (poorer prognosis). Painless lymphadenopathy. **T(11;14) mutation [cyclin D1].**
- **[4] Marginal zone:** small B cell proliferation surrounding the mantle. CD 20+. **t(11;18).** Low grade [usually due to B-cell hyperplasia from chronic immune or inflammatory states: (eg, Hashimoto's thyroiditis, Sjögren syndrome)]. 3 subtypes: **Extranodal (Mucosal-Associated Lymphoid Tissue) MALT**: Gastric MALT lymphomas **often associated with** *H-pylori* **infection.** 8%. Nodal: originate in lymph nodes. **Splenic:** originates in spleen or bone marrow (↑ **incidence with HCV).**
- **[5] Burkitt Lymphoma:** intermediate-sized B cell proliferation. CD 20+. **Associated with Epstein-Barr virus infection** (except sporadic). Presents as an extranodal mass. **Most commonly seen in pediatric/adolescent & HIV. Endemic (Africa): involves the jaw & facial bones (especially with Malaria). Sporadic:** GI & paraaortic involvement (may cause **abdominal pain or fullness). Immunodeficient:** seen with HIV or immunosuppression (eg, post-transplant). **Biopsy "starry sky" appearance.** Very aggressive but highly curable. **T(8;14) mutation [*c-myc* translocation].**
- **[6] Small lymphocytic:** spectrum of Chronic lymphocytic leukemia. Small lymphocytic usually found in the lymph nodes & spleen (whereas CLL is found in the bone marrow and the blood). 7%.

CLINICAL MANIFESTATIONS
- The clinical presentation varies tremendously depending on the type of NHL & areas of involvement.
- Local: **painless lymphadenopathy.** Indolent lymphomas may present with slowly growing lymphadenopathy. **Hepatosplenomegaly.**
- Extranodal involvement: common. **GI tract most common site of extranodal involvement.** Skin second most common site of involvement. CNS also common.
- **Systemic B symptoms: (fever, night sweats, weight loss) rarer in NHL**; may be seen if advanced.

DIAGNOSIS
- **Excisional lymph node &/or tissue biopsy: required for the diagnosis and classification of NHL.**
- **Staging: Combined CT/PET scan of chest, abdomen, and pelvis.**

MANAGEMENT
- **Standard management of indolent stage I and contiguous stage II NHL consists of radiation therapy alone.** Careful observation an option of asymptomatic indolent NHL.
- **Limited stage (Stage I and II): chemotherapy mainstay for limited disease: R-CHOP (Rituximab, Cyclophosphamide, Doxorubicin, Oncovorin, Prednisone)** alone or with radiation. Chlorambucil, Fludarabine, 2-CdA (2-chloro-2'-deoxyadenosine). Rituximab (monoclonal antibody against CD20+). Stem cell transplant in refractory cases. BTK inhibitors for Mantle cell lymphoma.
- **Intermediate-grade:** combination chemotherapy (R-CHOP) plus involved-field radiation therapy.
- High Grade (Aggressive): R-CHOP. BTK inhibitors for Mantle cell (eg, Ibrutinib, Acalabrutinib).

HODGKIN LYMPHOMA [HL]

- Germinal or pregerminal **B-cell malignancy** originating in the lymphatic system.
- <u>Bimodal distribution</u>: **peaks at 20 years (15-34 years) & then again >50 years (≥55 years).**
- <u>Risk factors</u>: **Epstein-Barr virus (EBV),** immunosuppression, smoking, Caucasians.

4 MAIN TYPES:
- **[1] Nodular sclerosing: most common type of HL overall** (64%). **Female predominance.**
- **[2] Mixed cellularity** 25%. Associated with Epstein-Barr virus. Prevalent in both children and elderly patients and commonly presents with advanced disease stage.
- **[3] Lymphocyte rich/predominant**: most common in males <35 years. **Best prognosis.**
- **[4] Lymphocyte depleted:** (4%). Most common in males >60 years. Usually associated with other systemic diseases. **Worst prognosis.**

CLINICAL MANIFESTATIONS
- **[1] Asymptomatic painless lymphadenopathy: most common presentation** (70%). **Usually painless but alcohol ingestion may induce lymph node pain within minutes.**
  Upper body lymph nodes: neck most common site (cervical &/or supraclavicular), axilla, shoulder, mediastinum, & abdomen. Usually rubbery in consistency, not fixed (does not adhere to the skin), & may fluctuate in size. Spreads in an orderly fashion to contiguous areas of lymph nodes.
- **[2] Mediastinal lymphadenopathy or mass: second most common presentation — incidental finding on chest imaging.** The mass may be large without producing local symptoms. If symptomatic — retrosternal chest pain, cough, or dyspnea may be experienced. Large mediastinal adenopathy is an adverse prognostic factor.
- **[3] Systemic "B" symptoms: fever** (>100.4°F), **night sweats, weight loss** (>10% of body weight over 6 months) — **B symptoms indicate advanced disease. Pel-Ebstein fever — cyclical fever** that recurs at variable intervals of several days or weeks and lasts for 1-2 weeks before waning. B symptoms are due to cytokine release by Reed-Sternberg cells.
- [4] <u>Other presentations</u>: fatigue, pruritus, intra-abdominal disease — **hepatomegaly, splenomegaly.** Cholestatic liver disease. **Nephrotic syndrome,** Hypercalcemia.

DIAGNOSIS
- **Excisional whole lymph node biopsy: Reed-Sternberg cell pathognomonic — large cells with bi- or multilobed nuclei ("owl eye appearance") & inclusions in the nucleoli.** Reed-Sternberg cells are derived from an abnormal germinal B cell in the early stage of differentiation with **CD15 & CD30 positivity.** T lymphocytes are often observed surrounding the characteristic neoplastic cells.

MANAGEMENT
- **Early-stage disease (stage I or II): combination of chemotherapy (eg, ABVD "gold standard" chemotherapy) followed by radiation therapy. "ABVD": Adriamycin (Doxorubicin), Bleomycin, Vinblastine, Dacarbazine.** The amount of chemotherapy and radiation dose varies in patients with favorable and unfavorable prognosis disease. Chemotherapy alone is an acceptable alternative in patients at increased risk of complication from radiation therapy.
- **Advanced stage (III to IV): combination chemotherapy is the main treatment (ABVD).** Radiation therapy may be used for some as consolidation. "MOPP": Mustine, Oncovorin/Vincristine, Procarbazine, Prednisolone.
- <u>Refractory</u>: second-line High-dose chemotherapy not used in original treatment, followed by an Autologous stem cell transplant is the standard of care for the majority of patients who are refractory or relapse post-initial therapy.

<u>Prognosis</u>:
- **Hodgkin lymphoma has an excellent overall prognosis** (~80% cure rate) compared to Non-Hodgkin lymphoma.
- Lymphocyte-predominant = best prognosis. Lymphocyte-depleted = worst prognosis.

WORKUP
- Laboratory tests include CBC, complete metabolic panel, erythrocyte sedimentation rate, Hepatitis B virus, hepatitis C virus, and HIV. Testing for HIV is recommended as the treatment of the infection can improve outcomes in HIV positive individuals.
- LDH levels correlate with the bulk of disease. Elevated levels of alkaline phosphatase may suggest liver or bone involvement.
- **Imaging for staging: chest radiographs and combined whole-body PET/CT scan of chest, thorax, abdomen, and pelvis.**

STAGING NOMENCLATURE (ANN ARBOR)
Staging used for both Hodgkin & Non-Hodgkin lymphomas.
- **Stage I: involvement of single lymph node region** (I) or one extranodal site (IE)
- **Stage II: ≥2 lymph node involvement all on the same side of the diaphragm** or local extralymphatic extension plus one or more lymph node regions same side of the diaphragm (IIE).
- **Stage III:** lymph nodes or structures on **both sides of the diaphragm.**
- **Stage IV: involvement of an extra lymphatic organ.**
- Disease staging is further categorized as "A" if patients lack constitutional symptoms or as "B" if patients have 10% weight loss > 6 months, fever, or drenching night sweats.

Staging of lymphoma

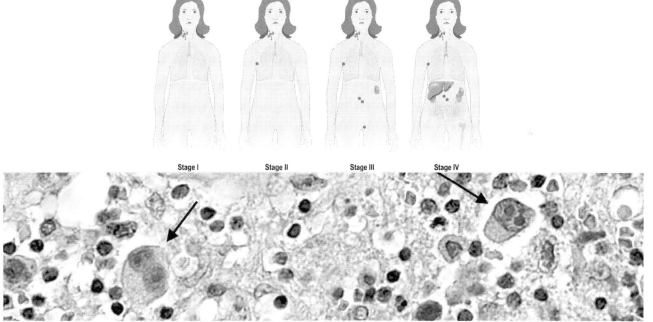

Reed-Sternberg cell pathognomonic of Hodgkin lymphoma – large cells with bi- or multilobed nuclei ("owl eye appearance") & inclusions in the nucleoli comprising the minority (1-10%) of the cellular population, admixed with a cellular environment of lymphocytes, eosinophils, histiocytes, neutrophils, plasma cells, fibroblasts, and collagen fibers. Reed-Sternberg (RS) cells are derived from an abnormal germinal B cell in the early stage of differentiation with CD15 & CD30 positivity.

- **EXAM TIP**
- Primary vs. Secondary erythrocytosis.
- **Primary erythrocytosis (PV): normal O2 saturation, decreased erythropoietin,** increased WBCs & platelets.
- **Secondary erythrocytosis (eg, hypoxemia): decreased O2 saturation, increased erythropoietin,** normal WBCs & platelets.

CHEMOTHERAPEUTIC AGENTS FOR CANCER

ALKYLATING AGENTS	
Cyclophosphamide Ifosfamide	• <u>Mechanism of action:</u> **inhibits DNA replication by alkylating DNA,** increasing programmed cell death. They require bioactivation by the liver. • <u>Indications:</u> leukemia, lymphoma, multiple myeloma, ovarian and breast cancer, rheumatoid arthritis, rapidly progressive glomerulonephritis. • <u>Adverse effects:</u> **hemorrhagic cystitis** (reduced by hydration, Mesna or N-acetylcysteine), GI mucosal damage (eg, nausea, vomiting, **stomatitis, diarrhea),** emesis, **alopecia**, myelosuppression, SIADH, **bladder cancer.**

PLATINUM AGENTS (Alkylating-like Agents)	
Cisplatin Carboplatin	<u>Mechanism of action:</u> • **Inhibits DNA synthesis similar to alkylating agents.** • The platinum atom binds to DNA and crosslinks DNA. This interferes with DNA synthesis & cellular metabolism, triggering cell death. <u>Indications:</u> • <u>Cisplatin:</u> advanced metastatic testicular, ovarian. and bladder cancers • <u>Carboplatin:</u> advanced ovarian cancer <u>Adverse reactions:</u> • **Neurotoxicity** – **ototoxicity (acoustic nerve damage** causes hearing loss usually bilateral & irreversible, tinnitus, vertigo), **peripheral neuropathy.** • **Nephrotoxicity** – Acute kidney injury may be reduced with hydration and Amifostine, a free radical scavenger. Cisplatin is most nephrotoxic. • **Highly emetogenic:** nausea, vomiting. Myelosuppression; Alopecia. • <u>Electrolyte disorders:</u> eg, Hypomagnesemia, Hypocalcemia. Monitor CBC.

ANTIMETABOLITES	
Methotrexate	• <u>Mechanism of action:</u> inhibits dihydrofolate reductase **(folic acid antagonist)** leading to decreased DNA and protein synthesis; inhibits lymphocyte proliferation. <u>Indications:</u> • <u>Chemotherapy:</u> non-Hodgkin lymphoma, trophoblastic tumors (eg, choriocarcinoma, hydatidiform mole), lung, breast, CNS, neck cancers, osteosarcoma. • <u>Inflammatory arthritis:</u> Rheumatoid arthritis, Psoriatic arthritis. • <u>Reproductive:</u> ectopic pregnancy and termination of pregnancy. <u>Adverse effects:</u> • **GI adverse effects most common** - **stomatitis,** nausea, vomiting, diarrhea. • **3 cardinal side effects** of Methotrexate involve the **liver, lung, & marrow: hepatitis, interstitial pneumonitis, & marrow suppression.** • **Leukopenia (prevented by administration of Leucovorin/Folinic acid).** • Neurotoxicity, thrombocytopenia, nephrotoxicity. <u>Drug interactions:</u> • **Penicillins may increase toxicity of Methotrexate** by decreasing elimination. • Aminoglycosides reduce GI absorption of Methotrexate. • Retinoids increase hepatotoxicity. • **Trimethoprim & sulfonamides increase hemotoxicity** (synergistic folate antagonism). • **Avoid NSAIDs with high-dose Methotrexate** (anti-neoplastic doses) due to increased toxicity from decreased renal excretion of Methotrexate. <u>Contraindications:</u> • **Pregnancy** (folic acid inhibition), **severe liver or renal disease.**

Fluorouracil (5-FU)	• Mechanism of action: antimetabolite - **pyrimidine analog** that inhibits RNA synthesis in cancer cells by uracil antagonism (uracil is essential for RNA synthesis). Inhibits thymidylate synthase, leading to decreased DNA and protein synthesis. Low emetogenic potential. Indications: • Topical: superficial basal cell cancer, actinic keratosis. • Metastatic colon and breast cancers, ovarian cancer, head or neck cancer. Adverse effects: • **GI** (eg, **nausea, vomiting, diarrhea**, anorexia, stomatitis) • Teratogenicity, **alopecia,** cardiotoxicity (eg, bradycardia, hypotension), ocular toxicity. • **Myelosuppression ("rescue" with Thymidine).** • Dermatitis & photosensitivity with topical.
Cytarabine	• Mechanism of action: inhibits DNA & RNA synthesis. • Indications: hematologic cancers (AML, ALL, blastic phase of CML), NHL. Poor activity vs. solid tumors. • Adverse effects: **CNS neurotoxicity** (cerebellar syndrome), myelosuppression, stomatitis, emetogenic, sloughing off of the skin on the palms & soles, **ocular toxicity, ototoxicity.**
Gemcitabine	• Mechanism of action: inhibits DNA synthesis. • Indications: advanced breast, ovarian, pancreatic & non-small cell lung cancers. • Adverse effects: emetogenic, hepatitis, myelosuppression.

MITOSIS INHIBITORS (TAXANES)

• Paclitaxel • Docetaxel	• Mechanism of action: **stabilizes microtubules, preventing mitosis and cell division** (prevent disassembly into tubulin monomers). Indications: • **Paclitaxel: advanced ovarian cancer (with Cisplatin),** advanced breast and non-small cell lung cancers. Second-line for Kaposi sarcoma. • Docetaxel: advanced & metastatic breast, prostate, gastric, squamous cell, head, neck, and non-small cell lung cancers. Adverse effects: • **Black box warning for hypersensitivity reactions and bone marrow suppression** (thrombocytopenia, neutropenia). • **Hypersensitivity reaction** (may need to pretreatment with Dexamethasone, Diphenhydramine and H2 blocker, such as Nizatidine, prior to infusion to reduce the incidence). **Immune-mediated pneumonitis.** • Alopecia, nausea, vomiting, mucositis, anorexia, brittle nails, change in taste, leukopenia, neutropenia, myalgia, weakness, and **peripheral neuropathy**. • **Hyaluronidase via the same IV line is the antidote for Paclitaxel toxicity due to extravasation.**

MITOSIS INHIBITORS

• **MOA:** destabilizes microtubules, preventing mitosis and cell division.

Vincristine Vinblastine	Indications: • Vincristine used for leukemia, Hodgkin lymphoma, non-Hodgkin lymphoma, solid tumors. Vinblastine used for lymphoma and testicular cancer. Adverse effects: • **Neurotoxicity most common side effect especially with Vincristine** (eg, **neuropathy such as foot drop,** cranial nerve palsies, demyelination, pain). • Myelosuppression, dermatologic (alopecia, rashes). • **Gastrointestinal: constipation,** nausea, vomiting, abdominal pain. • **Genitourinary:** eg, urinary retention, bladder dysfunction. • Oculotoxicity and hyperuricemia. • **If extravasation: stop drip, apply heat & local injection of Hyaluronidase.**

ANTHRACYCLINES

• Doxorubicin • Daunorubicin	**Mechanism of action:** • **Intercalating agents:** inhibit nucleic acid & protein synthesis by intercalating and binding with DNA. **Generate free radicals and inhibit topoisomerase-II** (antibiotics derived from *Streptomyces* fungus). Indications: • Hematologic malignancies: AML, ALL, Hodgkin lymphoma (the A in ABVD) • Solid tumors: endometrial, lung, breast, and ovarian cancer. Adverse effects: • **Cardiotoxicity: dilated cardiomyopathy, Myopericarditis.** • Gastrointestinal: nausea, vomiting, stomatitis. • Bone marrow suppression & alopecia. Monitoring: • **Echocardiogram or MUGA scan should be performed prior to initiation of therapy to document the ejection fraction.** **Prevention of cardiotoxicity** • **Dexrazoxane is a cardioprotective agent** against the toxic effects of anthracyclines used in select patients (prevents free radical formation).

OTHER AGENTS

• Bleomycin	**Mechanism of action:** • Glycopeptide antibiotic that affects the G2 phase of cell division, generates free radicals (oxidatively damages DNA), & inhibits DNA synthesis & replication, with lesser inhibition of protein and RNA synthesis. Indications: • **Hodgkin lymphoma** (the B in ABVD), non-Hodgkin lymphoma, squamous cell and testicular cancer. • Sclerosing agent for **pleurodesis in patients with malignant pleural effusions.** Adverse effects: • **Pulmonary toxicity: pulmonary fibrosis & pneumonitis** due to free radical production. Periodic chest imaging to assess for damage. • Dermatologic: alopecia, hyperpigmentation. • Raynaud phenomenon. • Myelosuppression not a significant side effect.
• Hydroxyurea	• **Mechanism of action: increases production of Hb F** (which does not sickle and has a higher affinity for oxygen), increases RBC water, **reduces RBC sickling**, alters RBC adhesion to the endothelium. Inhibits ribonucleotide reductase. • **Indications: mainstay of treatment** in SCD - **reduces the frequency and severity of pain episodes, decreases hospitalization rates and prolongs survival.** Because it takes weeks to months to take full effect, it is not used for acute episodes. • Uses: Sickle cell disease, Polycythemia vera, Essential thrombocythemia. • The combination of Hydroxyurea and L-glutamine can have additive benefits. • Adverse effects: myelosuppression, GI (anorexia, nausea). • **Contraindicated in pregnancy.**

R-CHOP Rituximab (antibody against CD20), Cyclophosphamide, Hydroxydaunorubicin, Oncovin/Vincristine, Prednisone. Used in non-Hodgkin lymphoma.

ABVD Adriamycin (Doxorubicin), Bleomycin, Vinblastine, Dacarbazine. Used in Hodgkin lymphoma

MOPP Mustargen, Oncovin, Procarbazine, Prednisone. Older regimen for Hodgkin lymphoma

GENERAL CHEMOTOXICITIES

Gastrointestinal
- **Nausea/Vomiting:** Doxorubicin, Cytarabine, Cyclophosphamide, Methotrexate, Cisplatin.
- **Mucositis:** 5FU, Methotrexate.

Cardiovascular
- **Anthracyclines (eg, Doxorubicin) cause dilated cardiomyopathy.**

Pulmonary: Bleomycin (fibrosis), Methotrexate.
Neurologic: Vincristine, Methotrexate, Cytarabine, Cisplatin.
Renal: high-dose Methotrexate, Cisplatin (renal failure), Cyclophosphamide (bladder cancer & hemorrhagic cystitis)

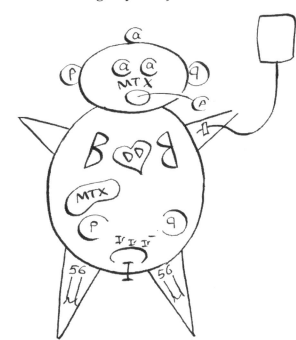

Ca = Cytarabine
- CNS toxicity, Ototoxicity

Cp = Cisplatin
- ototoxicity, highly emetogenic, renal failure

B = Bleomycin (pulmonary fibrosis)
MTX = Methotrexate
- Stomatitis, hepatotoxic,

D – Daunorubicin, Doxorubicin
- Dilated cardiomyopathy

C I = Cyclophosphamide, Ifosfamide
- Hemorrhagic cystitis

Irinotecan = acute & delayed diarrhea
Bone marrow toxicity:
5 = 5-FU; 6 = 6-Mercaptopurine, M = methotrexate
V of the arms & legs = Vincristine for peripheral neuropathy.

TUMOR MARKERS

TUMOR MARKER	MAIN ASSOCIATIONS
ALPHA FETOPROTEIN	• **Hepatocellular carcinoma** • **Nonseminomatous germ cell testicular cancer** • Decreased in Down syndrome "AFP is down in Down syndrome"
Beta-hCG	• **Nonseminomatous germ cell testicular cancer** • **Choriocarcinoma**, Teratomas • **Trophoblastic tumors** (eg, Hydatidiform molar pregnancy)
CA-125	• **Ovarian cancer**
CA 19-9	• **Pancreatic cancer** • GI – colorectal, esophageal, & hepatocellular cancers
CALCITONIN	• **Medullary thyroid cancer**
CEA	• **Colorectal cancer** • Medullary thyroid, pancreatic, gastric, lung, & breast cancers
PROSTATE SPECIFIC ANTIGEN	• **Prostate cancer** • Can also be elevated in BPH & Prostatitis

TRANSFUSION REACTION

- **Adverse events associated with the transfusion of whole blood or one of its components.**

[1] MILD ALLERGIC

- **Urticaria (hives) & or pruritus, without other allergic reaction symptoms hallmark.**
- <u>Mechanism</u>: Due to hypersensitivity leading to an antigen-antibody reaction to a foreign serum protein in the donor product.
- <u>Clinical manifestations</u>: **urticaria &/or pruritus within minutes of the transfusion.**

[2] ANAPHYLACTIC REACTION

- **<u>Type 1 hypersensitivity</u>: any other allergic reaction other than hives** (eg, angioedema, wheezing, pruritus, and/or hypotension, and can evolve into respiratory compromise and shock).
- **May start immediately (within seconds to minutes to 2-3 hours after initiation of transfusion).**

<u>Mechanism of reaction:</u>

- **<u>Allergic reaction due to IgE</u> antibodies in the recipient's blood due to <u>antigens in the donor plasma (eg, IgA)</u>.** IgE releases inflammatory mediators (histamine & tryptase from mast cells.

<u>Epidemiology:</u>

- **Commonly seen in <u>IgA-deficient individuals</u>** who make or have preformed IgA alloantibodies that react to the IgA in the transfused product (most transfused blood contains IgA antibodies). May have a history of recurrent respiratory & GI infections (hallmark of selective IgA deficiency).

<u>Clinical presentation:</u>

- **Rapid onset (within seconds to minutes to 2-3 hours) of any allergic reaction other than Hives (eg, angioedema, wheezing, stridor, pruritus, &/or hypotension);** can evolve into respiratory compromise and shock. Dyspnea, hypoxemia, and an abnormal lung examination.

<u>Management:</u>

- **[1] stopping the transfusion immediately, [2] <u>intramuscular Epinephrine</u> should be given** (0.01 mg/kg; maximum 0.5 mg), **[3] an H1-antihistamine (eg, oral Loratadine or oral Cetirizine 10 mg orally, or Diphenhydramine 25-50 mg oral or IV), and [4] Oxygen.** Corticosteroids may also be given. Vasopressors if severe.
- For severe bronchospasm, inhaled bronchodilators, continuous positive airway pressure (CPAP), and/or an H2-antihistamine (eg, Famotidine) may be needed.

<u>Prevention:</u>

- **Using washed blood products (removes IgA antibodies) can prevent this reaction in patients with selective IgA deficiency** because washing the blood removes the potentially harmful plasma proteins.

[3] FEBRILE NON-HEMOLYTIC

<u>Mechanism:</u>

- **<u>Cytokine release</u> — Most commonly due to inflammatory cytokines released from blood donor leukocytes in products that have not been leukoreduced.** May also be due to type 2 antibodies of the recipient blood targeting HLA antigens of the recipient's blood.
- There is no hemolysis and is mainly characterized by **fever following a transfusion.**
- Most commonly seen in children.

<u>Clinical presentation:</u>

- **Characterized by fever, chills, headache, & flushing in the absence of other systemic symptoms 1-6 hours after transfusion initiation.**
- Diagnosis of exclusion after the other causes of transfusion reaction have been ruled out.

<u>Management:</u>

- **The transfusion should be stopped, and antipyretics should be administered.**

<u>Prevention:</u>

- **Leukoreduced blood donor products.**

[4] TRANSFUSION-ASSOCIATED CIRCULATORY OVERLOAD (TACO)

- <u>Pulmonary edema</u> **due to volume overload from the transfusion: excess volume or circulatory overload** in patients who receive large volume of a transfused product over a short duration.
- **Often in the setting of <u>preexisting positive fluid balance</u> (eg, Heart failure**, cardiovascular disease, Chronic kidney disease, receiving large amounts of fluid prior to the transfusion).

Clinical presentation:
- **TACO should be suspected in a patient who develops <u>respiratory distress, hypoxia</u>, or <u>hypertension</u>* while receiving a transfusion or within 12 hours post-transfusion**.
- <u>**Cardiogenic pulmonary edema & cardiogenic shock:**</u> ≥3 of the following: **[1] respiratory distress (acute or worsening dyspnea, orthopnea, tachypnea), [2] evidence of pulmonary edema on examination or radiographs, [3] elevated brain natriuretic protein (BNP)** or [4] **elevated central venous pressure**. Less commonly associated with fever compared to TRALI.

Findings:
- **<u>Hypoxia, tachycardia, &/or Hypertension</u>** (due to hypervolemia & volume overload), tachycardia, a wide pulse pressure, and/or jugular venous distension. **S3 gallop**; lung examination often reveals rales and/or wheezing. TACO does not cause fever, hives, or angioedema.

Management:
- **Once the diagnosis is strongly suspected, the transfusion should be stopped + treatment of TACO is similar to treatment of Cardiogenic pulmonary edema from other causes: [1] fluid mobilization (<u>diuresis</u> with diuretics, such as Furosemide) & [2] supplementary oxygen**.
- Ventilatory support is rarely needed; Noninvasive positive pressure ventilation may be helpful if severe respiratory compromise; intubation may be required if NPPV is unsuccessful.

[5] TRANSFUSION-RELATED ACUTE LUNG INJURY (TRALI)

- **<u>Life-threatening form of acute lung injury (pulmonary edema)</u> when the recipient neutrophils are activated by the antigens & anti-leukocyte antibodies in the transfused donor product in an appropriately primed pulmonary vasculature** (the transfused product having either anti-leukocyte (HLA) or anti-neutrophil antibodies). **#1 cause of transfusion related deaths**.

Mechanism:
- 2 hit model: [1] first hit occurs before the transfusion when a stressor (eg, sepsis, shock, recent infection, recent surgery, inflammation, or trauma) causes neutrophils in the pulmonary vasculature to become recruited, primed, and sequestered in the pulmonary vasculature. [2] The second hit is the transfusion, where antibodies and bioactive lipids stored in blood products activate the primed neutrophils activate an inflammatory reaction (eg, cytokines, oxidases, and reactive oxygen species).
- **The recipient's immune system responds and causes the release of mediators that increase capillary permeability, leading to leakage of protein & fluid, resulting in <u>Noncardiogenic pulmonary edema (similar to ARDS)</u>.**

Clinical presentation:
- **TRALI presents with fever, chills, <u>Acute respiratory distress</u> (dyspnea, tachypnea, hypoxia), <u>hypotension</u>* within minutes to 6 hours after transfusion, and a new infiltrate on chest radiography** (similar to ARDS).
- TRALI presents very similarly to ARDS with signs of respiratory failure and **transient diffuse infiltrates (whiting out of the lungs) on radiography**. Transient leukopenia, thrombocytopenia, and normal pulmonary artery occlusion pressure due to noncardiogenic pulmonary edema.
- TRALI more often associated with hypotension and a normal pulmonary artery wedge pressure.

Management
- **Largely supportive and may include supplemental oxygen, intubation, mechanical ventilation, and vasopressor support**.

TACO vs TRALI

- **TACO is more often characterized by hypertension, TRALI is often associated with hypotension**.
- TACO symptoms are more often responsive to diuresis & associated with elevated BNP.
- TRALI is more often accompanied by fever; fever is not a classic feature of TACO.

[6] ACUTE HEMOLYTIC TRANSFUSION REACTIONS

- **Acute hemolytic transfusion reactions** can result in intravascular (or extravascular) hemolysis of transfused red cells, depending on the specific etiology.
- **Type 2 hypersensitivity: Immune-mediated reactions are often a result of preformed antibodies in the recipient to blood donor antigens (eg, ABO incompatibility due to clerical error causing transfusion of the wrong product) and attacks the donor cells (intravascular hemolysis of transfused RBCs).** Non-immune reactions are possible and occur when red blood cells are damaged before transfusion (eg, by heat or incorrect osmotic conditions).

Clinical presentation:

The entire "classic triad" of [1] fever, [2] flank pain, and [3] red urine (uncommon).

- **Presenting symptoms include fever, chills, rigors; flank, back or chest pain; hemoglobinuria (pink/red urine), tachycardia, tachypnea, hematuria, oliguria (Acute kidney injury), hypotension, or evidence of DIC (eg, epistaxis or oozing from IV sites) occurring during or within 24 hours of transfusion initiation.** May develop jaundice due to hemolysis.

Laboratory evaluation:

- **May show hemolysis** — schistocytes, increased indirect bilirubin, increased lactate dehydrogenase (LDH), decreased haptoglobin, decreased fibrinogen, plasma discoloration from free hemoglobin, spherocytes on the peripheral blood smear. **UA: hemoglobinuria.**
- **An acute hemolytic transfusion reaction can be diagnosed by a positive direct antiglobulin (Coombs) test and plasma free hemoglobin level >25 mg/dL.**
- A repeat type and crossmatch will show a mismatch.

Management:

- **[1] stop the transfusion, [2] hemodynamic support (eg, aggressive hydration with Normal saline),** and [3] contact the transfusion service.
- Assess for complications — rapid intravascular hemolysis can be associated with Acute kidney injury, hypotension (hemodynamic collapse), and Disseminated intravascular coagulation (DIC).

[7] TRANSFUSION-ASSOCIATED SEPSIS

- **Contaminated donor blood by bacteria or bacterial byproducts (eg, endotoxin).**
- Clinical presentation: initial findings may include fever, chills, rigors, and hypotension.
- Management includes broad-spectrum antibiotics and hemodynamic support.

- Fever/chills suggest an AHTR, septic transfusion reaction, transfusion-related acute lung injury (TRALI), or FNHTR.
- Respiratory symptoms characterize TACO, TRALI, and anaphylaxis.
- A significant drop in systolic blood pressure (by >30 mmHg) is characteristic of AHTR, TRALI, and sepsis.

ANTICOAGULANTS

UNFRACTIONATED HEPARIN (UFH)

- Large, sulfated polysaccharide polymer obtained from animal sources. Molecules of varying size (15,000–20,000).
- Heparin is highly acidic and can be neutralized by basic molecules (eg, Protamine).
- Heparin is given intravenously or subcutaneously to avoid the risk of hematoma associated with intramuscular injection.

Mechanism of action:
- **Indirect thrombin inhibitor: complexes with & potentiates antithrombin III.** By thrombin inactivation, prevents conversion of fibrinogen → fibrin. (Intrinsic pathway), indirectly inactivates both factors IIa (thrombin) & factor Xa. Because it acts on preformed blood components, heparin provides anticoagulation immediately.
- Heparins bind indirectly only to soluble thrombin (not thrombin enmeshed within developing clots).

Monitoring:
- **The action of Heparin is monitored with the activated partial thromboplastin time (aPTT) laboratory test.**

LOW MOLECULAR WEIGHT HEPARINS (LMWH)

Enoxaparin, Dalteparin, Tinzaparin, and Fondaparinux

Mechanism of action:
- **Binds & potentiates antithrombin III; works more on factor Xa than thrombin (Factor IIa);** more selective action on Xa than UFH (the short chain LMW heparin–ATIII and fondaparinux–ATIII complexes provide a more selective action).

Pharmacokinetics:
- **Subcutaneous injection.** Duration of action ~12 hours.
- **Compliant, low-risk patients can be discharged home during bridging therapy.**
- **No need to monitor PTT** (weight based – more predictable dosing).
- **Protamine Sulfate is the antidote** (not as effective as it is for UFH).
- **Lower risk of HIT:** higher anti Xa-IIa ratio means less potential binding with platelets.

Indications:
- Similar to Unfractionated Heparin.
- **Pregnancy: Because it does not cross the placental barrier, Low molecular weight heparin is the drug of choice when an anticoagulant must be used in pregnancy.**
- **Malignancy: LMWH preferred anticoagulant of choice for malignancy.**
- LMW heparins and Fondaparinux have similar clinical applications.

Contraindications:
- **Renal failure** (Cr >2.0) because LMWH excreted by kidneys. **Thrombocytopenia.**

FONDAPARINUX

- Small synthetic drug that contains the biologically active pentasaccharide present in unfractionated and LMW heparins. **Administered subcutaneously once daily.**

ADVERSE EFFECTS OF HEPARINS
- **Increased bleeding: is the most common adverse effect of heparin** and related molecules; the bleeding may result in hemorrhagic stroke. **Antidote for bleeding: Protamine sulfate** can lessen the risk of serious bleeding that can result from excessive unfractionated heparin. Protamine only partially reverses the effects of LMW heparins and does not affect the action of fondaparinux.
- Metabolic effects with prolonged use: Prolonged use of unfractionated heparin is associated with Osteoporosis.
- **Thrombocytopenia:** UFH causes moderate transient thrombocytopenia in many patients (Type I). UFH may cause severe thrombocytopenia + thrombosis (heparin induced thrombocytopenia, type II HIT) in a small percentage of patients who produce an antibody that binds to a complex of heparin and platelet factor 4. **LMW heparins and Fondaparinux are less likely to cause HIT.**

DIRECT THROMBIN INHIBITOR
Bivalirudin, Argatroban, Desirudin. <u>Oral</u>: Dabigatran

<u>Mechanism of action:</u>
- **Unlike the heparins, Direct thrombin inhibitors inhibit both soluble thrombin and the thrombin enmeshed within developing clots.** Bivalirudin also inhibits platelet activation.

<u>Clinical use:</u>
- **Heparin-induced thrombocytopenia (HIT)**: Parenteral Direct thrombin inhibitors are used as alternatives to heparin primarily in patients with Heparin induced thrombocytopenia.
- Bivalirudin is also used in combination with Aspirin during percutaneous coronary angioplasty.
- Like Unfractionated heparin, the action of these drugs can be monitored with the aPTT.

<u>Advantages of oral Direct thrombin inhibitors include:</u>
- predictable pharmacokinetics, which allows for fixed dosing.
- predictable immediate anticoagulant response (no need for routine monitoring) or overlap with other anticoagulants unnecessary.
- these agents do not interact with P450 interacting drugs.
- Dabigatran (by mouth) is approved for most indications of oral anticoagulation, including prevention of stroke and systemic embolism in nonvalvular atrial fibrillation & prophylaxis of venous thromboembolism (VTE) following hip or knee replacement surgery.

<u>Toxicity & reversal</u>
- <u>Bleeding</u>: Like other anticoagulants, the direct thrombin inhibitors can cause bleeding.
- **<u>Reversal agent</u>: Idarucizumab is a humanized monoclonal antibody Fab fragment that binds to Dabigatran and reverses the anticoagulant effect.**

FACTOR XA INHIBITORS
<u>Oral Xa inhibitors</u>: Rivaroxaban, Apixaban, Edoxaban, Betrixaban

<u>Mechanism and effects:</u>
- **These small molecules directly bind to and inhibit both free factor Xa (10a) and factor Xa (10a) bound in the clotting complex.**
- These drugs are given as fixed oral doses and do not require monitoring.

<u>Indications:</u>
- Rivaroxaban is approved for prevention and treatment of venous thromboembolism following hip or knee surgery and for prevention of stroke in patients with atrial fibrillation, without valvular heart disease.
- Apixaban is approved for prevention of embolic stroke in patients with nonvalvular atrial fibrillation.

<u>Toxicity & reversal:</u>
- Bleeding.
- **<u>Reversal agent</u>: Andexanet alfa is a modified recombinant inactive form of human factor Xa developed for reversal of factor Xa inhibitors.**

<u>Direct Oral Anticoagulants versus Warfarin:</u>
Compared to Warfarin, the direct oral anticoagulants (dabigatran, rivaroxaban) have consistently shown:
- equivalent antithrombotic efficacy
- lower bleeding rates when compared with warfarin.
- lack of need for monitoring
- fewer drug interactions

The new direct oral anticoagulants have replaced warfarin for many indications (except in Antiphospholipid syndrome).

VITAMIN K ANTAGONIST [WARFARIN (COUMADIN)]

- **Warfarin inhibit vitamins K epoxide reductase (VKOR), which normally converts vitamin K epoxide to reduced vitamin K.** The vitamin K-dependent factors include
  - **(1) Procoagulants: Thrombin [2a (IIa)] and factors VII (7), IX (9), X (10), and**
  - **(2) Anticoagulants: protein C and protein S.**
- Warfarin elimination depends on metabolism by cytochrome P450 enzymes.
- Monitoring: **The effect of Warfarin is monitored by the prothrombin time (PT) and INR.**

Clinical uses:

- Chronic anticoagulation in all of the clinical situations for heparin, except in pregnant women.
- **Warfarin: drug of choice for anticoagulation in Antiphospholipid syndrome if not pregnant.**

Toxicity

- **Bleeding** is the most important adverse effect of warfarin.
- **Early in therapy, a period of hypercoagulability** with subsequent dermal vascular necrosis can occur. This is due to deficiency of protein C, an endogenous vitamin K dependent anticoagulant with a short half-life. **Warfarin is often "bridged" by Heparin during this time.**
- **Teratogenicity**: Warfarin can cause bone defects and hemorrhage in the developing fetus and, therefore, is **contraindicated in pregnancy.**
- Narrow therapeutic window, its **involvement in drug interactions is of major concern.**

Drug interactions:

- **Cytochrome P450-inducing drugs** (eg, carbamazepine, phenytoin, rifampin, barbiturates) increase warfarin's clearance and **reduce the anticoagulant effect of a given dose.**
- **Cytochrome P450 inhibitors** (eg, amiodarone, selective serotonin reuptake inhibitors, cimetidine) reduce warfarin's clearance and **increase the anticoagulant effect of a given dose.**

WARFARIN SUPRATHERAPEUTIC LEVELS:

Patients with coagulopathy without bleeding:

- **INR <4.5 in a patient with no bleeding: observation and serial monitoring.** Hold Warfarin.
- **INR 4.5-10 without bleeding: Hold Warfarin** (eg, 1 or 2 doses), **with or without administration of a small dose of oral Vitamin K (1-2.5 mg).** oral Vitamin K administration reduces risk of anaphylaxis with IV vitamin K administration. Activity modification to avoid trauma.
- **INR >10 without bleeding: Hold Warfarin** until the INR falls into the therapeutic range. **Vitamin K oral dose 2.5-5 mg,** depending on the bleeding risk of the patient.

Patients with coagulopathy and active bleeding:

- **Minor bleeding (eg, epistaxis, bruising) administer vitamin K$_1$ orally** (eg, 2.5 mg orally) and hold the next dose of Warfarin. Alternatively, the patient could be instructed to hold Warfarin until the INR was rechecked and found to be in the therapeutic range.
- **INR ≥5 but ≤10:** omit 1 or 2 doses, monitor, and resume Warfarin when in therapeutic range. Another option is to omit the dose and administer oral vitamin K ≤5 mg orally if patient is at increased risk for bleeding. Oral Vitamin K can also be given if rapid reversal needed for surgery (reduction often occurs within 24 hours).
- **INR >10 + bleeding that is not significant: Hold Warfarin & administer higher dose of Vitamin K (2.5-5 mg orally)** which will reduce the INR significant within 24-48 hours. Resume therapy at lower dose when INR is therapeutic.
- **Serious bleeding + any elevation of INR: Hold Warfarin +** administer a 4-factor protein complex concentrate (PCC) [PCC contains **factors II, VII, IX, and X and activated proteins C and S; most effective for reversal] + administer Vitamin K slow IV infusion.**
- **Life threatening bleed:** [1] hold Warfarin, [2] **administer a 4-factor protein complex concentrate (PCC); if a PCC is not available, a plasma product such as Fresh Frozen Plasma (FFP), Thawed Plasma, or recombinant Factor VIIa should be given, and [3] administer intravenous vitamin K (10 mg slow IV infusion).** IV vitamin K$_1$ does **not** have an immediate effect on restoring normal coagulation. Patients with major bleeding warrant hospitalization and bed rest until their coagulopathy is controlled. Repeat INR as needed.

PHOTO CREDITS

CHAPTER 15 – PEDIATRIC PEARLS

CHAPTER 15 – PEDIATRIC PEARLS

ERYTHEMA TOXICUM NEONATORUM

- **Benign self-limited pustular disorder thought to be due to immune system activation seen in neonates in the first 72 hours of life.** More common in neonates with higher birthweight & greater gestational age.

CLINICAL MANIFESTATIONS
- **Small erythematous macules &/or papules (1-3 mm in diameter)** ⇨ **pustules on an erythematous base. Most common on the face, trunk, and proximal extremities.** Does not involve the palms or soles.
- They rash may be present at birth but typically appear within 24-48 hours.

DIAGNOSIS
- Clinical based on appearance. May be confirmed by microscopic examination of a Wright-stained smear of the contents of a pustule that demonstrates numerous eosinophils & occasional neutrophils.

MANAGEMENT
- Self-limited so no treatment is necessary. The rash usually resolves in 5-7 days, although it may wax and wane before full resolution.

MILIARIA (HEAT RASH)

- **Transient skin disorder due to blockage of the eccrine sweat ducts** (especially in hot, moist, and humid conditions). This leads to sweat into the epidermis & dermis.
- Increased counts of skin flora (*S. epidermis, S. aureus*).
- **Most common in neonates** (especially in 1-week-old neonates) and in hot environments.
- Most common on the trunk and intertriginous areas.

PATHOPHYSIOLOGY
- Occlusive clothing, fever while bedridden, and medications that promote sweat from the sweat glands (eg, Beta blockers, Opioids) may increase the risk.
- Plugging of the ostia of sweat ducts occurs, with ultimate rupture of the sweat duct, resulting in an irritating, stinging reaction.

TYPES
- Miliaria crystallina: tiny, friable clear vesicles form at the orifices of eccrine sweat ducts (due to sweat in the superficial stratum corneum). Most common in neonates.
- Miliaria rubra: most common form of Miliaria. Characterized by severely pruritic erythematous nonfollicular papules most common on the upper trunk. Deeper in the epidermis.
- Miliaria profunda: flesh-colored papules due to sweating in the papillary dermis (blockage deep within the duct). When damage to the sweat gland from miliaria profunda or miliaria rubra is severe, anhidrosis may develop in affected areas resulting in hyperthermia and heat exhaustion.

MANAGEMENT
- Management of Miliaria is based on reducing exposure to factors that stimulate sweating and blockage of eccrine sweat glands — wearing breathable clothing (eg, cotton), placement in a cooler, drier environment, avoidance of the use of occlusive material & antipyretics for fever.

MILIA

- Skin eruption due to keratin retention & sebaceous material in the pilosebaceous follicles within the dermis of immature skin.
- 1-2mm pearly white-yellow papules especially seen on the cheeks, forehead, chin, & nose.

MANAGEMENT
- None. Usually disappears by the first month of life (may be seen up to 3 months).

CAFÉ AU LAIT MACULES (CALM)

- **Uniformly pigmented (tan to dark brown) oval flat macules or patches with sharp demarcation a few millimeters to >15 cm in size.** They enlarge in proportion to the growth of the child.
- That may be present at birth or appear during early childhood, frequently initially. May be more noticeable following sun exposure.

PATHOPHYSIOLOGY
- Due to increased number of melanocytes and melanin within the dermis.

ASSOCIATIONS
- **Neurofibromatosis I** — ≥6 CALM (≥1.5 cm in adults & ≥0.5 cm in prepubertal children), **especially if associated with axillary or inguinal freckling)**
- Tuberous sclerosis
- McCune-Albright syndrome (a large, unilateral Café au lait macule). Bloom syndrome, Fanconi anemia.

MANAGEMENT
- They do not need to be treated but if treatment is desired, pigment-specific laser therapy is used.

PORT-WINE STAINS (CAPILLARY MALFORMATION, NEVUS FLAMMEUS)

- Capillary malformation of the skin due to superficial dilated dermal capillaries and postcapillary venules that are present at birth.
- May be part of malformation syndromes (eg, Sturge-Weber or Klippel Trenaunay syndrome).

CLINICAL MANIFESTATIONS
- Sharply demarcated, blanchable, pink to red macules or papules in infancy. **Over time, they grow & darken to a purple (port wine) color and may develop a thickened surface (nodularity) in adulthood.**
- Most commonly occurring on the face and may follow the distribution of the trigeminal nerve branches but can occur anywhere.

MANAGEMENT
- **Pulse dye laser if treatment is required** (best used in infancy for best outcomes).

STURGE-WEBER SYNDROME
- Congenital disorder associated with the triad of **[1] Facial port wine stains** (especially along the trigeminal nerve distribution area — forehead, cheeks), **[2] Leptomeningeal angiomatosis** & **[3] Ocular involvement** (eg, glaucoma).
- May develop hemiparesis contralateral to the facial lesion, seizures, intracranial calcification, or learning disabilities.

CONGENITAL DERMAL MELANOCYTOSIS (MONGOLIAN SPOTS)

- Congenital dermal melanocytosis due to mid-dermal melanocytes that fail to migrate to the epidermis from the neural crest.
- May be seen in >80% of Asians & East Indian infants. Increased in Hispanic and Black infants.

CLINICAL MANIFESTATIONS
- **Circumscribed blue or slate grey pigmented macules & patches with indefinite borders most commonly seen in the presacral, sacral-gluteal areas** but also can be seen on the shoulders, legs, back, posterior thighs, arms, abdomen, and thorax. May be solitary or multiple.

MANAGEMENT
- Usually fades over time in the first few years of life.

NEVUS SIMPLEX (STORK BITE, MACULAR STAIN, NEVUS FLAMMEUS NUCHAE)

- **Areas of surface capillary dilation.**

CLINICAL MANIFESTATIONS
- **Single or multiple blanchable pink red, irregularly shaped macular patches most commonly seen on the midline of the nape of the neck, eyelids, and forehead (glabella) of infants.**

MANAGEMENT
- <u>Observation:</u> most will fade & resolve spontaneously by age 2 and don't usually darken over time.
- Laser therapy can be used to reduce the appearance of persistent lesions.

STAPHYLOCOCCAL SCALDED SKIN SYNDROME (RITTER DISEASE)

- **Superficial skin blistering condition due to dissemination of *Staphylococcus aureus* exfoliative epidermolytic exotoxins A and B (especially *S. aureus* strains 71 & 55).**

EPIDEMIOLOGY
- **Most common in infants** (3-7 days of age) or young children <5 years of age.
- In adults, it often occurs in the setting of renal impairment, immunosuppression, or other comorbidities that decrease the immune response to bacterial infection.

PATHOPHYSIOLOGY
- Toxins cleave desmoglein-1, which breaks down desmosomes, resulting in detachment within epidermal layers. This results in the formation of flaccid, fragile bullae, & skin fragility.

CLINICAL MANIFESTATIONS
- **Erythema phase: fever, irritability, skin tenderness followed by rapidly progressive extensive cutaneous blanching erythema [erythroderma (often beginning at the mouth)** or intertriginous areas before becoming diffuse]. The erythema is worse in the flexor areas and around orifices.
- **Bullae phase: flaccid sterile blisters & bullae & erosions** occur about 1-2 days after the erythema, especially in areas of mechanical stress (eg, flexural areas, buttocks, hands, and feet). **Positive Nikolsky sign (gentle pressure applied to skin causes separation of the dermis and blister rupture).** Sheet-like desquamation. Patients also often develop thick crusting and radial fissuring around the mouth, nose, and eyes, as well as skin pain, fever, irritability, and poor feeding
- **Desquamative phase:** sheet-like skin desquamation that easily ruptures, leaving moist, denuded skin before healing. May develop thick crusting and fissuring around the orifices.
- Conjunctivitis may be seen but mucous membranes involvement is not involved.

DIAGNOSIS
- Clinical diagnosis. Cultures from blood or nasopharynx. Blisters are sterile.
- <u>Skin biopsy:</u> if diagnosis remains uncertain — splitting of the lower stratum granulosum layer.

MANAGEMENT
- The initial management of SSSS usually involves (1) hospitalization of the patient, (2) intravenous antibiotic therapy, and (3) supportive measures.
- <u>Antibiotics:</u> **IV Penicillinase-resistant Penicillins (eg, Nafcillin, Oxacillin).** May add Clindamycin. **Vancomycin if MRSA suspected or Penicillin allergy. Cephalosporins** are also alternatives.
- <u>Supportive care:</u> maintain the skin clean and moist, emollients to improve barrier function, fluid & electrolyte replacement.

<u>Prognosis:</u>
- With appropriate management, SSSS usually resolve completely within 2-3 weeks without long-term sequelae. Potential complications include secondary infection, hypovolemia, electrolyte imbalances, sepsis, and rarely death. Recurrence of SSSS is rare.

TURNER'S SYNDROME

- **Group of X chromosome abnormalities characterized by loss of part of, all of, or nonfunctional X sex chromosome.** Most common sex chromosomal abnormality in females.
- **TS results from the absence of one complete set of genes located on the X chromosome or a nonfunctioning X chromosome due to mosaicism (67-90%) – 50% of cells have a combination of X monosomy (45, XO** due to missing X chromosome), some cells are normal (46, XX), cells with partial monosomies (X/abnormal X), or cells with a Y chromosome (46, XY). Most aren't inherited.

CLINICAL MANIFESTATIONS

- <u>**Hypogonadism:**</u> 45, XO leads to **gonadal dysgenesis (rudimentary fibrosed streaked ovaries) that can cause early ovarian failure** (primary amenorrhea in 80% or early secondary amenorrhea), delayed secondary sex characteristics (eg, **absence of breasts**), **infertility.** Growth failure.
- <u>Physical examination:</u> **short stature, webbed neck,** prominent ears, low posterior headline, **broad chest with widely spaced nipples "shield chest",** short fourth metacarpals and metatarsals, narrow, high-arched palate, nail dysplasia, congenital lymphedema of the hands & feet in neonates.
- <u>**Cardiovascular:**</u> **coarctation of the aorta (30%), bicuspid aortic valve (30%),** mitral valve prolapse, aortic dissection, & hypertension.
- <u>Renal:</u> congenital abnormalities (eg, horseshoe kidney), hydronephrosis, & other malformations.
- <u>Endocrine:</u> **Osteoporosis** & fractures, hypothyroidism, Diabetes mellitus, obesity, dyslipidemias.
- <u>GI:</u> telangiectasias (may cause GI bleeding), inflammatory bowel disease, colon cancer, liver disease.

DIAGNOSIS

- <u>**Karyotype analysis**</u> — **definitive diagnosis. 45, XO mosaicism or X chromosomal abnormalities.**
- <u>**Primary hypogonadism:**</u> **low estrogen + high FSH and LH.**

MANAGEMENT

- Recombinant human growth hormone replacement (may increase final height).
- Estradiol-progestin replacement therapy should start if no breast development occurs at around 11-12 years of age to cause pubertal development.

KLINEFELTER SYNDROME (47,XXY)

- **Genetic disorder seen in males with an extra, inactive X chromosome (<u>47,XXY</u>)** karyotype (90%).
- Extra sex chromosome due to failure of separation of sex chromosome or translocation.
- Most common chromosomal abnormality associated with hypogonadism.

CLINICAL MANIFESTATIONS

- Normal appearance before puberty onset but may have hypospadias or micropenis in infancy.
- **Delayed puberty, followed by tall stature (thin & long-limbed with Eunuchoid features).** Scoliosis, ataxia, mild developmental delays, & expressive language-based issues.
- <u>**Primary hypogonadism:**</u> <u>**small testes, gynecomastia,**</u> infertility (azoospermia), scarce body hair (eg, pubic & axillary hair), female hair distribution, decreased libido, weaker muscle.
- <u>**Adulthood:**</u> **Obesity in adulthood.** Increased risk of Testicular cancer, Breast cancer, Extragonadal germ cell tumors and non-Hodgkin lymphoma.

DIAGNOSIS

- <u>**Prenatal or postnatal karyotyping**</u> definitive diagnosis — **47,XXY** or chromosomal microarray.
- <u>Labs:</u> **Primary gonadal failure — low or low-normal serum testosterone + increased FSH & LH** (FSH usually predominates over LH). Increased estradiol (due to loss of inhibition).

MANAGEMENT

- <u>Supplemental testosterone</u> may help with secondary sex characteristic of pubertal boys & adult men.

FRAGILE X SYNDROME

- **X-linked dominant genetic disorder associated with the loss of function of the fragile X mental retardation gene (FMR1).**
- **Most common gene-related cause of intellectual disability & Autism spectrum disorder.**
- <u>Pathophysiology:</u> loss of function of the fragile X mental retardation gene leads to lack of production of the fragile X mental retardation protein.

CLINICAL MANIFESTATIONS

- <u>Younger males:</u> strabismus, midface hypoplasia, arched palate, hyperextensible joints, hypotonia, soft skin, and flexible, flat feet, macrocephaly, and mitral valve prolapse.
- <u>Older males:</u> **long & narrow face, prominent forehead & chin, <u>large ears, macro-orchidism</u> (enlarged testicles)**, flapping hands. Frequent bouts of otitis media and sinusitis are often present.
- <u>Behavioral:</u> **expressive language deficits** [eg, delayed speech, poor expressive language skills) > receptive]. **Mild to moderate intellectual disability.** Hyperactivity, seizures.
- Females with the full mutation usually have milder features than males. 50% have normal cognition.

DIAGNOSIS

- <u>Genetic studies:</u> X chromosome in the q27 regions have an expanding repeating CGG segment

DOWN SYNDROME (TRISOMY 21)

- Genetic disorder due to 3 copies of chromosome 21 (**Trisomy 21**) or 3 copies of a region of the long arm of chromosome 21.
- **Most common chromosomal disorder and cause of mental developmental disability.**

CLINICAL MANIFESTATIONS

- <u>Head and neck:</u> low-set small ears, flat facial profile, flat nasal bridges, open mouth, protruding tongue, upslanting palpebral fissures, folded or dysplastic ears, brachycephalic, **prominent epicanthal folds**, excessive skin at the nape of the neck, short neck, **almond-shaped eyes.**
  Brushfield spots white, grey, or brown spots on the iris.
- <u>Extremities:</u> **transverse, singular palmar crease (Simian crease),** hyperflexibility of the joints, short broad hands, **wide space between the first and second ties (sandal gap deformity).**
- <u>Neonates:</u> poor Moro reflex, hypotonia, dysplasia of the pelvis, hypotonia, may develop transient neonatal leukemia.
- <u>Congenital heart disease:</u> **atrioventricular septal defects,** tetralogy of Fallot, patent ductus arteriosus.
- <u>GI:</u> duodenal or esophageal atresia, Hirschsprung disease.
- <u>Complications:</u> atlantoaxial instability (C1-C2), Acute lymphocytic leukemia, early onset of Alzheimer disease.

DIAGNOSIS

- Based on history, physical examination. Genetic testing used to confirm the diagnosis

PRENATAL SCREENING

- **Biochemical screening tests:** performed in the first trimester. **A low PAPP-A (serum pregnancy-associated plasma protein A) may be seen with Down syndrome.**
- **Nuchal translucency ultrasound: performed at 10-13 weeks. If increased nuchal fold thickness is present, fetal chromosomal abnormalities are usually diagnosed with chorionic villus sampling or amniocentesis.** Chorionic villus sampling can be performed at 10-13 weeks' gestation. >15 weeks is the testing range for amniocentesis.

MANAGEMENT

- The management of patients with Down syndrome is multidisciplinary.
- Treatment is basically symptomatic.
- Parental education regarding the management and associated conditions of Down syndrome.

EHLERS DANLOS SYNDROME (EDS)

- **Group of genetic disorders of collagen synthesis characterized [1] <u>skin hyperextensibility</u>, [2] joint hypermobility, and [3] fragile connective tissue.**
- Most often an autosomal dominant trait, but up to 50% of patients can present as a de novo mutation.
- Hypermobile EDS involves an autosomal dominant (AD) inheritance pattern and has no known associated gene mutation(s). Classical EDS involves an AD inheritance pattern, and associated mutated genes include COL5A1 &/or COL1A1, which code for Type V & Type I collagen, respectively.

Pathophysiology:
- **Abnormal collagen production** (especially type IV EDS) affecting tendons, ligaments, skin, blood vessels, eyes, and other organs.

6 major types:
- <u>**Hypermobile**</u>: **most common type** — large- & small-joint & spine hypermobility; joint dislocations (patella, shoulder, temporomandibular joint), joint pain, scoliosis, & premature osteoarthritis.
- <u>**Classical EDS**</u>: joint hypermobility but tends to affect the skin more (eg, skin laxity, stretchy skin, fragile skin, slow and poor-healing wounds).
- <u>**Vascular EDS:**</u> rare & most serious (can lead to life-threatening bleeding). No joint hyperextensibility.
- Kyphoscoliotic EDS, arthrochalasia EDS, and dermatosparaxis EDS.

CLINICAL MANIFESTATIONS
- <u>**Skin hyperextensibility**</u>: ability to stretch the skin >4 cm in areas such as the neck and forearm.
- <u>**Joint hypermobility:**</u> **hypermobility leading to repeated joint dislocation & subluxation,** leading to early osteoarthritis & chronic pain. Hypermobility may manifest as early as peripartum with hip dislocations in a neonate. Recurrent fractures may also occur. Pes planus, pectus excavatum.

<u>Fragile connective tissue:</u>
- <u>Cutaneous</u>: hyperextensibility, smooth and velvet-like texture & translucency of the skin, **fragility & easy bruising,** delayed & poor wound healing, thin atrophic scars after wound healing. Nodules.
- <u>Cardiovascular</u>: **mitral valve prolapse** and, less commonly, tricuspid valve prolapse. Aortic root dilation is also a common feature that can lead to rupture with or without trauma. **Other vessels may become aneurysmal, predisposing them to rupture (eg, aortic root, intracranial arteries, saccular berry aneurysms).** Capillary fragility — easy bruising & bleeding.
- Other tissues are subject to friability due to the underlying collagen dysfunction, including both hollow & solid internal organs (spontaneous & traumatic rupture or perforation). Hernias and rectal prolapse are common features. May develop myopia. Cervical insufficiency.
- Classic facies include down slanting palpebral fissures, epicanthal folds, blue sclera, the appearance of premature aging, and micrognathia.
- <u>Neurological</u>: hypotonia, which may manifest in the developing child as delayed motor milestones such as walking. Generalized pain, insomnia, and chronic fatigue are also common.

Physical examination:
- **Smooth, velvety (doughy) hyperextensible and fragile skin that bruises easily or may split with trauma, widened atrophic scars, delayed and abnormal wound healing.**
- <u>**Metenier's sign**</u> upper eyelid everts easily. Pes planus, pectus excavatum, and a high arched palate.

DIAGNOSIS
- <u>Clinical</u> — symptoms and signs consistent with EDS. Clinical diagnosis is the only way to diagnose EDS hypermobile type.
- <u>Molecular genetic</u> or biochemical testing confirms the diagnosis, except for EDS hypermobile type.

MANAGEMENT
- Treatment and management of patients with EDS should use a multidisciplinary approach that aims to slow down or prevent progression of disease and complications.
- Screening for cardiovascular abnormalities of the heart, such as aortic root and mitral valve abnormalities, are performed using echocardiography.

MARFAN SYNDROME

- **Autosomal dominant systemic connective tissue disorder that leads to cardiovascular, ocular, and musculoskeletal abnormalities**; involvement of the lung, skin, & CNS may also occur.

PATHOPHYSIOLOGY
- **Mutation of the fibrillin-1 gene (FBN1),** leading to transforming growth factor beta (TGF-beta) mutation & misfolding of the protein fibrillin-1, resulting in **weakened connective tissue.**

CLINICAL MANIFESTATIONS
Cardiovascular:
- **Mitral valve prolapse** (40-54%), which may be associated with **Mitral regurgitation.**
- **Progressive aortic root dilation leads to aortic regurgitation, aortic dissection, & aneurysmal dilation (eg, thoracic or abdominal aortic aneurysms) main cause of morbidity & mortality.** Echocardiography is recommended at initial diagnosis & at 6 months to assess the aorta in MFS.

Musculoskeletal:
- **Tall stature** due to excess linear growth of the long bones. **Abnormal US/LS & arm span/height.**
- **Arachnodactyly — abnormally long, slender, and lanky fingers, arms, and legs.**
- **Positive thumb sign** — the entire distal phalanx protrudes beyond the ulnar border of a closed fist.
- **Positive wrist sign** — the top of the thumb covers the entire fingernail of the fifth finger when wrapped around the contralateral wrist
- **Joint laxity**, reduced joint mobility. Pes planus (flatfoot deformity). Hindfoot valgus.
- Scoliosis & kyphosis, anterior chest deformities (eg, **pectus carinatum,** pectus excavatum), lumbosacral dural ectasia by computed tomography or magnetic resonance imaging.

Ocular:
- **Ectopia lentis** — malposition or dislocation of the lens of the eyes; **The lens is usually displaced** upward and temporally, leading to reduced vision and extreme nearsightedness (**myopia**).

Pulmonary:
- Lung bullae resulting from emphysematous pulmonary changes especially in the upper lobes, may lead to spontaneous Pneumothorax.

DIAGNOSIS
- Major criteria: include **ectopia lentis, aortic root dilatation/dissection** involving the sinuses of Valsalva or aortic dissection, lumbosacral dural ectasia by CT or MRI, family or genetic history, 4 of 8 typical skeletal manifestations. Perform yearly Ultrasound to assess the aortic diameter.
- Laboratory: **Testing for mutations in Fibrillin-1 (FBN1).**

MANAGEMENT
- Conservative: avoid high-contact sports & vigorous physical exercise. **Beta-blockers (first line) or Angiotensin II receptor blockers to halt the progression of aortic root dilation.**
- Surgical: aortic aneurysm repair or cardiac valve repair if indicated. Treatment targeted at symptoms.

PROGNOSIS
- **Decreased life expectancy occurs primarily due to aortic complications** — aortic root disease, leading to aortic regurgitation, aneurysmal dilatation, and dissection, is the primary cause of morbidity and mortality in MFS, in up to 60% - 80% of patients. Aortic dissection & rupture preventable by prophylactic replacement of the ascending aorta if diameter reaches 5.0 cm.

- **EXAM TIP**
- Both: joint laxity, hypermobility, scoliosis, & aortic aneurysms that may rupture.
- Marfan only: **tall stature, arachnodactyly** (overgrowth or long bones), **dislocation of the lens**, retinal detachment, pectus carinatum &/or excavatum, and high incidence of progressive aortic dilation.
- Ehlers-Danlos: **skin hyperextensibility and fragile connective tissue (eg, easy bruising,** hypertrophic scar formation).

FETAL ALCOHOL SYNDROME

- Syndrome due to maternal alcohol use during pregnancy.
- **Most common preventable cause of intellectual disability.**

CLINICAL MANIFESTATIONS
- Children are often born small and remain relatively small throughout their lifetime.
- Associated with developmental delays & congenital abnormalities of internal organs.

PHYSICAL FINDINGS
- **3 hallmark features** — **[1] thin upper lip (vermillion border), [2] long & smooth philtrum, and [3] short palpebral fissures.**
- **Microcephaly, and small distal phalanges.** Epicanthal folds, midface hypoplasia, short nose.
- Intellectual disabilities, developmental delays and abnormalities, & congenital abnormalities of internal organs. Prenatal and postnatal growth delays. Neurological developmental deficits.

SMOKING DURING PREGNANCY

ADVERSE EFFECTS
- Preterm birth, miscarriage, stillbirth, reduction in birth weight, placental abnormalities, congenital malformations (eg, congenital heart defects, cleft lip, cleft palate, **limb reduction defects**, digital anomalies, bilateral renal hypoplasia or agenesis, anal atresia, etc.).

NEURAL TUBE DEFECTS

Birth defects of the brain, spine, or spinal cord.
- **The 2 most common types are spina bifida & anencephaly.**
- **Increased incidence with maternal folate deficiency.**

PATHOPHYSIOLOGY
- Anencephaly: failure of closure of the portion of the neural tube that becomes the cerebrum.
- Spina bifida: incomplete closure of the embryonic neural tubule leads to non-fusion of some of the vertebrae overlying the spinal cords. This may lead to protrusion of the spinal cord through the opening. Most commonly seen at the lumbar and sacral areas of the spine.

TYPES OF SPINA BIFIDA
- **Spina bifida with myelomeningocele: most common type.** Meninges and spinal cord herniates thought the gap in the vertebrae. Often leads to disability.
- Spina bifida occulta: mildest form. No herniation of the spinal cord. The overlying skin may be normal or have some hair growing over it, dimpling of the skin or birthmark over the affected area.
- Spina bifida with meningocele: only the meninges herniate through the gap in the vertebrae

CLINICAL MANIFESTATIONS
- Sensory deficits, paralysis, hydrocephalus, hypotonia.

MANAGEMENT
- The back lesion should be surgically closed, preferably within the first 72 hours after birth if the infant is stable. For the next few weeks, the infant should be monitored closely for the development of hydrocephalus, using serial head circumference measures and head ultrasounds

SCREENING
- Increased maternal serum alpha-fetoprotein followed by **amniocentesis showing increased alpha-fetoprotein & increased acetylcholinesterase.**

PREVENTION
- **Folic acid supplementation decreases the occurrence and recurrence of neural tube defects** and is recommended in all periconceptional women **and** continued throughout the first trimester.

PRADER-WILLI SYNDROME

- **Genetic disorder characterized by prenatal hypotonia, postnatal growth delay, developmental disabilities, hypogonadotropic hypogonadism, & obesity after infancy.**
- Small deletion or inexpression of genes in the **paternal copy of chromosome 15** (15q11.2-13).
- **PWS is associated with hypothalamic dysfunction,** leading to several endocrinopathies (eg, hypogonadism, hypothyroidism, central adrenal insufficiency, with reduced bone mineral density).

CLINICAL MANIFESTATIONS

- **Neonates: severe hypotonia, floppy baby, weak cry, feeding difficulties,** trouble swallowing and suckling (nasogastric feeding may be needed). **Hypogonadism: cryptorchidism,** genital hypoplasia (small testicular & penis size). Very few females reach menarche. Depigmentation of the skin, eyes, excessive sleeping, strabismus.
  Physical examination: almond-shaped eyes, high/narrow forehead, thin upper lip with small, down-turned mouth; prominent nasal bridges. Small feet & hands (with tapering of the fingers). Soft skin that easily bruises (may have extreme flexibility). Excess fat (especially *truncal obesity*).
- **Early childhood: during the first year of life, muscle tone improves, and child develops voracious appetite (hyperphagia) including aggressive behavior related to eating, obesity.** Major milestone delays, behavioral and learning difficulties. Short stature (due to growth hormone deficiency), skin picking. Patients may have lighter hair and skin compared to other family members.
- Later childhood/adolescence: delay of secondary sex characteristics, increased incidence of epilepsy & scoliosis. Women are often infertile. Sleep disorders, hypopigmentation, thick viscous saliva, high pain threshold, decreased vomiting, temperature instability, scoliosis/kyphosis, Osteoporosis.

DIAGNOSIS

- **DNA testing** DNA-based methylation studies.
- **Genetic karyotyping,** molecular testing with DNA methylation. Chromosome analysis with FISH.

MANAGEMENT

Growth hormone replacement, obesity control by monitoring food intake. Diet and exercise.

BECKWITH-WIEDEMANN SYNDROME

- **Abnormal gene expression affecting the chromosome 11p15.5 region.**
- **Hallmark features: omphalocele (exomphalos), macroglossia, & macrosomia (gigantism).** Large for gestational age, organomegaly, hypoglycemia in infancy, earlobe creases & pits, asymmetric limbs. **Increased risk of hepatoblastoma & Wilm's tumor.**

NEUROBLASTOMA

- **Peripheral sympathetic nervous system cancer** associated with **amplification of N-Myc oncogene.** 90% diagnosed by age 5y. **Most common in adrenal medulla (40%)** & paraspinal region.

CLINICAL MANIFESTATIONS

- Most common in the abdomen (firm, irregular, nodular abdomen or flank mass). Unlike Nephroblastoma, **Neuroblastoma can cross the midline.**
- **Ataxia, opsoclonus myoclonus syndrome (hypsarrhythmia/rapid "dancing eyes" & myoclonus/"dancing feet" – jerky movements),** hypertension (especially diastolic), diarrhea.
- **Proptosis, periorbital ecchymosis ("raccoon eyes"),** Horner syndrome (miosis, ptosis, anhidrosis), paraspinal mass, localized back pain, weakness, palpable nontender subcutaneous nodules.

DIAGNOSIS: **CT scan: tumor often seen with calcification & hemorrhaging. ↑vanillylmandelic acid.**

MANAGEMENT

- Surgical resection &/or radiation therapy & chemotherapy. Select patients: stem cell transplant.

NEUROFIBROMATOSIS TYPE 1 (von Recklinghausen's disease)

- Multisystem genetic disorder with manifestations that include pigmentary changes, benign tumors of peripheral nerve sheaths (neurofibromas), increased risk of central nervous system (CNS) gliomas and other malignant tumors and learning disabilities.
- **Autosomal dominant neurocutaneous disorder due to a <u>mutated NF1 gene (chromosome 17q11.2 region)</u>** encoding for the protein neurofibromin (a tumor suppressor).
- **Most common type** (90%).

PATHOPHYSIOLOGY
- Loss of neurofibromin ⇨ increased risk of developing benign and malignant tumors.
- Mutations are highly variable between patients with NF1 and can appear at any age.

CLINICAL MANIFESTATIONS
- ~50% with sporadic NF1 meet clinical criteria for diagnosis in the first year of life, and nearly all do so by 8 years of age.

Requires at least 2 of the following:
- **≥6 café-au-lait spots**: flat, uniformly hyperpigmented macules that appear during the first year of birth and increase in number during early childhood. >5 mm prepubertal; >15 mm postpubertal.
- **Freckling:** Usually appear in intertriginous areas/skin folds [**especially axillary freckling (Crowe sign) or inguinal freckling**] & the neckline. Not usually present at birth but often appears by age 3 to 5 years.
- **Lisch nodules of the iris: raised, tan-colored hamartomas of the iris seen on slit lamp examination.** Large nodules on a light-colored iris can be seen with a direct ophthalmoscope, but slit lamp examination is more reliable. Uncommon before the age of 6 years.
- **≥2 neurofibromas or ≥1 plexiform neurofibroma: Discrete cutaneous neurofibromas are the most common type of neurofibroma in NF1.** Cutaneous neurofibromas usually appear just before or during adolescence, although small lesions can be seen in younger children. Neurofibromas are focal, benign peripheral nerve sheath tumors (often a combination of Schwann cells, fibroblasts, perineural cells and mast cells) described as small, rubbery lesions with a slight purplish discoloration of the overlying skin. Neurofibromas typically involve the skin but may be seen along peripheral nerves, blood vessels and viscera. Plexiform neurofibromas are located longitudinally along a nerve and involve multiple fascicles (may produce an overgrowth of an extremity).
- **Optic pathway gliomas**: may involve the optic nerve, optic chiasm, and/or postchiasmal optic tracts. Most commonly occurs in younger children (eg, <6 years of age). May develop an afferent pupillary defect. If the tumor is large and involves the hypothalamus, it may be associated with delayed or premature onset of puberty.
- Less common tumors include sarcomas, glomus tumors, hematologic malignancies, and breast cancer.
- Other manifestations: **osseous lesions: scoliosis is common** (especially thoracic spine), sphenoid dysplasia, long bone abnormalities. First degree relative with NF1 or short stature.

NEUROIMAGING
- **MRI**: unidentified bright objects = hyperintense T2-weighted signals (may be due to demyelination or focal areas of increased water content). Seen most commonly in the basal ganglia, brainstem, cerebellum, and subcortical white matter. There are no associated neurologic deficits. Increased brain volume often seen.

MANAGEMENT
- The management approach depends on the tumor type, location, and associated complications.
- Optic pathway glioma: regular annual ophthalmologic screening. If any symptoms occur, an MRI of the brain & orbits should be performed. Surgical resection may be needed.
- Neurofibromas: not removed unless there are associated complications.

NEUROFIBROMATOSIS TYPE 2

- **Autosomal dominant associated with multiple CNS tumors [bilateral CN VIII tumors** (also known as schwannomas, vestibular neuromas, or acoustic neuromas)], spinal tumors & intracranial tumors.

PATHOPHYSIOLOGY
- Mutation of the NF2 tumor suppressor gene (normally produces the protein schwannomin aka merlin).

CLINICAL MANIFESTATIONS
- **Neurologic lesions:**
  - BILATERAL VESTIBULAR SCHWANNOMAS **(95%).** Most develop by 30 years of age — hearing loss (usually gradual & progressive), tinnitus, and balance disturbances. Over a period of time, they can expand, causing hydrocephalus & brainstem compression.
  - **OTHER CNS TUMORS: Meningiomas:** often multiple (especially in childhood), spinal & intramedullary tumors, **Ependymomas,** neuropathy.
- **Optic lesions: juvenile cataracts** (eg, visual impairment early in childhood), retinal hamartomas.
- **Skin lesions:**
  - Cutaneous tumors, skin plaques (slightly raised and may be hyperpigmented), subcutaneous tumors that presents as nodules. Café-au-lait spots are seen with less frequency in NF2.

MANAGEMENT
Vestibular schwannomas:
  - Surgery may be needed for complicated or symptomatic tumors.
  - Bevacizumab: may cause shrinkage of the tumor and improvement in hearing.
    MOA: monoclonal antibody against vascular endothelial growth factor (VEGF).

TAY-SACHS DISEASE

- Rare, autosomal recessive genetic disorder most common in Ashkenazi Jewish families of Eastern European descent, Cajuns in Southern Louisiana, & French Canadians.

PATHOPHYSIOLOGY
- **Lysosomal storage disorder: Mutation of the HEXA gene on chromosome 15 ⇨ deficiency in β-hexosaminidase A ⇨ accumulation of GM2 gangliosides within the lysosomes of nerve cells in the brain ⇨ premature neuron death & progressive degeneration of neurons.**

CLINICAL MANIFESTATIONS
- **Infantile onset: increased startle reaction, loss of motor skills. At 4-5 months of age ⇨ decreased eye contact, hyperacusis (exaggerated startle reaction to noise),** paralysis, blindness, progressive developmental delays & dementia.
- Second year: seizures & neurodegeneration. **Death usually occurs between 3-4 years.**
- Juvenile onset: symptoms occur between the ages of 2-10y ⇨ cognitive and motor skill deterioration, dysphagia, ataxia, spasticity. Death often occurs between the ages of 5-15y.
- Adult onset: usually develops symptoms during the 30s & 40s. May have unsteady, spastic gait and progressive neurological deterioration (leading to speech, swallowing difficulties), psychosis.
- Physical examination: **Retinal examination: cherry-red spots with macular pallor.** Macrocephaly.

DIAGNOSIS
- **Enzymatic assay** — infantile form is associated with no or extremely low level of beta-hexosaminidase A enzyme activity (0-5%) in addition to normal or elevated levels of Beta hexosaminidase B isoenzyme levels (HEX B isoenzyme). Juvenile or adult forms associated with low level of beta-hexosaminidase A enzyme activity (10 to 15%).

MANAGEMENT
- No effective treatment. Various supportive measures to ensure patient survival includes anticonvulsant therapy, nutritional, and hydration support except for metabolic therapy.

TYPES OF VACCINES

1. LIVE, ATTENUATED VACCINES:

Contains a live, weakened version of the organism. Because it is the safest, closest thing to actually having the infection, it induces a good immune response of both *humoral (antibody) immunity & cell-mediated immunity.* No booster usually need. Cons: they are unstable & must be refrigerated. Because they may become virulent, **live attenuated vaccines are not given to immunocompromised or pregnant patients.**
- **MMR.** The only live, attenuated vaccine that can be given to HIV patients (if CD4 >200/μL).
- **Chicken pox (Varicella Zoster), Rotavirus.**
- Smallpox, yellow fever, oral typhoid, *Franciscella tularensis*, oral polio.

2. KILLED (INACTIVATED) VACCINES:

Killed organisms. These stimulate a weaker immune response compared to live attenuated vaccines so they only induce a humoral (antibody) immunity - may need booster shots.
- **Influenza, Rabies, Polio Sal<u>K</u> (K= killed** - this is the primary form used in US), Vibrio cholerae, **Hepatitis A Vaccine.**

3. SUBUNIT CONJUGATE VACCINES:

Presents only the essential antigens needed to induce an immune system response (instead of giving the whole organism). Often contain multiple antigens that are linked or "conjugated" to toxoids or antigens that the immature immune system will recognize to identify bacterium that use their polysaccharide outer coating as a defense. **Made of capsular polysaccharides** so often used for many **encapsulated organisms** "SHiN".
- **<u>S</u>. pneumococcal** (infant version is conjugated so induces a helper T cell response).
- **<u>H</u> influenza** (capsular polysaccharide), **<u>N</u>. meningitidis,** PCV13 (pneumococcal vaccine).

4. SUBUNIT RECOMBINANT VACCINES:

A type of subunit vaccine in which recombinant DNA technology is used to manufacture the antigen molecules. Genes that encode for the important antigens are placed into Baker's yeast. The yeast reproduces the antigens that are processed & purified.
- **Hepatitis B vaccine** (HBsAg), **HPV vaccine** (6,11,16, & 18).

5. TOXOID VACCINES:

Chemically modified inactivated toxins from toxin-producing organisms to allow the body to recognize the harmless toxin. Later it has the ability to attack the natural toxin if exposed to it.
- **Tetanus, Diphtheria, Pertussis**

VACCINE CONTRAINDICATIONS

- **<u>Baker's yeast:</u> Hepatitis B** should be avoided (Think <u>B</u> for <u>B</u>aker's yeast & Hepatitis <u>B</u>).
- <u>Gelatin:</u> avoid varicella, influenza vaccines.
- <u>Thimerosal:</u> preservative used in vaccines so should be avoided in multi-dose vaccines.
- **<u>Neomycin & Streptomycin allergy:</u> MMR** (Measles Mumps Rubella) & **inactivated Polio vaccine** should be avoided (Neomycin & Streptomycin are preservatives in these vaccines).

<u>PREGNANCY</u>
Only vaccines safely given in pregnancy: diphtheria, tetanus, inactivated influenza, HBV, rabies, meningococcal.
Avoid live vaccines:
- <u>Live vaccines:</u> MMR, Varicella, Polio.
- <u>Live attenuated vaccines:</u> intranasal influenza vaccine.

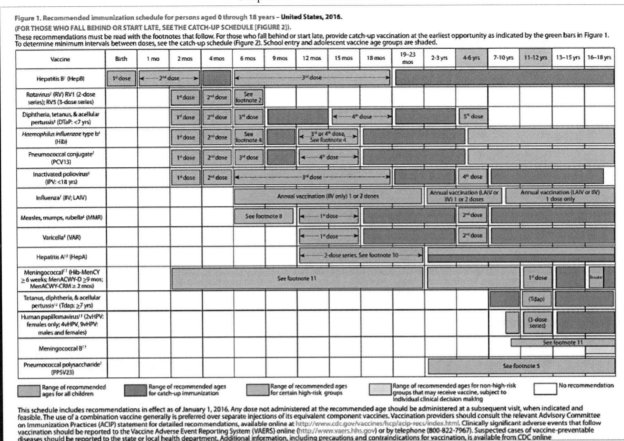

Figure 1. Recommended immunization schedule for persons aged 0 through 18 years – **United States, 2016.**

(FOR THOSE WHO FALL BEHIND OR START LATE, SEE THE CATCH-UP SCHEDULE [FIGURE 2]).

These recommendations must be read with the footnotes that follow. For those who fall behind or start late, provide catch-up vaccination at the earliest opportunity as indicated by the green bars in Figure 1. To determine minimum intervals between doses, see the catch-up schedule (Figure 2). School entry and adolescent vaccine age groups are shaded.

TANNER STAGE	2	3	4	5
Males	Age 11 - 12	Age 13	Age 14 – 15	Age 16-17
Pubic hair	Straight pubic hair at the base of penis	Coarse dark and curly pubic hair	Hair is almost completely full	Pubic hair achieves adult appearance
Females	Age 11	Age 12	Age 13	Age 14-15
Pubic Hair	Minimal straight pubic hair (long, downy)	Increased pubic hair (dark & coarse) lateral extension	Adult-like extends across pubis	Adult appearance (extends to medial thighs)
Breast	Breast buds palpable, areola enlarge	Elevation of areola contour, areola enlargement	Secondary mound of areola & papilla	Adult breast contour

TANNER STAGES

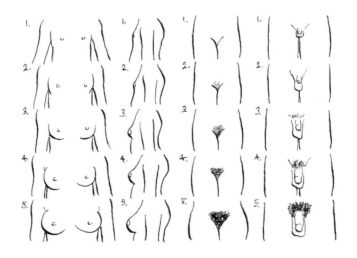

PANCE PREP APP

TRY OUR SWEET APP :)

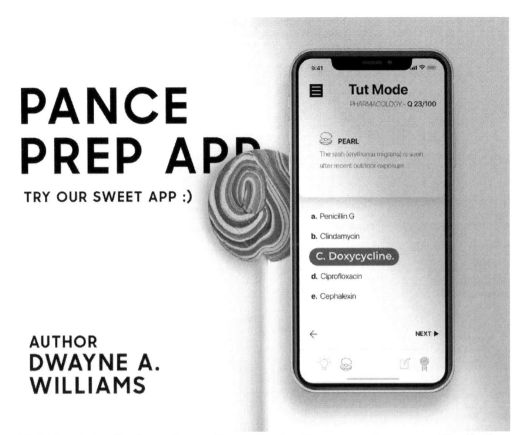

AUTHOR
DWAYNE A. WILLIAMS

Over 15,000 clinically-based practice examination questions specifically formulated to enhance clinical skills and improve performance on examinations, such as the PANCE, PANRE, OSCES, USMLE, end of rotation examinations and comprehensive medical examinations.

Special clinical pearls, disease review, explanation of the answers, test taking strategies and much more.

3 modes,
Timed mode to simulate the exams
Tutor mode that allows you to review the disease states in addition to the questions and **improve mode** to enhance your weak areas.

For every question in tutor mode, there is a feature for a hint to see if you are going in the right direction, answer explanation, a clinical pearl, and a bonus questions. Create your own examination based on organ systems or task areas. The ultimate study and exam preparation app!

PANCE PREP QUESTION APP
EARN 20 CATEGORY 1 SELF-ASSESSMENT CME CREDITS

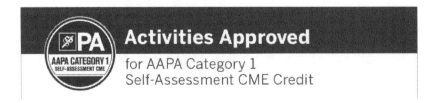

ALSO AVAILABLE

CYTOCHROME P450 INDUCERS

John was **wort**hy when referred & <u>**inducted**</u> into sainthood for giving up **chronic alcohol** use & placing him**self on a real** fast, **fend**ing off **greasy carbs**, leading to **less warfa**re with **theo**logians.

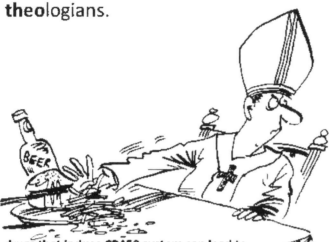

drugs that induce CP450 system can lead to decreased levels of certain drugs ex. warfarin (less warfare), theophylline (theologians) and phenytoin

INDUCERS OF THE P450

* **St. Johns Wort**
* **rifampin** (referred)
* **chronic alcohol use**
* **sulfonylureas**
   (self on a real)
* **Phenytoin**
* **Phenobarbital** (fend)
* **Griseofulvin** (greasy)
* **Carbamazepine**
   (carbs)

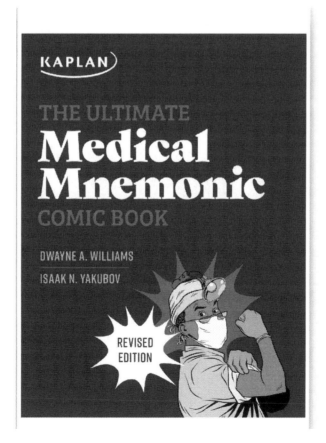

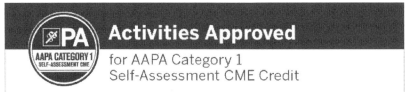

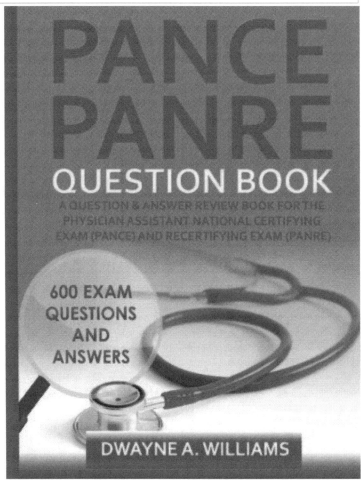

COMING SOON IN 2024: PANCE PREP QUESTION BOOK SECOND EDITION!

Made in the USA
Coppell, TX
03 October 2024

38114071R00258